What People Are Saying About *Great Expections*: *Your All-In-One Resource for Pregnancy & Childbirth:*

"If you are searching for one book for your pregnancy or for that one book to refer *all* of your expectant clients to, this book is by far the greatest achievement in childbirth education reading material! Sandy Jones and her daughter Marcie Jones have included absolutely *everything* an expectant woman and her family needs to know. This book should be on everyone's recommended reading list!"

— CONNIE LIVINGSTON, BS, RN, FACCE (DONA), CCE, CLD,
www.birthsource.com

"*Great Expectations* really is great! I told a girlfriend of mine that, 'it's so good it makes me want to get pregnant all over again.'"

— JENNIFER JAMES, EDITOR, MOMMY TOO! MAGAZINE

"Emotions, physical changes, lifestyle changes, baby development, it's all there. Get ready: This book will get dog-eared from all your reading and then passed along to your best friends and sister."

— PEG MOLINE, EDITOR-IN-CHIEF, FITPREGNANCY

"*Great Expectations* is the perfect resource for moms-to-be. Sandy and Marcie Jones speak to the expectant mother of today in a friendly, approachable tone, and present their thorough information in a way that's great for both quick look-ups and in-depth reading."

— STACIA RAGOLIA, VP, COMMUNITY & PARENTING, IVILLAGE.COM

"*Great Expectations* is terrific. The style of writing is clear, warm and very supportive. It's a great reference for any question that might arrive in pregnancy."

— ANN STADTLER, MSN, CPNP, DIRECTOR OF THE BRAZELTON TOUCHPOINT
CENTER AT CHILDREN'S HOSPITAL IN BOSTON

"Consumer friendly book filled with great women's quotes, helpful information and tips for pregnant women and new families."

— MAUREEN CORRY, EXECUTIVE DIRECTOR, THE MATERNITY CENTER ASSOCIATION

"Accurate, comprehensive, empowering, and current. I see this as being the new Dr. Spock for pregnancy.... This is definitely a book I will recommend to my clients who are planning a pregnancy or currently pregnant."

— CHERIE C. BINNS, RN, BS, MSCN

"Lots of good info and advice for moms and dads...a book that's fun, readable and full of good information...a great combination. I especially liked the embryology/ fetal development sections that make it easy to envision how the baby is growing. Helps to make the normal discomforts of pregnancy worth the bother!"

— SHARON SCHINDLER RISING, MSN, CNM, FACNM, FOUNDER AND EXECUTIVE
DIRECTOR, THE CENTERING PREGNANCY & PARENTING ASSOCIATION

G·R·E·A·T EXPECTATIONS

Your All-in-One Resource for
Pregnancy
& Childbirth

Sandy Jones & Marcie Jones
with Peter S. Bernstein, MD, MPH, FACOG and
Claire M. Westdahl, CNM, MPH, FACNM

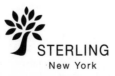

STERLING
New York

STERLING
New York

An Imprint of Sterling Publishing
387 Park Avenue South
New York, NY 10016

STERLING and the distinctive Sterling logo are
registered trademarks of Sterling Publishing Co. Inc.

© 2004 by Sandy Jones and Marcie Jones
Illustrations by Stephen Tulk and Nicole Kaufman

ISBN 978-0-7607-4132-0

Library of Congress Cataloging-in-Publication Data Available

Distributed in Canada by Sterling Publishing
c/o Canadian Manda Group, 165 Dufferin Street
Toronto, Ontario, Canada M6K 3H6
Distributed in Great Britain by GMC Distribution Services
Castle Place, 166 High Street, Lewes, East Sussex, England BN7 1XU
Distributed in Australia by Capricorn Link (Australia) Pty. Ltd.
P.O. Box 704, Windsor, NSW 2756, Australia

While the publisher believes the information used in creating this book to be reliable,
the medical field changes rapidly and there are new developments almost daily.
The publisher cannot guarantee the accuracy, adequacy, or the completeness of
the information contained in this book and must disclaim all warranties, expressed
or implied, regarding the information. The publisher also cannot assume any
responsibility for use of this book, and any use by a reader is at the reader's own
risk. This book is not intended to be a substitute for professional medical advice, and
any user of this book should always check with a licensed physician before adopting
any particular course of treatment.

For information about custom editions, special sales, premium, and corporate
purchases, please contact Sterling Special Sales Department at 800-805-5489
or specialsales@sterlingpublishing.com

Printed in China

10   9

DEDICATION & ACKNOWLEDGMENTS

We are a mother-daughter writing team, and we would like to dedicate this book to Virginia McWhorter Freeman, our wonderful mother and grandmother, who passed on during the year we wrote this book. Over the course of her meaningful and remarkable life, Virginia imparted to us the skills of listening, serving others, and raising children with room to grow.

Sandy would also like to acknowledge the help of her brother, James, and his wife, Barbara, for their support during the past year so that this giant book could be completed.

Marcie would like to dedicate this book to Zoë and extend special thanks to Claire Rusko-Berger, who helpfully became pregnant during the writing process and never hesitated to graphically describe her discomforts; to Paul Jones, ultimate dad and bastion of love and stability; and to the Reverend Matthew Brennan.

Acknowledgments to the great contributions of Dr. Brian Woolf, Kathleen Sloane and Mary Knauer, CNMs, Susie Creamer and the office of Dr. Beth Aronson, Dr. Steve Matanle, Dr. Neil Kleinman and the research of Dr. James F. Clapp III, Robin Baker, and the excellent medical reporting of Eric Nagourney.

Our agent, Faith Hamlin, a true professional, was indispensable in making this book become a reality and ensuring that it got the attention it needed to be born and to thrive.

This book would not have been possible without the wonderful support and intense devotion of Senior Editor Laura Nolan of Barnes & Noble, whose upbeat, "can-do" attitude, positive input, and sense of humor saved the day time and again.

We also would also like to offer our deepest thanks to all of the people at Barnes & Noble who made this book a reality: Steve Riggio, Alan Kahn and Michael Fragnito. We also extend our appreciation to Jeff Batzli, Charles Kreloff and Charles Donahue, who helped to design the book, and Nicole Kaufman and Stephen Tulk, M.D., who produced the wonderful illustrations for it.

We also are deeply indebted to Peter Bernstein, MD, MPH, FACOG, Claire Westdahl, CNM, MPH, FACNM, and Miriam Schecter, MD, who ensured the book was accurate and provided invaluable insights. And to the hundreds of pregnant women and new moms who took the time to share their hopes, their dreams, and their day-to-day realities with us.

CONTENTS

CHAPTER 1
Your Pregnancy Week-by-Week

CHAPTER 3
Your Guide to Giving Birth

Chapter 4
You and Your Baby

A Word from the Authors

CONGRATULATIONS—YOU'RE
PREGNANT!
Three little words, or a line on a little
wand, and you'll find yourself in a
strange new world.

There's no way to be prepared
for carrying another person inside
of your body, someone you are
responsible for, body and soul, as
long as you both shall live—even if
this isn't your first pregnancy.

While the changes in your body
may be easy to see and feel, the
changes that happen to you as a
person, in your heart, mind, and
hormones are just as momentous.
We wrote this book as a travel
guide to this journey.

A lot of pregnancy books seem
to be written by people who have
never been pregnant before, or who
have forgotten what it's really like.
The books we studied seemed to go
no deeper than the message "don't
worry, you're normal." While you
probably shouldn't worry, and
chances are you are normal, we
wanted to give you more than simple
reassurances. We assumed that, like
us, you wanted to know why and
how things happen, and that you
would rather know more than is
necessary, rather than less.

Equally as important, we wanted
you to have a book that would give
you information without being
judgmental about it. We know
all too well there's nothing more
annoying than the chorus of people
telling pregnant women what they
should do. The terrible truth about
being pregnant (or being a parent)
is that no matter what choice you
make, there will always be someone
who thinks your choice is wrong.
You can't please everyone—try as
you might to be the "perfect" pregnant woman with the "right" kind
of delivery. But if you've done your
research, you can separate real
risks from imagined ones and
make choices based on evidence,
not opinion.

Finally, we have tried to create a
book that would present pregnancy
as realistically as possible. There's
a lot more to pregnancy than just
glowing! Sure, it's a miracle and
everything, and you're probably
excited about having a baby, but
sometimes, frankly, pregnancy can
be uncomfortable, undignified, and
yucky. It can feel like a boot camp
of learning how to surrender to discomfort and unpredictability, and
find balance between self-caring
and self-sacrifice. No matter what
other books tell you, it's okay to not
enjoy the experience all of the time.

Even when pregnancy isn't fun,
it is always meaningful. You will
never be the same after this. It may

feel like an endless sacrifice, but in the final analysis, what you will have lost in muscle tone, you'll gain tenfold in heart, courage, and humanity. You can do it, you will do it, and we're rooting for you, no matter how you do it!

INSIDE OUR BOOK

Our first section, **"Your Pregnancy Week-by-Week"** (pages 3–107), is an easy-to-navigate map that says "You Are Here" and carries you from the first day you discover you're pregnant through your final weeks until labor. It shows you how you and your baby change and grow and directs you to all the information you'll need when you're most likely to need it.

The second section, **"Managing Your Pregnancy"** (pages 109–253), gives practical solutions for the head-to-toe aches and pains of pregnancy and offers solid information for navigating the medical and emotional aspects of pregnancy. Want to know how to deal with so-called morning sickness that's happening all day? Go to page 129. Are you worrying about your weight and wondering what's the best nutrition for pregnancy? See page 145. Wonder when to tell your boss you're expecting? See page 250.

Section three, **"Your Guide to Giving Birth"** (pages 255–357), helps you prepare for birth with confidence by giving you the most up-to-date, comprehensive information available in a single reference. You'll learn all about the process of labor, what your pain relief options are, and the latest research on the most commonly used medical interventions. We offer you both the benefits and the risks of routine procedures such as epidurals, induction, labor augmentation, and cesarean sections, and tell you how they feel.

Section four, **"You and Your Baby"** (pages 359–451), will help you in recovering physically and emotionally from pregnancy and childbirth. It also offers hundreds of practical suggestions for taking care of your newborn during the first six months.

The fifth section, **"Baby Gear Guide"** (pages 453–535), is an A to Z guide to buying safe, durable baby products. It will guide you in what to buy and what to avoid, and give you the skinny on all major baby product categories, including cribs, car seats, and strollers.

Section six, our **"Resource Guide"** (pages 537–570), is chock-full of lots of great Internet pregnancy and baby sources. And our final section, the **"Pregnancy Dictionary,"** is a basic reader on hundreds of pregnancy and medical definitions that have been translated by us into easy-to-understand concepts. It also offers page references throughout the book for more discussion on a given topic.

We have gathered the information presented in *Great Expectations* from hundreds of recent medical studies; from the wealth of wisdom and knowledge in the fields of obstetrics, family practice, midwifery, and nursing; and from the shared experiences of childbirth educators and doulas. In addition, we have incorporated wisdom from the numerous mothers who have shared their pregnancy, birth, and childrearing experiences with us.

And of course, we have used our own experiences of pregnancy, labor, and infant care to guide us.

FINDING YOUR WAY AROUND

Great Expectations is designed to be a "thirty-second" reference book for busy mothers just like you. We want you to have the choice of dipping into topics based on your specific concerns or to read the book from cover to cover.

Beginning with its detailed table of contents, the book shows you where to go inside to find what you need at any given moment and where you are in the book. Each of the seven sections in the book also has its own "Look and Go" guide on the first page to help you access information quickly without wasting time on topics that aren't of interest.

Throughout the text of each section, you'll find references to specific pages elsewhere that discuss the topic you are currently exploring. Medical terms throughout the book are set in italics and bold the first time they appear in any section. That signals that you'll find them defined in the "Pregnancy Dictionary."

The "Index" at the end of the book gives more than 1,000 topics and page numbers to speed your journeys into the book. Throughout, we've translated the latest, most comprehensive research findings into easy-to-follow "flash facts" that will help you be an informed consumer.

When it comes to talking about your baby, we've tried to remain "gender neutral," by giving equal weight to the possibility of your baby being a "she" or a "he." So, you will find that we have alternated throughout the book by referring to both possibilities for the sex of your baby.

YOUR HEALTHCARE PROVIDER

Also, because nearly one-third of pregnant moms don't have husbands, we refer to your companion as your "partner," who may be your husband, your baby's father, a dear friend, your mother, or someone else you've chosen to accompany you through your pregnancy experience.

While this book is the most comprehensive out there, you're going to need more help and human support than any bound volume can offer during your pregnancy. That's why we consistently recommend that you seek the advice of your healthcare provider throughout the book.

Although most women in the U.S. use obstetricians for prenatal care and delivery, we purposely refer to the professional you've chosen to help you with your birth as "your healthcare provider." We recognize that you have the option of delivering your baby with a family care practitioner, midwife, or nurse-midwife too.

An experienced healthcare provider can play an important role in supporting you and guiding you through your birth and delivery. At best, he or she will be present to assist you in weighing a wide range of options every step of the way; will keep your preferred strategies for pain relief and your birth preferences in the forefront; and will refrain from recommending any medical tests or interventions that aren't totally in the best interest of you and your baby. (Information on how to choose a healthcare provider can be found on pages 166 and 167.)

Also, we can't overstress the importance of having someone in the room during birth to support and assist you. Recent research shows that women who have active support during labor feel less pain, have less anxiety, and experience better outcomes, such as fewer cesarean sections. We suggest using a combination of both your chosen birth partner and a labor assistant (doula) to accompany you through labor.

A NOTE ON EVIDENCE-BASED MEDICINE

We have based much of the factual findings on medical practices during pregnancy and birth on evidence-based medicine, the use of research from a variety of clinical studies of large numbers of pregnant women and babies, in order to recommend only practices that have been solidly proven to be beneficial.

Thanks to this exciting revolution in medicine, tests or interventions that have been shown to be of limited benefit, or no benefit at all, are being discontinued. However, sometimes there can be a time lag between the publishing of scientific findings and changes in the practices of healthcare providers, particularly when findings contradict routine procedures.

Healthcare practitioners, who are only human, tend to rely on what they've been taught and to trust routines they've become used to. And like everyone else in the world, they're more likely to believe information that seems to confirm what they already believe and find flaw with things that conflict with these beliefs. If you or your baby's safety and well-being are at stake, we suggest being a well-informed medical consumer, which may include seeking a second opinion.

ABOUT US

Great Expectations: Your All-in-One Resource for Pregnancy & Childbirth has been created by two mothers for all mothers.

Veteran writer Sandy Jones has a Master's degree in Psychology and has been authoring books and articles for parents for thirty years. She is the author of six other books on babies and child care, including *To Love a Baby; Crying Baby, Sleepless Nights;* and *The Guide to Baby Products* from Consumer Reports. She is the mother of Marcie Jones. Marcie Jones is a freelance writer, writing teacher, and mother, with a Master's degree in Publications Design.

Our ultimate hope is that *Great Expectations* will make the process of moving through your pregnancy, having your baby, and taking care of yourself and your baby easier and less intimidating. Our plan from the beginning has been that the book's progressive design and clarity will make it easy for you to access exactly the right piece of information you need when you need it.

We're very aware that the research that has formed the basis of our book is ever changing and expanding. Inevitably, research will come to light after our book has been published that expands and changes what is known and done in this field.

Our best remedy for the constant change and evolution of knowledge in obstetrics, family medicine, midwifery, and nursing is to issue new editions in the years to come. We welcome your comments and feedback that we will use to update future volumes of this book. You can write us in care of our publishers.

Sandy Jones & Marcie Jones

A Note from Dr. Peter Bernstein

In 1989 a United States Public Health Service expert panel issued a report on prenatal care in the United States. While they acknowledged the progress made over the past century in the modern medical care of pregnant women and their newborn children, they also indicated that there were significant areas that needed greater attention, specifically the psychological, social, and educational aspects of pregnancy. *Great Expectations: Your All-in-One Resource for Pregnancy & Childbirth* by Sandy Jones and Marcie Jones goes a long way to answer this need.

While modern medicine has made great advances in prenatal care, more and more research is demonstrating that those expectant couples who educate themselves and actively partner with their prenatal care provider have the best outcomes. The more fully informed a pregnant woman is, the more she can completely participate in her care. Unfortunately, too often care providers do not have the time to educate their patients on many important components of prenatal care, such as good nutrition, the importance of breastfeeding, contraceptive options, and caring for newborns.

Here's an example of the power that knowledge can provide to a pregnant woman. For a woman who is uninformed about the natural process of labor, every contraction can be a terrifying experience, making her feel like her body is out of control. All the fear she experiences can even make her labor more painful. For the woman who is prepared, the onset of contractions signals that labor has begun, which is exciting, less scary, less painful, and more fulfilling.

Great Expectations: Your All-in-One Resource for Pregnancy & Childbirth provides the expectant couple with many of the tools they'll need to prepare for the pregnancy, delivery, and initial care of their newborn.

I like the systematic and complete way this book approaches all aspects of pregnancy. It carefully covers pregnancy from start to finish and beyond, as well as from head to toe. It helps women to understand what is happening to their bodies, prepares them emotionally for changes of pregnancy, and gives them the knowledge they need to be active participants in their prenatal care. And then the book goes one step further by helping the new mother to prepare for the early days of parenthood. This is all done in a clear and easy to understand way.

Pregnancy is an exciting time for a woman—but it is also an important opportunity for her to refocus on her own health and the health of her family. Armed with the knowledge contained in this book, she will be in a great position to make a genuine difference in creating a strong foundation for herself and her family.

Peter S. Bernstein, MD, MPH, FACOG
Medical Director of Obstetrics and Gynecology
The Comprehensive Family Care Center at Montefiore Medical Center

Associate Professor of Clinical Obstetrics & Gynecology and Women's Health
Albert Einstein College of Medicine

Pregnancy for the 21st-Century Woman

My life as a midwife began over 30 years ago in the "good old days" when women were vocal and demanded change in their care during pregnancy and birth. This cultural revolution in pregnancy and birth pioneered family-centered care, which placed an emphasis on natural childbirth and a home or home-like surroundings for family bonding and the comfort of the mother. Common discomforts and complications of pregnancy and birth were also treated through nutrition and herbal remedies.

Pregnancy and birth became seen as spiritually meaningful life experiences for women that tapped into their deep resources of power, providing them with the energy necessary to nurture a newborn. In addition, women were taught to trust their bodies and to trust the process. Besides becoming a midwife during this time, I gave birth to my sons and also experienced the creation of myself as a mother.

Today, the experience of pregnancy and childbirth is very different. Advances in technology such as routine ultrasounds; electronic fetal monitoring; genetic testing; amniocentesis; routine induction of labor; and the widespread use of epidural anesthesia have altered the experience of a "normal" pregnancy and birth. Most women expect to know the gender of their baby about the time their pregnancy begins to show. Women can choose a "painless birth"; their baby's birthday; and whether to be delivered by induction or cesarean section. Breast pumps are *de rigueur* for the woman too busy to nurse.

Nowadays, pregnancy and birth are viewed as medical events that must be monitored, measured, and controlled, and as complicated events fraught with danger and risk. Women are afraid of what they can't control or understand. For example, as the expectant mother moves through her pregnancy, she successfully passes one set of medical tests only to face another battery of tests for another set of possible conditions. Danger and risk lurk in the background and the mind of the woman and her care provider. There is no time for the pregnant woman to relax, feel free, powerful, and mighty. Pregnancy and birth are "normal" only in hindsight. So where does this leave the pregnant woman in the 21st century? From my experience of listening to hundreds of pregnant women, I can attest to the fact that women lack confidence in their own natural ability to grow, birth, and nurture their baby. *Great Expectations: Your All-in-One Resource for Pregnancy & Childbirth* meets the needs of today's pregnant woman. Sandy and Marcie Jones demystify modern medical practices while also suggesting holistic options for the various stages of pregnancy and childbirth. During pregnancy, women are encouraged to learn all they can about fetal development, nutrition, maternal physiology, and physical science. *Great Expectations* provides that foundation for the woman who wants to be informed, knowledgeable and who wants to actively participate in the decision-making process affecting her pregnancy, birth and parenting style.

This is a book I will gladly recommend to the women I care for. It provides the most up-to-date medical information about the complexities of modern pregnancy and birth care, but most importantly, communicates the belief that women are powerful; pregnancy is a joyous time; and that birth can be an empowering experience. This is a message that pregnant women desperately need to hear.

Claire M. Westdahl, CNM, MPH, FACNM
Director, Nurse Midwifery, Emory University School of Medicine

G·R·E·A·T
EXPECTATIONS

Your All-in-One Resource for
Pregnancy
& Childbirth

Your Pregnancy Week-by-Week

n this section, organized by week, you'll find out how many days you've been pregnant, how many days you have to go, and details our baby's height, weight, and physical and mental development. You can read about what's happening to your body, what should worry about, and what's normal. Every week, you'll find information about risks you should be aware of, choices you can make, and situations you may find yourself in as your pregnancy progresses.

This section serves as a way to get oriented and is also a gateway into the rest of the book. This guide was designed to keep you from losing your place—you can read each week as it applies to you, just to find out about your pregnancy's progress, or you can use this section as a way to find the subjects in this book that you want to read more about, by following the references to other sections. Specific medical and pregnancy terms will be highlighted in bold and italic, which will let you know that a more thorough and specific definition can be found in the *Pregnancy Dictionary* on page 574.

You can begin reading the Week-by-Week Guide at the specific week you're in in your pregnancy if your care provider has given you a due date. Or if it's too soon to even have a due date—you're waiting until it's soon enough to test, or you have a feeling you might be pregnant but you aren't sure—you can start reading right here!

Are You Pregnant?

You feel like you have PMS, but your period won't come.

Missing a period may seem like an obvious sign, but many women have irregular periods and don't make note of the date every month. Early pregnancy symptoms feel a lot like PMS: cramps, bloating, achy or sensitive breasts, fatigue, and crankiness. You may even experience light blood spotting.

Your sense of smell is sharper.

For some women, the first sign of pregnancy is their ability to suddenly detect odors that they couldn't before. The stink of exhaust fumes, cigarette smoke, incense, or other airborne odors may offend you to the point of queasiness. This reaction will intensify as your hormone levels rise and may last your entire pregnancy.

You feel bloated.

Your underwear, rings, and bracelets may feel like they've shrunk, and you have to suck in to zip up the tighter clothes in your wardrobe.

Something's different about your breasts.

Your breasts may simply feel tender, as they would if you had PMS. But pregnancy breasts are more extreme: they suddenly appear larger, fuller, and perkier, as if you were wearing a push-up bra. Some women may even experience tingling.

Your home pregnancy test is positive.

If you take a home pregnancy test, and it's positive, you can believe it. Pregnancy tests detect the presence of *human chorionic gonadotropin* (*hCG*), a hormone produced by the fertilized egg and, later, the human placenta during pregnancy. It takes about four days for the fertilized egg to begin secreting any amount of hCG. Unless you've misread the test results, or have been taking very specific fertility drugs that contain hCG, it's virtually impossible to get a false-positive result.

What If I Think I'm Pregnant, But the Test Is Negative?

Pregnancy-test false negatives are really common, in spite of what test packages say. Recent research published in the *American Journal of Obstetrics and Gynecology* found that only one of eighteen brands tested were sensitive enough to detect pregnancy at four weeks from *LMP (last menstrual period)*.

If you get a negative result on a home pregnancy test, but your period is still late, test again a day or two later. A pregnant woman's hCG levels will double every two to three days in early pregnancy. Plenty of pregnant women will not have levels of hCG high enough to be detectable by over-the-counter tests until as late as six weeks after their last periods.

The Test Is Positive, Now What?

If you get a positive pregnancy-test result, you'll want to call your family doctor, gynecologist, healthcare provider, midwife, or clinic right away to receive independent confirmation of your results, to have your health evaluated, and to get your due date calculated. Care providers

can also be great to talk to about some of the early concerns you may have before you tell your partner, family, and friends.

You may also decide that you want your baby to be delivered by a different care provider than the obstetrician/gynecologist who performs your checkups or that you'd like to be cared for by a *certified nurse-midwife (CNM)*. It's okay to make prenatal appointments with your current doctor now and to politely cancel them if you find a different care provider. (See *Managing Your Care* on page 162, for details on different types of care providers.)

Hearing the News

Women's reactions to positive pregnancy tests can range from total denial to unmitigated glee to hyperventilating horror. Don't blame yourself for your emotions—there's no wrong way to react to such big and shocking news. It's also okay to be happy about the baby, but not thrilled about the prospect of pregnancy, labor, and birth. Everyone's different, and you have nine months (and eighteen years!) to figure out how you feel about parenthood.

Whom Should You Tell?

Your Partner

After a pregnancy test confirms that you're pregnant, you get to tell your partner, unless he was standing next to you as you stared at the stick. Will you say two words, or put on an elaborate production number? As you try to decide, keep in mind that a reaction of disbelief, shock, and terror is as common as whoops of joy. Your partner is normal if he doesn't believe it at first ("Are you sure?") or expresses his misgivings

> *"I told my mom by mixing a sonogram picture in with our vacation pictures. It was so funny watching her figure it out!"*

Things to Ask on Your First Prenatal Visit

About Your Care Provider

How long has he been in practice?

What kind of training does she have, and from where?

What is his general philosophy concerning pregnancy and birth?

Which hospitals/birth centers is she affiliated with? Why did she decide to become a doctor or midwife?

How many babies does he deliver per week/month/year?

Who are the other people in the practice? Will you have visits with them also? Who will deliver? How long have the others been in practice?

Do you have a choice about whom you see in the practice?

What's the rotation schedule?

How often will visits be during your pregnancy?

What happens during a typical visit?

What kind of pain relief options will be provided to you in labor?

What is his definition of a high-risk pregnancy?

How does she feel about partners being involved at prenatal exams and during labor and birth?

How does he regard written birthing plans?

What's her c-section rate?

Will he be in town when you're due?

What tests does she recommend, and when should they be scheduled?

Does he recommend ultrasound tests? When, and how often?

Does she recommend certain prenatal classes?

About You and Your Pregnancy

What is my due date?

Should I follow specific recommendations concerning weight gain, exercise, and diet?

What foods and activities should I avoid?

What kind of options do I have for prenatal vitamins?

Should I be concerned about anything that I was exposed to before I knew I was pregnant?

("How are we going to afford it?"). This reaction is just as legitimate as one of joy, and it doesn't mean your partner won't blossom into a wonderful parent.

Your Friends and Family

Of course you'll tell your best girlfriends, parents, and close relations right away, no matter what any pregnancy book tells you to do. However, you may want to wait until you're sure how you (and your partner) feel about the pregnancy. Also, it's important to take into account that one in every five pregnancies results in miscarriage during the first trimester. You may want to tell only those people who would be sensitive to any negative development that came along. Remind your partner that he faces the same issue, and to not tell his every friend, client, and co-worker.

At Work

If you work, it's good sense to wait to make your announcement until the first trimester has passed, and you've done some quiet research about your company's leave policies and treatment of previous pregnant employees. (We go into more detail on this topic on page 249 of the *Managing Your Finances* section.)

Your First Visit to Your Doctor or Midwife

After you get a positive test result, you'll want to make an appointment for your first prenatal visit to your care provider, to confirm your pregnancy and be checked for infections, conditions, and other issues that may need to be dealt with. Your healthcare provider will want to take a full medical history and assess your lifestyle. If you've switched providers, make sure your new provider has your previous records.

The first part of your prenatal visit will involve filling out lots of forms and answering plenty of questions about your personal and family history. Your clinician will ask you questions about your health and lifestyle, your menstrual history, past pregnancies or miscarriages (if any), medication use, recent birth control methods, allergies, and your partner's health and medical history.

Your care provider will also want to find out if you have any preexisting conditions, a family history of genetic disorders, allergies, or dangerous habits. Some of the questions may seem a bit intrusive. Some care providers, for instance, will ask how old you were when you first had intercourse, or if any of your previous pregnancies ended in abortion. It's okay to ask your care provider why the information is necessary or to leave the question blank. Also, if you find you don't feel comfortable telling your care provider the truth, consider it a sign that you should investigate the possibility of finding someone else to deliver your baby.

After a review and discussion of your medical history, your care provider will

1. Create a chart that will be checked at every visit to make sure that you're gaining enough weight.

2. Manually measure the height of your uterus to confirm how far along you are and to create a growth chart for your uterus.

3. Take a blood sample from your arm in order to

- Determine your blood type and whether or not you are Rh negative. If so, this means that you have a blood type that may be incompatible with your baby's, and you'll need an injection during your pregnancy to prevent potential complications. (See "Rh Factor Screening" in *Testing: Risks and Benefits* on page 188.)

- Check the *hemoglobin* levels in your blood. If they're low, you may be anemic and will need to take iron supplements or prenatal vitamins with iron to stay healthy. (See more on *iron* on page 150 of *Managing Your Nutrition* and *anemia* in the *Pregnancy Dictionary*.)

- Check for the presence of infections that may have no symptoms but can complicate your pregnancy and harm the baby if they aren't treated or managed, such as syphilis, Hepatitis B, and HIV. (See *Managing High-Risk Conditions* on page 211.)

- See if you have antibodies to *rubella* (German measles). If you were vaccinated or had the disease as a child, there's no need to worry. If you don't have antibodies, however, you'll need to be careful to avoid exposure to anyone with the infection, because it can cause birth defects. (See *Immunizations and Vaccines* on page 204.)

- See if you're potentially a carrier for certain genetic disorders such as **sickle-cell anemia**, **Tay-Sachs disease**, or **cystic fibrosis**. If you have a family or personal history, extra blood will be taken for a test called hemoglobin electrophoresis. If you are a carrier of a genetic disease, then your baby's father should also be checked. If both of you are carriers of one of these disorders, then your baby has a twenty-five percent chance of developing it. (See more under "Genetic Disorders" in *Testing: Risks and Benefits* on page 179.)

- Some care providers also may check to see if you have immunities to **toxoplasmosis**, especially if you have a preexisting infection such as **HIV**. If you're not immune, you may be tested for the infection during your pregnancy and should avoid contact with soil, unwashed produce, and the cat box—anywhere that you may come into contact with cat or vermin feces. (See page 642 of the *Pregnancy Dictonary* for more about toxoplasmosis.)

If your care provider doesn't have a lab on site to draw and test blood, ask him to recommend a diagnostic lab where the phlebotomists are experienced enough to draw blood with the first stick. You may have quite a few vials drawn from you during the first trimester, so a good technician can make the experience much more tolerable.

Your care provider will also take a *urine* sample to check your levels of protein, sugar, and bacteria. Protein and/or the presence of red and white blood cells could be a sign of high blood pressure or a urinary tract or kidney infection. Later in pregnancy, protein can be a sign of *preeclampsia*, also known as toxemia. Your care provider will probably check your urine at every visit. (For more information, see "Toxemia" in *Managing High-Risk Conditions*, page 215.)

You'll also receive a physical exam, where your care provider will

1. Measure your height, weight, and blood pressure.

2. Assess your eyes, teeth, and skin.

3. Listen to your heart and lungs to check for abnormalities or congestion.

4. Palpate your abdomen for abnormalities.

5. Conduct a pelvic exam. Your caregiver will inspect the color of your *cervix* and the size of your *uterus*. If you're pregnant, your cervix will have a bluish tint, and your uterus will be heavy and firm. The size and position of your uterus can also be used to estimate fetal age. Your care provider may also take swabs from your cervix for a Pap test to screen for cervical cancer and to check for infections and *sexually transmitted diseases (STDs)*, such as *chlamydia* and *gonorrhea* that can be harmful to an unborn baby.

Last but not least, your care provider will give you a *due date*. If you have no idea when your last menstrual period was, or if your periods tend to be irregular, your care provider may order an ultrasound to help determine the age of your embryo. There is controversy about the safety of ultrasounds. (For more information, see *Testing: Risks and Benefits*, page 188.)

How Your Due Date Is Calculated

Establishing an estimated due date is important, not only for your own peace of mind, but so that your care provider can make sure that your baby isn't threatening to arrive dangerously early or late.

For consistency, healthcare providers (and many pregnancy books) start counting how many weeks pregnant you are by the date of the first day of your most recent menstrual period (last menstrual period, or LMP). This is used to calculate your baby's *gestational age.*

When you visit your caregiver, he will probably use a forty-week medical standard as a timetable for the length of your pregnancy. That means that according to most week calculations, you're already two weeks pregnant on the day you conceive.

Why? Because the last menstrual period is an easy and reliable outward sign from which to calculate a due date. The forty-week standard is a way doctors calculate the length of pregnancy that predates *sonograms* and goes back to the early days of medicine. (See pages 648–649.)

In reality, your actual pregnancy will last about 266 days, thirty-eight weeks, or nine-and-a-half months as measured from the day you really conceive. This way of calculating how far along you are is called your baby's fetal age.

Care providers can measure the fetal age of your baby with a sonogram after about six weeks of pregnancy and figure out your baby's true age with a fair amount of accuracy, and many women are able to determine exactly when they conceived, but even with the accuracy of these new imaging tools, the forty-week gestational calendar remains in use by medical professionals. This can get confusing, especially if your periods are irregular. When your care provider says you're ten weeks along, will that mean that your fetus is ten weeks old, or only eight?

In this book, we use the forty-week convention so that you'll be able to be on the same page with your caregivers, but we'll also provide fetal age in smaller type so you'll know exactly how old your baby is at any given time.

Your Due Date

Only about one in twenty women delivers on her exact due date. Unless you're planning to have a scheduled C-section, what day, hour, and minute your baby will be born is one of life's great intangibles. Your due date actually just suggests a five-week window for when it would be healthy for your baby to be born. The week surrounding your due date is when he is *most likely* to be born. Babies born before thirty-seven weeks or after forty-two weeks gestational age are thought to be more at risk for physical problems. (See discussion of past-due babies at week forty on page 106.)

When you have a due date established, you can get a calendar and number the weeks, months, and trimesters.

> *"I bought a big blank book for my husband and me to write in about anything and everything—appointments, cravings, how we're feeling. I put it on the kitchen counter and doodle in it while I'm on the phone. It's fun!"*

Making Your Own Pregnancy Calendar

As you count down to that magic due date, it's impossible to resist the urge to create your own pregnancy calendar. Do you *need* one? Not really. But it's fun to know what trimester you're in, how many days you've been pregnant, and how many days you have left. You can use calendar software on your computer or have one generated by a Web site. A paper calendar that you've written on yourself will also make a great memento. Day-by-day calendars that give you enough space for comments are ideal. You can not only use them to mark the time but also to keep your baby-related to-do list, write down what you eat, keep track of how often you exercise, note any symptoms or discomforts you experience, and write down questions you have for your care provider.

Whatever sort of calendar you pick, customize it by simply counting back 266 days (thirty-eight weeks) from your estimated due date. This will give you the fetal age. Count back two more weeks to calculate the age of your pregnancy according to medical convention. (You may want to have two sets of numbers on your calendar.) Then, keep a running tally of your pregnancy. If you're curious to know how long it is until your baby gets born, you can count the weeks backward from your due date, as in: "I've got twenty-three more weeks to go."

After you have your weeks written down, go back and add trimesters, each of which is twelve weeks (or about 88 days) long. And voilà, now when someone asks you how far along you are, you can say, "Ninety-two days, or fourteen weeks by a 280-day medical calendar, or four days into my second trimester."

The First Trimester

Weeks 1 through 13

Fetal age: 1 to 13 weeks

During these next twelve weeks, your future child will grow from a single fertilized egg that would fit on the head of a pin into a recognizably human shape that's about the height of a tube of lipstick!

For your baby's first twelve weeks of existence, she will be building basic body structures according to a standard genetic blueprint. While all of the genes for individual characteristics are there, in the formative first few weeks, your baby will look like the embryo and fetus of any animal. Yet by the end of the first trimester, she will look unmistakably human, with a head, arms, legs, and the beginnings of all major organ systems.

For you, the first trimester can feel like a real roller coaster ride.

As your baby develops during the first trimester, your body changes dramatically to sustain and support her. You'll lose the shape of your waist, and your breasts may grow an entire cup size. Your ribs and hips will widen. By the end of the first trimester, you'll feel and look more padded all over, though probably not so much that people on the street will know your condition. Your body and head hair, complexion, and the pigment on your nipples and body will be different three months from now. Your breasts will be preparing to make milk for the first time, with systems that have been in place since you yourself were a fetus. During this trimester, you may even find that your breasts begin to leak drops of *colostrum*, though usually not enough to soak through your bras or shirts.

Believe it or not, by your second trimester, you'll almost be used to being pregnant. Your hormone levels will have stabilized, your condition will be known, and your friends and family will be well on the way to adjusting to their new roles. By the time you go into labor, you'll probably feel *more* than ready for the baby's arrival! That may seem like a pretty far-fetched notion right now, though.

Some women love the physical experience of pregnancy. They love the excitement, anticipation, attention, and healthy glow, and the feeling of growing a little life inside. When it's over, they can't wait to do it again. Other women hate everything about pregnancy, dreading labor and feeling ugly and oppressed by their tiny slave driver downstairs. Your genes, family's attitude, home situation, and outlook on life will all play a part.

Love or hate pregnancy, lots of women find the first trimester the most difficult, for a number of reasons.

You feel awful.

Eighty percent of women experience nausea and/or vomiting. Even if you can keep your food down and aren't in a constant state of disgust, you still will certainly experience fatigue, bloating, crabbiness, and achy breasts.

It's the biggest news of your life, and you have to keep it secret.

You don't have to, but most women do, because of the risk of miscarriage during the first twelve weeks. If you're not used to keeping secrets, it can be hard to keep the cat in the bag.

Your relationships are changing and being tested.

Your "husband" or "boyfriend" is now your "baby's father," your mother is "grandma." You're now closer to some friends, and others you have a harder time relating to. If you aren't married to your baby's father, you may be wondering if you should be. (See more about single parenting in *Managing Family and Emotional Issues*, page 246.)

Your future has changed.

You were going one way, now you're headed to parts unknown. Any plans you had for moving to a foreign country or touring small clubs with your rock band are now on hold for the time being.

You're moody.

Combine the mental stress of pregnancy with your surging hormones, and you can feel like you're losing your mind. One minute, you may feel great elation at the idea of having a baby, and the next minute, deep despair and concern about what's happening. It can be hard to know if what you're feeling is real or if it's just a by-product of what's going on with you physically. Drops and jumps in your blood sugar and blood pressure can make you nauseated. Aches and pains can make you cranky. All of the extra estrogen in your system can make you feel weepy and sensitive. If you're unlucky enough to be slowed down by physical symptoms, it can be easy to get depressed.

You feel "out of it."

As your veins expand, and your blood pressure goes down, there actually is less blood than usual making it to your brain. You may find yourself feeling "fuzzy minded," as though getting pregnant has altered your ability to think clearly and make decisions.

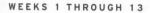

What to Avoid During Your Pregnancy

For quick reference, here's a rundown of things you should start avoiding right now. (More details about dangers and risks can be found in *Managing Other Risks,* **page 225.)**

Definitely unsafe:

- **Alcohol.** As little as a glass and a half of wine a week can cause serious damage to the fetus and kill fetal brain cells.[1] (See page 205*)*

- **Cigarettes.** (See pages 21–22 of the *Week-by-Week Guide* for more on why smoking is dangerous and how to quit.)

- **Frequent exposure to secondhand smoke.**

- **Taking any drug, topical cream, vitamin, or herbal supplement** without talking to your care provider. Seemingly harmless drugs, such as Naproxen (Aleve®), have been linked to birth defects in animals. (See *Managing Your Medicine Cabinet* on page 195 of the *Managing Your Pregnancy* section for more details about the safety of over-the-counter medications.)

- **Cured or smoked meats,** hot dogs, deli meat, lunch meats, raw milk, unpasteurized cheeses, unpasteurized juices, or raw leafy vegetables or sprouts, because of the risk of exposure to listeria bacteria. (See ***listeriosis*** on page 616 of the *Pregnancy Dictionary* for more information.)

- **Baths, hot tubs, saunas or using electric blankets** hotter than 102 degrees. Heat exposure during the first trimester has been linked with an increased rate of miscarriage. (See page 230 of *Managing Other Risks* for more information.)

- **Being on a strict vegan diet without taking vitamin supplements.** (See more on vegetarian diets in *Managing Your Nutrition* on page 152.)

- **Exposure to baby-harming infections.** Chickenpox, rubella and hepatitis B can hurt your baby, as can sexually transmitted infections such as Chlamydia, genital herpes, HIV and hepatitis. Refrain from exchanging bodily fluids with infected persons and use a condom.

- **Ingesting more than 150 mg. of caffeine a day.** (See more about caffeine on page 205.)

- **Handling dirty cat litter**, soil, or dead rodents without gloves. (See more under toxoplasmosis in the *Pregnancy Dictionary* on page 642.)

- **Eating shark, swordfish, king mackerel, or tilefish** (also called golden or white snapper). Mercury can be harmful to a fetus's growing brain, and these large ocean fish contain more mercury than the FDA considers safe for pregnant women. Also, limit your intake of tuna and farmed salmon to twelve ounces or less a week. You may wish to consider purified fish oil capsules as a source of DHA. (See more about mercury in the *Pregnancy Dictonary*, and more about DHA on page 619.)

You don't know what's safe and what's not.

It's a scary reality that the world is full of dangers that you can't see and that have the potential to harm your baby. You don't have to go crazy purging your house of chemicals, but do clean out your medicine cabinet, and get rid of suspect drugs (for a complete list, see *Managing Your Medicine Cabinet: Common Drugs* on page 195), acne medications, scented feminine hygiene products, herbal supplements, and anything expired. Also give yourself license to throw away anything in the refrigerator that's old or smells funny.

So what CAN you do during the first trimester? Here's a list of ideas:

Nap

The first trimester is for resting. Sleep as much as you need to. It'll keep your mood up.

Eat right

Now is the time to focus on healthy eating habits. Remember to eat small, low-sugar high-protein snacks during the day. Avoid big sugar bombs such as soda, candy, pastries, and doughnuts. (See *Managing Your Nutrition*, page 145.)

Research

You'll be seeing your care provider about once a month until your last month of pregnancy, when you'll see him once a week. Use your appointments to ask plenty of questions—the more you know and the more confidence you feel in your provider's abilities, the less frightening the whole pregnancy, birth, and labor process will be. Also don't be afraid to call the office for any question you may have, even if you just want advice about nutrition or safe foods.

Adjust your lifestyle

Does this describe you? You're of ideal weight. You eat five different fruits and/or vegetables every single day, drink nothing but milk or water, don't touch caffeine, exercise for at least an hour five days a week, and never smoke or so much as look at a white wine spritzer. You're so healthy you don't even need to keep aspirin in your medicine cabinet. If you're like most of us, you're in for some major lifestyle changes if you want to give your baby the best start in life. It's really hard to change your every habit overnight, but small changes can make a big difference.

Keep a journal of your habits

As you probably already know, smoking and drinking are bad, exercise and a nutritious diet are good, and you want to gain enough, but not too much, weight. But how do you translate this information into real-life action?

One way is to start keeping a journal. To establish better habits, you have to know what your current habits are. For a week, write down everything that you put in your mouth and every physical activity you engage in. Do you need to eat less candy, get more calcium, drink more water, or exercise more often? Write it down.

Set small and manageable goals, and phrase them positively. Don't try to stop eating candy forever, for instance. Instead, set a goal to eat smaller portions less often, and think of ways to substitute better alternatives to your habits. Try to isolate exactly what it is about a bad-habit food that you love so much, and see if you can satisfy your craving in a healthier way. For instance, if you notice that you can't go a day without potato chips, think of ways to feed the craving for a salty crunch without the calories, like vegetable chips, or carrot sticks or celery with low-fat dip.

After you've looked over your lifestyle in black and white and thought about alternatives, start a fresh section of your journal, and assess every week—are you achieving your goals?

Don't worry about individual days, but whether by the end of the week, you're eating and living a little bit healthier on average than you did before. Your pregnancy can be an opportunity to establish lifelong healthy habits.

Start or continue exercising

Pregnancy, labor, birth, and your baby's infancy and toddlerhood are physically difficult, and the more fit you are, the easier they'll be for you. Women who are in shape and keep fit during pregnancy have shorter labors, fewer complications, and quicker postpartum recoveries. Fit women are less likely to suffer depression during pregnancy and after birth.

If you're already exercising regularly and feel up to it, pregnancy itself is no reason to change your routine or cut back. Just use common sense to avoid dehydration, overheating, and injury.

If you're out of shape or have never exercised before, start gently when you feel physically up to it. Try a simple thirty-minute walk, swim, or stretch or yoga session three times a week, adding more frequency and intensity as you progress. (See more about exercise in *Managing Your Weight and Fitness* on page 157.)

Prepare emotionally

It makes sense to wait until at least the end of the first trimester to make practical plans about work, money, and nursery decorating. There's a one in five chance of miscarriage during these first weeks (though only about a one in ten chance after the pregnancy is detected, and a heartbeat is heard). The rate is high enough that it puts you and your family in a kind of emotional limbo, hoping for the best, preparing for the worst, talking out scenarios and what-ifs, and making lists of baby names.

Weeks 2 and 3

Fetal Age: 1 to 14 days
38 to 37 weeks, 266 to 252 days until your due date

YOUR BABY

Size

Fits on the head of a pin.

Development

Though some women swear that they were aware of the moment of conception, most are oblivious. The radical hormonal changes of the first trimester don't kick in until implantation, which happens between three to five days after conception. Meanwhile, your uterus is like a high-school biology film come to life. Here's what happened:

At the moment of conception, two single cells, his sperm and your egg (otherwise known as gametes) merge. The conditions that allow this to occur are extremely specific. Twelve to twenty-four hours prior to conception, your estrogen levels will have reached their monthly peak, triggering a release of an egg from one of your ovaries. Your cervix softens and lifts and begins to secrete a slick fluid that contains microscopic fernlike ladders. Before ovulation, the cervical mucus is dense and impenetrable to the sperm. But during ovulation, the mucus becomes more watery, and the sperm travel up the ladders it forms, swimming upward at a rate of seven inches in half an hour.

Sperm work in teams and are somehow aware of one another. They organize into scouting parties to find the egg. If another man's sperm is around, some sperm will form a kamikaze army and beat them back, fighting to the death for domination.[2] Like bicyclists in the Tour de France, sperm form protective, defensive groups that help each other maintain speed and edge out competitors.

If there's no egg, the sperm will rest their heads on the walls of the fallopian tubes, waiting like groupies. A strong sperm can wait for up to forty-eight hours.

If a group of sperm finds an egg, the sperm get "hyperactivated," and the ramming begins. Sperm whack at the egg's outside with their thick, enzyme-coated heads. The enzymes actually can weaken and dissolve the egg's outer shell (called the zona). The winning sperm, the one in two hundred million, is the one whose head first penetrates the egg's outside. At that nanosecond, the egg absorbs the winning sperm's head, the egg shuts down completely, and no more sperm will be admitted.

Inside the egg, the two sets of cell nuclei lie side by side. Each cell has half of a set of chromosomes, and the moment of conception is the moment they fuse together and unite them. Your future baby has been assigned a gender, eye color, hair color, and at least two hundred other characteristics. The cell that results is called a zygote.

Over the next few days, as the zygote divides, it creates a blastocyst, a tiny fluid-filled ball of cells that travels down the fallopian tube and into the cavity of the uterus and lands along the uterine wall.

After about three to five days, the blastocyst will implant, or burrow, into the lining of the wall of the uterus and will be known as an *embryo* from that point until the end of the first trimester, when it earns the title of *fetus*, Latin for "little one." About sixty percent of fertilized eggs do not successfully implant, and are instead passed within twelve days of conception.

YOU

What's happening to you

In spite of the drama going on in your cervix and uterus, you probably won't feel any different. Some women report intuitively knowing that they're pregnant, but if you were clueless until you saw that line on the stick, you're in the majority.

How you feel about it

If you've been trying to get pregnant, you may be waiting on the edge of your seat until a test can confirm your pregnancy. If you weren't trying, you may be on the edge of your seat for the same reason.

What you can do

Now, if not before you start trying to conceive, here's what you should do.

- Quit smoking. (See box.)

- Avoid alcohol.

- Avoid drugs: the legal, the illegal, those labeled "herbal supplements," and those that come as skin creams (such as acne medication) and in beverages (like caffeine). Don't swallow, drink, snort, inject, or apply anything until you've talked to your care provider about it. Immediately tell your care provider about any prescription or other medications you currently take or were taking at the time you conceived.

- Avoid taking large amounts of vitamins: an over-the-counter prenatal or even daily chewable (like a Flintstone) is enough and is recommended for all women who are trying to conceive or could possibly become pregnant. And excessive amounts of some vitamins (such as vitamin A) can be dangerous. Don't assume that if a little is good, a lot is better!

- If you have any kind of medical appointment with a doctor or dentist, inform them that you may be pregnant. You'll want to avoid X-rays or any unnecessary medical tests or vaccinations.

- Eat five servings of different fruits and vegetables daily.

- Drink plenty of water—it will prevent headaches, help your body make blood and eliminate waste, and make your skin more radiant. Drinking water will also make you less likely to retain water.

Smoking

No doubt you've already heard how bad smoking is for your baby when you're pregnant. Still, in America, about one in ten women continues to smoke while pregnant.[3]

There continue to be studies that inform us of the effects of smoking on the fetus, the most recent reporting that smoking while pregnant can make your child have lasting mental and behavioral problems that can endure throughout childhood and adolescence.[4]

Smoking while pregnant increases your baby's risk of being born prematurely, being stillborn, or dying from SIDS. Children whose mothers smoked while pregnant are also more at risk for a wide range of adult problems.

Of all times in your life to quit, this is the best and the easiest time. Here's why:

- **You want your baby to be healthy.** In addition to everything mentioned earlier, children of smokers are more than twice as likely to smoke themselves. What's a little withdrawal compared with saving your baby's life?

- **It stinks.** Your body is already causing you to have aversions to certain odors. Use this extra support to help you kick the habit.

- **You're making other changes.** You've probably already started changing your eating habits and daily routines.

- **Avoid dirty looks.** As you get visibly pregnant, you'll have plenty of peer pressure. Exceptionally self-righteous perfect strangers will give you dirty looks and lectures and may even snatch cigarettes from your hands and put them out.

- **Weight gain won't matter.** What's an extra few pounds at this point?

- **Vanity.** You'll have less acne, fewer blackheads, and fewer wrinkles on your face and body (a great thing, considering how much stretching your skin is going to get!). Smoking cuts off blood flow to the capillaries in your face, and quitting will make you look as if you had a facelift.

- **Vitality.** As more oxygen gets to your cells and brain, you'll have more energy.

- **Money.** Smoking isn't cheap—and good luck finding someone to bum cigarettes from when you're pregnant! Save your money, and use it to buy something nice for yourself—a pedicure or massage, for instance.

- **Pleasure.** Food will taste better.

- **An easier labor.** With stronger lungs and better oxygenation, you'll have an easier labor.

- **Fitness.** You'll have an easier time getting up stairs at the end of your pregnancy, when your baby is squashing your lungs.

- **A longer, healthier life.** If you quit now, you'll get to spend more years of your life with your child. Half of all smokers will die from their addiction.[5]

- Start exercising, or keep up whatever fitness routine you have, to get in shape for your body changes and birth and labor.

- Get someone else to change your cat box! (See toxoplasmosis in the *Pregnancy Dictionary* on page 642.)

Tips to Help You Quit Smoking

- **Get help.** People who attend smoking-cessation programs have twice the success of people who try to quit alone. Ask your doctor for a referral.

- **Postpone.** If you have the urge, make yourself wait fifteen minutes, and distract yourself somehow. Often the urge will pass.

- **Don't bring them home.** Just don't buy them.

- **Use a visual aid.** Every time you light up, your baby smokes too, whether he wants to or not. Copy one of the pictures from your baby's sonogram, and put it inside the cellophane of your pack as a reminder of what you're doing.

- **Smell it, and taste it.** Try using your brain to convince your body that you just smoked. Imagine the taste in your mouth. Breathe deeply, and imagine that your lungs are already full of tar.

- **Go where the nonsmokers are.** Hang out where you can't smoke: the gym, the pool, the mall, etc.

- **Chew, chew, and chew.** Keep that mouth working! Carrot and celery sticks, gum, licorice, straws, rawhide, whatever works for you.

- **Write it down.** Make lists of your reasons for stopping. Tape one on your bathroom mirror at home, and post the other one next to your computer at work.

- **Take in fresh air.** Breathe deeply, and hold air in your lungs for a few seconds when the urge hits.

- **Hydrate yourself.** Drink lots of water (and seltzer, milk, iced tea, etc.) to flush out the chemicals in your body as quickly as possible.

- **Think clean.** Take a bath or a shower when you get a craving, or brush your teeth.

Week 4

Fetal Age: 2 weeks (15 to 21 days)
36 to 35 weeks, 251 to 245 days until your due date

YOUR BABY

Size

Barely visible to the naked eye.

Development

During the short window of time that implantation in the uterus is possible, the zygote, or mass of cells, has a coating of protein called selectins, which latch onto carbohydrates.

After ovulation, the lining of the uterus develops carbohydrate molecules that reach out to these selectins.

The synchronization of these two events means that when the zygote descends into the uterus, it can firmly take hold of the uterine wall, burrow beneath the surface, and start forming a placenta using tiny, fingerlike projections called *villi* to dig in and set up the baby "nest." A majority of pregnancy losses occur during this very sensitive implantation process. After implantation, the zygote is called an embryo.

Within your embryo, cells are lining up to create a central streak that will turn into the neural tube.

YOU

What's happening to you physically

The fertilized egg burrowing into your uterus can make you shed a few spots of blood.

Any pregnancy symptoms you have will be barely, if at all, noticeable. If you're very sensitive, you

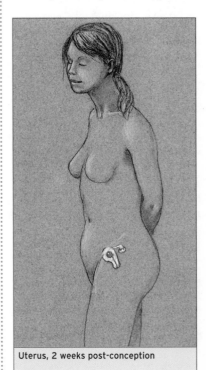

Uterus, 2 weeks post-conception

may notice feelings of fatigue, queasiness, bloating, and breast tenderness, and changes in your skin and hair.

If you take a super-sensitive test, such as a blood test at your doctor's office, it's possible to get a positive result a week after conception. If you test at home this early, know that it's possible to get a false negative at this stage.

How you feel about it

It can seem difficult to believe the news, especially if you look and feel completely normal.

You may be worried about the living it up you did before you knew you were pregnant. Don't worry. Stress is bad for your baby. Many care providers and researchers subscribe to the "all or nothing" theory: If anything you ingested was toxic enough to harm your pregnancy, the zygote would not have implanted, or the embryo would have been lost early on.

What you can do

If you took a pregnancy test, and it was negative (very likely at this stage), but your period hasn't come, and you feel like you have PMS that just won't go away, then take another test.

TIP

Buy glasses that hold sixteen ounces. That way, if you drink two glasses of milk (or calcium-enriched orange juice or soy milk), you'll know you have your calcium needs satisfied for the day.

When you get the news that you're pregnant, accept your emotions, and don't worry about how you "should" feel. No one knows what you're going through but you. (For more on dealing with your new relationships, see *Managing Family and Emotional Issues* on page 233.)

Oysters? Alfalfa sprouts? Hair dye? Genetic testing? Pregnancy can be maddening, because so many things are labeled risky, even if the risk is just a theoretical one. The world can seem like one big accident waiting to happen while you're pregnant. The best you can do is to research, talk to your care provider or check up-to-date reliable online resources. (See our *Resource Guide* on page 538.)

TIP

Use measuring tape to take your measurements, so you'll be able to see yourself grow.

Week 5

Fetal Age: 3 weeks (22 to 28 days)
35 to 34 weeks, 244 to 238 days until your due date

YOUR BABY

Size

The embryo is about two millimeters long, about the size of a grain of sand.

Development

Your baby transforms into a bundle of cells organized in a C-shape with a top, bottom, front, and back. A groove has developed on the embryo's back, which will seal and develop into the neural tube (which later will become the spinal cord). At this point, the tube already has a wider, flatter top that will grow into your baby's brain. A bulge has developed in the center of the embryo, which will soon become a tiny U-shaped tube which will form the heart. This tube will start beating between days twenty-one and twenty-four, and is circulating the embryo's own blood. On about day twenty-six, arm buds form, looking like knobs on the side of the body. Your embryo is encased in protective membranes and attached to a yolk sac, which manufactures the embryo's unique blood cells.

YOU

What's happening to you physically

Now and for the next six weeks, your body is producing large amounts of pregnancy hormones. Hormones are chemical signals that circulate in your body fluids and cause physical effects in your cells. Hormones are the unsung heroes of pregnancy. They actually affect the cells in your body—changing you at the most elemental level. Their powerful effect includes

- Keeping your uterus from shedding the embryo as it naturally would during your monthly cycle.

- Stimulating your breasts' milk production.

- Widening your blood vessels, which brings more blood to the baby and less to your brain—making you feel dizzy. (See more on dizziness under "Circulatory System" in *Managing Your Body* on page 122.)

- Making your digestion more efficient by slowing down your metabolism. (See "Intestinal Tract" on page 132.)

- Affecting your brain chemistry, causing mood swings. Estrogen, in particular, will make you feel weepy, sensitive, and vulnerable.

- Sharpening your sense of smell. (See "Nose" on page 116.)

- Making the ligaments in your hips soften to make room for pregnancy and birth. (See "Muscles," on page 125.)

How you may be feeling

Here's what you may feel now and for the rest of your first trimester.

Emotionally

- **Excited.** No matter what happens, you can't claim that your life is boring.

- **Moody and emotional.** You may feel a whole range of emotions, from elation and pride to doubt and insecurity. Some are caused by hormones, some are just circumstantial. It's natural to feel anxious in the face of the unknown. Just take it one day, or one hour, or one diaper commercial at a time.

- **Happy.** Pregnancy can feel like a joyous blessing, especially if you've been trying. The thought of making a contribution to the future of the human race can be awe-inspiring and humbling.

- **Cautious.** Sharing your news is always fun, but most people suggest waiting to tell anyone but your closest friends until you've been pregnant for three months. If you manage to keep it quiet for three months while racing to the bathroom to throw up, you've got some amazing discretion.

- **Stupid.** You may experience an inability to concentrate and periods of forgetfulness. It's a by-product of low blood flow to your brain and swings in your blood sugar. Plus, you now have more important things on your mind than where you left your keys! Date books and Post-it™ notes can be lifesavers. And if you feel stupid because you're one of the one-quarter of all pregnant women whose pregnancy is the result of contraceptive failure, you aren't alone. Put a Post-it in your date book to talk to your doctor in nine months about birth control options.

- **Worried.** You may be concerned that you're not up to the task of pregnancy, birth, and parenthood, or you may be afraid that you might miscarry or that you won't be able to deal with the discomforts or physical stress.

  You can soothe your anxieties by learning as much as you can about the physical process of pregnancy and by talking to other pregnant women and moms. Your baby's father may be helpful—or he may be in his own world of worry. It's a good thing that pregnancies are about 266 days long— you and your newly expanding family will have lots of time to adjust to this new and radical life change and work through your feelings.

- **Feisty.** The first trimester can feel a lot like horrible PMS, and it's not unusual to pick fights with your spouse, family, co-workers, or people in the parking lot of the grocery store. You may also find yourself feeling enraged at your partner. He doesn't know what you're going through, he's not helpful enough—you name it.

- **Crazy.** Do you feel like you have no control over your emotions, like you're in over your head, like your life is careening out of control, and your body is rebelling against you? You're normal, not nuts.

Physically

- **Tired.** Your body is spending a lot of energy adjusting to pregnancy. Don't feel guilty about taking as many naps as you feel like—the dishes can wait. Or better yet, somebody else can do them.

- **Crampy in the pelvis.** Generalized pain in your pelvis, akin to menstrual cramps, is normal. One-sided sharp pain is a warning sign and should be reported to your doctor.

- **Bloated.** Your clothes may feel unusually tight. To people who see you in clothes, though, your body will appear the same until at least the second trimester.

- **Obsessed with food.** You may be having strange cravings for and aversions to foods that you never used to think about.

- **Disgusted by smoke, alcohol, odors, and/or caffeinated beverages.** Your disgust can be expressed in any number of ways: feeling short of breath, feeling nauseous, feeling dizzy, having dry heaves, or just throwing up. Your body's baby-protecting mechanisms have kicked in. Avoid being exposed to whatever disgusts you—even if it doesn't make sense to you at the time, your body's clearly trying to tell you something.

- **Nauseated.** At any time of the day or night, you may have a vaguely queasy stomach or full-on vomiting bouts. Keep your stomach lined with small, healthy meals. If your prenatal vitamins are making you sick, stop taking them, and talk to your doctor. A children's chewable can often supply your vitamin needs just as effectively. (See our nausea discussion under "Stomach" on page 129.)

- **Like you gotta go.** Pregnancy hormones can make your bladder seem to shrink in half, as increased blood flow to your kidneys increases the amount of urine you make. In about two months, the pressure will ease. Lean forward when you pee to empty your bladder completely. The good news is that increased blood flow to the pelvis can also make sex more fun, though you may be too tired and uncomfortable to care.

- **Chesty.** Your breasts can get seriously uncomfortable, tingly, and achy as they swell. Your nipples are also sensitive and tender. If going down the stairs, running, or jumping hurts, try a snug sports bra, or even two, one on top of the other. Many women even sleep in a bra, French style, to avoid having their nipples rubbed by a nightgown or bed sheets.

- **Drooly.** Pregnancy makes you produce more saliva. It's not uncommon to wake up from a nap and find a puddle on the pillow. You may also start to spit when you talk.

> "It's weird to walk around like everything is normal, knowing that I'm pregnant and about as far from normal as you can get."

- **Gassy.** Nothing complements spitting when you talk like having copious amounts of gas, which is the by-product of your slowed-down intestinal tract. Some foods may cause more gas than others. (See "Intestinal Tract" on page 132 for more on this.)

What you can do

Eat salads, fortified breakfast cereals, and other foods rich in folic acid, which helps your baby's neural tube to close. (Even if you only feel well enough to lie in bed and eat Twizzlers for the time being.)

Think about choosing a health-care provider: If you're pregnant, you're going to need a healthcare provider who knows something about delivering babies. The person who prescribed your pills and diaphragms may not necessarily be the one you want to be dealing with for the next nine or so months and on your delivery day. You can't anticipate every complication or make your baby's birth follow a schedule, but you can certainly do what you can to make sure you have a team you believe in.

Take an afternoon to schedule consultations with obstetricians and midwives. Also take time to tour the hospitals or birthing centers where they practice. If they don't offer free consultations or have time to talk to you, scratch them off the list.

Your health insurance company, if you have one, will have some suggestions for providers and places to deliver. This is also a good time to find out exactly what they plan to pay for. Some companies may not cover procedures such as an elective c-section or circumcision. As unpleasant of a phone call as it may be, it's important to know the details of your coverage. Take and save notes during this conversation.

As soon as you choose your provider, make an appointment for your first prenatal visit. (See *Managing Your Care* on page 162.)

Week 6

Fetal Age: 4 weeks (29 to 35 days)
34 to 33 weeks, 237 to 231 days until your due date

YOUR BABY

Size

The embryo and yolk sac are about the size of an M&M's candy.

Development

A month after conception, your embryo looks something like a newt or a tadpole, and it has gills like a fish! Right now, the embryo of your future baby looks much like the embryo of any other animal—a bird, rabbit, or monkey. It has two tiny cups of pigment on the side of its head that will develop into eyes. Tiny buds that will form the lungs have appeared. The neural tube has closed. One end is flattening and expanding to become the brain, and the other end will become the spine. It's already 10,000 times larger than the fertilized egg. The embryo doesn't have gender characteristics yet, but has little dots where the nipples will be, whether it's a boy or a girl.

The heart, a tiny U-shaped tube, will start beating between days twenty-one and twenty-four and is circulating the embryo's own blood. It has a small mouth and lips and fingernails are forming.

YOU

What's happening physically

Your production of pregnancy hormones (hCG) continues to increase, making you susceptible to nausea and fatigue. Your blood pressure is lower than it was before you were pregnant, which can make you lightheaded and dizzy. (Read more about how pregnancy changes your circulatory system on page 122.)

Miscarriages can and do happen during these early weeks. If you've had miscarriages before, your doctor may monitor your hCG levels. (See "Miscarriage" on pages 30–31 for more information on what happens and what to do if you think you may be losing the embryo.)

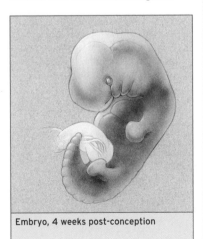
Embryo, 4 weeks post-conception

Miscarriage

Should you worry about having a miscarriage?

Miscarriages are common. Your chances of having one increase as you age: A Danish study[6] in 2000 found that about 9 percent of recognized pregnancies for women ages twenty to twenty-four ended in miscarriage. The risk rose to about 20 percent at age thirty-five to thirty-nine, and more than 50 percent by age forty-two. Worrying won't help; most miscarriages cannot be prevented.

What is a miscarriage?

A miscarriage is a pregnancy that ends before the twentieth medical week. After the twentieth week, the loss of the fetus is classified as a stillbirth or a preterm delivery. Eighty percent of miscarriages happen in the first trimester. They commonly occur around the time the woman's menstrual periods would have—around the fourth, eighth, twelfth, and sixteenth medical weeks of pregnancy. Miscarriages that happen in the first few weeks of pregnancy are referred to as **blighted ovums**, or **anembryonic gestations**, which means that the fertilized egg simply fails to develop for unknown reasons.

Many women miscarry more than once in their life. About one in thirty-six women will have two miscarriages due to nothing more than chance. Most often they are unpreventable, and no cause is found. Having a miscarriage does not affect your ability to carry a baby to term in the future.

Why do they happen?

Most of the time, for no reason other than bad luck, some chromosomal or genetic information is lost during conception. When the needed genetic information is not there at the developmental point when the fetus needs it to continue growing, the fetus dies, and you will miscarry. By eliminating about ninety-five percent of fertilized eggs or embryos with genetic problems, it's nature's way of ensuring that any offspring you have will have the best possible chance for long-term survival. Certain infections may also play a part in some miscarriages.

What happens?

Miscarriages early in pregnancy often happen in the form of a heavy, late period, and if you don't know that you're pregnant, you may not even be aware you're having one. Spotting and light bleeding is common in early pregnancy, but the longer the bleeding lasts and the more cramps you feel, the more likely it is that you're experiencing a miscarriage. The bleeding associated with miscarriages lasts for about seven to ten days.

What to do

If you suspect that you're having a miscarriage, call your care provider immediately.

Your practitioner will probably perform an ultrasound exam. If you have indeed miscarried, your doctor will determine if the miscarriage is complete (all fetal tissue has been passed) or incomplete.

If you haven't miscarried, your doctor may test the hormone levels in your blood and will continue to monitor you with ultrasound. Some doctors may order bed rest. (See "Coping with Bed Rest" on page 223.) If your proges-terone levels are low, you may be given suppositories of progesterone to help maintain your pregnancy, although this is of no proven benefit.

Incomplete miscarriages, when some but not all of the pregnancy tissue is passed, are more common the longer you've been pregnant. In the case of an incomplete miscarriage, your doctor may order a D&C (**dilation and curettage**). This procedure reduces the likelihood of infection. If you have an incomplete miscarriage and are under the supervision of a midwife, you'll be put under the care of her attending obstetrician for this procedure. During a D&C, you will be given general or local anesthesia, your cervix will be dilated, and any retained fetal or placental tissue will be removed. The D&C doesn't weaken your cervix or make you more likely to miscarry in subsequent preg-nancies. Very rarely, a D&C can cause an infection in your uterus, which is treated by a course of antibiotics.

An alternative, which many doctors are starting to use, involves the use of certain medications that trigger the uterus to start cramping and cause the remaining tissue from the pregnancy to be expelled.

How does a miscarriage feel?
Any of the following symptoms may signal that you are going into premature labor and possibly having a miscarriage: your abdomen rhythmically tighten-ing and releasing (**contractions**) every ten minutes or more often; a feeling of pelvic pressure as though your baby is pushing down; a low, dull backache; abdominal or menstrual-like cramps with or without diarrhea; and fluid, blood, or clots being discharged from your vagina.

Emotionally, things may be difficult, particularly if you've been trying hard to get pregnant, or a lot of people know your baby news. It can take a long time to recover from the grief, and family and friends may not know how to react in a supportive manner. Since miscarriage is so common, there are a lot of women out there who share your pain. Internet support groups can be a great resource. Some hospitals hold support groups for women who have lost their pregnancies.

If you worry that drinking, smoking, or staying out late caused your mis-carriage—don't. Unless you're a chronic alcoholic, or you smoke five packs a day, your behavior alone is unlikely to be the cause.

A note on ectopic pregnancy
In about one out of one hundred pregnancies, the ovum doesn't implant in the wall of the uterus where it should, but migrates and implants in the wrong place, such as the side of a fallopian tube, or extremely rarely, in the abdomen. If the embryo is in the fallopian tube, this can cause the tube to rupture. Removal of the embryo often requires surgery (although it is sometimes possible to treat this condition with a medication called methotrexate). In such cases, saving the pregnancy is not possible. The signs of an **ectopic pregnancy** are severe abdominal pain, bleeding, and severe cramps, and you may possibly experience faintness, nausea, dizziness, and vomiting.

By the way, remember the cramps you had with your last menstrual period? They may well have been the last period cramps you'll ever experience. Not only can you put your tampons on a high shelf for the next year, but after your baby's born, your cramps will be milder and may even disappear altogether. Unfortunately, you'll still bloat.

How you're feeling

The extra progesterone and other hormones may be making you feel tired, achy, nauseous, and cranky, or you not may be feeling much different than normal.

You might have an ultrasound as early as this week to determine fetal age or if you've had multiple miscarriages in the past.

You'll start noticing babies more and wondering if yours will be as funny-looking as the ones you see on the street. Don't worry, your baby will be the cutest ever born (or at least, you'll think so).

Should you join a gym?

Maybe. You certainly don't need an expensive membership somewhere to get exercise. But sometimes paying for something will force you to keep your commitment. Gyms also offer community and support that can make it easier to adopt and keep a healthy lifestyle. If you are considering joining a gym, here's what to look for:

A swimming pool. If you can find, and afford, a gym with a pool, go for it! During the second half of your pregnancy, you'll really appreciate the relief from gravity that water offers. Swimming is also a great low-impact exercise and is

> ### EXERCISE TIP
>
> There's no need to stop exercising or curtail your activities, unless you want to. In fact, keeping active will help your body be more able to cope with the stress of carrying around the extra weight you'll be gaining.

perhaps the safest way to exercise while you're pregnant.

Child care. If you can find the gym with the best babysitting facilities in town, you'll probably also find plenty of classes and features geared toward pregnant women and new moms. Not to mention lots of fit moms, who can be great role models. And after the baby's born, reliable child care will also mean that you have a place to go to take long showers.

Prenatal classes. Find a place that offers prenatal aerobics, yoga, or stretching classes that work with your schedule.

Prenatal and postpartum personal trainers. Ask if the gym has personal trainers on staff who are certified to work with pregnant women.

Nutritionists. Some higher-end gyms have on-staff nutritionists, and your insurance company may even foot the bill for you to consult with them!

A flexible contract. Make sure that you can cancel or modify your membership if medical issues or complications arise that make it unsafe or inadvisable for you to work out.

Week 7

Fetal Age: 5 weeks (36 to 42 days)
33 to 32 weeks, 230 to 224 days until your due date

YOUR BABY

Size

Your baby enters its second month of development, weighing no more than a chocolate chip or a berry. It's about five to thirteen millimeters long (less than half an inch), and weighs less than a gram (0.8g), or less than one-twentieth of an ounce.

Development

It has only been a little more than a month, and the human blueprints are already visible. Your child still has a tail but is also beginning to form a digestive tract, lungs, nostrils, hands and feet, and a bump of a mouth. The liver, tongue, and lenses

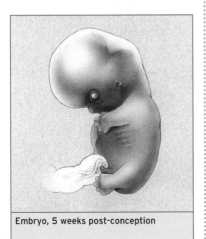

Embryo, 5 weeks post-conception

of your baby's eyes are forming. There are beds for your baby's fingernails, and the buds of teeth are forming in the gums. If you could take a picture, your baby would look more like a baby and less like a reptile. The baby's nerve channels and muscles are connecting, and the body can wiggle when the cells communicate. In just two days, from days thirty-one to thirty-three, the brain becomes one-quarter larger.

If you were to have an ultrasound, it would be able to detect the beating heart, which shows up looking like a tiny flashing light.

YOU

What's happening to you physically

The mucus on your cervix is thickening, forming a plug that will keep your uterus sealed until you give birth.

You may not notice any difference in your body, or you may notice that you're beginning to lose your waistline. Every pregnant woman's body changes at a slightly different pace. If you've had a child before, you may start to look pregnant sooner than you did with your first child.

How you're feeling

You might be feeling tired, achy, and cranky—or not. You might be feeling queasy, or you may never feel queasy. A lack of symptoms doesn't mean that there's anything wrong with you or the baby.

If you are already feeling sick, tired, and miserable, it may comfort you to know that lots of symptoms mean that pregnancy hormones are working hard to support your pregnancy.

You've probably experienced one of pregnancy's first psychological changes: You relate everything you eat, drink, or experience to how it may affect your condition. Your baby is smaller than a fingernail, so she doesn't need lots of calories right now, but she does need to have certain nutrients available for cell division and communication. Prenatal vitamins will help prevent deficiencies, but your body uses nutrients most efficiently if you get them through the foods you eat. A diet with plenty of fiber, vegetables, and fluids will also help keep you from gaining weight that may be hard to lose later. Fortified cereal, big salads with colorful vegetables, and vegetable soups are good choices that will help you get enough folic acid and B vitamins as well as calcium and fluids. (See more about prenatal vitamins and what to eat on page 146 of *Managing Your Nutrition*.)

Things to organize

Your Refrigerator
If you're not feeling too queasy, now is a good time to clean out your refrigerator. Pregnancy gives you a free pass to throw away any food that's old, unappealing or

suspect. Food-borne bacteria are never something you want to take lightly, and avoiding food poisoning is particularly important while you're pregnant because there are harmful bacterial strains that can make both you and the baby sick.

Bad bacteria can come into your life on raw food products, especially meat and dairy, though produce can also be contaminated. They can also thrive in cooked food that's been improperly heated and stored.

Kick off your new, food-safety-conscious lifestyle with a fridge party with a big new garbage bag.

Patrol the shelves for:

- Any foods older than the "use by" or expiration date, or a week or more past the "sell by" date

- Leaky containers

- Shellfish more than a day old

- Raw or smoked fish, poultry or ground uncooked meat more than 2 days old

- Cooked leftovers, cold cuts, salads made with mayonnaise that are more than 3 to 5 days old

- Uncooked fresh beef, pork or lamb chops, steaks or roasts more than 3 to 5 days old

- Fresh vegetables more than a week old

- Mayonnaise and dressings more than 2 months old

Probably needless to say, never test a suspect food by tasting it. Give it the smell test, and heed the adage, "if in doubt, throw it out."

When you're finished purging, clean the refrigerator shelves with warm soapy water and sanitize them with a solution of 1 teaspoon of bleach to a quart of water. While you're in there, leave a thermometer so you can make sure that the refrigerator is maintaining a temperature between 34 and 40 degrees. Colder temperatures don't kill bacteria, but do make them reproduce more slowly.

Other ways to avoid food-borne illness:

When you go grocery shopping:

- avoid produce that is slimy, wilted or smells funny

- Check sell-by and use-by dates on packages to pick the freshest food

- Avoid undated meat and dairy products

- Check bread, produce and dairy for signs of mold

When you cook:

- thoroughly rinse all of your produce, even the pre-washed kind.

- avoid transferring bacteria by keeping your hands, utensils and food prep surfaces clean.

- rinse surfaces with bleach-and-water solution after they come into contact with raw meat or dirt from vegetables.

Bacteria multiply most quickly in food at a temperature of 40-140 degrees and are killed at 165 degrees, which is why it's risky to eat from a buffet that's more than three hours old, and a good idea to use a meat thermometer when you're cooking hamburgers or roasts. Bacteria are also transmitted by poor hygiene, a good reason to avoid eating at restaurants with dirty bathrooms.

Recommended Exercise

It's never too soon to start doing Kegel exercises! This miraculous exercise, invented by California gynecologist Arnold Kegel, strengthens urogenital and pubococcygeus muscles, which support the pelvic floor. If you keep these muscles in shape you can prevent urinary incontinence, promote good blood flow to your pelvic floor, and more quickly recover your tone after childbirth.

To do a Kegel, you tighten the same muscles you would use to stop the flow of urine. Practice on the toilet, and after you get the hang of them, you can practice your Kegels while you're driving, at work, or even standing in the grocery line— no one will know what you're up to. Work on contracting the muscle as many times in a row as you can, contracting as tightly as you can, and holding the move for as long as possible. If you Kegel during every red light, boring phone call, and TV commercial, later in your pregnancy and after birth, you'll be less likely to leak urine as you laugh or cough.

Week 8

Fetal Age: 6 weeks (43 to 49 days)
32 to 31 weeks, 223 to 217 days until your due date

YOUR BABY

Size

Your baby is now about the size of your thumbprint: one-half to three-quarters of an inch.

Development

Six weeks is barely enough time to start a magazine subscription, but it's enough time for your fetus to develop limbs, tiny fingers and toes, the beginnings of external ear structures, eyelids, an upper lip, the tip of a nose, and intestines! The outer cells of the embryo have grown links to your blood supply.

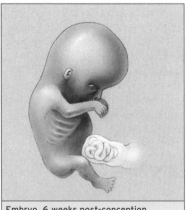

Embryo, 6 weeks post-conception

YOU

What's happening to you physically

If you're going to get pregnancy-related nausea (aka morning sickness), it probably will have kicked in by now. Researchers don't know its exact cause, but it's certainly related to your surging hormones.

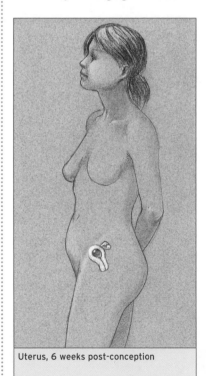

Uterus, 6 weeks post-conception

Your hormone levels and your level of nausea will rise and fall together, and women pregnant with multiples tend to feel more nauseated. We know that a vitamin B6 supplement can help ease some women's nausea, but the nausea doesn't appear to be related to a deficiency.

A pregnant woman's increased sensitivity to odors also seems to play a part, as does how sensitive her stomach is to begin with. Whatever the cause, it does seem as if the nausea and vomiting serve a purpose— the sicker you feel, apparently, the less likely you are to miscarry (which is not to say if you don't feel sick, you'll miscarry; you could just be lucky). (For a complete list of remedies for morning sickness, see "Stomach: Nausea and Vomiting" in *Managing Your Body* on page 129.)

It's common at this stage to have sharp pain on either side of your pelvis, especially when you twist or stand up after sitting for a while. Your uterus is becoming heavy, and this can strain your round ligaments, the muscles that hold your uterus in place. Tell your care provider if you're concerned.

It is not uncommon to have pink or brown discharge at this stage.

> *"As soon as I stop feeling sick, I'll start eating the way I'm supposed to. But right now, all I can stand is grilled cheese sandwiches."*

Report it to your care provider, but only page him or her in the middle of the night if the blood is bright red, heavy, or clotted.

You may experience gastrointestinal problems, such as constipation and/or diarrhea. The constipation is related to the slowing down of your digestive tract (see "Stomach: Constipation" in *Managing Your Body* on page 132), and the diarrhea appears to be your body's way of quickly moving out any food that isn't good for your system.

How you're feeling

Because of nausea and vomiting, you may worry that you're not getting enough vitamins to your baby. Unless your sickness is so severe that you can't keep down anything for more than a day or two, or if you can't stay hydrated, you have nothing to worry about. Your embryo is tiny and doesn't need a lot of calories at this point. Eat what you can stand, and never force yourself to eat anything you don't want. If you can only stand one or two foods for a week or two, your baby will be no worse for it. Try to take a vitamin supplement if you can stand to. (See *Managing Your Nutrition* on page 145.)

Have you discovered online "expecting clubs" yet? Just a few years ago, you'd have to look high and low to find a woman who was due the same month as you. Now you can find thousands at any time of the day or night! You can anonymously and endlessly type about all of the things too weird to ask your care provider or too personal to tell your partner and get advice from women going through the same thing. One warning though: Online

> ## "I just discovered pregnancy bulletin boards this week! It's great to have somewhere to talk about what's going on."

bulletin boards by nature have many more posts from troubled moms-to-be than from pregnant women who are doing fine. It's easy to get the idea that complications and health issues are much more common than they actually are. Still it's sometimes nice to know that however badly you may have it, somebody out there has it worse.

How you're feeling emotionally

Worried. Are you worrying about all of the living it up you did before you knew you were pregnant?

You probably have nothing to worry about. If you'd done any damage at this early stage, the embryo probably would not have survived to this point. However, do stop consuming alcohol immediately. Researchers are constantly discovering links between maternal drinking and long-term mental disabilities in children. A protein which is critical to the developing fetal brain is directly affected by alcohol, and as little as a drink and a half a week can lead to a baby with symptoms of *Fetal Alcohol Syndrome*, such as being born shorter than

average and with a smaller head circumference.

If you've been trying to conceive for a long time and have had miscarriages in the past, this can also be a harrowing time. Do your best to relax and think positively, as difficult as that may be. Even if your doctor offers a weekly ultrasound and frequent blood tests to check your hormone levels, consider that this plan won't prevent or stop an impending miscarriage and is likely to increase your stress level.

What you can do

As soon as your underwear is tight, treat yourself to stretchy cotton bikini-style maternity underwear. You don't want a *urinary tract infection (UTI)*. Toss your thongs—they help *E. coli* bacteria migrate to your urinary tract and vagina, which can cause potentially dangerous (and painful) UTIs and vaginal bacterial and yeast infections. Thongs made of synthetic materials can also cause tiny cuts, which provide a place for bacteria to grow. You're more susceptible to infections while you're pregnant, and any infection is potentially dangerous to the baby.

While you're at it, also toss any scented toilet papers, perfumed bubble baths, or feminine deodorant sprays you have. Soaps, sprays, and scented products can upset the balance of "good" bacteria in your vagina, making you more prone to yeast infections, vaginitis, and UTIs.

It is normal to have more discharge than usual during pregnancy, but nothing in your vaginal area should hurt, burn, or have a foul odor. Discharge that smells funny, has an unusual texture, or is any color but white is not healthy. (See more on discharge in the *Managing Your Body* section on page 137.) If you do get a yeast infection or experience any kind of vaginal itching, burning, or experience unusual discharge or painful urination, tell your care provider right away, and don't try to self-diagnose or medicate. Many yeast infection treatments shouldn't be used during the first trimester. And urinary tract infections can only be treated with prescription antibiotics.

Recommended exercise

One of the best things you can do now to prevent injury, muscle pulls, and fatigue in the future is to work on strengthening the muscles in your back. Back muscles may not be the ones that you show off at the beach, but you need them to keep you upright, support your growing belly, and keep you stable as your center of gravity shifts. They'll also come in handy for lifting and carrying your child. A certified personal trainer can help you design a program with weights, or you can swim laps to help you build strength, endurance, and flexibility.

Week 9

Fetal Age: 7 weeks (50 to 56 days)
31 to 30 weeks, 216 to 210 days until your due date

YOUR BABY

Size

Your baby is now about three-quarters of an inch long.

Development

As the embryo enters its fiftieth day of existence, it becomes known as a fetus. A membrane lid covers your baby's eyes. Your baby's muscles are beginning to develop, and she can make tiny movements. Your child's limbs are growing, but her arms and hands are forming more quickly than her legs and feet. The hands are actually still known as "hand paddles"

and look just like they sound. Ridges have formed on the paddles, which

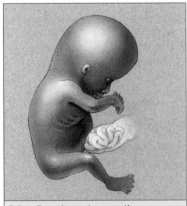

Fetus, 7 weeks post-conception

TIP

The Chinese cure for morning sickness is lots of shredded fresh ginger boiled in water to make tea, sweetened with sugar or honey.

will soon become well-defined fingers. Your baby is developing little dimples where her knees and ankles will go, and her elbows are becoming visible. This week is when sex characteristics begin to assert themselves, and ovaries or testes will soon appear (though an ultrasound won't be able to detect specific sex organs for another two months or so). Your baby's brain waves can now be detected.

YOU

How you're feeling physically

Your nauseating hCG levels are at their peak this week. The good news is that starting next week, as your hormone levels stabilize, you'll start feeling a lot better. The bad news is that this week is probably going to be rough. If you're throwing up a lot, drink plenty of water to keep yourself from dehydrating. (See page 129 for more tips on coping with nausea.)

Your uterus has doubled in size and is now about the size of a tennis ball. The area under your navel is definitely firmer than usual. Most women report being uninterested in sex at this stage, though some women also report being more interested than usual.

You may begin to notice changes in your hair and skin. Your hair might feel thick and lustrous—or greasy, thin, and limp. Resist the urge to try to dye, perm, or highlight your hair—it may not take to the chemicals evenly. Do switch your shampoo and conditioner to suit your new hair texture.(See hair in the *Managing Your Body* section for more tips on page 112.)

How you may be feeling emotionally

It's tough to be upbeat while you're feeling sick. It's also hard to keep your pregnancy a secret at work if you're constantly nauseated. Take care of yourself and have faith—you'll feel better soon. If you're lucky, you have a co-worker you can trust to keep your secret, who can cover for you on your many trips to the bathroom.

It can also be tough to keep your pregnancy a secret if you were once a drinker, and suddenly you aren't. If your work or social life is punctuated

"I think that my pregnancy hasn't hit home for my husband yet. He doesn't seem excited or like he wants to talk about baby stuff at all. I guess to him, if you can't see it, it isn't real."

by lots of drinking occasions, and you want to keep your pregnancy under wraps, think in advance of ways to excuse away your club soda. It can be fun to tell everyone you're on a diet, then confuse them as you pack on weight at a rapid pace. Or order juice at the bar, and tell everyone it's a screwdriver.

Pregnancy can make you feel like you're all alone in the world, no matter how many billions of women have been in your condition. It also doesn't help that your condition is invisible to your partner—he just sees that you're moody, tired, and queasy and may be wondering when you're going to be back to your old self again.

Things to organize

If you haven't already visited your care provider, make an appointment now. The earlier you can be tested

---

EXERCISE TIP

You probably don't feel like exercising much this week, but do try to take walks—they'll help your food move on down.

---

for certain conditions and infections, the more likely you are to deliver a healthy baby. Your first *ultrasound* may be performed as early as this week. While you may be anxious to get an ultrasound, remember that they are expensive medical tests. You probably won't be offered one unless you can't remember when your last menstrual period was, if multiple births run in your family, or if you've had unusual bleeding.

It's important to note that much is still unknown about the effects of ultrasound. Some scientists believe

---

What Makes a Care Provider Good?

Are you not sure that your current care provider is the right person to deliver your baby? If you're having doubts, it's best to address them sooner rather than later. Talk to your insurance company about your options, and schedule consultations with other care providers. You have choices!

• You feel comfortable discussing intimate subjects with her.

• You feel comfortable asking questions, and your questions are answered thoroughly and with respect.

• He explains what's happening during every exam or procedure.

• You like the other doctors, midwives, and nurses in the practice.

• Your care provider offers options that you want during labor, such as letting you eat or drink during labor if you want to.

• Someone is available at all times (at least by phone) to address any health concerns you have.

• You don't feel rushed during visits.

For more about choosing a care provider, see *Managing Your Care* on page 162.

that it causes small bubbles in a baby's body fluids to vibrate, which may affect brain development.[7]

The U.S. Food and Drug Administration says this: "Ultrasonic fetal scanning, from a medical standpoint, generally is considered safe if properly used when information is needed about a pregnancy. Still, ultrasound is a form of energy, and even at low levels, laboratory studies have shown it can produce physical effects in tissue, such as jarring vibrations and a rise in temperature. Although there is no evidence that these physical effects can harm a fetus, the fact that these effects exist means that prenatal ultrasounds can't be considered completely innocuous."

For this reason, ultrasounds should be performed only by trained medical professionals and only when necessary for medical reasons. For more on ultrasound, see "Testing: Risks and Benefits" on page 188.

Week 10

Fetal Age: 8 weeks (57 to 63 days)
30 to 29 weeks, 209 to 203 days until your due date

YOUR BABY

Size

Your baby is now about an inch long and weighs five grams, or one-sixth of an ounce, roughly the size of a garden beetle.

Development

This end of the two-month mark is a landmark date for your baby. It's looking more human all the time. If you could look inside, you'd see a thumb tip–size, translucent creature that's unmistakably human. Kidneys, lungs, genitals, and the gastrointestinal tract are all present, though far from fully formed. Your baby's bones begin to form in his limbs, a process called ossification. The floor plan for your baby's structure has been laid down, and the next thirty weeks will be about expanding and developing on this blueprint.

If your baby is a boy, his testes are already producing testosterone.

A Doppler handheld device can usually detect a fetal heartbeat

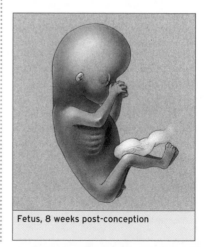

Fetus, 8 weeks post-conception

by this point. Once the heartbeat is detectable, your chances of miscarrying in the first trimester are immediately lower: between five and ten percent.

YOU

What's happening to you physically

Congratulations, your uterus has swollen to the size of a softball! Looking in the mirror, your shape has definitely changed: less waist and more chest.

If you're over 35 or have a family history of genetic disorders, over the next two weeks, your care provider may offer a test called *chorionic villus sampling (CVS)*, which uses a sample of tissue to screen for hundreds of genetic disorders. This test is highly accurate, but carries a significant risk of miscarriage. See "Testing: Risks and Benefits" for more information.

You may develop little white bumps on your nipples, called Montgomery glands, or *Montgomery's tubercles* (named after the Irish obstetrician who "discovered" them). These bumps secrete a white lubricant, which will help make breastfeeding more comfortable.

> *"I got to hear the baby's heartbeat for the first time with the Doppler at my appointment this week. Amazing!"*

You may notice changes in your pigmentation: your moles, freckles, and nipples may darken. They'll go back to normal after birth.

How you may be feeling emotionally

Your hormone levels may be producing emotional effects, that is, making you feel crazy, angry, sad, euphoric, and irritable, sometimes all in the same ten minutes. No one ever likes feeling like their body and fate are out of their control, but pregnancy is an exercise in acceptance, rolling with the punches, and just doing the best you can. It helps to avoid thinking more than a few weeks into the future and rehearsing a lot of what-if scenarios.

How you may be feeling physically

Your weight gain may be picking up—though don't worry if you haven't gained any by now. If you've begun eating a healthier diet and exercising, you may have even lost weight. Bottom line, if your care provider isn't concerned about how much or little you've gained, you shouldn't be either. Regardless of what the scale says, keep a journal of your diet to determine what nutrients you're getting, what supplements you may need to take, and how much of your diet is empty calories. If you gain extra weight during your pregnancy, don't try to diet it away—just make sure that you aren't going overboard on the sweets and processed foods. (See more in *Managing Your Nutrition* on page 145.)

Still sick, tired, and cranky? It's not your imagination, it won't last

Nine Coping Tips to Get You Through

1. Scale down stresses. Cut back on what you're doing to give yourself more downtime for resting and relaxing. Try to avoid negative people and situations.

2. Sleep whenever you can. Getting enough sleep can make the difference between being able to cope and being miserable. Don't be afraid to take naps at odd times if you need to.

3. Be candid about your needs. Don't expect people to read your mind. Be honest about what they can do to help you feel better.

4. Get peer support. Consider joining a support group for pregnant women, such as a neighborhood La Leche League group, so you can make new friends with women who are also pregnant or rearing babies and toddlers. It's a great way to not feel alone.

5. Seek professional help, if your negative feelings overwhelm you, or you've got the classical symptoms of depression. (See *Managing Family and Emotional Issues* on page 233.)

6. Keep learning. Nothing's scarier than the unknown. Read all the parenting books and magazine articles you can lay your hands on. Consider enrolling in a course on child development at a local college. Any preparations you do now are bound to be useful later and will make you feel proactive instead of like a sitting duck.

7. Practice deep breathing and relaxation. If you don't have the time to take naps during the week, you can teach yourself refreshing deep breathing techniques that will send your baby and your body oxygen. Buy some good relaxation tapes or soothing music for your portable CD, or watch an instructional video to get yourself started.

8. Maintain your journal. Writing down your experiences will help you put them in perspective over time. One simple journaling trick is very useful: divide your journal page into two columns. In the left column, write down every negative thought you have about being pregnant, and don't stop until you've gotten every feeling out. In the right column, force yourself to write down the exact opposite of those feelings. If you're afraid the baby will be born deformed or die, the positive column should say that the baby is healthy, beautiful, and perfect. You'll soon discover that positive thoughts can be powerful too.

9. Don't try to be perfect. If you've spent your life being a perfectionist, a pleaser, or a control freak, pregnancy is a great time to relax your reins and coast. Your baby-to-be won't care if you don't have the perfect, color-coordinated nursery. She will just want to be rocked, held, and fed by you.

forever, and it doesn't mean that you are or will be a less-than-ideal mom. Don't feel guilty or let others make you feel guilty—now is the time to nap, relax, and take things one day at a time.

What you can do

- Nap, eat, relax, and refuse to feel guilty.

- Snack on foods rich in calcium, potassium, and magnesium. Try a smoothie made with skim milk, vanilla yogurt, and bananas.

- Brush and floss for two. Make sure you have a nice, soft-bristled brush, some appealing dental floss, and an antibacterial mouth rinse.

Your gums may be softening and be more likely to bleed while you brush and floss. You also may be producing more saliva. Use a soft-bristled brush, brush frequently (after every meal, if you can), floss daily, and avoid sticky sweets that can stay in the crevices of your gums.

Now is a good time to make a dental appointment for a checkup and cleaning. Women with gum disease may run a greater risk of delivering a premature baby of low

> *"I don't make any plans for more than twenty-four hours in advance. I never know when I'm going to be completely exhausted."*

birth weight. Besides, you won't want to worry about going to the dentist for a cleaning in the next six months; you'll have other things to think about! (For more about changes in your teeth, see page 116.)

Wear your seat belt. This is the single most important thing you can do for you and your baby's safety. Before the car even starts, buckle your belt around your hip bone. Wear it even if you're just going on a short trip. If your shoulder belt rubs your neck, buy a seat belt adjusting clip or panel (available in any auto-parts store, and at most major discount stores), and use it to adjust the belt so it fits across your shoulder.

FLASH FACT

Is it true that a heart rate of more than 140 beats per minute means the fetus will be a girl? No. Unfortunately, there's no reliable way to predict the gender of your baby, other than genetic testing. Even ultrasound is really unreliable when it comes to making a gender call.

Week 11

Fetal Age: 9 weeks (64 to 70 days)
29 to 28 weeks, 202 to 196 days until your due date

YOUR BABY

Size

Your baby is about 1³/₄ to 2¹/₂ inches long and weighs about a third of an ounce, the size of a peanut.

Development

This is a big week for your baby's growth—she'll double in height. At the end of the week, her head and body will be roughly equal in length.

This week also starts an active phase for her—she can turn somersaults, roll over, flex her fingers, hiccup, and stretch. You won't be able to feel her movement for another month and a half. She's floating in lots of amniotic fluid. Her limbs are developing from

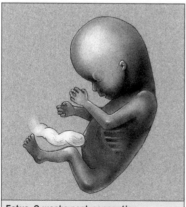

Fetus, 9 weeks post-conception

webbed paddles into arms and legs that have well-defined fingers and toes. Fingernails, toenails, and hair follicles are also beginning to form.

Your baby's testes or ovaries have developed, though the sex probably won't be visible on a sonogram for at least another month.

Intestines have developed at the place where the umbilical cord meets your baby's body. The intestines are able to make constricting movements, though there won't be anything to digest until later.

YOU

What's happening to you physically

Your body's expanding, inside and out. The next ten weeks will be a period of rapid growth for you and the baby.

You'll need more water as you produce more blood, sweat, oil, and amniotic fluid. You may feel desperately thirsty at times. It's a good idea to carry a beverage with you wherever you go, to keep your fluid levels up. Drink plenty of water, decaf iced tea, and milk, but steer away from carbonated beverages, sodas, and fruit juices that may contribute to extra weight gain and swelling.

The volume of blood in your body is increasing. An average woman with nine pints of blood will have an extra 1.8 pints by the time she gives birth—a blood volume increase of almost twenty percent. As you make more blood, your blood pressure will return to normal, which will mean less dizziness, fatigue, and mental confusion.

It's also common to have headaches caused by dehydration or sinus congestion. Your body needs a lot of water to make blood and amniotic fluid for the baby, and your sinuses have swollen to provide extra defense against germs. Other common causes of headaches are hunger and stress. If water, food, and relaxation don't work, remember to take acetaminophen (Tylenol), not aspirin. (See more on headaches in *Managing Your Body* on page 113.)

You're burning calories in a hurry—up to twenty-five percent faster than you did before you were pregnant.

What you can do

Do you have the urge to eat dirt, cornstarch, cigarette ashes, or other weird non-foods? The urge is not as unusual as you might think. If you have weird cravings, tell your doctor—it may be pica and signify a vitamin or mineral deficiency. Similarly, if you crave raw meat,

---

NUTRITION TIP

Are you feeling tired and weak? Try eating a high-iron food, such as linguine with clam sauce, a glass of prune juice, milk with a few tablespoons of blackstrap molasses, liver and onions, or a well-done hamburger.

It's OK to be Active

If you're in training for a marathon, ride horses, participate in contact sports, or even skydive, there's no reason to curtail your activities now. You don't need to worry about engaging in contact sports until your uterus tops your pelvic bones. Your baby is well protected by your abdominal muscles, your pelvis, and her amniotic fluid right now. With any sports activity, listen to your body. If you're just too tired, or feel faint, weak, or sick, skip the kickboxing tournament, and crawl under the covers. Next trimester, as your uterus emerges from your pelvis, sports that risk trauma to your abdomen won't be safe unless you're exceptionally experienced and well padded.

---

you may be anemic. (See more on iron requirements in *Managing Your Nutrition* on page 150.)

As your appetite increases, keep healthy snacks in your purse so you won't get ravenous and gorge on vending-machine food.

YOUR RELATIONSHIPS

According to your friends and family, you may be eating too much of the wrong things and too little of the right things, exercising too much or too little, and working too hard or not enough. If you're finding your family or friends too opinionated or intrusive, you may find yourself reexamining your relationships. (See *Managing Your Family and Emotional Issues* on page 233.)

Week 12

Fetal Age: 10 weeks (71 to 77 days)
28 to 27 weeks, 195 to 189 days until your due date

YOUR BABY

Size

Your baby's crown-to-rump height is 2½ inches, or about as tall as a squash ball. She may weigh as much as half an ounce.

Development

This begins the age when the fetus starts to look really cute in those womb pictures. If you had a womb camera, you'd be able to see your baby's proportions changing, with the growth of the head slowing down to let the rest of the body catch up. Arms, legs, and fingers are also growing out and tapering to look more like a newborn's, and your baby's posture becomes less curled and more upright.

Isn't it amazing that every person in the world was once the size of your thumb? And for that matter, for every person alive, some woman went through a pregnancy!

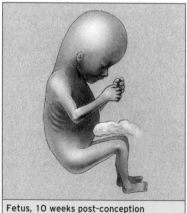

Fetus, 10 weeks post-conception

YOU

What's happening to you physically

This is about the time the muscles of your stomach slow down, making your stools harder and drier and making you gassier. (See "Stomach" on page 129.)

Your uterus has gotten too big to fit in its usual spot—your pelvis. It's now pushing into your abdomen, though not yet in any uncomfortable way.

Your heart rate may speed up because of the extra volume of blood in your body.

As you breathe in, you're taking forty to fifty percent more air into your body than normal. Your rib cage has expanded, which may mean your bras need to be a size larger than usual.

As your ligaments soften, you may experience pain in your tailbone (coccyx), especially if you spend much of your day sitting down. Your hips are actually widening to make more room for your uterus to grow. Apply heat or ice (whichever feels

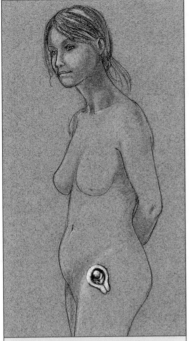

Uterus, 10 weeks post-conception

"I've found that sitting on a birth ball really helps my tailbone pain."

your condition, if they haven't figured it out already.

Take brisk walks, eat high-fiber foods, and drink plenty of water to help keep your intestinal tract moving. If you find yourself exceptionally gassy, check your food journal, and see what you ate earlier in the day. You may be able to pick out certain "trigger foods" to avoid.

If you feel your sex drive coming back, take advantage now, because your partner's sex drive may decrease as the weeks go by! (See "Couvade Syndrome" in *Managing Family and Emotional Issues* on page 244.)

better) to your tailbone area for fifteen minutes at a time, or try a warm bath.

How you may be feeling emotionally

With one week to go in your first trimester, you may feel more like your pregnancy is real.

For many couples, pregnancy is a very intimate time. Your emerging bump may bring out a protectiveness and sensitivity in your partner that you've never seen before.

What you can do

The magic end of the first trimester is at hand, which means it'll soon be time to let your boss, co-workers, and distant relatives know about

EXERCISE TIP

Your breasts may become so uncomfortable that you have to consider changing your exercise routine to avoid activities that aggravate them. Consider swimming, riding a stationary bike, stair-stepping, or using a cross-country ski machine, or if you're in good shape already, a rowing machine.

Week 13

Fetal Age: 11 weeks (78 to 84 days)
27 to 26 weeks, 188 to 182 days until your due date

YOUR BABY

Size

Your baby is 2$\frac{1}{2}$ to 3 inches long, the size of a medium goldfish. She weighs about one ounce.

Development

Your baby is shorter than a finger, but her face is already showing individual features and characteristics!

Her ears are now developed enough that she may be able to hear when you sing, hum, or talk. And her vocal cords will form this week—soon she'll be able to sing back.

Your baby spends her time in your womb flexing her new and developing muscles and joints. Bouts of prenatal hiccups are strengthening your baby's diaphragm, which is preparing her respiratory system for breathing.

Less glamorous but highly necessary organ systems for making hormones, absorbing nutrients, and filtering waste are also in place this week. The pancreas, gall bladder, and thyroid have developed, the kidneys can make urine, and her bone marrow is making white blood cells to help fight infection after she's born.

YOU

What's happening to you physically

Good news—at this point you'll start to feel less sick and more energized with each passing day as your placenta takes over hormone production. In two weeks or less, you could be nausea-free.

However, you may still have several weeks of nausea before you get relief. Your smell and taste aversions will probably stick with you for the rest of your pregnancy, but unless you're very unlucky, the spontaneous throwing up will ease. Tell your care provider if it doesn't. If you haven't felt queasy by now, you've probably successfully avoided morning sickness altogether.

It may be time for a shoe check—shoes that fit pre-pregnancy will start feeling tight as your feet swell. Now is a good time to invest in a pair that can accommodate your widening feet. Soon it won't be easy to tie your shoes, and you'll appreciate a pair that slips on and off easily. Shoes made for doctors and nurses are good for pregnant feet. They're designed to be lightweight and to support you while standing. Cork-soled sandals, pool shoes, and canvas sneakers are also comfortable. Avoid high heels and platform shoes, because your sense of balance will start to be thrown off by your changing weight. (See "Feet" on page 143.)

Recommended Exercise

If you're starting to feel better, this can be a good time to try a new exercise. There are activities out there for every body type and temperament. Try a variety of activities, so you'll have options if the weather is bad, the pool is closed, or you simply get bored with your existing routine.

If you haven't tried swimming lately, check out why many care providers call it the perfect pregnancy exercise. Swimming is safe for your joints, it works a lot of muscle groups, and it will improve your flexibility and cardiovascular endurance. Swimming will strengthen your upper body, which will come in handy for carrying the baby. And as your pregnancy progresses, you'll appreciate the way the water takes the pressure off your back and legs.

The practice of yoga is another low-impact activity that can help you feel better. The balancing postures can help you cope with a shifting center of gravity, and other postures can prevent back strain and lessen your everyday aches and pains. Certain yoga poses should be avoided by pregnant women. Choose an establishment that offers a specialized prenatal yoga class. (For more on exercise, see *Managing Your Weight and Fitness* on page 157.)

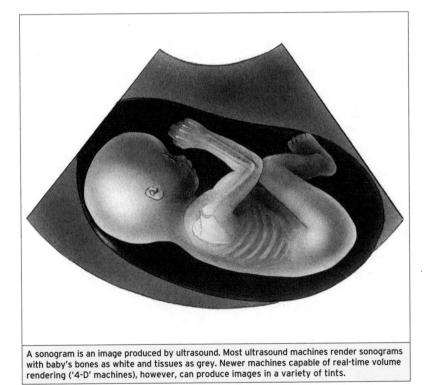

A sonogram is an image produced by ultrasound. Most ultrasound machines render sonograms with baby's bones as white and tissues as grey. Newer machines capable of real-time volume rendering ('4-D' machines), however, can produce images in a variety of tints.

The Second Trimester

Weeks 14 through 24

Most moms agree that the second trimester is the highlight of the pregnancy experience. Your chances of carrying your pregnancy to term have gone from 80 percent to higher than 97 percent. Your nausea eases, you have almost as much energy as a non-pregnant person, and some women report that their sex lives during these three months are better than ever. (For more information about Sex and Pregnancy, see *Managing Your Body* on page 136.)

You start to look pregnant instead of just padded, but you're not so pregnant that it's become difficult to put on your socks or get out of a car. You may even get the "glow of pregnancy," a kind of radiance that comes from extra blood flow to the capillaries of your skin, and if you were plagued with acne, it may ease up. The second trimester is a great time to travel, to decorate, and to take care of projects that need your attention. As you enter the third trimester, weight and fatigue may slow you down again.

The second trimester is also a great time for your baby. Organ systems are fully in place, and by the end of the trimester, they'll be developed to the point that the baby could possibly survive outside of the womb with medical intervention. In the meantime, your body will nourish, protect, and keep her clean as she goes from being the size of a fist to the size of a football. She already looks human and will grow from being scrawny with a huge head to looking more like a newborn.

Another highlight of the second trimester is feeling movement—if you've had a baby before, you may feel wiggling any day now. If this is your first child, you may have to wait for another month or so before you feel anything. What starts as a feeling of wiggling will turn into poking, and even sharp kicking, by the end of this trimester.

The odds of your baby being born healthy are tremendously in your favor, even if your pregnancy has been labeled high risk.

It may seem like you have a long time left to wait, but considering what goes on, pregnancy is so brief as to defy belief. Most cities can't get a pothole filled in nine months. Unlike the department of public works, there's never an idle moment in your uterus. Waste is moving in and out, neurons are forming, bones and tissues are building, and the baby is in almost constant motion.

You can comfortably operate on the assumption that six months from now, someone's going to send you home from the hospital with a healthy baby.

In other words, you can begin painting that nursery.

The start of the second trimester is also a good time to find a child-birth class. Plenty of people don't take classes and go on to have a fine birth experience, but taking a class has some definite advantages:

Classes can calm your fears.

Nothing is scarier than the unknown, and the more you know about birth and labor, the less anxiety you'll feel.

You'll make friends with other parents-to-be.

It's easy to become friends for life with people in your birthing class, because they know exactly what you're going through. Even if you don't make friends, you'll get an idea of how other people are dealing with their pregnancies.

You'll be an educated consumer.

You'll learn what to expect from, and how to communicate with, your care provider and/or hospital.

Ask your care provider for child-birth class recommendations. You can take a one-day seminar at a local hospital, or a very detailed thirteen-week-long Bradley class. The advantage of a longer class is that you'll have more of a chance to get to know other parents and to build confidence in the process. The downside is that these classes may not be covered by your insurance. (See page 171 of *Managing Your Care* for a list of common birth classes and their philosophies.)

The second trimester is ideal for travel, because you have plenty of energy, your nausea has abated, and you don't have to worry about going into labor when you're far from home. It's going to be pretty hard to schedule a romantic interlude in the coming years, so take some time to enjoy your partner and friends while you can focus on them exclusively.

Week 14

Fetal Age: 12 weeks (85 to 91 days)
26 to 25 weeks, 181 to 175 days until your due date

YOUR BABY

Size

Your baby weighs about 1½ ounces now and is about three to four inches long—about as wide as your fist.

Development

Your baby's face continues to look more human, with individual characteristics becoming more pronounced all the time. Teeth have formed in your baby's gums.

Your baby's skin is very thin. If you took a photo, you would be able to see her developing blood vessels. Hair is growing on her head and eyebrows and may even have pigment in it if she has the genes for dark hair.

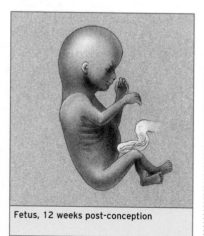

Fetus, 12 weeks post-conception

Her bone marrow has begun to produce blood cells, a chore previously performed by the yolk sac.

Your baby rarely sits still. She's often wiggling fingers and toes; stretching, yawning, and hiccupping. However, you probably won't be able to feel the movements for another month or so.

YOU

What's happening to you physically

Between now and the next five weeks, you can opt to have blood drawn for the Quad Screen test (sometimes also called the AFP test).

This test detects levels of the hormones **AFP**, hCG, inhibin and **estriol**. High levels of AFP may mean that the baby has a neural tube defect, and lower-than-normal levels may indicate Down syndrome. Your decision to test or not may depend on your age and how important it is to know the result. (For a complete discussion of the Quad Screen and other screening tests, see "Testing: Risks and Benefits" on page 188.)

The amount of amniotic fluid that your baby is floating in increases dramatically this week, to about a quart. This is why amniocentesis may be performed during the coming weeks.

Most moms find that their nausea, mood swings, exhaustion, and other hormonally related annoyances are easing up, though symptoms may not completely disappear until after the baby is born.

Has the news of your pregnancy reached the far ends of your office and family yet? Almost certainly. As far as gossip goes, pregnancy is everyone's favorite news. Now that everyone knows, you have an instant excuse to not do anything you don't want to do. For once, no one will be offended if you turn down socializing by saying, "I just don't feel up to it."

If you still feel tired this week, make sure you're getting enough iron. The National Institutes of Health recommend that expectant moms take a daily iron supplement containing thirty milligrams. Try to get your extra iron from other sources besides iron supplements, because the mineral is much better absorbed through food. Eat clams, red meat, liver, leafy green vegetables, and acidic foods such as tomato sauce that is prepared in an iron frying pan. (The acids actually erode the pan a little bit, so that you get extra iron in your diet.) Take iron supplements with a glass of orange juice, because acid breaks down the iron so it is absorbed more readily.

If you've started suffering from pregnancy-related heartburn, however, acidic juices and sauces may not be what you want. This annoying symptom can kick in as your digestive system slows down. (For more detail, see "Heartburn" on page 132.)

You probably have plenty of cravings and food aversions by now. Give into cravings, but with moderation. If you crave meats, dairy, or vegetables, consider that your diet may be deficient in certain vitamins or minerals, so by all means send your partner out in the driving snow for that pork chop or milkshake.

What you can do

It's not too soon to think about your birth philosophy and give some thought to who will be on your birth team. You've probably already picked out an obstetrician or midwife to deliver your baby, but who else do you want in the room? What do you want your baby's birth to be like? What will your partner's role be?

You're probably now wearing the more forgiving items in your wardrobe. You may as well shop for maternity clothes as soon as you feel like it—or at least maternity underwear and big cotton bras. If you can borrow from your relatives, friends, or husband, so much the better. You'll only be wearing this stuff for the next six to nine months, and you're going to get a whole lot bigger, so a custom-tailored suit is not a good purchase right now.

"For my first pregnancy, I had tons of energy the second trimester. Not this time. I'm not anemic or anything, I just want to sleep all the time."

Loose dresses, big shirts, and stretchy pants are good values. If you're planning to breastfeed, opt for button-down shirts that you can wear after the baby arrives.

Week 15

Fetal Age: 13 weeks (92 to 98 days)
25 to 24 weeks, 174 to 168 days until your due date

YOUR BABY

Size

About 4 to 4½ inches and about 1¾ of an ounce.

Development

If you could see your baby's face, you might be able to see her wince and grimace, because her facial muscles are developing and flexing.

All of her tiny organs, nerves, and muscles are starting to function. The intestines have moved farther into the baby's body; her liver begins to secrete bile, which will later aid in the digestion of fats; and her pancreas begins to produce insulin, a hormone which turns sugar into energy.

YOU

What's happening to you physically

Your womb is now starting to grow up and out of your pelvis, so you may have a neat and noticeable bump below your belly button. Now that you're becoming visibly pregnant, you may also find yourself a topic of discussion.

Beware of belly-touchers: colleagues and relatives who would never so much as pat your shoulder before, but who now want to reach out and rub your stomach. Announcing your pregnancy to others may also elicit intrusive questions ("Have you stopped drinking?" "Are you going to breastfeed?"). Or you may receive compliments that are also insults ("My, you've blossomed. You're really eating for two, aren't you?"). How you handle these situations depends on your personal style.

It is now your baby's turn to go through rapid growth and adjustment, while yours is to coast. In three months, the baby will be the one relaxing, putting on weight, and developing its brain, while your body prepares to give birth.

Your milk glands may already be kicking into production. You may sometimes notice what looks like water sitting on the tips of your nipples, or nipple-level wet spots on your sheets when you wake up in the morning. If you need to, put breast pads (or trimmed pantiliners) inside your bra. Your body is practicing making colostrum, a protein-rich fluid that is great for newborns.

You may begin to feel **Braxton-Hicks contractions**, which get your uterus in shape to give birth. These "practice" contractions feel like a tightening in your uterus or abdominal area. You may get them more frequently after exercise. If you have regular contractions (more than four or five an hour), uncomfortable pelvic pressure, or discharge lots of fluid or mucus, contact your care provider.

When you have an orgasm, you may notice that your uterus hardens for several minutes. This has always happened, but now that your uterus is bigger, you can feel it.

Emotionally

Although your hormonal roller coaster ride has slowed down, you'll probably still feel vulnerable, sensitive, and more easily annoyed than you did before you were pregnant.

What you can do

Let your partner or friends help you with pregnancy crafts that you can show your child later.

Some ideas:

- Start a scrapbook, and save mementos of your pregnancy.
- Make a journal out of a big, blank book.
- Start a monthly video diary.
- Videotape your friends and relatives delivering messages to your baby.
- Take weekly photos of your expanding stomach.

- Knit booties, socks, or caps.
- Sew stuffed animals, clothes, or light baby blankets.
- Build baby furniture.

CHOOSING YOUR BABY'S PEDIATRICIAN

A pediatrician is a medical doctor who has completed four years of college, followed by four years of medical school and three years of supervised residency (on-the-job training) for providing medical care for babies and children. Some pediatricians also have advanced training in neonatal care, child cardiology, or other specialties.

> *"Whenever someone reaches out for the belly rub, I simply take a step back, put my hand up, and very calmly say, 'Please don't.' Almost every time, they pull their hand back. And then I say, 'Please don't take it personally, I'm just not comfortable with all the belly rubbing.'"*

If the initials FAAP follow the pediatrician's name, that means that he or she has passed a written exam, is considered to be board certified, and has become a fellow of the American Academy of Pediatrics. You can check on any doctor's board certification by going to: www.certifieddoctor.org.

It's important to find someone with whom you feel comfortable. The physician you choose should be not only versed in treating childhood illnesses, but also knowledgeable in child development and child health. Determine if you want a male or female doctor, since some children feel more trusting of same-sex providers. Also decide whether you will be more comfortable in a small, office practice or a larger group practice.

The ideal physician is warm, caring, and a good listener, and one with whom you feel confident sharing thoughts and concerns. If you feel cut off, rushed, or diminished from your interactions, then you should probably move on.

You can speed up the doctor screening process by telephone. Some simple but important questions to ask are: whether the office accepts your health insurance; the doctor's hospital affiliations; the office hours; if the doctor has regular, daily call-in times; if there is more than one office, and how the doctor splits his time between them; how many other providers there are in the practice; and how weekend and night calls are handled; whether there is a separate waiting room for sick children; and if the office has laboratory facilities and can provide hearing and vision screening on site.

If you're satisfied with the answers, ask if there is a charge for

> **QUICK TIP**
>
> Keep a notebook in your purse to write down any questions that you want to ask your care provider at your next visit.

an initial, get-acquainted interview, and how soon you can get an appointment. If there will be a fee charged for your visit, ask if it can be applied to a future office visit, since it's not likely your health insurance will pay for it.

The first interview is a good time for you and your partner to assess the pediatrician and his or her practice to see if they are aligned with your values and needs.

As a new parent, you'll need someone with whom you feel completely comfortable and who will be there to support you should your baby become ill. Take a few minutes to converse with the support staff, too, since they are the persons you will most often encounter first when you call with concerns or to make appointments.

Questions to ask

1. Will you be the person we see each time we bring our baby in? (Or is there an assistant or other physician who will also be providing medical care?)

2. Will you be examining our baby in the hospital?

3. When should we schedule our first appointment after our baby is born?

4. What is your preferred immunization schedule for infants?

Can you give us some literature about that and what side effects we can expect?

5. How often should our baby visit you during his first year?

6. How far in advance do you recommend we make appointments?

7. On average, how long will we have to sit in the waiting room before we get see you? Can you recommend certain days or hours when your schedule is less crowded?

8. How much time do you typically spend with a baby and family on a routine visit?

9. How quickly can we expect you to return telephone calls?

10. What do you suggest we do if there is an emergency?

11. How do you feel about parents seeking a second opinion on medical decisions?

12. (If you're having a son) What are your recommendations about circumcision and whom do you think should perform it? Are there any side effects or risks that we should know about?

13. (If you plan to breastfeed) Does the office provide the services of a lactation consultant?

Let your baby's pediatrician know if you have special circumstances. For example, if you are concerned about the overuse of antibiotics, or you are in favor of complementary or alternative health approaches, then you may want to test out his, or her, acceptance of them. If you have important cul-

How to Find a Pediatrician

The best time to choose the pediatrician for your baby is by the beginning of your third trimester, or seventh month, of pregnancy, unless your pregnancy is considered at-risk. In that case, you may want to have your baby's pediatrician on board much earlier. Plan to meet with several pediatricians until you find one that feels right to you and your partner. There are several people and sources you can consult with about choosing the right pediatrician.

Friends and family members. Ask people you trust who have babies and young children whom they would recommend and why.

Your insurance company. Contact your insurance plan to find a list of preferred providers; many plans have Internet Web sites where you can do the search.

The best hospital. Check with the nearest hospital that offers neonatal intensive care. Many hospitals offer physician referral services to the public.

Your current healthcare provider. Your obstetrician, midwife, or family care physician may have suggestions for trustworthy pediatricians.

Internet locators. The following sites may have referral services by location to help you create a list of potential providers: American Board of Pediatrics: www.abp.org; American Academy of Pediatrics: www.aap.org; American Medical Association: www.ama-assn.org; The Health Pages: www.thehealthpages.com; The Doctor Finder: www.docfinderplus.com.

tural, religious, or moral tenets that could affect your decisions about your baby's care, or if you are gay, or a single parent, or your baby is adopted, or is known to have predisposing conditions, then you will want to get a sense of his, or her, sensitivity to these issues. You should walk away from the appointment feeling that you have a trusted ally on whom you can rely when you have any need or concern about your baby, no matter how insignificant it may seem.

Week 16

Fetal Age: 14 weeks (99 to 105 days)
24 to 23 weeks, 167 to 161 days until your due date

YOUR BABY

Size

Your baby weighs about 2.8 ounces (79 grams) and is about 4½ inches from crown to rump—roughly the size of a small gerbil.

Development

At any time, you will begin to feel fetal movement as your baby's bones harden, and she starts a big growth spurt. Your baby has plenty of room: At this point, she could fit in the palm of your hand. This is a great time to be a fetus. At any given time, she might be playing with the umbilical cord (which she's now able to grasp), putting her thumb in her mouth, or kicking at the amniotic sac.

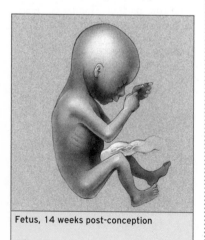

Fetus, 14 weeks post-conception

YOU

What's happening to you physically

Since you have almost a cup of amniotic fluid in your uterus, your pelvic area will feel heavy and firm. You're also carrying all the extra poundage your body's putting on that can be attributed to extra blood and fluid volume, your placenta and baby's support systems, and enlarging breasts.

Extra blood and mucous will make you more prone to nasal congestion and nosebleeds. Try a humidifier or warm shower to open up your sinuses. Treat nosebleeds by pinching your nose with a tissue and tilting your head back.

It's normal to be gaining a pound a week at this point.

If you have an appointment this week, your care provider may recommend or offer these screening tests to detect the possibility of genetic defects.

Ultrasound. This painless test uses inaudible sound waves to create video images of your baby's anatomy. A radiologist or obstetrician uses these images to make sure your baby's organ systems are in place and to screen for signs of certain genetic defects. The test is usually best performed at eighteen to twenty-two weeks, though some care providers give you the option of taking it earlier.

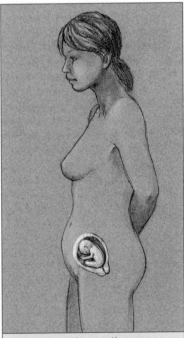

At 16 weeks post-conception, your uterus is outgrowing your pelvis.

> *"I'm 37 and will have an amnio because I just have to know that everything's all right. I know I'm not equipped to handle a child with a genetic disorder."*

Amniocentesis. This screening test is offered to women over thirty-five, to women who have a family history of genetic disorders, or to women whose ultrasound or Triple Screen results revealed a possibility of a defect. This test analyzes a sample of your baby's genetic material, extracted from your amniotic fluid, for defects. Amnio is usually performed between this week and week eighteen.

To test or not is entirely up to you. See "Testing: Risks and Benefits" on page 188 for more information on these tests. Some tests, such as an ultrasound and the Triple Screen, have no known risks and offer a lot of information. Others, such as amniocentesis, have some risks and should only be undertaken if you feel it's important to know the results. Only you can decide if the risk involved to obtain the information is worth it.

What you can do

If you're relatively young and have no family history of genetic defects, getting an ultrasound feels like more fun than a medical test should be.

For a lot of parents, the ultrasound is the first time that it really hits home that there's a little person in there. But the test can be stressful. For one thing, it's really hard to figure out what you're looking at. The image is gray and usually grainy, and the technician (called a sonographer) will be zooming in, out, and around. The blurriness has made many a mom shriek, "Oh my God! He has no hands!"

What can also be distressing is that most of the time your sonographer won't be able to make any diagnosis, unless he or she is also a perinatologist or radiologist. So though you may be frantically asking "Is the baby okay?" the person performing the test won't be able to tell you one way or the other. Instead, you have to wait for a radiologist, perinatologist, and/or your care provider to review images from the scan, which usually takes a few days. However, do ask the technician to point out body parts to you. And don't forget to ask for pictures, which make great illustrations for baby announcements.

If you want to know your baby's gender, wait as long as possible before getting an ultrasound. Making a gender call isn't an official part of the ultrasound test, but most technicians will humor you and try to catch a peek at the baby's parts if you ask. Figuring out the baby's gender via ultrasound is a matter of seeing if there's a penis or not. But it's not easy. The part in question is about the size of a grain of rice, and the baby has to be positioned just so. Even if your sonographer announces a gender with great confidence, don't print up the pink or blue baby announcements just yet.

Week 17

Fetal Age: 15 weeks (106 to 112 days)
23 to 22 weeks, 160 to 154 days until your due date

YOUR BABY

Size

She is about as wide as your palm, about six inches tall, and weighs about four ounces—about as much as a bar of soap. She now weighs more than your placenta.

Development

Your baby is now covered with a downy layer of **lanugo**, which swirls in fingerprint-like formations over her whole body. Her skin is still thin. Brown fat, a special type of fat that plays a role in body heat generation, is being deposited. In the next few weeks, your baby's eyes will begin to move beneath

Eight Indications That You Should Change Care Providers

- You spend a long time in the waiting room at every visit—a sign that your provider has more patients than he or she can comfortably handle.

- Exams are rough or uncomfortable.

- Your care provider dismisses, challenges, or demeans your questions, or responds with "Why do you want to know?"

- You feel like you can't be honest with your provider about your activities. (You're afraid to talk to her about smoking, drinking, or drug use, for instance.)

- When you telephone with a question, your call isn't taken or isn't returned promptly.

- You don't like the other care providers in the group practice.

- The hospital where your care provider delivers doesn't have features that you want, such as water birthing facilities.

- The hospital where your care provider delivers has a cesarean rate of more than 25 percent.

their fused lids in a side-to-side sweeping motion.

YOU

How you may feel physically

As your breasts grow, they'll be sensitive and tender and sometimes just plain painful.

Your placenta is now a fully functional, well-established network of blood and tissue, distributing nutrients and removing waste. Now that this major construction project is complete, you'll have a lot more energy.

Your heart is now pumping twenty percent more blood. Your uterus is now about two inches below your navel and easy for you to feel.

When you move around, you may experience brief sharp pains around the front and side of your uterus, about where the leg holes of a high-cut bathing suit would be. These are called *round ligament pains* and are a result of your growing uterus straining the muscles that hold it in place. If the pain persists after a short rest or goes on when you're not moving, call your care provider.

How you feel

Your sex drive, which probably took a backseat to your fatigue and nausea during the first trimester, may start coming back as you start to feel better. Many women report that sex during the second trimester is the best of their life! All of the extra blood flow to your pelvis may make arousal more frequent and intense than ever.

But, like a great cosmic joke, for hormonal and psychological reasons, many men have feelings of apprehension about having sex with a pregnant woman. *Couvade syndrome* is the medical term for when your partner starts showing pregnancy symptoms along with you. This isn't just a psychological phenomenon—men who spend a lot of time with their pregnant partners can actually undergo hormonal shifts. The changes are in no way as dramatic as the ones you undergo, but your partner may indeed experience some nausea, indigestion, heartburn, loss of appetite for food, weight gain, and, notably, a loss of interest in sex.

Beyond hormonal changes, some men worry that they might hurt the fetus or that the fetus might be watching them (all untrue, but nevertheless not very arousing notions). Men can be unsettled by the realization that sex is for making babies, and breasts are for feeding them. Plus, because of hormonal changes, your vagina is darker-colored, has more discharge, smells different, and has more hair, which may make your partner feel like someone snuck in and redecorated his favorite room in the house. (For more about what your partner is going through, see "Fatherhood" in *Managing Family and Emotional Issues* on page 240.)

What you can do

It's okay to use vibrators or sex toys during pregnancy—just keep them clean, use as directed, and never, ever, insert anything in your vagina that's been used for anal penetration. *E. coli* bacteria can cause dangerous urinary tract infections.

Don't deprive yourself of orgasms, though; they keep your uterus and PC muscle toned and give the baby a happy hormonal rush (though of course the baby hasn't a clue what the source is).

By the way, if your care provider has told you to avoid sex because you're at risk for preterm labor, be sure to ask exactly what he or she means by sex and which acts may be off limits.

Week 18

Fetal Age: 16 weeks (113 to 119 days)
22 to 21 weeks, 153 to 238 days until your due date

YOUR BABY

Size

She's about 5 to 5½ inches long from top to tail and weighs a little more than five ounces, about the size of a lobster tail.

Development

While in earlier weeks, your baby may have been able to sense sound with her primitive ear structures, this week, the bones of the ear become fully formed along with the part of her brain that processes signals from his ears.

There's no evidence that playing music, language tapes, or any other sounds to your baby will make her a genius, but then again, it can't hurt.

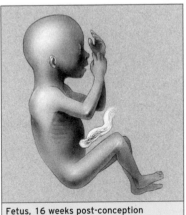

Fetus, 16 weeks post-conception

Studies have suggested that babies will remember sounds that they have heard *in utero* and that they have a preference for known sounds. So a song you play for her now may help soothe her to sleep after she's born.

There's still plenty of room in your uterus, so your fetus can be quite active with her new muscles. She may change positions frequently, cross her legs, recline, suck her thumb, and turn somersaults.

Her retinas have become light sensitive, and your baby may be able to detect a glow if you shine bright lights at your belly (even though her eyelids are sealed).

YOU

How you're feeling physically

During this week and the next few weeks, you may feel your baby's first movements—a fluttery sensation in your pelvis. Called quickening, many cultures believe that this is when life begins.

You may have aches and pains in your legs, tailbone, and other muscles.

Emotionally

At some point during your pregnancy, you and your partner should take time to talk about how your house will be managed in the future.

In the first few months after the baby's born, and in fact, until your child goes to day care or school, it's going to be impossible for you to care for the baby and take care of household chores by yourself. For the first few weeks, until you establish a routine with your new baby, you'll be too occupied to cook meals, take care of pets, open the mail, pick up the phone, or do anything but breastfeed, soothe the baby, and sleep. We hope your partner is up to the challenge. If not, prepare to move your mother or another relative in for a time. Also consider hiring a postpartum doula or a baby nurse to help out.

Week 19

Fetal Age: 17 weeks (120 to 126 days)
21 to 20 weeks, 146 to 140 days until your due date

YOUR BABY

Size

Your baby is between five and six inches long and weighs about seven ounces—about the size of an apple.

Development

If the baby is a girl, early ovaries contain follicles with forming eggs. Soon, half of the genetic material for your potential future grandchildren will be formed.

Pictures of babies at this age show them touching the membrane of the amniotic sac, touching their own faces, reaching for the umbilical cord, pedaling their legs, and sucking their thumbs. If you're carrying twins, they may already be swatting at each other. Your baby may already have a preference for the left or right hand.

In the brain, areas of nerve cells that serve the senses of touch, taste, smell, sight, and hearing are becoming specialized and are forming more complex connections.

Loud sounds as well as any feelings you may have of stress or alarm may be communicated to the baby. The baby responds to these stresses by becoming more active. Practicing yoga and meditation can be good for your sense of calm and balance.

YOU

What's happening physically

You may experience shooting pains if your baby puts her weight on your sciatic nerve. (For more information, see "Remedies for Back Pain" on page 128.)

You may be popping out all over, with bigger breasts and a bulge above your pelvis.

You may experience back pain as the weight of your uterus makes your back work harder to keep you upright.

What you can do

Make sure that your diet contains plenty of B vitamins and good fats to support your baby's developing brain cells.

When you exercise, work on your cardiovascular endurance. Take long walks outside, walk on a treadmill with an incline, ride a stationary bike, or use an elliptical trainer. The endurance will come in handy during labor and will make you more able to carry your new baby around with you everywhere.

If your legs are restless at night, or you get sharp calf cramps, make sure that your diet and/or your prenatal vitamin contains magnesium. (For more on how nutrition can help ease your health concerns, see *Managing Your Nutrition* on page 145.)

If you find yourself getting irritable for what seems like no good reason, try a snack. Low blood sugar can make you tired and crabby.

What's happening emotionally

Even though in the second trimester, your odds of carrying a healthy baby to term are quite high, you may find that you can't force yourself to stop worrying that something will go wrong with your pregnancy. As normal as worrying is, if you feel like it's taking over your emotional life, then it may be time to pinpoint your worries, examine how likely they are to be true, and consider what you might do if they were. (For more on worry, see page 232.)

Week 20

Fetal Age: 18 weeks (127 to 133 days)
20 to 19 weeks, 139 to 133 days until your due date

YOUR BABY

Size

Your baby is between 5¹/₂ and 6¹/₂ inches crown to rump, and between nine and ten inches from head to toe. She weighs about nine ounces. Over the next month, she'll gain about a pound! Right now, she is about the size of a mango.

Development

Your baby's permanent teeth are already starting to form behind her

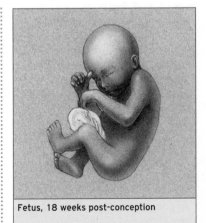

Fetus, 18 weeks post-conception

baby teeth. These permanent teeth won't be mature for several years.

By this point, your baby can move her eyes, though not always in tandem. What were sweeping left-right eye motions last week are turning into eye rolls that will last through her teenage years. Eyebrows have formed, and hair is beginning to form on your baby's scalp.

She's begun to produce vernix, a white, creamy substance that protects her developing skin in utero.

From this point on, the baby seems to be able to differentiate between mornings, afternoons, and nighttime and starts to become active at certain times more than others.

Your baby also has all of the neurons in his brain that she'll need, and the process of myelination begins in the brain. This is the growth of myelin, a substance that acts as an electrical insulator of the systems that send messages between parts of the brain. Much like the covering of an electrical wire, the coating of myelin keeps the wiring of the brain from crossing signals or shorting out. This is a slow process, starting now and continuing on through the first years of your baby's life. The myelin is made of about eighty percent fat and twenty percent protein and is why pediatricians recommend a high level of fat in babies' diets until about age two.

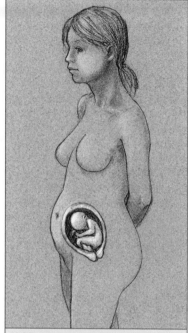

At 20 weeks, your belly may be outpacing your cleavage.

YOU

How you're feeling

Can you believe it, you'll be halfway there at the end of this week!

Have you settled on a name yet? If people keep asking, you can always make up a temporary nickname to satisfy their curiosity.

Your belly may be horizontally outpacing your cleavage.

Your care practitioner will now monitor your growth by measuring the height of your uterus with fingers or a tape measure. Your uterus is now about in line with your belly button. From now on, the top of your uterus will grow toward your rib cage at a rate of one centimeter a week.

What you can do

Now is a critical time for your baby's brain and a good time to make sure you get enough fat and cholesterol. You need to make sure that there's some amount of real, non-hydrogenated fat in your diet.

Omega-3 fatty acids, found in oily fish such as salmon, tuna, and sardines, are great for your baby's brain. Some fish may be high in mercury, however, so consider limiting your intake of oily fish to about twelve ounces a week and taking an omega-3 supplement instead. (See page 146 of *Managing Your Nutrition* for more about fish and mercury.) Also good are the fats in nuts, avocados, and olive oil—and the fats in dairy products! So help yourself to half-cup servings of butter pecan ice cream. Try to limit your fat intake to one-third of your total daily calories.

Week 21

Fetal Age: 19 weeks (134 to 140 days)
19 to 18 weeks, *132 to 126 days until your due date*

YOUR BABY

Size

She weighs about 10½ ounces, and her length from head to rump is seven inches, about the length of a spoon. Ten and one-half ounces is also the size bear cubs are when they are born.

Development

Your baby has begun her main project for the rest of your pregnancy: putting on weight.

She regularly drinks amniotic fluid for hydration and nutrition, urinates in the fluid, and breathes it in and out. Fortunately, the fluid pool is constantly changing and refreshing itself every three hours.

Her eyebrows and eyelids are fully developed. Taste buds are forming on her tongue.

Her eyelids are still sealed, but her eyes are active.

YOU

What's happening to you physically

Some women report feeling better and more energized at this stage of pregnancy than they have at any point in their life. We hope you're one of them!

Your uterus is about a half an inch above your navel.

As your baby lays down her layers of fat, you're probably not going to be able to hide your expanding form. You need about three hundred extra calories a day to support your active metabolism.

If you look in the mirror, especially if you're light-skinned, you'll be able to see your blue veins all over your chest.

Emotionally

Strollers, swings, play mats, diaper disposal systems…it's easy to see how parents can spend thousands of dollars on baby gear before the baby is even born! It's not necessary to go broke outfitting your nursery. It also makes sense to wait to buy anything until after your baby shower, which is traditionally held around the thirtieth week of your pregnancy.

For gear-buying tips, see the *Gear Guide* on page 455.

What you can do

Continue to eat (fortified cereal, crackers, and toast), drink (milk), and be merry to avoid the nausea that may still sometimes show up from having an empty stomach. If you wake up in the middle of the night to go to the bathroom, have a snack available just in case.

Things to organize

Your closet. Now is a good time to shop for versatile clothes that you can wear in both the next months and for a few months postpartum. You'll most likely be the size you are now for about the first two months after the baby's born.

Good clothing buys include

- Jeans or pants with elastic in the sides. If you buy pants now, make sure you have at least two inches of room in the hips to allow for second-trimester pelvic spread. As you get larger, pants with a tummy panel may become more comfortable.

- Comfortable cotton bras with a flap that converts them into nursing bras. If you're large-breasted, look for supportive wide straps. Only buy one or two bras at a time, because your breasts will continue to grow.

- Button-down shirts long enough to cover your pants' elastic and panels. (You can unbutton bottom buttons if the shirt gets tight.) These shirts can also be used for nursing later.

- Maternity dresses with drawstrings in the back to loosen or tighten the fit.

- Bikini-style maternity underwear.

- Maternity hose or an adjustable garter belt with stockings.

- Small hats and sunglasses to protect your face from the sun.

- Flat-soled, slip-on shoes.

Bad buys include

- Non-maternity plus sizes—they'll fit your stomach, but will drape badly everywhere else.

- Thong-style underwear, which can enable urinary tract infections.

- Over-the-stomach underwear, which tends to be too big for postpartum use.

- Bras made of synthetic fabrics, which can cause skin problems such as eczema and nipple irritation.

- Normal, non-pregnant panty hose or tights, which are sure to roll down at the waist or bag at your ankles.

- Shirts too short to cover expandable panels on maternity pants.

- Wide-legged pants, which will make you look wide all over.

- A-line tops, which will start to look like tents as months go on.

- Finger and toe rings, anklets, and cuff bracelets—if they fit now, they'll be too small in a few months and too big after the baby's born. Besides, you don't want to draw attention to how swollen you are.

- New piercings or tattoos—they'll bleed more and be more prone to infection.

Week 22

Fetal Age: 20 weeks (141 to 147 days)
18 to 17 weeks, 125 to 119 days until your due date

YOUR BABY

Size

Your baby is about 7½ inches from crown to rump and weighs between thirteen and sixteen ounces—about the size of a small grapefruit.

Development

Your baby is entering her fifth month of existence.

Her fingernails are almost fully

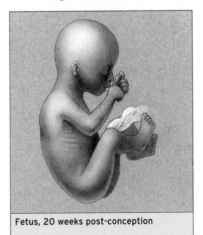

Fetus, 20 weeks post-conception

grown, and her organ systems are becoming more functional and specialized. She has a distinct pair of lips, and her first canines and molars are developing from hard tissue below her gum line. She looks like a miniature newborn.

Blood is traveling through the umbilical cord at four miles an hour, fueling her growth with oxygen and nutrients.

YOU

How you're feeling physically

Your uterus is certainly growing, but you can probably still bend over, sit, drive, and function fairly comfortably.

You may have increased vaginal discharge as your pregnancy progresses. Yeast infections during pregnancy are quite common. Symptoms include redness and itchiness around your vagina and a yeast-smelling discharge, but douching during pregnancy is not advised. Yeast infections are discussed on page 138.

What you can do

This is a good time to have your iron levels checked and to make sure you're drinking enough water, given how much your blood volume has increased over the past few months. As many as 20 percent of pregnant women are anemic, and anemia can put you at serious risk if you hemorrhage during your delivery.

Your care provider will also continue to monitor you for high blood pressure. Women who have no history of high blood pressure can develop what's called *pregnancy-induced hypertension (PIH)*, which is dangerous if left untreated and may require medication. Tell your care provider if you experience dizziness, blurred vision, or swelling in your hands and feet. These all may be signs of PIH. (For more, see *Managing High-Risk Conditions* on page 214.)

As pressure increases on your rear end, you enter the danger zone for constipation and *hemorrhoids*. Drinking water and getting enough fiber in your diet can help you avoid these annoyances. (See our discussion of constipation on page 132.)

Don't let your pregnancy isolate you. Make friends with other pregnant women online, in your childbirth class, in your care provider's waiting room, or in the grocery store. Thanks to the Internet, if you want someone to commiserate about hemorrhoids with at four a.m., you can find her.

Week 23

Fetal Age: 21 weeks (148 to 154 days)
17 to 16 weeks, 118 to 112 days until your due date

YOUR BABY

Size

Weighing in at about a pound, and at eight inches long, your baby is starting to really look like a baby! You can compare her size to a box of sugar or a bag of coffee beans.

Development

Her skin is filling out as the first layers of fat are deposited and her muscles grow. During the next month, her weight may almost double.

YOU

What's happening to you physically

Your care provider should be monitoring your expanding uterus and weight. You should be feeling movement at this point. If you haven't, talk to your care provider. No feeling of movement could be a sign that your placenta is in front of the baby. It may also take more time to feel movement if you're overweight.

As your size expands, you may want to keep an eye on your sodium intake, which can make you swell and bloat. Care providers recommend a limit of three grams of sodium a day. If you experience rapid bloating, call your care provider.

As your baby gains weight, so do you. You've probably gained at least fifteen pounds by now. Some women enjoy the fact that pregnancy is a chance to gain weight without worry or guilt. For others, weight gain can inflame body-image issues.

As you expand, you may begin to itch. There's no need to buy moisturizers made especially for pregnancy. Any product that absorbs well and has an inoffensive smell will do.

EXERCISE TIP

It's important that you stand, walk, and sit with good alignment. You want your lower back to be well supported and your back to be more straight than curved. Check out your work station, and make sure that you aren't contorting yourself, hunching over, leaning to one side, or putting pressure on your wrists. If you lift weights or do aerobics, position yourself by a mirror to keep a constant eye on your stance.

"It's so exciting to feel real movement! It started as little flutters, and now I feel it several times a day."

What you can do

Are you thinking of decorating? Now is a good time, while you have the energy.

If you live in a house built in the 1970s or earlier, you need to have a professional painter get rid of any chipping, flaking, or peeling paint as soon as possible. Lead paint chips and dust are poisonous to humans and especially dangerous to small children and infants.

If you plan to paint the baby's room or refinish the floors, wear an industrial-quality mask, and open plenty of doors and windows for ventilation. The same goes for laying new carpeting, putting up vinyl-coated wallpapers, or sanding down windowsills and doors. Try to have your project completed by the end of this month, so there will be enough time for the paint's chemical fumes to air out. Wall-paint fumes aren't dangerous, but their intense odor can make you feel dizzy and sick. Don't climb up more than a few rungs on a ladder—your balance has shifted, putting you at risk for falls.

Week 24

Fetal Age: 22 Weeks (155 to 161 days)
16 to 15 weeks, 111 to 105 days until your due date

YOUR BABY

Size

Your baby weighs a little over a pound and is about 8½ inches long—the size of a banana.

Development

Your baby's skin becomes less translucent as pigment is deposited, and it looks wrinkly because her body is making her skin more quickly than it makes the fat to pad underneath it.

Your baby's unique hand- and footprints are forming.

You may feel jumps as she has bouts of hiccups. In fact, it may seem like the baby is in perpetual motion.

Some babies now kick in response to sounds and touch from outside the womb. Encourage your partner to talk to the baby, and see if she kicks in response!

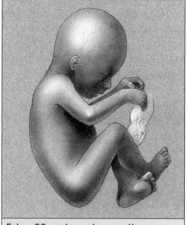

Fetus, 22 weeks post-conception

YOU

How you may be feeling

Your uterus is about 1½ to 2 inches above your belly button, and your bump is definitely apparent and hard to disguise!

You may be suffering from heartburn, muscle aches, sore feet, fatigue, and dizziness.

Call your care provider if you feel dizzy often or if you faint; it may be a sign of anemia. Dizziness is often caused by low blood sugar or by standing up too fast. Rise slowly, and eat regularly.

What you can do

Have you picked out a name yet? Bestowing a name is so much fun— and so much responsibility! You could name your child anything— even a one-letter initial or a symbol. Whatever it is, remember that the baby inside your stomach will have it for life (or until she's 18 and can legally change it). So pick wisely!

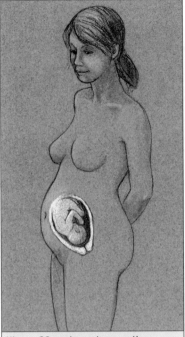

Uterus, 22 weeks post-conception

Some tips:

Avoid misspellings of traditional names. Your child will spend much of her life spelling out the name and correcting those who are confused. Studies have shown that kids with a "misspelled" name are often perceived as being less intelligent and are less likely to land job interviews when they grow up![8]

Beware of initials that spell out words. If your son is David Olsen Grant, you'll deny him the pleasure of monogrammed luggage.

Remember nicknames. If you can't stand "Liz," then don't name your daughter Elizabeth. Nicknames are bestowed on the playground, and you'll have no control over them. Try to think of any unflattering variations that six-year-olds could come up with.

Check your name's popularity. Your kid might like finding a key chain with her name on it every so often, but she would probably feel a little generic if five other kids in her class share her name, causing confusion and making her use a last initial.

If you really can't decide, remember that there's no law that you have to have your baby named by the time you leave the hospital.

Your relationships

Religion matters. If religion has or will ever matter to you, it will matter now more than ever as you and your partner consider how you want to raise your child. You're making sure that the baby's emotional and spiritual environment is the healthiest one you can create.

If you're in a mixed-faith relationship, or have family members and in-laws who are vehement about their chosen religion, the disagreements about how your child will be raised will probably crop up as you near your delivery date.

"My husband felt movement for the first time! I was sleeping, and he was curled up behind me, holding my tummy. It was like the baby was communicating just to him!"

"I was all set on a name until I found out how popular it was last year! I want something that's unique and not trendy. Back to the drawing board."

As much as a faith can be a matter of conflict, it can also be an infallible source of support.

If you and your partner have religious leanings but aren't practicing, you may want to check out various religious establishments to find a place where you share beliefs and feel at home. Even if you're an atheist, it's worthwhile to find a group of like-minded people who can serve as a consistent point of reference during the often-disorienting years ahead. (For more on religion, see *Managing Family and Emotional Issues* on page 247.)

The Third Trimester

Weeks 25 through 40

Waiting is definitely the hardest part of the third trimester. You have only three months to go before a new member joins your family—but the suspense can make it seem like a lot longer. Every day, you're just a little bit bigger and more prepared to finally meet your baby.

As you may have already noticed, more weight brings more discomfort. If you're still working a desk job by the end of this trimester, you'll have the urge to lie under that desk with your feet up to ease back pain. Standing jobs will start to put serious pressure on your knees and ankles. You're probably having trouble sleeping because there simply isn't a comfortable position that works. As the trimester goes on, you may experience any variety of symptoms such as periodic contractions, heartburn, lower back pain, or shooting leg pain when your baby gets into position over your sciatic nerve.

If you need to run to the bathroom several times a night, you're a groggy mom-to-be. These discomforts seem to be designed so that as the trimester progresses, any fear of labor you may have had is transformed into a strong desire to get the baby out by any means necessary. It's normal to become increasingly disenchanted with being pregnant.

But as some grandma once noted, "Babies are easier to take care of in there than out here!" And your baby is definitely being well taken care of. She'll go from being the size of a football to a six- to-nine-pound newborn this trimester. She develops lungs, grows hair, adds fat, and builds up connections in her brain. She can hear your voice, see light and dark, and sense taste in the womb. Over the past three weeks, the swirl of amniotic fluid has molded her unique fingerprints, and her fingers can sense touch.

Week 25

Fetal Age: 23 weeks (162 to 168 days)
15 to 14 weeks, 104 to 98 days until your due date

YOUR BABY

Size

Your baby weighs 1¼ pounds and is a little more than 11 inches long, about the size of a small bag of sugar. In the last third of pregnancy, she'll double and triple her weight.

Development

Your dexterous baby can touch and hold her feet and make a fist.

You may be able to hear your baby's heartbeat with a simple stethoscope. Your partner may be able to hear it by pressing his ear against your belly.

Your baby has a regular sleep schedule now and active and inactive periods. You may or may not be able to discern when these periods are.

Her nostrils, which have been plugged, open up.

YOU

How you may be feeling

Welcome to the third trimester! You're two-thirds of the way there when your fetus is 177 days old. You're really in the homestretch now.

While reaching the third trimester feels like great progress, with it comes a return to fatigue, dizziness, and constant trips to the bathroom.

Your belly can't be disguised. Your uterus is the size of a soccer ball, and your ribs, diaphragm, and stomach are becoming compressed. This compression forces acid back up into your esophagus, which can give you heartburn (see "Heartburn" on page 132) and make you feel full after eating only a little food. Antacids are safe to take while you're pregnant.

"I really recommend the hospital tour. As a first-time mom who has only ever been in a hospital three times (when I was born; when one of my siblings was born; and to visit an ill relative), I didn't really know what to expect. I have a mild fear of hospitals, so seeing everything beforehand was really useful."

Taking a Hospital Tour

If you'll be delivering in a hospital, taking a tour of the maternity wing before the big day is standard. Here are some suggestions for how you can make the trip as informative as possible:

- Time your trip to the hospital. Take notes on the quickest route to get there, and note any alternate routes in case of traffic jams or construction.

- Ask where to go to be admitted when you arrive and if there is a different procedure for after hours.

- Ask if you can complete pre-admission forms before you leave, so you'll be admitted more quickly when you're in labor.

- Find out where you and your visitors can park, during regular and late hours.

- Find out how many visitors you can have in your room and in the waiting room, during birth and after.

- Check out both the birthing suites and the recovery rooms. Some hospitals offer a few palatial birthing suites to entice new customers, but only tiny and considerably less-deluxe postpartum rooms, which is where you'll be spending most of your in-hospital time.

- Ask what the ratio is of certified labor and delivery nurses to patients, and if there's an upper limit to how many patients a nurse may be assigned to care for at one time.

- Inquire about the NICU (Neonatal Intensive Care Unit) and how its capabilities compare with that of others in the area.

- Locate the hospital cafeteria, and get a lead on where the closest convenience stores, delis, and restaurants offering take-out are, in case hospital food turns out to be unappealing.

- Ask about what kind of security procedures are in place to keep unauthorized visitors out of the maternity ward.

- If your hospital is a teaching hospital, find out if, and how, medical students and residents will be involved in your care.

- Ask what the hospital procedure is if you need a cesarean. Will your partner be permitted in the operating room with you?

- Ask whether the birthing wing has its own anesthesiologist, and whether you will be given an opportunity to interview him about your pain relief preferences or special conditions before you go into labor.

- Ask where the hospital performs circumcisions, who performs them, and what kind of pain medication they use. (If you're not sure whether or not you want to have your son circumcised, see our discussion on pages 402-406.)

As your weight gain increases, you may become one of the twenty to fifty percent of pregnant women who develop hemorrhoids.

What you can do

Now is a good time to get into the habit of doing back stretches. They probably won't help with delivery, but they can help with your aches and pains throughout the day. It's also a good time to be walking, swimming, and practicing yoga. Now is not a good time for weightlifting or kickboxing—exercises that might injure your softened ligaments. (See *Managing Your Weight and Fitness* on page 157.)

You may have cramps in your calves, back, tailbone, and even arms, as your ligaments soften. Calcium and magnesium, found in cow's milk and vitamin supplements, may help. (For more on your vitamin and mineral requirements, see page 146.)

If you're considering breastfeeding, this is a good time to start attending La Leche League meetings. These informal sessions will supply you with solid, practical information on how to breastfeed and tips on good nutrition and the process of childbirth. La Leche League groups often are listed in the white pages of the telephone book, and you can also find a local group by calling the organization's national number or by visiting their Web site. (See the *Resource Guide* on page 538.) Most groups offer a leader on call for support 24/7 if you're having problems after your baby is born.

If you haven't toured the place where you'll be giving birth, now is a good time to make an appointment to do so. Most hospitals have free guided tours of their birthing centers scheduled for future parents.

Week 26

Fetal Age: 24 weeks (169 to 175 days)
14 to 13 weeks, 97 to 91 days until your due date

YOUR BABY

Size

Your baby weighs about 1⅓ pounds and has undergone a growth spurt in the past few weeks. From weeks twenty to twenty-eight, she almost doubles in height and now would be about a foot tall if she could stand.

Development

This week marks a major milestone in your baby's hearing and sight.

Your baby's hearing system (cochlea and peripheral sensory end organs), which began fine development during week eighteen, is now completely formed, and over the next few weeks, she'll become increasingly sensitive to sound. In about a month, you'll feel her jump if she hears a sudden loud noise.

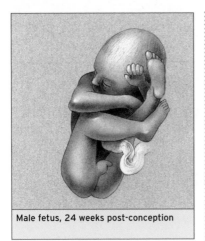

Male fetus, 24 weeks post-conception

Sound passes easily into your uterus, which helps her ears to develop.

Her eyes are almost fully formed. Did you know that all babies have blue eyes in the womb, no matter what their genetic inheritance is? A baby's eyes don't get their final color until a few months after they are born.

The air sacs of the lungs, called alveoli, will be developed by the end of this week and will begin to secrete a substance called **surfactant** that keeps the lung tissue from sticking together.

YOU

What's happening to you physically

Sleeping is definitely getting uncomfortable. Try sleeping on your left side. Your baby has to battle with your backbone when you're lying on your back, and sleeping on your back will also position your uterus over a major artery, cutting off blood flow. If this happens, you may feel light-headed. If it helps to sleep on the floor, give it a try.

Pregnancy-related **carpal tunnel syndrome** affects one in four pregnant women. It's most common with, but not limited to, women who type on keyboards or otherwise work with their hands and wrists all day. The extra fluid in your body can accumulate in your wrists and cause sharp pains that can run up your arm, or numbness in your fingers and hands. Take as many typing breaks as you can, use a wrist rest at the computer, and consider wearing a plastic splint at night and sleeping with your wrists elevated. (For more on this see "Fingers and Hands" on page 127.)

Between now and the next three weeks, you may be tested for **gestational diabetes** with a **glucose tolerance test.** This test requires you to fast for twelve hours and then drink a glucose-rich liquid usually in the form of a syrupy orange-flavored drink. After an hour, a blood sample is taken. If you have a positive test, you'll be given another, longer, three-hour diagnostic test. This is a similar procedure, except that your blood is

> *"You really need someone to drive you home from the glucose tolerance test. I could drive safely but I felt sick and sorry for myself. It would have been nice to have someone there."*

Things to Ask Your Doula (Labor Assistant)

- How many births have you attended?
- What type of childbirth classes do you recommend? (Some doulas may require that you take certain classes.)
- What are your feelings about the use of drugs in labor?
- At what point should I call you when I go into labor?
- Will you be available on my due date?
- Have you worked with my care provider before? If so, what were your impressions of him or her?
- What kind of relaxation techniques do you know?
- What do you think about women eating, drinking, and getting out of bed during labor?
- Do you usually bring accessories, like a birth ball, massaging foot roller, aromatherapy oils, or other relaxation devices?
- Are you also a licensed massage therapist?

checked before you drink the glucose cocktail, and again once every three hours afterward. If you do have gestational diabetes, you'll be advised to adopt a low-carbohydrate diet. Gestational diabetes is a temporary condition, which goes away after the baby's born. For more on the glucose tolerance test, see page 186.

How you may feel

You may feel like your body has been taken over: It's weird to have another person sharing your body with you, especially one who kicks so much! Nature has taken over, and there's not a whole lot you can do about it but cope, rest, relax, and marvel. You probably wish that you could take a vacation from your pregnancy sometimes. Floating in a swimming pool with your eyes closed may be as close as you can get.

Things to organize

If you're planning a home or hospital birth, now is a good time to look into hiring a labor assistant or doula if you are planning to do so. Your care provider, hospital, or childbirth educator can help you locate one, or you can find an assistant yourself by contacting DONA (Doulas of North America) or the International Association of Childbirth Educators (ICEA, at www.icea.org). The person you call will set up a meeting with you and your partner prior to labor to talk about your birth philosophy and what kind of services you may find helpful.

Are you preparing for a home birth? Your attending midwife will certainly give you detailed lists of what you'll need. Now is a good time to pack your clean linens, nightgowns, plastic sheeting, and so on, into a large box that you can keep in a safe place until you need them. If you've decided on a home birth, be sure to do your research— read every home-birthing book, and watch every video you can get your hands on. (See page 165 for more about home birth.)

Week 27

Fetal Age: 25 weeks (176 to 182 days)
13 to 12 weeks, 90 to 84 days until your due date

YOUR BABY

Size

Your baby weighs about two pounds and is about 12 to 15 inches long, about the size of a small pot roast.

Development

If your baby were born now, he would have an excellent chance (85 percent) of surviving.

He still isn't fully formed and would probably not be able to breathe by himself. He would need to stay in an incubator to keep his body temperature regulated, and he would have a weak liver and immune system.

(Fact: Babies have more taste buds at birth than they will have later in life. Newborns can sniff out and tell the difference between their mother's milk and someone else's.)

YOU

What's happening to you physically

The weight of your baby is putting pressure on your back, which can cause shooting pains (sciatica) in your lower back and legs. Lifting, bending, and walking can make the pain worse. Warm baths, ice packs, and changing positions may help. (For more on sciatica, see "Back" on page 127.)

Your cholesterol levels may rise. Cholesterol is used by you and your baby's placenta to help make progesterone, a hormone with wide-ranging effects, such as preventing preterm birth, helping maintain cells' oxygen levels, and regulating metabolism.

The volume of your **amniotic fluid** is reduced by about half. With less cushioning to block the view, you'll be able to see bony knees and elbows poking out of your stomach when the baby kicks and turns. Her kicks may be vigorous—others will be able to see them if they stare at your stomach.

As you grow, you may start to see stretch marks on your breasts and abdomen. (See "Stretch Marks" on page 120.) You may also have a hard time bending over and tying your shoes. Your heart rate may have increased, causing you to feel flush and look winded with less exertion.

What you can do

Have you thought about getting a pregnancy massage? It can be the most comfortable hour of your month! Massages may even be covered by your health insurance. Here are some other safe indulgences:

A manicure. Your nails are long and strong, so take advantage. Get them polished at a salon that's hygienic and well-ventilated.

A pedicure and foot massage (though don't get a leg massage if you have varicose veins). Your poor feet will be subjected to five hundred pounds of pressure or more every time you take a step, so treat them well!

A warm bath in a dim room with soft music playing. Treat yourself to new sponges, loofahs, a waterproof bath pillow, gently scented glycerin soaps, and bath oils.

A home facial. If you have dry skin, mix up papaya, avocado, and a few teaspoons of oatmeal. Leave the mask on for fifteen to twenty minutes, then massage your face and rinse. The fruits are rich in natural oils, and the oatmeal will slough off dead skin.

If you have oily skin, substitute cornmeal for oatmeal; the gritty grain will help you exfoliate. (For more about skin care, see "Skin" on page 118.)

Week 28

Fetal Age: 26 weeks (183 to 189 days)
12 to 11 weeks, 83 to 77 days until your due date

YOUR BABY

Size

Your baby has doubled her weight in the past month and is the size of a bag of flour. She now weighs almost $2^{1}/_{2}$ pounds. Her total length is nearly fifteen inches.

Development

Your baby's lungs are now capable of breathing air! This is big news. It means if the baby is born from now on, she'll be able to survive with less medical intervention.

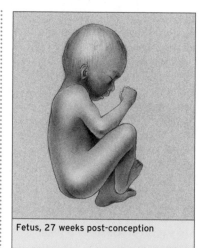

Fetus, 27 weeks post-conception

Your baby's main job right now is to put the finishing touches on major organ systems, such as her brain, lungs, and liver. As you can probably tell, she's also working on gaining layers of fat. Her body fat is about 2 to 3 percent.

Your baby's eyes, which were covered by her eyelid folds at the sixth week of development, are capable of opening this week. Her sucking and swallowing skills are improving.

YOU

What's happening to you physically

You're getting larger, and as you grow larger, you become more uncomfortable. Your legs may ache or cramp, it's hard to get a good sleeping position, and the baby is big enough to give you some sharp kicks to the ribs!

Your perspiration can get trapped in the folds of your skin, which can be irritating and make you feel grubby. Try applying talcum powder under your breasts before you put your bra on, and in any other nooks and crannies you may have developed. If you're going to get stretch marks, you probably have them by now.

Remember that hot weather, standing for long periods of time, or low blood sugar can make you prone to dizziness and fainting. Drink water, and stay in the shade if you're pregnant in the summer.

Emotionally

If you know you're having a boy, you and your partner may be battling over circumcision. Consider doing research on the procedure (see pages 402–406), talking to your baby's future pediatrician for her views, and talking to other parents to see how they resolved the issue.

What you can do

With twelve weeks to go until your baby is officially due, you may start having more regular visits to your care provider. If you're Rh negative, you should get the RhoGAM™ shot this week (for more information, see "Testing: Risks and Benefits" on page 188) to prevent complications at delivery.

Between now and the next few weeks, you'll be given blood tests for your iron levels and offered a glucose tolerance test if you haven't already had one.

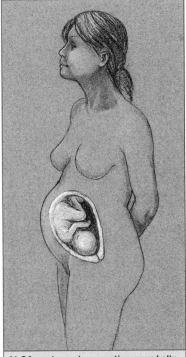

At 26 weeks post-conception, your belly announces your condition to the world.

What you can do

Feel your belly to see if you can find the baby's head, knees, and elbows! Try finding your baby's position inside your belly by lying in a semi-upright position on your back. Your baby's head will feel like a hard mass with a distinctive round, smooth texture. Put your palms on either side of your belly, and try gently pushing back and forth—the side where your baby's backbone is will feel firmer and offer more resistance to moving. Or simply walk your fingertips across your abdomen—your baby's back will be firm, and the arms and legs will be knobby. Once your baby moves into the head-down position, you may feel your baby's heel kicking around your ribs. It will be a small, mobile knob the size of a large bubble-gum ball pressing out just below your rib cage.

Week 29

Fetal Age: 27 weeks (190 to 196 days)
11 to 10 weeks, 76 to 70 days until your due date

YOUR BABY

Size

Your baby is about two and a half pounds and would be between fifteen and seventeen inches tall if she could stand.

Development

Your baby's adrenal glands are producing a chemical which will be made into estriol (a form of estrogen) by the placenta. This estriol is thought to stimulate the production of **prolactin** by your body, and the prolactin makes you produce milk. So even if your baby comes early, you'll still be able to breastfeed.

Each passing week improves the likelihood that your baby will be born strong and healthy. Her brain can direct rhythmic breathing and control body temperature, so she's less likely to need breathing assistance should she be born early. She's growing eyelashes, adding fat, and developing her brain.

Because of brain wave activity, researchers have speculated that babies can even dream at this time!

YOU

How you're feeling physically

As the levels of prolactin increase in your body, your breasts may secrete colostrum, which can dampen your bra. Prolactin also has a sedating effect, and you may feel the need to take naps the way you did in the first trimester.

Your uterus is now in a position where it exerts pressure on your bladder. Your frequent trips to the bathroom may also remind you of the first trimester. The tubes that link your kidneys, bladder, and urethra are also compressed, which means you can't empty your bladder as efficiently. You may also leak urine when you laugh or cough.

Exercise

If you can, keep up your swimming, walking, yoga, or other non–weight bearing exercise, though you're not feeling as energetic (and as comfortable) as you did last trimester. Exercise can help relieve your back, hip, and leg pain and help you have

a speedier physical recovery after childbirth. If you've been lifting free weights or using weight machines, you don't have to stop, but keep the weight level and the repetitions and range of motion at maintenance level. Don't try to add muscle mass or increase your range of motion, because your ligaments are relaxed and more prone to injury.

One exercise you don't want to slack off on is the Kegel, especially if laughing or coughing is already making you leak urine. Don't forget to Kegel! It will keep your pelvic floor toned.

Week 30

Fetal Age: 28 weeks (197 to 203 days)
10 to 9 weeks, 69 to 63 days until your due date

YOUR BABY

Size

Her length is about 16 inches—about as long as a laptop computer—and she measures almost 11 inches from crown to rump. She weighs approximately $2\frac{1}{2}$ to 3 pounds. From now until delivery, every baby will gain weight at a more individual rate.

Development

Your baby has doubled in height over the past six weeks, and from now until delivery, she'll gain only a

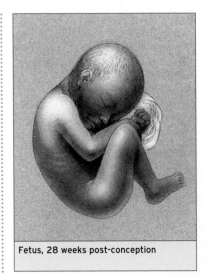

Fetus, 28 weeks post-conception

few more inches in length. Don't worry if she's in a strange position (what your care provider might call a *transverse lie*). There's still plenty of time for her to get settled into a head-down (*cephalic*) position for birth. She's floating in about 1½ pints of amniotic fluid and has some room to move.

Your baby's most important organ, her brain, continues to develop at a rapid pace. Her eyes are able to track light, and some researchers have theorized that exposing your belly to light may stimulate development. Try moving the beam of a flashlight slowly over your belly in a dim room, and see if she reacts.

YOU

What's happening to you physically

If you have light skin, you may notice enlarged veins (see "Varicose Veins" on page 144) on your legs or all over your body. Avoid staying in one position for very long. Take walks, and move around to improve circulation. Wear loose clothes, including loose socks, to keep your circulation from being restricted. Some doctors have suggested buying support hose and putting it on before you even get out of bed to

> **TIP:**
>
> The damage that can be done by continuing to smoke increases as you get closer to term. If you and your partner haven't quit, give it another try.

> *"I've started to get out of breath just from walking up a flight of stairs or up a little hill! It really makes me sympathetic to people who are out of shape."*

keep your veins from having the chance to pop out. Or you can just ignore them. Enlarged veins are just a cosmetic problem, not a sign that anything's wrong.

You've now been officially pregnant for seven months, and the home stretch is in sight. You're big now, no doubt about it! Your belly is about the size of a watermelon. Tying your shoes is a challenge, and you may already have adopted the pregnant "waddle." You may feel your heart pounding and have shortness of breath as you exert yourself. If you've been exercising and are in good shape, you may experience this less.

Did you know that hormones cause your lung capacity to expand during pregnancy, making you breathe more frequently and deeply? During this trimester, you may really feel it, especially if you're an ex-smoker or not in the best cardiovascular shape. If you feel short of breath, take slow, relaxed, and deep breaths.

You may have the urge to nest. You may feel like you have to get everything done now, while you still can—from tying up loose ends at work to refacing your cabinets. You do have more energy now than you will in the remaining months, but you also have a lot less than you normally do. Our advice is to take advantage of your pregnant form to get other people to pitch in.

Your abdominal muscles have stretched and loosened, so when you're lying down, you can't get up as quickly as you used to. Practice getting up by rolling to one side.

Things to organize

Your birth plan. You can't anticipate everything that's going to happen during labor and delivery, but you can certainly make a wish list of how you want things to go. A birth plan is a tool to facilitate a conversation between you and your care provider. Don't expect that your labor and delivery nurses will

have an opportunity to read it. Depending on the time of day and the hospital, your labor and delivery nurses may have to be tending to as many as seven other contracting women at a time.

Instead, view your birth plan as a way for you to figure out for yourself what kind of birthing environment you'd like, how you want to manage your pain, what kind of interventions you want (and which to avoid), and what your friends and family's roles will be. Then use your plan as the start of a discussion with your care provider about what you can expect during labor. Also be sure to involve your partner in the plan, so he'll be prepared to express your wishes if you're too busy.

Many Web sites, such as www.childbirth.org and www.parentsplace.com offer interactive programs that let you generate your own birth plan.

Week 31

Fetal Age: 29 weeks (204 to 210 days)
9 to 8 weeks, 62 to 56 days until your due date

YOUR BABY

Size

She weighs between 2¹/₂ and 3¹/₂ pounds. She continues to gain weight at a faster pace than she lengthens, which will give her those cute chubby cheeks. She's about fourteen to sixteen inches tall, although individual growth rates vary.

Development

Your baby begins to run out of room as she puts on weight. You should feel about ten kicks an hour. Some care providers suggest keeping a "kick chart" by writing down how many kicks you can feel in an hour, so that you are aware if there's a decrease in activity. Other care providers may advise that as long as it feels like the baby's active, there's

Some Ideas of What to Include in Your Birth Plan

1. Your strategy for pain management:

Do you want to be offered

- An epidural?

- Narcotics, sedatives, and/or opiates?

- The use of a tub or shower?

- The opportunity to walk around?

- The coaching services of a labor assistant or doula?

- Low lights, soft music, or a specific ambience?

- Labor accessories, such as a birth ball, birthing stool, or beanbag?

- Acupressure, acupuncture, or guided relaxation techniques?

If you know you want an epidural, ask your care provider when you can expect it to be administered to you and how many hours of relief you can expect. For more, see "Coping with Labor Pain" in the *Guide to Giving Birth* on page 298.

2. Your hospital experience:

What levels of intervention are you comfortable with?

- Do you mind having a routine IV for fluids or a heparin lock? Hospitals have different policies on IVs—some will routinely insert a heparin lock in the back of your hand as soon as you're admitted, making it easier to administer intravenous medication or fluids. Others will just give you an IV if you have an epidural or a need for extra fluids.

- Will you be shaved or given an enema? Believe it or not, some care providers and hospitals still do these things. (See page 239 of the *Guide to Giving Birth* for more).

- Are there interventions you want to avoid for religious reasons, such as blood transfusions?

- If you've previously had a cesarean delivery, do you want the opportunity to deliver vaginally this time? (See "Vaginal Birth after Cesarean" in *Managing High-Risk Conditions* on page 222.)

- What circumstances would make labor **induction** or **augmentation** necessary? Induced labor is more painful and tiring than regular labor, subjects you and the baby to drugs and their side effects, and is more likely to end in a c-section or cause you injury. Still, sometimes inductions become necessary. Ask how many days past term you can go before your care provider will consider induction, and how many hours the hospital will give you to go into labor after your water breaks. (For more on induction, see page 335 of the *Guide to Giving Birth*.)

- Can you eat and drink in labor? Some hospitals forbid eating and drinking during labor—it's ice chips only. You probably won't feel like eating, but you may appreciate being allowed to drink when you're thirsty.

- Who do you want to have in the room with you? Tell your care provider if you want to have extra people in your room, such as your labor assistant or children.

- Who do you want kept out?

- What's the policy on fetal monitoring? Some hospitals require that your contractions and your and your baby's heart rates be electronically monitored at certain intervals (such as once an hour). Having to stand still or lie down to be monitored when you're in labor can be aggravating.

3. Delivery:

How do you want to participate in the birth? Do you want to

- Be told when to push, or to push as you feel the urge?

- Touch the baby's head as it crowns?

- Watch the birth in a mirror?

- Have your partner catch the baby or cut the umbilical cord?

- Have the baby be placed on your chest immediately after delivery?

- Have newborn procedures such as weighing and fingerprinting be performed in the room, or in the nursery?

If a cesarean is necessary,

- Will you be awake?

- Will your partner be allowed in the room?

- Do you want the drape removed when it's time for the baby to be lifted out?

4. Recovery:

- How soon after delivery will your care provider check up on you?

- Will the baby be in your room around the clock, only when you're awake, or just for feedings?

- If you're planning to breastfeed, ask how the hospital supports breastfeeding. Will the baby be placed on your chest for feeding immediately after birth? Is there a lactation consultant on staff? If the baby has to go to the NICU, will the hospital help you pump milk?

- How long will you stay in the hospital?

no need to keep notes. If you do sense a decrease in activity, try drinking a large glass of juice. If that doesn't make the baby energized, or makes her less energized than she usually would be, call your care provider.

YOU

How you're feeling

- **Bloated.** If your blood pressure is normal, and you don't have protein in your urine, your puffy face, hands, legs, and feet are probably normal.

- **Tired.** If you are working, you probably keep a secret calendar in your desk that counts the days, hours, and minutes until your maternity leave starts.

- **Clumsy.** Extra inches and a shift in your center of gravity can make you bump into furniture, knock things over, and be more prone to accidental falls. (See "Accidents" on page 226.)

Things to do this week

Add to your baby registry! If you're going to have a baby shower,

> "I think the baby's running out of room. I used to feel more kicks, but now it feels more like squirmy knots in there."

it'll probably be between the thirtieth and the thirty-sixth weeks. Guests want to see you in all of your pregnant glory, and you want to be spry enough to enjoy your own party!

Here are some registry tips:

- Refer to the *Baby Gear Guide* on page 454, and take stock of what you have and what you'll need.

- Pick at least one big store to register in, so friends and family from out of state will also be able to send gifts.

- Select items from every guest's price range.

- Test out items in the store, and choose carefully. You can always return stuff, but it's best to get what you want the first time!

- Venture out of the baby department. Consider adding towels, washcloths, clothes hampers, unscented detergent, or an extra trash can or two. You'll need that stuff too!

Week 32

Fetal Age: 30 weeks (211 to 217 days)
8 to 7 weeks, 55 to 49 days until your due date

YOUR BABY

Size

She weighs about four pounds and is about fifteen to seventeen inches tall.

Development

Photographs of babies in utero at this stage show their skin becoming less translucent and pinker, as layers of fat are deposited under the skin.

Her skeleton is rapidly ossifying (turning from cartilage into solid bone), which means that kicks will be stronger. Kicks may even become visible through your shirt as the trimester progresses. Well-placed kicks under your ribs can take your breath away!

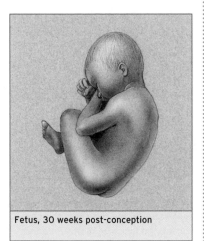

Fetus, 30 weeks post-conception

YOU

What's happening to you physically

From now until delivery, you'll be gaining about a pound a week. About half of that gain is the baby's, the rest is fluid retention. Consider giving up wearing heels, not only because balancing is difficult, but because your feet will swell over the course of the day. You may also

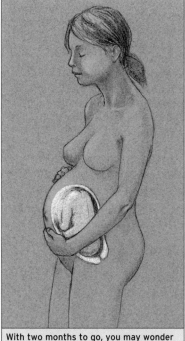

With two months to go, you may wonder how much bigger you can possibly get!

want to give up on wearing rings on your fingers from now until about a month after delivery; they won't fit well and may get stuck. Fight bloat by avoiding high-sodium foods and carbonated beverages. (For more on fluid retention, see "Swelling" in *Managing Your Body* on page 141.) Call your care provider if you suddenly feel puffy in your face or hands; this is a symptom of preeclampsia.

Have you given any thought to whom you want in the room with you while you're in labor? First-time moms' labor lasts an average of twelve to fifteen hours. Even your partner will need to take a break at some point.

Hospitals may have different policies on visitors, so it's worthwhile to ask about those policies on the hospital tour, especially if you're planning on bringing a film crew. Be sure to review your hospital's visiting hours and policies.

Week 33

Fetal Age: 31 weeks (218 to 224 days)
7 to 6 weeks, 48 to 42 days until your due date

YOUR BABY

Size

Your baby's crown-to-rump length is about $11^1/2$ inches. She weighs about $4^1/2$ pounds and gains about eight ounces every week.

Development

Your baby has probably moved to the head-down position and may descend into your pelvis at any time in the next six weeks and begin to press into your cervix. This position not only prepares her for birth but allows blood to flow to her developing brain. The dark quiet of your womb is perfect for this activity.

Right now, your baby is also in the process of receiving your antibodies. If she were born right now, her immune system would be immature, and extra care would need to be taken to keep her in a sterile environment.

YOU

What's happening to you physically

You continue gaining weight at the rate of a pound a week, and it probably seems impossible that your body will find somewhere to fit six more pounds. Your amniotic fluid has reached its maximum density of two to six cups.

How you may be feeling

Anyone who says, "Wow, you only have six weeks to go!" doesn't understand how time slows down during the last weeks of pregnancy.

If you're still working, you're probably already counting the minutes until your maternity leave starts. During the next six weeks, you may be trying to decide if you'll be one of the sixty percent of moms who will return to the workforce in the year after having a baby, or if you'll be among the forty percent who stay home.

What you can do

If you know that you don't want to go back to work after the baby's born, or you're undecided, now is a good time to update your résumé. Collect a copy of your job description and samples of your work. Write down all of your duties and accomplishments now, while they're fresh in your mind. Copy down important phone numbers from your Rolodex, and save a list of the e-mail addresses stored on your work computer. (For more about work issues, see *Managing Your Finances* on page 249.)

Week 34

Fetal Age: 32 weeks (225 to 231 days)
6 to 5 weeks, 41 to 35 days until your due date

YOUR BABY

Size

Your baby weighs five pounds or more, about the size of a bag of sugar. She will continue to gain about two or more pounds in the next six weeks.

Development

Now that your baby's brain has formed billions of neurons, it must accomplish the even more complex feat of hooking the neurons and synapses together. Your baby's brain is forming trillions of connections, making it possible for her to learn in the womb.

All of this brain development may be the reason that your baby sleeps frequently at this stage. She may even be dreaming—her eyes dart around rapidly just as an adult's might in REM sleep.

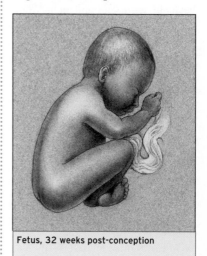

Fetus, 32 weeks post-conception

Your child's brain development is in no way complete at birth. In the first year after birth, a baby's brain triples in size and becomes three-quarters of its adult size.

YOU

What's happening to you physically

The volume of your uterus is five hundred to one thousand times larger than before you got pregnant, so it's safe to say you're feeling huge and slow.

You're still running to the bathroom frequently and probably will be from here on out. Try to drink a lot of water early in the day, so you don't get thirsty at night and make things worse.

What you can do

If your partner wonders what it feels like to be pregnant, try filling a backpack with as many pounds as you've gained (dried beans or bags of sugar make good weights) and have him wear it around on his front.

Things to organize

Your car seat.
If you haven't purchased your baby's car seat and installed it facing rearward in the backseat of your car yet, do it now. Your baby might come early, and the hospital staff won't let you drive your baby home without one. And there's nothing worse than watching from a hospital wheelchair as your partner goes nuts trying to install it while he's parked in the fire lane. (See our discussion of car seats in the *Baby Gear Guide* on page 491.)

Your hospital bag.
Yes, it's a little early yet, but think about what you want to bring with you to the hospital. Perhaps find a corner of your closet to start piling things in. Don't forget a newborn-size and photogenic outfit for the baby to wear home, and a blanket to swaddle her with. (The nurses can show you how to swaddle.) Hospitals are quite good at providing everything you'll need while you're there. Some even give you disposable underpants. Still, it's nice to have things from home.

Here are some things you may want to include when packing for the hospital.

Don't forget these items:

- Your health insurance card.

- Baby car seat, installed facing rearward.

- An outfit for the baby to wear home.

- Address book with phone numbers of relatives and friends to be notified.

- Your cell phone, though you'll have to leave it off until you are in a recovery room—it may interfere with monitoring equipment.

- Deodorant, brush, and comb, toothbrush and toothpaste.

- Maternity underwear (hospital may supply, but just in case).

- Socks. (The kind with non-slip soles are best.)

Optional items:

- Your birth plan.

- A CD player with extra batteries and your favorite music.

- Snacks for you, your partner, and guests after the baby's born.

- Bottles of juice or sports drinks.

- A legal pad and pen for taking notes for recording things you want to remember.

- A folder to take your hospital documents home in.

- A bathrobe and slippers.

- A lightweight blanket for your partner.

- Makeup: foundation, blush, lipstick, nail polish, hand or face cream. Sounds vain, but you'll probably be taking a lot of pictures, and you'll feel better if you know you look good!

- Lip balm.

- Hair clips, elastics, and/or a headband.

- Your favorite maternity outfit to wear home. (You'll be about ten pounds lighter, so bring what was comfortable last month.)

- Camera and film.

- Change for snack an machines.

- Natural childbirth pain relief supplies.

- Your birthing ball.

- A two-level footstool for supporting your feet as you sit in a chair or on the toilet.

- Back massage supplies, such as a tennis ball.

The following will be supplied by the hospital (but bring if you prefer your own):

- Your favorite pillow with a colored pillowcase (so it doesn't get lost).

- A nightgown with front openings for nursing (something that you don't mind getting stained).

- A box of disposable breast pads. (Check a source such as epinions.com to see what brand nursing moms like best.)

- Heavy-flow sanitary napkins.

When to Contact Your Care Provider

- Blurred vision
- Severe headaches
- Severe swelling
- Sudden weight gain

These symptoms can indicate high blood pressure, which is more common in the second half of pregnancy and can be a sign of preeclampsia.

Week 35

Fetal Age: 33 weeks (232 to 238 days)
5 to 4 weeks, 34 to 28 days until your due date

YOUR BABY

Size

At more than five pounds and between sixteen and twenty inches, your baby is becoming more ready for birth with every passing hour. She's the size of a small roasting chicken.

Development

Her nervous system and immune system are still maturing, and she's adding the fat that she'll need to regulate her body temperature. But everything else, from her toenails to the hair on her head, is fully formed. If she were born now, she'd have more than a ninety-nine percent chance of surviving.

YOU

What's going on physically

You're just huge, and your size is probably making you really uncomfortable. You're carrying so much extra weight and fluid that simple things can be tiring.

If your job requires sitting all day, it's probably getting hard to work.

You should take frequent breaks to walk around and stretch your legs (if you have the privacy to lie down for a few minutes or do stretches on your hands and knees, even better). Change your sitting position frequently, and bring in pillows to support your back.

You'll be seeing your care provider once every one to two weeks now.

What you can do

If you have other children, this can be a poignant time, because it is the last few weeks of being a family in the way that you're used to. It can seem hard to imagine that there will be enough of you to go around, and you may wonder if it will ever be possible for you to love a new baby as much. You may feel guilty about the sacrifices your other children will have to make to accommodate the new baby. No matter how many children you have, each new baby is a leap of faith that the sacrifices will be worth it. (For more on preparing siblings for a new baby, see page 236.)

Don't forget to arrange care for any children or pets for the two to three days you'll be in the hospital. Ask a neighbor to collect your newspapers and mail. You probably will send your partner home to check on things at some point, but you don't want to have to worry, especially if the hospital or birthing center is far from your home.

Week 36

Fetal Age: 34 weeks (239 to 245 days)
4 to 3 weeks, 27 to 21 days until your due date

YOUR BABY

Size

With one month to go, she weighs about six pounds and is fattening. Her full length from crown to feet is about $20^{1}/_{2}$ inches.

Development

Has your baby's movement slowed down? If so, you shouldn't worry. Five to ten percent of all mothers report that babies start to slow down as they grow larger and get more cramped for space. Still, you should be able to feel your baby move more than ten times a day. If you're concerned, try drinking a sweet beverage, such as orange juice, and then lying on your side for a while.

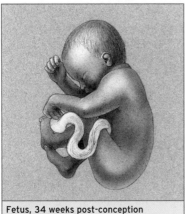

Fetus, 34 weeks post-conception

Most babies will wake up and start to move. If you're still concerned, contact your healthcare provider.

YOU

What's happening to you physically

As women in the grocery store may have already told you, you look like you could go any minute. And they might be right—your due date just suggests a time when the baby's likely to be born. In reality, you could go into labor any time between now and six weeks from now!

Your belly button is becoming flattened or may even stick out like a wine cork.

You may feel a lightening sensation on your ribs and organs as your baby descends into your pelvis. Breathing and eating will be easier, but you'll be running to the bathroom more often than ever, and the change in pressure may cause shooting pains in your groin and leg.

What you can do

If you're aching (and we don't see how you couldn't be), indulge in a pregnancy massage from a professional masseuse, or find a pool, and take a swim. At home, try sitting on an exercise ball (also known as a birth ball). This will take pressure off your back because it forces you to sit straight and with good balance, using your legs to support and stabilize you. This is good practice for labor.

If you'll be breastfeeding, you'll want to stock up on nursing bras and shirts that button down the front (or are specifically made for breastfeeding). This is a particularly good time to buy nursing bras, since your breasts are about the size they'll stay for the duration of your nursing experience. Make sure that your bras fit well, don't itch, and are made of natural, breathable materials (synthetics may cause a rash!).

Some women report going into an intense and obsessive nesting phase in the hours before labor began—cleaning out closets, sorting socks, or baking cookies with a zombie-like intensity. If you find yourself doing this, double-check that your bag is packed while you're at it!

Week 37

Fetal Age: 35 weeks (246 to 252 days)
3 to 2 weeks, 20 to 14 days until your due date

YOUR BABY

Size

Extra large! Your baby has likely hit the six-pound mark by now, and her length is approximately twenty-one inches. The weight on your abdomen probably feels like twice that.

Development

Your baby is practicing her breathing, but she has increasingly less space to practice stretching and kicking. Your baby's intestines are also building up meconium, a greenish-black substance made of baby by-products such as dead cells, shed lanugo, and amniotic fluid. It'll become your little darling's first bowel movement, hopefully after she is out of the womb.

Her body fat has increased to about eight percent. By birth, it'll be about fifteen percent.

If your baby is a boy, his testes will have descended into his scrotum.

While your baby could be born at any time, the longer she stays in, the more time she has to develop the connections in her brain in the pleasant peace and quiet of your womb. At this point, she can do all the things a newborn can, with the exception of breathing air and pooping in a diaper. Just as you're feeling stretched, your baby is being squeezed on all sides.

Some of your antibodies are crossing the placenta, giving your baby's immune system some support for her first days in the world. If you breastfeed, you'll later be giving her immunities in your milk.

YOU

What's happening to you physically

The hormone *relaxin* is causing all of the smooth muscle in your body to unclench. You'll feel like you have loose "rag-doll" joints. Even tall, fit women will start to get a waddling gait as ligaments soften. Inside, the smooth muscle layer of your uterus is flattening and relaxing to accommodate your baby's weight gain. You may have round ligament pains (sharp muscle cramps around the place where your bathing suit's leg holes would be) as these ligaments are softening and being pulled by the growing weight of the baby. (For more about the role of smooth muscle tissue, see page 125.)

You're probably having Braxton-Hicks contractions, which you may or may not notice. How can you tell these contractions from the real thing? If you have to ask, they probably aren't. Real contractions grow progressively stronger, more intense, and more regular. They may start and stop in a series over a day or night before they get down to business. Use a timer to see how far apart they are and how long they last. If they become regular, let your care provider know.

You may expel *bloody show,* also known as your *mucus plug,* at any time. This is a blood-tinged mass of mucus which has been covering your cervix for the past nine months. It doesn't mean that you'll go into labor right away—it can take as long as two to three weeks after bloody show before labor begins. (For more about this, see page 263 of the *Guide to Giving Birth.*)

How you may be feeling

As you approach your due date, you'll start to get frantic calls from well-meaning friends and relatives who just want to check and see if you're in labor yet. Of course, only five percent of moms deliver on their due date. Any care provider who can tell you when you're going to go into labor is lying or planning to induce you.

Waiting for labor can make you feel discouraged. Make plans every day, go to the movies, walk outside, and enjoy the last few days of quiet.

What to do for the next three to five weeks

Keep your car filled with gas, and make sure you can always get in touch with whoever is designated to drive you to the hospital.

Write down the phone number of a local taxi or ambulance service in case you go into labor when you're home alone.

If you're impatient, take plenty of walks and keep swimming. The activity may or may not move things along, and you'll feel better.

> *"I asked my midwife when she thought the baby would be born, and she said, 'If I could tell that, I wouldn't be a midwife, I'd be down betting at the track."*

Stay rested, nourished, and hydrated to prepare for labor.

In addition to waiting for serious contractions to start, be on the alert for the rupture of your membranes (water breaking). You'll have a lot of discharge now as your vaginal canal cleans and prepares itself for the big event, but your water breaking is usually hard to miss. It'll be a gush or a rapid trickle that smells like the ocean. Sometimes, but rarely, the fluid can leak out and seem like a heavy, watery discharge. Only one in ten moms experiences her water breaking before labor begins. If this happens to you, call your care provider right away, but don't panic unless you also have contractions. You may or may not go into labor immediately. If you don't, your care provider may wait for twenty-four to forty-eight hours for labor to start naturally and then will probably induce you out of concern for the possibility of infection.

Week 38

Fetal Age: 36 weeks (253 to 259 days)
2 to 1 weeks, 13 to 7 days until your due date

YOUR BABY

Size

The average newborn has a length of 21$\frac{1}{2}$ inches and weighs 7$\frac{1}{2}$ pounds.

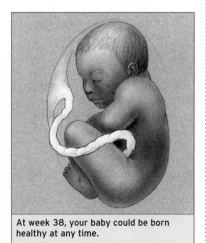

At week 38, your baby could be born healthy at any time.

Development

She is fully developed, though still adding connections between neurons in the brain (this continues well after birth).

Her nails have been growing and now reach to the ends of her fingers and toes. Her movements are quite restricted by her close quarters.

YOU

What happens to you physically

A whole lot of back and neck strain, lots of fatigue, and not much relief! You continue to add a pound a week and have an increasingly hard time getting around gracefully.

How you may be feeling

Next to the waiting, the uncertainty of when labor will begin is the hardest part of the third trimester. Your due date may very well come and go, especially if you're a first-time mom, and the current recommendation is that doctors wait at least two weeks after a due date passes before considering induction unless there's a medical problem.[9]

What you can do

Don't be tempted to try to induce labor with herbs or castor oil, no matter what it says on the Internet. Herbal supplements are unregulated by the FDA and can contain highly variable concentrations and unlisted

ingredients. Their effects can be nonexistent, unpredictable, or dangerous, and no herbal supplement has been tested for safety for pregnant women by the FDA. (For more on herbs and castor oil, see *Managing Your Medicine Cabinet* on page 195.)

Keep eating frequent small, nutritious meals, and if you think that your contractions may be the real thing, eat something. The calories will help fortify you for the job at hand. Also keep yourself hydrated with water, tea, milk, or juice. Avoid carbonated beverages, which can increase bloating.

For two to four weeks postpartum, you'll need more help than just your partner can provide, especially if he'll going back to work soon after the baby's born. Finalize arrangements for someone who can cook and do chores to live in or drop in for several hours a day. If you have a school-age child, you may also need additional babysitting help.

Are you still working? We understand that starting your leave early means less time with the baby, but even so, you may want to seriously consider starting your leave soon. If you sit all day, you could be plagued with back pain, hemorrhoids, varicose veins, swollen ankles, carpal tunnel syndrome, or all of the above. If you do a lot of standing or walking at work, your muscles will be easily and seriously fatigued as they strain to keep supporting your frame.

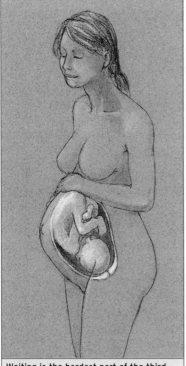

Waiting is the hardest part of the third trimester.

Week 39

Fetal Age: 37 weeks (260 to 266 days)
6 to 0 days left until your due date

YOUR BABY

Size

Your baby is newborn size—any-where from seventeen to twenty-three inches tall and from six to ten pounds or more.

Don't be too frightened if your care provider says that your baby is large. It's extremely difficult to judge a baby's weight from the outside.

Development

Your baby is adding neural con-nections and growing hair and still gaining weight. Researchers have theorized that when babies are ready to be born, they send a chemical signal of androgens to the placenta, which increases the pro-duction of estrogen and leads to labor.[10] If so, it's proof of the old saying that "only a baby knows when it's ready to be born."

YOU

How you may be feeling

"Like a dump truck."

"Like I'm doing nothing but waiting."

"I wish people would quit calling to ask if I'm in labor."

"One minute I want labor to start, the next I'm worried about labor and what I'll do with him when he gets here."

Self-care tip

To get some relief from your weight and aches, do plenty of hands-and-knees cat stretches and pelvic tilts. Soak in a warm bath, swim, or just float in the pool to take a break from gravity.

Things to organize

Is your partner prepared to take over your household duties?

Help prepare him by writing a list of any phone numbers he may need and taping it by the phone:

* numbers for your doctor, mid-wife, and/or labor support person or doula

* your kids' pediatrician

* household repair people

* your mechanic

* grocery delivery service

* cleaning service

* veterinarian

* dentist

* any other medical specialists you use (dermatologist, psychiatrist, podiatrist, etc.)

Make a to-do-list of anything that you think he should take care of for the next two months: routine car maintenance, household repairs, changing the sheets in the guest room for your mother, and so on.

Make a file of important documents:

- receipts for products and services
- vehicle maintenance records
- contact information and policy numbers for any insurance policies you have
- mortgage or rental contract documents for your home

Create a mail area in your house, if you don't already have one. Get a box to put bills in that's furnished with stamps, envelopes, and pens that work. Put a trash can nearby to keep junk mail from accumulating and a place to keep magazines until you can get to them.

Get a calendar with lots of room to write, if you don't already have one, and record trash days, recycling days, upcoming appointments, birthdays, and other occasions that you'd usually keep track of in your head.

Stock up on nonperishable goods so you'll have less shopping to do later:

- paper towels and napkins
- canned, jarred, and frozen foods
- extra-absorbent maxi pads
- paper plates and plastic flatware and cups (so you'll have fewer dishes to wash)
- trash and recycling bags
- batteries

Collect an envelope of local carryout and delivery menus, and circle what foods you like (and cross out ones you don't).

Yes, we know, it sounds like you're hunkering down for a hurricane. But trust us, any rare spare time you get in the near future, you'll want (and deserve) to spend relaxing, not shopping and washing dishes and getting the car fixed! People want to help, but they need to be instructed. You and your helpers will appreciate clear signals about what needs to be done and how to do it properly.

Call Your Care Provider If You Experience Any of These Symptoms:

- Vaginal bleeding
- Pain or burning when you urinate
- Very bad or frequent headaches
- Severe vomiting

- Pelvic pain or cramps
- Increasing pelvic pressure
- Decreased fetal movement

Week 40

Fetal Age: 38 weeks, days 266 and beyond

YOUR BABY

Size
Huge.

Development
Fully formed.

YOU

If your due date has come and gone, your pregnancy is officially post-date. If you're still pregnant two weeks from now, then your pregnancy will be post-term. Anywhere from three to twelve percent of pregnant women may go post-term. The good news is that the baby is going to come out at some point—the bad news is that it may be as long as two weeks from now.

In the meantime, your care provider will check your dilation (how open your cervix is, if it all) and effacement (how thick your cervix is), to try to predict when labor will begin.

There are plenty of methods of attempting to induce labor, such as stripping the membranes (page 339), herbs, and cervical massage, but unless your care provider has a real concern that you or your baby's health is compromised, you shouldn't try any of them. And

needless to say, inductions should only happen in a well-equipped medical facility because of the pain involved and the potential to cause injury.

We understand that you are bigger and more uncomfortable than you ever thought possible. We know you can't sleep or do much more than watch television, read, and make trips to the bathroom.

These are tedious times, but do try to enjoy the peace and quiet. Don't feel guilty about just sitting around. Do try to stretch your legs and encourage labor with daily walks. Walk while talking to your baby about how you're ready for her, or try singing "Get Down Tonight" or "Happy Birthday to You," or whatever you find encouraging. Relax yourself and your abdominal muscles as you walk.

So what if labor just doesn't happen? If you hit forty-two weeks, your doctor will assess the baby's health with a non-stress test. Your care provider may use ultrasound to see if your baby has enough amniotic fluid. If the baby seems fine, you and your care provider can discuss when to schedule induction of labor.

No matter what, one way or another, somehow, that baby is getting out!

To read more about how, turn to the birth and labor guide.

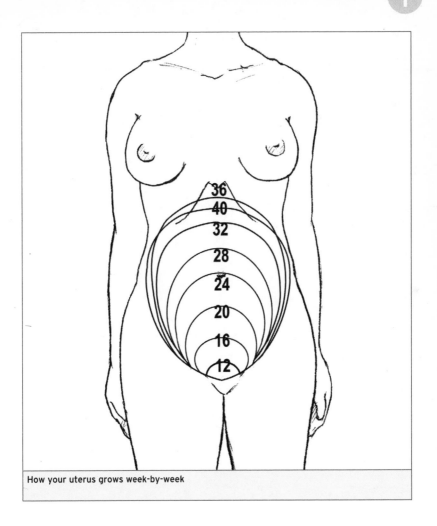

How your uterus grows week-by-week

Managing Your Pregnancy

Pregnancy is a whole-body, whole-life makeover. The shift in your reality can seem so extreme, you may feel as if you've been suddenly relocated to an alien planet. Not only is it not clear what foods and activities are safe, but gravity itself has shifted. Even the daily routines that you've taken for granted, like getting out of bed and getting dressed, will present new challenges. It's not easy to get adjusted to the pregnant lifestyle (and as soon as you do, it's almost over). Probably the hardest adjustment is in accepting all of the changes you can't control, while making good decisions about the things you can. That's what this section is about.

In **Managing Your Body**, we'll take a look at all the physical changes you undergo from head to toe. If you have strange hairs, nagging aches, or physical symptoms, this is where to look. We've arranged the chapter anatomically, so you can immediately locate the precise place on your body you're concerned about.

In **Managing Your Nutrition**, we provide the most up-to-date information on your prenatal vitamin and mineral needs. Not only is nutrition important for basic health, but what you eat can actually help ease your aches and pains, prevent complications during birth, and develop your baby's brain.

The next chapter, **Managing Your Weight and Fitness**, will help you find ways to work with your body to be healthy and fit for birth. With healthy weight gain and a little exercise, you may actually be able to experience a shorter, easier labor and a faster recovery.

In the next chapter, **Managing Your Care**, we introduce you to the various people and places that can help you manage your prenatal care and deliver your child. We discuss the different kinds of care providers, the facilities where they deliver, and how your choice of where and with whom you deliver can affect your experience. We also discuss childbirth classes: their major philosophies and what you can expect to learn. Next, we tell you what you need to know about prenatal tests: when and why they're taken, if they pose any sort of risk to you or your baby, and what you may experience when you take them.

Managing Your Medicine Cabinet provides a rundown on the safety of commonly used over-the-counter, prescription, and recreational drugs. This information is not meant to replace your care provider's advice. He will have the most up-to-date information on the safety of medications and will know how certain drugs may affect health concerns specific to you.

The next section, **Managing High-Risk Conditions**, discusses physical conditions that may or may not apply to your pregnancy: advanced age, medical conditions, multiple births, and prenatal complications.

Managing Other Risks covers some of the everyday choices and situations of pregnancy that may worry you. Should you have your baby's cord blood stored? Is it safe to use pesticides in your home? Should you be concerned if you became pregnant while using birth control? We provide you with information to help you make decisions about situations you may face, so you'll know what's risky and what isn't.

Managing Family and Emotional Issues offers tips on how to deal with your changing relationships with your partner, parents, and friends.

And finally, **Managing Your Finances** will give you an overview of current laws relating to pregnancy and the workplace and other financial considerations.

When you're pregnant, there's a lot to think about. If you didn't worry a little bit, you wouldn't be normal. But if you can arm yourself with the information you need to make informed choices, you can work toward replacing your worry with great expectations.

Managing Your Body

Do you remember adolescence? How your body that you knew so well became less familiar, and it took you a while to get used to it? Well, that was nothing compared with the changes of pregnancy! While the hormones may be similar (with the notable exception of hCG, the human pregnancy hormone), pregnancy changes can be so quick and extreme, it can feel like you've gone through six years' worth of puberty in six weeks! Plus you can throw in some nausea, fatigue, dizziness, body aches, and a whole menu of new symptoms.

Pregnancy affects everything. It's not just that your chest and belly expand; in fact, every single cell in your body is somehow affected by your pregnancy.

Here's a rundown of the head-to-toe changes you experience, with tips on how to cope.

Head

HAIR

Thanks to your pregnancy hormones, you'll have more hair from head to toe, and your hair will have a different texture. You may notice that your hair is different as soon as you find out you're pregnant, or changes may take a few weeks. Some women have such extreme changes that their curly hair straightens, or their straight hair gets waves!

Normally, the hair on your head grows for about seven years, stays on the scalp for about six months, and then falls out. But during pregnancy, this growth pattern is interrupted, and the old hair isn't shed. Your hair will feel thicker and stronger and may be easier to style. For most women, the second trimester begins the best hair days of their lives, when the "no-shed" effect becomes noticeable.

Your body hair undergoes the same change of cycle. Even your pubic hair will appear to grow longer and more quickly. In the months after birth as your hormone levels return to normal, you'll lose the extra hair, though thankfully, not all at once.

Your scalp condition may also change while you're pregnant. Depending on your genetic makeup, your oil-producing glands may either speed up or slow down production in response to hormonal changes. So your hair may be drier or oilier than normal.

Change your shampoos and conditioners for the next nine months to suit your new hair texture. If your hair is dry, shampoo once only every few days. Use deep-conditioning packs or hot oil treatments once a week. If it's oily, wash once a day, applying conditioner only when needed to detangle.

With oily or dry hair, get a trim every six weeks to get rid of split ends or breakage, and brush your hair gently and only when necessary.

For your body hair, shave, or trim with scissors. Waxing or depilatory creams may irritate your skin and follicles.

Can you curl or dye your hair?

Hair dye hasn't been linked with any human birth defects, but tests have shown that some ingredients in dyes can cause cancer and chromosomal damage in animals in large doses. For this reason, and because of the strong fumes of dyes and relaxers and the hair-texture changes most women experience, many care providers suggest that you avoid any hair-styling procedure that allows chemical cocktails to sit on your scalp for long periods of time, especially in the first trimester. However, other experts, including the American College of Obstetricians and Gynecologists, say that a review of the literature shows no reason for anyone to alter hair dyeing habits on account of pregnancy.

Because chemicals are absorbed into your body through your scalp, no-risk alternatives are coloring or styling methods that have low scalp exposure, like highlights or semi-permanent color. These less-drastic measures may also be a better idea on a practical level, because your new hair texture may make dye shades turn out unevenly, especially if your hair is drier than usual.

The same is true for perms and hair relaxers. Chemicals can enter your bloodstream, and your baby's bloodstream, through your scalp. And while no researcher has linked these products to any defects or damage in a fetus, no one can say for certain that they're harmless. And again, the chemical process can "take" unevenly, leaving you with a lopsided hair "don't." Consider braiding, or just going natural, or finding other solutions for taming your mane.

If you choose to dye, perm, or relax, make sure you have plenty of ventilation. Even if you're used to processing your hair at home, consider going to a well-ventilated salon to avoid your exposure to the fumes and chemicals.

HEADACHES

Headaches are common and likely during pregnancy, especially in the first trimester, because your body is trying hard to get blood to your head while your blood pressure is low. More rarely, severe headaches in later pregnancy can be a symptom of preeclampsia (discussed on page 215).

Other over-the-counter medications for headaches you may have used before you were pregnant, such as aspirin and ibuprofen (commonly known as Advil® or Motrin®), shouldn't be taken unless your healthcare provider gives you the go-ahead.

If needed, the Food and Drug Administration's (FDA) drug ratings appear to show that the use of acetaminophen (Tylenol®) during pregnancy is not considered harmful when used in the doses described in the package inserts. (See FDA charts, page 196.)

MIGRAINES

Migraines are not normal headaches. These are throbbing, debilitating episodes, apparently caused by an inherited disorder in the central nervous system. Pregnancy is known to change their occurrence—you may have one for the first time, especially during the first half of pregnancy. Or if you suffer already, they may become more severe, or they may disappear.[1]

The headaches feel horrible, but they don't appear to cause any long-term damage to you or your fetus. The cause of migraines is unknown, but they may be caused by inherited abnormalities in certain areas of the brain. Many women who suffer from migraines also suffer from depression, suggesting that there may be some biochemical link.

A migraine's hallmark is the side effects that the blood vessel dilation brings on. About ten to thirty minutes before an episode, sufferers may experience fatigue, nausea, and possibly vomiting, visual effects (called "aura") such as blurred vision or flashing lights, a tingling sensation in their hands or legs, and/or a sensitivity to light and noise, followed, of course, by a hellish pounding in the head.

Contact your healthcare provider if you get a headache that's unusually bad and/or comes with nausea or visual effects—you may be experiencing symptoms of high blood pressure, which can be quite dangerous for you and your baby. Plus, your healthcare provider can help you find ways to relieve your pain.

Things you can do for a migraine

Experienced migraine sufferers may know if their headaches are set off by certain triggers and combinations of environmental factors, such as certain foods, medications, weather conditions, stressful situations, odors, or bright or flickering lights. Obviously, you want to avoid known triggers to the best of your ability.

Studies have shown that magnesium supplements may help reduce or eliminate migraines,[2] so make sure that your prenatal supplement contains 450 to 600 milligrams. (Magnesium may also reduce premature labor and helps with leg cramps and indigestion.)

Some migraine medications, such as zolmitriptan (Zomig®), have been associated with fetal abnormalities in lab animals[3] and should be avoided. If your migraine is mild enough, over-the-counter medications may work, but talk to your care provider before attempting to medicate your migraine. The standard treatment advice for pregnant migraine sufferers is to simply lie in a dark, quiet room with a cool washcloth on your forehead until the pain subsides in four to seventy-two hours.

Alternative Headache Cures

Some headaches may be cured faster and more effectively without medication. Here are some remedies that may make the pain disappear:

- **Drink water.** Dehydration is a common cause of headaches, particularly in early pregnancy. Your body needs a lot of water to make extra blood, amniotic fluid, and all of your new extra bodily fluids. Prevent these headaches by getting your eight glasses of water a day, plus one glass for every caffeinated beverage you drink. (See "Caffeine" on page 205 for tips on how to break your addiction.) Before you try anything else, try a pint of water. If dehydration is the problem, the water will get rid of the headache almost instantly.

- **Check when you last ate.** Low blood sugar can also cause headaches, so stock your purse, pocket, or car with a packet of peanut butter crackers, a box of orange juice, or some other little nosh in case you have to go a stretch without a meal, or you lose the one you had.

- **Clear your sinuses.** Sinus congestion is another pregnancy-headache culprit. If the pain is sharp or feels like pressure behind your eyes or in your cheeks, or it gets worse when you move your head, or won't go away with a regular painkiller, you may have a sinus headache. Breathing steam, either in a warm shower or with a facial steamer, can help unclog the stuffiness. If your congestion is bad and won't go away, consider running a humidifier in your room while you sleep. Over-the-counter decongestants, such as Sudafed®, are considered safe to take during pregnancy.

- **Lower your stress level.** Stress headaches are also common. If certain people or situations tend to bring them on, for the sake of you and your baby's health, you'll need to find a way to reduce, eliminate, or work through the tension. Yoga or other moderate exercise can help keep your stress level in check and your blood sugar levels steady. A head and neck massage can help, as can having someone massage your big toe—it's an acupressure point for head pain.

DIZZINESS

Pregnancy lowers your blood pressure, which can lead to dizziness, particularly if you stand up quickly or are on your feet a lot. If you skip meals, low blood sugar may also contribute to your dizziness.

If you often feel faint to the point of passing out or seeing spots, or if you feel like you could nap for more than a couple of hours a day, call your care provider. Excessive dizziness and fatigue can be a sign of anemia.

By the start of the second trimester, when your placenta is up and running, and your hormones aren't surging quite as much, your dizzy fatigue may be less frequent. It may return in the third trimester when you are, once again, getting less oxygen to your brain.

You can calm your dizziness by rising slowly from a sitting or lying position, and by keeping food in your stomach. If you're often dizzy when you get up in the morning, keep crackers or fruit by your bed, and have a snack before you get up.

EYES

Occasionally, the hormonal changes of pregnancy lead to a temporary increase in nearsightedness, which normally goes away after the baby is about six months old.

This change usually happens at the end of the second trimester, though the time frame can vary. It's caused by the thickening of the jelly-like substance in the middle of your eye.

If you wear contacts, you may find they become more uncomfortable or don't seem to fit well. That's because your eyes are drier. Lubricate your contacts often. Some contact lens brands may better retain liquid than others—ask your optometrist for a recommendation.

If your contacts tend to bother you, keep a comfortable pair of glasses in your purse. Many women switch to glasses in the last trimester.

NOSE

Constant sniffling, congestion, and sinus headaches are common in pregnancy. Your body is making more mucus than usual, to defend itself against germs and allergens. So your eyes may water, your nose may itch and run, and you may get sharp headaches that water and your healthcare provider's recom-

mended painkiller don't fix. (See "Headaches" on page 113, and page 196 for more about the safety of various over-the-counter painkillers.)

You can help most mild sinus problems with hot herb tea or warm steam from a bath, a humidifier, or a hot towel. If those remedies don't work, most over-the-counter antihistamines are considered safe.

Decongestants such as Benadryl® and Sudafed® are most often recommended for pregnant women. (For more information about over-the-counter drugs and pregnancy, see page 195.)

MOUTH

During pregnancy, your body defends itself from harmful bacteria and foreign material by making your gums more puffy, more sensitive, and more likely to bleed. This condition is known as pregnancy gingivitis, and it will go away after the baby's born. If you already have gum disease, pregnancy can make it worse. You may need to switch to a soft-bristled toothbrush and gentler floss, such as a waxed-ribbon variety.

Morning sickness can endanger your teeth. The acids from vomiting can break down enamel. Plus, you're eating more food, may be eating more sweets, and may be too distracted to remember to brush. It's important not to neglect your mouth, because research has shown that moms with poor oral health are more likely to have low-birthweight babies. This may be because bacteria and bacterial secretions can enter the bloodstream through the gum line. Here

are ways to take care of your teeth
and gums during pregnancy:

- **Brush frequently.** Brush two
times a day, and floss at least
once daily. Use an antibacterial
rinse if you can stand it.

- **Floss or wipe.** If sticking a toothbrush in your mouth makes you
feel sick, floss gently after every
meal, and use a damp, warm
washcloth to wipe down your
teeth, followed by an antibacterial
mouth rinse.

- **Visit your dentist.** If you haven't
had a dental appointment for an
exam and cleaning in the past six
months, make one now.

- **Good nutrition.** A diet rich in
calcium, vitamins C, D, and A in
the amounts found in prenatal
vitamins can help to maintain
healthy gums and teeth, as will a
diet low in sugars.

When you go in for any dental
work, be sure to inform your dentist
or hygienist that you are pregnant
and how many weeks along you are.
Most dental X-rays can be postponed
until after your baby arrives. If not,
then be sure to request both a lead
apron and a neck collar to protect
your baby from radiation.

There's no evidence that having
your teeth whitened with peroxide
or microbrasion is harmful to your
pregnancy. Like so many things,
there's no solid evidence that it's
safe, either, but it seems unlikely
that anything could be absorbed
into your body through your tooth
enamel.

SNORING

Even if you've never snored before,
you may start while you're pregnant,
especially in the second half of your
pregnancy. Increased nasal congestion is to blame, and if you gain
extra weight, fat may accumulate
in the lining of your nasal tissue,
believe it or not. These blockages
cause the unladylike honking and
gurgling sounds.

Ask your partner to tell you if
you make gasping sounds in your
sleep or seem to stop breathing.
If so, inform your care provider.
You may have sleep apnea, which
pregnant women seem especially
prone to. This is when breathing is
obstructed, making you wake up
to catch your breath. It can really
keep you from feeling rested and
can even become dangerous,
causing heart and blood pressure
complications.

But if you're just sawing a log,
there's not much to be done. Sleep
on your side (as you probably do
anyway), and try the nasal strips
that you tape to the bridge of your
nose. Reassure your partner that the
snoring will go away after birth as
your tissues and weight return to
normal.

FATIGUE

Pregnancy makes you tired, especially in the first trimester and in the
last month before you give birth.

During the first trimester, your
fatigue is urgent: "I have to take a
nap this second!" You'll find that you
can nap in places where you never
could before: in a bedroom while a

party's going on, on the bus, or a couch in the ladies' room. These are no catnaps, either: You're out like a light.

Your fatigue is a by-product of all the work your body is doing. Your brain is getting less oxygen, your blood pressure is down, you're growing a whole new organ (the placenta), and your waste system is working twice as hard from your sweat glands to your kidneys. Plus, the fluid you're retaining is rapidly adding extra weight for you to carry around.

If you're having a hard time holding down food, then you may also have low blood sugar. Make sure that your body's getting what it needs to do its job: at least thirty mg. of iron in your diet daily (it may or may not be in your prenatal vitamin), an extra three hundred calories' worth of nutritious food, and plenty of water. If you're regularly sleeping more than twelve hours in a twenty-four-hour period, and/or your fatigue doesn't ease up by about the fourteenth week of your pregnancy, ask your care provider to test you for anemia. Generally, the only cures for your first-trimester fatigue are time and naps.

By your third trimester, your dizziness and fatigue may come back. While first-trimester fatigue is urgent, third-trimester fatigue is the kind of sluggishness that comes from not being able to get a good night's sleep and lugging around twenty-plus pounds of extra weight. What's more, as your baby grows, he puts pressure on major blood vessels, once again making less oxygen available to your brain.

If you've kept up an exercise routine, this is when it will pay off, because your body will be better able to deal with the extra weight. However, even the fittest moms will feel more tired than usual, with nights of tossing, turning, and running to the bathroom every hour. Needless to say, sleep when you can! Avoid becoming overheated, standing quickly, and lying flat on your back, which may put more pressure on a large artery.

Skin

If you haven't noticed already, a pregnant woman's skin can change from head to toe. Your skin is made up of three layers of many different types of specialized cells, and its job is much more than simply attractively covering your muscles. Its functions are as varied as maintaining your body temperature, protecting you from germs and environmental dangers, and gathering sensory information from the environment.

Depending on your skin's genetic makeup, your facial skin may react to the extra estrogen in your body by becoming drier or oilier. If your skin is dry, cleanse it only once a day, and apply a moisturizer to your damp skin before you go to bed, so that your skin oils will have a chance to replenish. Most dermatologists recommend mild or low-detergent soaps regardless of your skin type, such as products from Dove, Aveeno, or Burt's Bees, which are gentler and less likely to strip off your skin's natural and necessary oils. If your skin is oily, cleanse twice a day, in the morning and evening, and apply astringent to remove extra oil and soap residue.

Though your skin may be drier or oilier, it probably also looks smooth and dewy. This is because water retention smooths the spaces between skin cells, and the cells themselves become rounder. The rosy look comes from small dilated blood cells under the skin's surface.

ACNE

About 2 to 5 percent of women may develop acne-prone skin, especially in the first trimester. More production from your oil glands may mean that you have acne like a teenager again, or blackheads, whiteheads, or cysts on your back or chest. If you're using Accutane® or Retin-A®, stop immediately—there is a concern that they may be associated with birth defects.[4]

Also, products with benzoyl peroxide, salicylic acid, retinols, or steroids may have side effects that could harm your baby. Avoid them now and after your baby arrives if you're breastfeeding. Also avoid using topical vitamin A creams, such as Differin® or Tazorac®, because of research that appears to link excessive vitamin A with fetal damage. On the other hand, products containing glycolic acid and other alpha-hydroxy acids are considered safe. Consult with your healthcare provider about any preparation you apply directly to your skin.

CHANGES IN SKIN COLOR

Strange colorations in your face and body are common in pregnancy. They can range from a dark "mask" on your face called *chloasma* (particularly common during the start of the second trimester in brunettes), to new or darker freckles anywhere and everywhere on your body, to a dark line that runs from your navel to your pubic bone, called the *linea nigra*. These coloring changes are a harmless sign that pregnancy hormones are affecting your skin cells and will gradually fade after your pregnancy is over.

Your moles may darken and get larger. Tell your care provider about any new moles, or any that bleed or darken, have uneven sides instead of being round, or turn to a blackish color.

Warts are also more common in pregnancy. You may grow funny little wart-like "skin tags" in your armpits. These usually go away after delivery, and if they don't, your doctor or dermatologist can freeze them off.

To avoid promoting wrinkles and discoloration, dermatologists agree that pregnant women should take extra care to stay out of the sun and to wear sunscreen and a hat when exposure can't be avoided. Definitely avoid tanning booths, and self-tanning sprays, which may distribute unevenly. Overactive pigment cells may make you extremely sensitive to ultraviolet light, particularly if you're pale and freckle easily to begin with.

The areola around your nipple will also become dark and larger as your pregnancy progresses. Your exterior genital area may darken too. Both changes are temporary and will fade after delivery.

You may also notice the appearance of **spider veins** (**spider nevi**). As their name implies, they resemble little red spiders on your nose and cheeks (and sometimes back, chest, or arms). They are small, dilated blood vessels, which usually disappear by six weeks after delivery.

ITCHINESS

You're retaining extra fluids, you have an extra pint or two of blood circulating in your body, and your growing belly and breasts are making your skin stretch everywhere on your body. This stretching skin can itch, and your skin is also more sensitive to stimuli, such as rubbing from synthetic fabrics. You may find it more comfortable to wear natural fibers, since synthetics can chafe and may not be able to absorb your new, increased sweat load. You also want to keep your skin from getting too dry, because stretched, dry skin is itchy and uncomfortable and may lead to wrinkles. So moisturize, moisturize, moisturize, if your extra skin oil production isn't enough to keep your skin supple. Try sampling lotions in the store until you find one that leaves your skin soft and has an inoffensive odor.

STRETCH MARKS

You can't prevent stretch marks, even if you slather on the world's most expensive lotion five times a day. Stretch marks are caused by broken collagen fibers under your skin's surface, where no lotion can reach. The strength of your skin's collagen is genetic—if your mom got them, congratulations, you probably will too. But there's good news: They do fade, sometimes within a few months after birth, and you can make them less severe by keeping your skin hydrated and healthy and doing what you can to avoid rapid weight gain.

SUNSCREEN AND SUNLESS TANNERS

Sunscreen is safe to use during pregnancy and is recommended. Do pick one that's PABA-free, however, since PABA is known to cause skin irritation in some people.

Sunless tanners are also considered safe. However, they may not be a good idea. Even if you apply them perfectly even, skin pigment changes and your increased sweat and oil production make you more susceptible to a blotchy result.

Neck

The weight of pregnancy can change your posture, and this can make your neck spasm as you use muscles in a different way. Pregnancy is also stressful, and a lot of people react to stress by hunching up their necks and shoulders. Keeping your neck in good shape with stretching or exercise can prevent spasms and help relieve the kinks.

If you stare at a computer all day or don't move around a lot on your job, plan to take breaks every fifteen minutes to turn your head and roll your neck around to help avoid tension headaches and muscle pains.

Also check your posture periodically to make sure you're sitting up straight, not bent over or leaning to one side. If your work chair has a flexible back support, exchange it for one that is rigid to give better support to your spine. Sit completely back in the chair, use a pillow for the small of your back, and support your feet with a small footrest or a stack of books. Neck pain can also be caused by an awkward sleeping position or by the inactivity that comes with bed rest. Gentle applied heat and stretches may help.

Ask your healthcare provider to suggest the best pain reliever by brand, what strength to take, and for how long.[5]

THYROID

The thyroid is a small gland located on either side of the voice box. The thyroid has a powerful role in controlling metabolism, the way the body uses energy.

Low thyroid *(hypothyroidism)*

Sometimes pregnancy and nursing can exaggerate a low thyroid condition.

If you have low thyroid levels, you may have some or all of these symptoms: cold hands and feet, low-grade fatigue, a hard time getting up and started in the morning, headaches, leg cramps, dry skin, brittle nails, puffy eyes, and easy weight gain regardless of what you eat.

Having a low thyroid level may affect your baby's brain growth. If you are concerned that your thyroid levels may be low, ask your healthcare provider about blood tests to obtain TSH and "Free T4" levels. These tests monitor the amount of thyroid in the bloodstream. If they are abnormal, then you may need to take thyroid supplements.

If you are given thyroid hormone replacement medication, careful monitoring will be important because the body is very sensitive to even small changes in thyroid hormones. Thyroid replacement needs change frequently during pregnancy, and iron supplements may affect the absorption of thyroid hormones. Be sure not to take more than the recommended dose of your medication. If you take more than your body needs, you may experience symptoms such as shakiness, rapid heartbeat, irritability, and sweating. If this happens, ask your healthcare provider about reducing your dose.

Circulatory system

An average-size woman has 9 pints of blood, and an average pregnant woman adds 1.8 pints during pregnancy. By the time you give birth, your heart will be pumping as much as 20 percent more blood with every stroke. Much of that excess blood is lost during childbirth.

BLOOD VESSELS

A week into your pregnancy, after the fertilized egg has implanted in your uterus, your entire circulatory system increases its capacity, as if you traded your garden sprinkler for a fireman's hose. Your body spends the first trimester working to fill the extra room in your blood vessels. Your circulatory system gives priority to providing blood to your developing placenta, nourishing the baby, and removing waste that would interfere with growth.

The side effects of this process of relaxing and expanding are to blame for many of your bodily discomforts, including these:

- Dizziness when you stand or sit up quickly—there's simply less blood and oxygen getting to your brain.

- Thirst and headaches from dehydration as your system retains water.

- A sweaty, flushed feeling from the increased blood flow to your skin.

- Frequent urination, because your kidneys have more blood to filter, and make extra urine to eliminate the extra waste.

By the second trimester, your circulatory system will have finished making the extra blood and will have adjusted to accommodate the volume, which will make your symptoms ease.

Lungs

If you feel short of breath, it's okay to put your arms over your head to expand your rib cage, so you can take in some really deep breaths. If you're pregnant, right now you're breathing 40 to 50 percent more air into your body than you ever have. Your lungs are operating at peak efficiency to get oxygen in to your baby and get carbon dioxide out.

Your rib cage has even widened to help you breathe for two! In the third trimester, as your baby gets larger and heavier and begins to nest just under your rib cage, you may find yourself becoming out of breath more easily.

Practicing deep breathing during pregnancy can send a surge of oxygen to your baby and help you feel less fatigued. It will come in handy during birth too. Once your baby drops as you near your delivery date, called **lightening**, you'll discover the luxury of being able to take deep breaths again.

Breasts

They're big, they're firm, they're sensitive, and they're working hard to get the dairy open in time. The breasts of pregnancy are sure signs that what you have is more than a simple case of PMS. If you were to have nude portraits taken periodically during your pregnancy, you'd see your breasts grow, your nipples get larger and darker, and your whole décolletage move farther south. Your breasts may even develop stretch marks. Your breasts will stay voluptuous during your pregnancy and for as long as you breastfeed. Then, after weaning (and even if you don't breastfeed at all), they'll be flatter and less pert than before.

Your breast changes are due to the effects of powerful hormones such as estrogen, progesterone, and prolactin.

A pregnant woman's breasts contain many complex things: a network of nerves that sensitize the breasts to the stimulation of a baby's suckling; fatty tissue to protect breasts from injury; glandular tissue; branching milk ducts that perform the work of converting proteins and fats from blood into milk; and ducts that deliver the milk to your nipples. Human milk is more than a beverage; it's living tissue loaded with antibodies that protect the baby from infection.

While you're pregnant, your areolas will grow larger and darker and will develop what looks like white goose bumps (Montgomery's tubercles) on the surface. These bumps are openings to tiny glands that produce oils to lubricate your nipple and areola. The oils change the acid/alkaline balance of your skin surface to slow down the growth of bacteria. So don't wash your nipple area with soap. Doing so will remove the protective oils.

Most women have a discharge from their nipples as early as twelve to fourteen weeks after pregnancy begins, and as late as days before delivery. It's a precursor to milk-making called colostrum, a high-protein substance that is especially healthy for newborns.

If you're planning to breastfeed, there's no need to worry about how big or little your breasts get during or after pregnancy. Milk-making is more a matter of demand and supply than it is of breast size.

While well-endowed women may have more milk storage capacity, moms with small breasts can still make all the milk their babies need. The speed of production may be different: big breasts that store more milk tend to make milk more slowly, while breasts with less storage capacity make it quickly. Most breasts, regardless of size, are able

Piercings

The major body changes of pregnancy can cause problems with your piercings, especially those in places that are tender and may stretch, such as your navel or nipples. Our advice is to remove any neck-down piercings to reduce the risk of infection and pain, especially if the site isn't completely healed yet.

Getting pierced (or tattooed, or doing anything that adds extra stress and pain to your life) while pregnant is also probably not such a good idea. You'll bleed more and may be more prone to infection. If any of your piercings hurt, swell, or smell bad, remove them immediately, and call your doctor.

Remember to wash your hands with a liquid antibacterial soap before removing the jewelry or touching the piercing. Also, be sure to keep your jewelry on a clean surface.

Tongue. All of the extra blood running through your veins can cause piercings in veiny places to start to hurt and bleed.

Navel. You almost certainly want to take out a navel piercing toward the end of your pregnancy or whenever it begins to annoy you. Your expanding stomach will make the hole stretch, which won't look so great. Your belly probably won't be looking rock-star toned for a time after your pregnancy anyway. You can always get it redone later.

Nipples. Nipple piercing does not prevent lactation, and having a piercing should not interfere with breastfeeding, provided you remove your jewelry first. Besides getting in your baby's way and increasing your discomfort, rings and beads can pose a choking hazard to infants if they come loose accidentally with the motion of feeding. If you're pregnant, trying to conceive, or nursing and are interested in getting a nipple piercing, our suggestion is to wait until you are finished breastfeeding.

Genital. Your care provider will most likely instruct you to remove any genital piercings because of the risk of tearing or stretching.

to make a lot more milk than a baby actually needs. If you bottle-feed, then your milk-making will slow down and stop in a few weeks.

If you have *inverted nipples*, it means your nipples turn inward instead of coming to salute when touched or exposed to cold air, and that may make it harder for your baby to nurse. If this is the case, try to find a lactation consultant to offer gentle stretching exercises for your nipples, or get guidance on the use of a manual breast pump to help pull the nipple into an outward position.

Treating your nipples roughly, brushing them with a towel, or wearing a plastic, doughnut-shaped shield have not been proven to be successful in changing inverted nipples.

Regardless of your nipple shape, don't try to toughen up your nipple skin in anticipation of nursing. Never treat your nipples roughly. The first week of breastfeeding can frequently be quite uncomfortable as your breast adjusts to the friction and suction of your baby's mouth. Irritating your nipples may make things worse.

(For more information on breast-feeding and alternative feeding methods, see page 408, and for information on how to choose maternity and nursing bras, see our clothing advice starting on page 70.)

Muscles

You have three types of muscles in your body: skeletal, cardiac, and smooth. Muscle changes have wide-ranging effects on your pregnancy, causing everything from constipation to vision changes.

Pregnancy has the most significant affect on your smooth muscles. This is the type of muscle that isn't under your voluntary control; it relies on nerve signals to activate it. You have smooth muscle in your uterus, stomach bowels, the walls of your blood vessels, in the iris of your eye, and in your hair follicles. They move your food down and out, focus your gaze, give you goose bumps, and will eventually birth your baby.

Some smooth muscle cells relax their functions during pregnancy. The ones in your bowels, for instance, receive signals to slow down and allow you to absorb more nutrition from your food. The smooth muscles in your arteries and veins also let go, making your blood vessels wider, in turn lowering your blood pressure and allowing for greater blood flow to your placenta.

Other groups of smooth muscle will regulate your contractions during labor. In the final two months of your pregnancy, you'll be able to feel the muscle groups "training" in the form of Braxton-Hicks contractions. (See discussions on pages 266, 270, and 298.)

Your skeletal muscles are the ones that generally move only when you tell them to. They keep you up and moving. In the first trimester, they may become strained as a by-product of the increase in your blood volume and the softening of your ligaments.

During pregnancy, your skeletal muscles are forced to continuously support and transport much more body weight than they're used to. If you haven't been doing weight-bearing exercises in the past few years, your muscles will be tighter and more rigid, and therefore more prone to injury. Stretching them and building them with sustained weight-bearing exercise will lessen your everyday aches and also make you less likely to get hurt if you have an accident.

The softening of ligaments in your hip and pelvic area can also strain your surrounding muscles, particularly in the first and third trimesters. Nighttime muscle cramps and spasms in your calves (see "Leg Cramps" on page 141) may be caused by a mineral deficiency. (For more information on exercising and muscle building during pregnancy, see *Managing Your Fitness*.) Round ligaments, which help support your growing uterus, are also often painfully strained in the first and third trimesters. If you feel sharp pain between your hip bone and uterus, around where the leg holes of a very high-cut bathing suit would be, then round ligament pain is probably to blame.

ABDOMINAL MUSCLES

As your uterus grows, it pushes forward into the skeletal muscle group that reaches from your rib cage to your public bone, known as your *rectus abdominus*. While these muscles may once have given you a rippling six-pack, as your uterus grows, they work to hold it in position.

As your pregnancy progresses, your abdominal muscles get pushed out and to the side. You may be able to feel them separating when you run your finger from the center of your ribs to your pubic bone, especially if you're lying on your back with your head tilted up.

You should avoid exercises that encourage this separation, such as leg lifts and sit-ups. During the final months of your pregnancy, you won't be able to sit up by contracting them as you normally do. Roll over on your side to get up from a lying-down position.

Arms

Around the fifth or sixth month of pregnancy, you may experience pain, numbness, tingling, and burning in your wrists, fingers, and sometimes up your arm. This is most likely a case of pregnancy-related carpal tunnel syndrome.[6] This annoyance is caused by the extra fluid you're retaining pressing against the median nerve in your arm and wrist.

Fortunately, these symptoms almost always go away after your baby is born. In the meantime, you may want to try wearing a wrist splint, elevating your arms and hands periodically to help drain the fluid in your tissues, and soaking your wrists in warm water or resting them on a heating pad at night.

If you work on a keyboard or cash register, take frequent breaks to flex your wrist and hand. If you use a mouse, consider switching to a trackball. Some studies[7] have shown that people who get adequate vitamin B6 are less likely to develop carpal tunnel, so make sure that your diet or prenatal vitamin offers an adequate supply. (See the discussion of prenatal vitamins on page 146.)

While you're pregnant, you shouldn't take the nonsteroidal anti-inflammatory drugs and steroids that you may have taken for carpal tunnel before you got pregnant.

Fingers and hands

Some mothers find that their palms redden during pregnancy. This is thought to be an effect of increased levels of estrogen. They usually return to a normal color within a week after the baby is born.

Finger swelling is common during the latter months of pregnancy. If it is accompanied by severe swelling in your face and ankles, or with strange vision changes and severe headache, notify your health-care provider; this may be a sign of preeclampsia.

To help reduce swelling, try raising your hands over your head periodically to help fluid return to your heart. Your swelling is likely to worsen in the latter months of pregnancy until you deliver, so store your rings in a safe place, and don't be tempted to put them back on.

To remove a ring that's stuck on your finger, wrap your entire finger in a length of cotton cord or dental floss. Then "unscrew" the ring along the string.

NAILS

Strong, fast-growing finger- and toenails are a nice perk of pregnancy. A manicure or pedicure makes a great pregnancy indulgence. If you go to a salon, pick one that's well ventilated. Make sure that their instruments are cleaned and sterilized between clients. If you have varicose veins, skip the calf massage.

Back

Back pain is common, especially during the last half of pregnancy. There are a number of things that can lead to back discomfort: extra weight that shifts your body's center of gravity, being less active as you get larger, and not being able to fully stretch and straighten out your back.

At the same time, the hormone relaxin is softening your joints. This means you're likely to suffer harmless but unpleasant back and tailbone pain.

Severe back pain can signify an infection or impending miscarriage, so let your doctor know about any

Remedies for Back Pain

Here are some simple remedies for soothing back pain:

- **Move around.** During the day, change positions frequently (at least every half hour).

- **Swim or soak.** Swimming or soaking in a mildly warm bath can help alleviate the pressure.

- **Change sleeping positions.** When you sleep, try positioning yourself on your left side with a pillow between your knees, which will increase blood flow to your uterus and help keep it off your nerve. A third pillow to prop up your upper arm will help to prevent pain in your upper back.

- **Alternate legs.** If you stand a lot during the day, consider using a step stool to place one foot about six to eight inches higher than the other, alternating frequently.

- **Get a good chair and pillow.** Use a chair with a rigid back, and sit all the way back. Place a small pillow behind the arch of your back for support.

- **Use a footstool.** When sitting, use a footstool to raise your knees slightly above your hips.

- **Stretch your back.** Anything that tilts your pelvis forward and flattens your lower back will help prevent back pain. When you've had a hard day and your back is tired, try getting down on your hands and knees like a cat and alternately arching your back, then letting it relax.

- **Keep active.** If you've had back problems in the past, they may be made worse by the weight and swelling of pregnancy. Keep active, with low-impact activities such as swimming. Stretching exercises can sometimes help too, to keep your back from kinking up. (See *Managing Your Weight and Fitness* on page 154.)

- **Get help.** Many pregnant women find that acupuncture, massage, or chiropractic treatments are able to help them with normal pregnancy aches and pains.

- **Put on a belly bra.** Sometimes a support belt designed specifically for pregnant women, a "belly bra," can help to redistribute the strain from the back muscles to a wider area of the body. But don't try to use back support belts designed for heavy lifting. They put undue pressure on the abdomen.

- **Change your shoes and purse.** Change to low shoes that offer good arch support. Also, instead of bearing the heavy weight of your purse on one shoulder, consider replacing your purse with a lightweight backpack.

sharp, gnawing, or unrelenting pain that doesn't ease up. Excruciating back pain in early pregnancy, especially when it's accompanied by abdominal pain, pain in the pelvic region, shoulder pain, bleeding, and faintness, may be a sign of the rupture of a pregnancy that has implanted outside of the uterus, or an impending miscarriage—contact your healthcare provider immediately.

Sometimes sharp lower-back pain can also be a less-serious sign of a urinary tract infection, which should be treated promptly to avoid harm to the baby.

If you have sharp, shooting pains down your lower back and down the back of one or both of your legs, particularly in the late second to early third trimester, your baby's probably literally getting on your nerves. Pressure from the baby's weight can pinch your sciatic nerve, causing some seriously unpleasant, knife-like pain. The nerve is so large that taking a painkiller is unlikely to offer you much relief. Your best bet is to find ways to relieve the pressure, by stretching or changing positions.

If you have upper back pain, it may be caused by the weight of your breasts. Try a bra that is comfortable and adds extra support.

Stomach

NAUSEA AND VOMITING

In the first trimester, if you're nauseated, you're normal. Between 70 and 85 percent of all pregnant women experience bouts of nausea, and about half experience vomiting as well. Approximately one in three working pregnant women loses work time because of so-called morning sickness.

Pregnancy-related nausea tends to kick in after about five weeks' gestation and gradually eases up as the second trimester starts. Although about thirteen percent of mothers in one study reported they still had it after twenty weeks of gestation. (See "Your Pregnancy Week-by-Week," page 4.)

The "morning" label is a misnomer. Only about seventeen percent of mothers-to-be experience nausea only in the morning. However, because it seems to be triggered by an empty stomach, mornings can indeed be worse. Other women are sick around the clock or at other times of day. Some lucky women don't experience nausea and vomiting at all. That's perfectly normal too. While some research shows that nausea is less common in women who experience miscarriages, this doesn't mean that if you don't experience nausea, something's wrong with your pregnancy.

The origins of morning sickness aren't known, but there are plenty of plausible theories. Researchers do know that the nausea has some relationship to hormone levels. The higher they are, the sicker women

Strategies for Coping with Nausea

B6. With the approval of your clinician, try to take ten to twenty-five milligrams of B6 three times a day.

Ginger. Drink ginger-infused tea, or eat ginger snaps. Ginger has been found to suppress vomiting. Contrary to popular belief, most ginger ale sodas do not contain real ginger, so drinking them won't help.

Seltzer. Sip on seltzer water or club soda.

Lemon. Make lemon zest from the peel of a whole lemon, keep it in a baggie, and sniff it when nauseous feelings start to rise. Lemon-flavored hard candies may also help.

Yogurt. Eat yogurt to encourage the friendly bacteria in your intestines.

Licorice. If you like licorice, try strings, twists, or drops.

Bouillon. Sip on a cup of warm beef or chicken bouillon or miso soup. Bouillon can be soothing and contains sodium, which may be useful in replenishing your stores after bouts of vomiting.

Sports drinks. Sip on a glass of cold Gatorade®, Accelerade®, or Cytomax®.

Water. Stay hydrated by sipping water throughout the day. Drink between meals and not with meals to prevent your stomach from becoming overfull.

Crackers. Try saltines or other crackers.

tend to feel. Nausea and vomiting are more common with women carrying twins.

If nausea and vomiting are a big problem for you, try our suggestions above. Contact your healthcare provider if you haven't been able to keep down any food for more than a day.

What to do for nausea

Some mothers find that keeping something in their stomachs at all times helps them to avoid the

Acupressure. Wear acupressure bands, usually displayed in pharmacies next to the seasickness medications. One brand is Sea-Band®. The bands fit around your wrists and have a small knob on the underside that presses into the area beneath your thumb about one inch below the inside of your wrist bone. This specific pressure point is thought to curtail nausea (and seasickness).

Avoid caffeine. Cut out coffee, tea, chocolate, and soda.

Eat first. Eat dry toast or crackers in the morning even before you sit up in bed.

Indulge. Give in to food cravings in moderation.

Change vitamins. If your prenatal vitamins make you sick, take them at night–or not at all. There's no need to tolerate a vitamin that's making you ill, and there's nothing magical about the prenatal label. Children's chewables with iron work too, as long as the vitamin contains a B-complex, folate, and iron. Be sure to let your healthcare provider know if you decide to stop or switch brands.

Go for protein. Avoid processed sugars, and eat frequent small, high-protein meals instead. The protein will help keep your blood sugar levels steady.

Sleep. Nap frequently. Fatigue only makes stomach upset worse.

Close your nose. Stay away from offending odors. For example, some mothers gag at the smell of frying fish or bacon.

nausea that comes when saliva hits an empty stomach. One simple strategy is to keep peanut butter or saltine crackers on your bedside table, and eat one or two right away before you stand up.

If you wake up in the middle of the night, have a snack or a glass of milk. During the day, eat healthy snacks and small meals frequently. Try to avoid snacks loaded with sugar.

Intestinal Tract

HEARTBURN

Heartburn, also known as indigestion, sour stomach, or acid reflux, is a common nuisance during pregnancy. It's caused by a backflow of acid from the stomach into the esophagus. The muscles that close off the upper stomach become lax, allowing stomach juices to enter the esophagus and irritate its lining. Plus, your growing baby may put pressure on your stomach, giving it less room. Your heartburn may be severe enough to keep you up at night and make you cough and choke. Usually, heartburn feels worse at night or when you're semi-reclining than when you're active and moving around during the day.

Practical heartburn remedies

- **Eat less, and more often.** Eat smaller meals every few hours instead of big meals, and especially control portions at dinnertime.
- **Avoid irritating foods.** You can sometimes prevent heartburn by avoiding acidic foods such as citrus fruits and juices, carbonated beverages, and tomatoes. Foods that combine onions with tomatoes and green peppers are often the culprit, such as chili, pizzas, and pasta sauces. Also avoid combinations of acidity and sugar, such as fruit pies.
- **Add a pinch of baking soda** to acidic foods like tomato sauce and chili.

- **Drink differently.** Avoid caffeinated beverages, such as sodas, coffee, and tea, because they can slow how quickly your stomach empties. Drink a large glass of water thirty minutes before a big meal, and then don't drink anything during your meal. This can help avoid acid reflux caused by having a full stomach.
- **Take a walk after you eat.** Moving around can help to stimulate your digestion.
- **Prop up at night.** Sleep in a semi-reclined position using pillows so your chest is higher than your hips.
- **Ask for help.** If your heartburn is severe, your healthcare provider may prescribe a pregnancy-safe antacid. However, take any antacid in moderation, such as only at night and only for a limited amount of time. Antacids can hinder the absorption of nutrients, and they neutralize all the acid in the stomach, including acids needed for digestion. Over-the-counter antacids such as Tums®, Rolaids®, Maalox®, and Pepcid AC® are the most common remedies people use for heartburn.

CONSTIPATION

Constipation during pregnancy is common. The extra progesterone in your body relaxes the smooth muscles in your intestinal tract (see "Muscles," page 125), and any iron supplements you may be taking will also have a binding effect. Other causes are the pressure your baby puts on your intestines, a sluggish thyroid, and not getting enough fluid or fiber in your diet. The result can be hard stools that are difficult to pass.

If you don't have a bowel movement in three days, you are having stomach cramps along with constipation, or your constipation gets severe enough that you find spots of blood on the toilet paper, ask your doctor to recommend a pregnancy-safe stool softener or suppository. Don't take any laxatives without first checking in with your healthcare provider.

Constipation aids

- **Fiber.** Most healthcare providers recommend making sure that you get plenty of fiber in your diet. Good sources for fiber are apples, celery, and whole grain breads with flax.
- **Liquids.** Sip water throughout the day.
- **Exercise.** A brisk walk will keep you toned and also help keep your bowels moving.
- **Prunes and prune juice.** The old-fashioned standby, prunes, now sometimes sold as "dried plums," and prune juice work well, as does drinking a combination of two tablespoons of prune juice mixed with two tablespoons of Milk of Magnesia before going to bed.
- **Take extra magnesium.** Magnesium carbonate or magnesium citrate supplements can help bowels to move. Ask your healthcare provider first.

HEMORRHOIDS

Hemorrhoids are swollen veins around the anus that can cause itching or pain. Sometimes they may even bleed, in which case you should contact your care provider. They can look like a bump or a small cluster of grapes. Sometimes they protrude after a hard bowel movement. They happen most often when a woman becomes constipated because of the slowing down of her digestive system.

Treating constipation can help, and so can gentle witch hazel compresses or wipes; pain-killing ointments; rinsing off your bottom with warm water after each bowel movement; and sitting in a warm bath.

Hemorrhoids are made worse by the pressure of birth, but they often disappear as you recover postpartum.

DIARRHEA

When you're pregnant, your body is more reactive to toxins in foods, in the form of bacteria or chemical additives. At the slightest suggestion, your body will probably expel food as quickly as possible to keep out harmful foodstuffs. Your bowels may naturally loosen as labor nears, which is not diarrhea, but the bowels cleansing themselves before the work of labor begins.

Mild diarrhea is nothing to worry about. It should go away after the offending matter has been expelled. But food poisoning and serious cramps and diarrhea can be dangerous because they cause your body to lose precious fluids, bringing about an electrolyte imbalance in your system. This can rob your body of valuable nutrients. In the worst-case scenario, dehydration could cause you to have premature contractions.

Contact your healthcare provider if diarrhea doesn't go away in twenty-four hours or if you feel abdominal pain and cramping that you believe is not related to gas.

GAS AND BLOATING

Your digestive tract has slowed down to allow your body to get maximum nutrition from your food and bacteria, and enzymes in your stomach now have more time to process whatever you eat. A side effect of this change is burping, a bloated feeling, and passing more gas than you usually would.

Keeping a food journal can come in handy. If you find yourself unusually gassy, you can look back and

see what you ate a few hours ago. You may discover that certain vegetables cause more gas than others. If milk products are causing your problem, you may suffer from lactose intolerance (which means you're allergic to some of the sugars in cow's milk).

In later pregnancy, your growing uterus will crowd your abdominal cavity and put pressure on your stomach, which can further slow digestion, making you feel even more bloated after eating, and more gassy.

Over-the-counter products containing simethicone are considered safe to take during pregnancy, but activated charcoal tablets are not.

Ask your practitioner for advice, and call right away if your gas discomfort ever feels more like abdominal pain or cramping or is accompanied by blood in your stool, severe diarrhea or constipation, or more vomiting than usual.

Reproductive organs

PLACENTA

The placenta is an organ that exists only during pregnancy and serves as a support system for your baby. The word is from the Greek term, plakoenta, meaning flat surface. After your baby is born, your body will expel the placenta. The birth of the placenta is called the third stage of labor. (You'll find more information on the stages of labor on page 281.)

The placenta becomes fully functional about the thirteenth week of your pregnancy (eleven weeks after conception). Using the umbilical cord, the placenta sends nutrients, oxygen, minerals, fluids, blood, and vitamins to your growing fetus. It also removes wastes such as carbon dioxide from the fetus' body, so that your own body can dispose of them. The placenta also produces heat and keeps your baby about one degree warmer than your own body.

While the placenta can filter out infections and certain harmful materials, it can't dispose of certain chemicals, such as caffeine, alcohol, cocaine, opiates, or cigarette by-products. A mother's stress hormones also cross the placenta to her baby.

At different times during pregnancy, the placenta secretes a variety of hormones, such as hCG in the early months. Later, it will make less hCG and will begin to secrete more estrogens and progesterone. The placenta also produces *human placental lactogen (HPL)*, also called *human chorionic*

somatomammotropin (HCS), which works with estrogens and progesterone to prepare a mother's breasts for lactation.

If the placenta is abnormally positioned over the cervix, it can result in potentially serious bleeding during mid- or late pregnancy, and during labor, it can block a baby from being born. This condition is called *placenta previa*. It is usually discovered by ultrasound during the first two trimesters of pregnancy. In some cases, the placenta may move out of the way as the uterus grows and stretches upward. If you've been diagnosed with placenta previa, your care provider will probably advise another ultrasound closer to the time of delivery to see if its position has shifted. If the placenta continues to block the opening for your baby's birth, delivery by cesarean section may be required.

Placental abruption, or *abruptio placentae*, is when the placenta separates from the uterine wall prior to labor, which cuts off oxygen flow to the baby. If the abruption is small, and you and the

Danger Signs

- Pain, tenderness, or cramping in your uterus.
- Contractions that don't stop.
- Bleeding, sometimes, but not always. It can vary from light to heavy, with or without clots.

baby are healthy, then you may be sent home and will be monitored closely for the rest of your pregnancy. If it's severe, then you may need immediate labor induction or a cesarean.

UTERUS

For the thirty-eight weeks of pregnancy, your uterus is your baby's home. It starts out the size and shape of a pear and then grows five hundred to one thousand times until it reaches the bottom of your rib cage. The uterus has three major layers: an outer layer made of connective tissue, an inner layer made of about four sub-layers of smooth muscle and elastic tissue (see "smooth muscle," above), and a lining, which, when you aren't pregnant, is shed every month.

Sex and pregnancy

Almost all pregnant women experience a change in their attitudes about sex during pregnancy, often for the better. The famous Masters and Johnson study, which surveyed 101 women, reported that most women's interest in sex decreased or stayed the same during the first trimester.

It was a different story by the second trimester though. Eighty-two of the women reported that their sex drives were in high gear, and the sex was the best of their lives. By the third trimester, however, interest had decreased again.

For men, however, desire may slow over the course of your pregnancy. Men who live with pregnant partners produce less testosterone and more of other hormones such as cortisol and prolactin. (See "Couvade syndrome" on page 244.) While this may make a man more relaxed and nurturing, it may also inhibit his sex drive.

Your partner may notice also that you aren't the same down there. You may look and smell different because of hormonal changes, which he may find off-putting. He may also feel weird about there being a baby living so close to the action.

Good communication is the key to working through the ups and downs of your respective sex drives. Take advantage when your desires meet, and be respectful of limits and sensitivities. Avoid any positions or activities that are uncomfortable or don't feel right.

Vibrators and sex toys made for vaginal insertion are completely safe during pregnancy. Just keep them clean, and use as directed.

IS SEX SAFE?

Intercourse or sexual activity won't harm the baby or induce miscarriage—in fact, orgasms are healthy for the baby. The baby is totally unaware of the cause, but she will get the same hormonal rush that you do.

An orgasm always brings on minor contractions of the uterus, and now that your uterus is larger, you can feel them more. This is not preterm labor, unless it continues for more than an hour.

Many positions may become impractical and uncomfortable in late pregnancy. Consider any position that keeps you off your back and is comfortable, such as those that position you on your side with your partner behind you.

Vagina

APPEARANCE

Your vagina is getting more blood, which may give it a swollen appearance. It may also look darker because of blood flow and pigmentation changes.

DISCHARGE

While you're pregnant, you'll have more discharge than usual. Normal vaginal discharge during pregnancy is called *leukorrhea*. It is white and slightly acidic. This discharge is made up of secretions from the cervix and vagina, shed skin cells, and normal and helpful bacterial flora. Pregnancy discharge serves to protect the birth canal from infection and helps maintain a healthy balance of bacteria. Any itching, burning, discomfort, or unusual discharge should be reported to your doctor.

As your labor approaches, the amount of discharge increases. If you discharge something that looks like a big and possibly blood-tinged wad of mucus, you may have passed your mucous plug.

If you notice an increase in discharge before thirty-seven weeks, especially if it's watery, mucus-like,

Molar Pregnancy

A molar pregnancy is an abnormality of the placenta, caused by a problem when the egg and sperm join together at fertilization. Molar pregnancies are rare, occurring in less than one out of every one thousand pregnancies. Molar pregnancies are also called *gestational trophoblastic disease* (GTD), hydatidiform mole, or simply referred to as a mole. Complete molar pregnancies have only placental parts (there is no baby) and form when the sperm fertilizes an empty egg. The placenta grows and produces the pregnancy hormone hCG. An ultrasound will show that there is no fetus, only a placenta.

or bloody (even if it's just tinged with pink or brownish old blood), call your practitioner right away. This can be a sign of preterm labor.

The color and consistency of the discharge may help your healthcare provider determine whether it is simply a normal thing or if it is a sign of a yeast infection, a sexually transmitted infection such as chlamydia, or other infections that could affect your pregnancy and your baby.

Although women stop having their periods once they are pregnant, some continue to have spotting particularly during the first trimester. Usually, slight bleeding is not a sign of something more serious.

More rarely, some women experience spotting or light bleeding, or what may seem like a normal menstrual cycle during the first few months after getting pregnant, but carry their babies to term.

It's very important to discuss any bleeding with your healthcare provider. You may need an exam to rule out vaginal or cervical infections. Early pregnancy bleeding may indicate an ectopic (tubal) pregnancy.

Heavier, menstrual-like bleeding can be an early sign that you're about to lose your baby. (See "Miscarriage" on page 30.) Your doctor or midwife may recommend blood tests and a sonogram just to make certain everything is okay.

Bleeding that doesn't stop and an internal exam that shows that the cervix has started to open may be signs that you have an incompetent cervix, one that may not be strong enough to hold your baby inside, or that you may be in the process of having a miscarriage.

YEAST INFECTIONS

The chances of your getting a vaginal yeast infection during pregnancy are high, due to hormonal changes that can affect the balance of bacteria. Fortunately, yeast infections are not associated with any kind of pregnancy complications or birth defects.

It's normal to have increased vaginal discharge during pregnancy. But if your discharge becomes thick, white, and creamy, and resembles cottage cheese, and you feel intense itchiness and irritation in your vaginal area, you may have a yeast infection. You also may have a different sort of infection, so it's important that you see your care provider.

Over-the-counter remedies such as Gyne-Lotrimin®, Mycelex G®, Femstat®, or Monistat® are generally thought to be safe in the last two trimesters of pregnancy, but manufacturers recommend that they not be used during the first trimester.

In the first trimester, most healthcare providers opt for the antifungal antibiotics Nystatin® and Mycostatin®, which are not always as effective as the over-the-counter remedies. In any case, don't medicate yourself without first talking with your clinician.

To prevent yeast infections, eat plenty of yogurt made from live lactobacillus bacteria cultures. This good bacteria promotes a healthy vaginal (and intestinal) environment. Wear loose, breathable cotton underwear, and avoid panty hose and synthetic fabrics. Steer clear of foods loaded with sugars, which encourage bacterial growth, and avoid long, hot baths, which create the perfect environment for the yeast to flourish. Try showers instead.

If you do get the dreaded first-trimester yeast infection, you can help ease the misery by applying cool compresses of witch hazel or plain yogurt with live lactobacillus to inflamed tissues. Also try a ten-minute soak in the bathtub with a combination of two cups of corn-starch and half a cup of baking soda.

VAGINITIS

Vaginitis is the term for any infection that causes unusual discharge or redness, soreness, or itching around the vagina. While most vaginal infections are yeast infections, they can also have a number of other causes, including a strepto-coccal infection (see "Group B Strep," page 188) or a reaction to a product such as a soap or bubble bath. So if you have itching or unusual discharge, see your care provider, rather than trying to treat the problem yourself.

Bacterial vaginosis is an infection caused by an overgrowth of bad bacteria in the vagina. If the infection isn't treated, you may develop an itchy discharge that can have a fishy smell. Because many women experience no symptoms, during your first pregnancy visit, your care provider may use a cotton swab to take a sample of your discharge, and check the sample to make sure that your vaginal bacterial balance is healthy.

Perineum

The perineum is the area between your vagina and anus. It undergoes considerable stress during birth. Many midwives and birth instructors believe that regular perineal massage in the later months of pregnancy will help reduce tearing and aid in your post-birth recovery. Others believe it makes no difference.

If you want to try perineal massage, you can massage yourself, or have your partner help you.

First, select non-perfumed, non-petroleum-based oil, such as wheat germ or almond oil. Wash your hands thoroughly, and make sure your nails are trimmed. Sit in a warm comfortable area, spreading your legs apart in a semi-sitting birthing position.

Become familiar with your perineal area with a mirror for the first few massages. Insert your thumbs as deeply as you can inside your vagina, and spread your legs. Press the perineal area down toward the rectum and toward the sides. Gently continue to stretch this opening until you feel a slight burn or tingling.

Hold this stretch until the tingling subsides, and gently massage the lower part of the vaginal canal back and forth.

While massaging, hook your thumbs onto the sides of the vaginal canal, and gently pull these tissues forward, as your baby's head will do during delivery.

Finally, massage the tissues between the thumb and forefinger back and forth for about a minute.

Urinary Tract

Your urinary tract consists of your kidneys, ureters, bladder, and urethra. Kidneys filter waste from your system, creating urine by mixing waste with water. The ureter carries urine to the bladder, which stores it. A ring-shaped muscle, the urinary sphincter, holds it in. When your bladder runs out of room (most women's bladders hold about ten ounces), you run to the bathroom, relax the urinary sphincter, and pass urine through the urethra. During the first trimester, your urinary tract is working overtime to filter waste from your blood, requiring that you take in and send out greater amounts of liquid. This means frequent, and urgent, trips to the bathroom. As inconvenient as this may be, don't be tempted to cut down on water, because your body and baby need to get rid of waste to grow.

URINARY TRACT INFECTIONS

Your urinary tract runs from your urethra to your bladder and then up to your kidney. Urinary tract infections (UTIs) are caused by bacteria that get caught in your urinary system and multiply. Some women

appear to be more vulnerable to infection than others.

Pregnant women are at a higher risk for UTIs due to the softening of the urethra as a result of hormonal changes. When UTIs do occur, they tend to be more serious, possibly due to a variety of changes in the urinary tract.[8] UTIs in pregnancy are more likely to develop into kidney infections, and kidney infections can increase your risk of preterm delivery. If you've had more than one UTI in the past, you're much more likely to get one in the future.

The classic symptom of a urinary tract infection is feeling like your bladder's constantly full, yet you're unable to pass much fluid when you get to the bathroom. Unfortunately, this is also a classic pregnancy symptom.

You may also have pain; a burning sensation when you urinate; bloody, cloudy, or foul-smelling urine; lower back or abdominal pain; or a low fever. Not everyone with a UTI has symptoms, however, which is why your care provider will periodically check your urine for signs of bacteria. It's important to treat UTIs right away because minor infections can lead to major kidney infections, which are painful and require hospitalization.

You can help prevent UTIs by practicing good hygiene.

- Wipe from front to back to keep bacteria out of your urethral area.
- Wear cotton underwear. This will help absorb vaginal secretions. Avoid thong underwear—the thong part can create abrasions where *E. coli* bacteria can breed and helps bacteria migrate to the urethra.
- Avoid irritating products. Steer away from perfumed toilet paper, bubble bath, perfumed soaps, douches, or feminine hygiene deodorants.
- Urinate frequently. Urinate whenever you get the urge, to keep urine from standing still in your bladder. And be sure to urinate as soon as possible after having intercourse to rinse out your urinary opening.
- Nix caffeine. Avoid caffeinated beverages. Caffeine is an irritant to the urinary tract.

Legs

MUSCLE CRAMPS

Pregnant women are prone to muscle spasms in their calves and feet at night. No one knows the exact cause, but many healthcare providers believe that it may be a result of a calcium or magnesium deficiency. Make sure to drink at least two pints of milk a day, or some equivalent, such as calcium-enriched orange juice or soy milk, and check that your prenatal vitamin has 450 to 600 milligrams of magnesium. It may help prevent leg cramps to wear socks to bed at night to keep your feet and legs warm.

SWELLING (EDEMA, OR WATER RETENTION)

In pregnancy, the changing levels of hormones affect the rate at which fluid enters and leaves the tissues, just like a massive case of PMS-related bloating. *Edema* is a fluid imbalance in your body, which can cause mild to severe swelling in one or more body parts.

Your circulatory system transports fluid within the body via its network of blood vessels. Your lymphatic system also absorbs and transports this fluid. The fluid carries oxygen and nutrients needed by the cells into the body's tissues. After the tissues use the nutrients, fluid moves back into your blood vessels. Normally, your body maintains a balance of fluid, but with edema, either too much fluid moves from the blood vessels into the tissues, or not enough fluid moves from the tissues back into the blood vessels.

Edema is extremely common in the latter months of pregnancy. You may find that swelling is worse in the late afternoon and evening. The retained fluid could be nature's way

Ways to Reduce Swelling

- **Magnesium.** Sometimes fast-absorbing capsules of magnesium (found in health food stores) taken with meals can help to reduce edema. Ask your healthcare provider.

- **Natural fluid reducers.** Natural diuretics that help the body to excrete excess fluid include watermelon, parsley, cilantro, dill weed, and cucumbers.

- **Prescription diuretics.** Your healthcare provider may prescribe a pregnancy-safe diuretic to help reduce very severe swelling, but never take an over-the-counter diuretic drug.

- **Keep off your feet.** Try to avoid standing for long periods of time. Keep your feet elevated at work so the pressure is taken off the back of your legs.

- **Lie down.** Lying on your side can help your body reabsorb extra fluid by taking pressure off your main veins.

- **Warm bath.** Taking a bath in warm water can help to compress your tissues and reduce swelling.

- **Swimming.** This is a great way for pregnant women to get exercise, and the pressure from the water helps squeeze the extra fluid back into your circulatory system.

- **No constriction.** Wear clothes and shoes that are loose and won't restrict any part of your body.

- **Eat more protein.** Increase the protein in your diet by including four servings of lean protein and four servings of soy milk or dairy products per day. The increase in protein will increase the protein pressure (osmotic pressure) of your blood and draw the fluid from your tissue back into your bloodstream.

Sometimes excessive swelling toward the end of pregnancy can be a sign of oncoming *preeclampsia,* sometimes called *toxemia.* The symptoms are sudden weight gain (more than two pounds per week), a swollen face and hands, a rise in blood pressure, and protein in your urine. Serious symptoms may also include severe headache, blurred vision, or severe abdominal pain. Contact your healthcare provider immediately. (See the discussion of preeclampsia on page 215.)

of making sure a mother is protected if there's nothing to eat or drink during labor. Since some labors can last for many hours, or even more than a day, the reserved body fluid can serve to help keep a mother hydrated. You may find that the excess fluid collects in your fingers so you can't get your rings off, or in your ankles. The edema usually decreases overnight because elevating your legs helps the fluid get back into your circulation.

Your healthcare practitioner will constantly monitor the level of your swelling by pressing into a bony area (usually your leg or the bony part of your ankle) to see what kind of indentation the pressure leaves. If the indentation stays for a few seconds, then you probably have edema.

VARICOSE VEINS

Varicose veins appear as a swollen, purple, knotted network just under your skin. Usually they appear on your calves or thighs, but some women may have them on their vaginas. Varicose veins seem to be genetic, so if your parents or grandparents have them, there's a good chance you will too.

These swollen veins may rupture if they're injured and bleed and are the most likely place for blood clots to form. So be kind to them, and don't try to massage them away.

Feet

Your feet are under more pressure than any other body part, and now they're being stressed like never before. The weight of your body, the softening of your ligaments, and the force of walking can make the bones in your feet spread. About eighty percent of women go up a half shoe size during pregnancy—usually permanently. Swelling or edema in your feet may also temporarily change your foot dimensions so that your favorite pair of shoes doesn't fit anymore.

Making sure that your feet get proper arch support and cushioning can save you a lot of discomfort in your later weeks of pregnancy. If you can get away with wearing running shoes to work, suspend your fashion sense, and do it. But, even with the greatest of care, foot pain and injury during pregnancy is common. If you have a tendency toward being flat- or high-arched, you are at greater risk for problems.

FOOT REPAIR

- **Stretch and massage.** Stretch your feet in the morning and before you exercise. Take regular walk-and-stretch breaks throughout the day to promote circulation.

- **Avoid impact.** Vigorous dancing, gymnastics, or jumping down from a high seat can put sudden and unusual pressure on your foot ligaments and cause an injury. Be gentle.

- **Get off them.** Elevate your feet as often as possible. If you have to sit for long periods of time, prop your feet on a footrest or stool by your chair.

- **Check your shoe size.** Have your feet measured and your foot width checked several times throughout your pregnancy. Your shoe size may change, and it's important to wear shoes that fit properly and don't constrict your circulation.

- **Keep moving.** Don't avoid activities like walking, jogging with a smooth gait, or swimming, which can help strengthen and tone feet. Walking on sand is particularly good for keeping your foot muscles in shape.

- **Keep hydrated.** Drink plenty of water.

- **Get slip-ons.** Invest in some comfy slip-on, flat-soled shoes. As your pregnancy progresses, you'll be happy to not have to bend over to tie laces. Look for cork insoles that will customize your fit as your feet grow.

Help for Varicose Veins

Keep off your feet. Avoid standing for long periods of time, and sit with your feet elevated as often as possible. Keep your office chair in its lowest position, and use a footstool to take pressure off the back of your legs.

Uncross your legs. Avoid sitting with your legs crossed. It only increases pressure on your veins.

Exercise and stretch regularly. Gentle stretching of your body can help blood to return to your heart so it doesn't pool in veins.

Wear support hose. If the swollen veins are in your legs, you may want to try maternity support hose. Put them on in the morning before you get out of bed, while your legs are less swollen, to help to keep your veins from popping out.

Avoid massage. Don't massage your veins or legs, which will push more blood into them and make them worse.

Managing Your Nutrition

Every culture has its own ideas and superstitions about pregnancy nutrition. In West Africa, women are instructed to eat specially prepared types of clay. In traditional Chinese medicine, each month of pregnancy has specific dietary recommendations, with the fourth month for rice and fish broth and the sixth for the meat of muscular fowl and fierce beasts.

In America, we tend to be superstitious about prenatal vitamins, believing that they're a magic antidote to a diet of doughnuts and fast food. Not so. Your body best absorbs vitamins and minerals from food sources and needs a variety of foods to stay healthy.

But eating a balanced diet is easier said than done—especially if you crave candy twenty-four hours a day. Here are some tips to make it easier.

"I gained 60 pounds with my first pregnancy, just letting myself eat any and everything, and it was really hard on my body. It took me three years to lose the extra weight. I'm going to try to avoid that this time around. It's so easy to gain extra weight when you're pregnant—and hard to lose it postpartum."

Vitamins and Minerals 101

WHAT'S IN A PRENATAL?

If you compare labels, you'll see that there's nothing magical about the ingredients of prenatal vitamins. They typically contain a B-complex, four hundred micrograms of folate, and some quantity of iron. Many over-the-counter vitamins do too, so if you find your prescription multivitamin makes you feel queasy, consider switching brands, perhaps to a liquid formula or a children's chewable with iron and folic acid (folate).

If you eat a healthy diet that contains fortified cereals or breads, meat, and four or five varieties of fruits and vegetables a day, you may not need to take a supplement at all. Talk with your healthcare provider.

If your diet consists of not much more than fast food, soda, and vending machine snacks, or if you don't eat any meat or dairy products, it's probably best that you take a vitamin as insurance.

CALCIUM

Pregnant women need a lot of calcium, at least one thousand milligrams a day. Your baby builds her bones from the calcium in your diet, not from the calcium already in your bones or teeth. Your muscles also need calcium to react to nerve stimuli. If you dislike or can't tolerate dairy products, your growing baby will be fine without milk, as long as you devise an alternative way to get the recommended amount of calcium.

Recommended Daily Allowances of Vitamins and Minerals for Pregnant Women[9]

Calcium 1,000 milligrams (mg.)
Folate 400 micrograms (mcg.)
Magnesium 320mg.
Iron 30 mg.
Niacin (B3) 18 mg.
Protein 60 grams (g.)
Riboflavin (B2) 1.6 mg.
Selenium 65 mcg.
Thiamine (B1) 1.5 mg.

Vitamin A between 4,000 and 5,000 International Units (I.U.)
Vitamin B6 2.2 mg.
Vitamin B12 2.2 mcg.
Vitamin C 60–300 mg.
Vitamin E 10 mg.
Vitamin K 65 mcg.
Zinc 15 mg.

Tips for Pregnancy Nutrition

- **Figure out what a calorie is.** You only need an extra three hundred calories a day while you're pregnant, which is not very many. Get in the habit of reading labels so you can decide if the calories in a certain food are "worth it."

- **Keep a journal.** The easiest way to monitor your diet is to put a journal in your kitchen (and take it with you when you go to work), and write down what you eat. Consider keeping a calculator with it, because serving sizes on labels are often quite confusing. A journal will let you see in black and white if you're getting enough vitamins and minerals and if you're going overboard with the empty-calorie snacks.

- **Aim for a good week.** It's nearly impossible to have every day's diet be exactly balanced. Instead, try to have a balanced week.

- **Pay extra attention to iron and calcium.** These minerals are best absorbed in food form.

- **Give in to cravings, but with moderation.** Don't deny yourself anything you want, but watch your serving sizes! Scoop some ice cream into a bowl instead of digging into the carton. Have a small fast-food burger with a side of skim milk, not a double-bacon cheeseburger with super-sized fries and a Sprite. Your craving will be satisfied, and so will your protein and calcium needs.

- **Plan your meals around the vegetables.** When you shop, hit the vegetables first with the plan of making them the entrée of your meals. Fill half of your dinner plate with vegetables and let your meat and starches serve as the accessories.

- **Up your fiber.** If you eat all of the fiber the USDA recommends (twenty-five grams a day), you won't have much room in your stomach for junk food. Fill up on beans, oatmeal, bran cereal, strawberries, apples, and pears.

- **Exercise.** Running, swimming, walking, weight training, and yoga are all good for keeping your weight gain from getting extreme. If you can't commit to a routine, just walk as much as you can.

VITAMIN A 4,000–5,000 I.U. A DAY

This essential vitamin helps your vision and increases your resistance to viruses. It can be found in animal products, such as liver and butter, and in plant products that contain carotene, which your body converts into vitamin A. Carotene-rich vegetables are dark green, deep yellow, and orange: broccoli, greens, green peppers, sweet potatoes, carrots, pumpkins, winter squash, apricots, carrots, papaya, cantaloupe, spinach, pumpkin, sweet potatoes, and mangoes.

Sources of Calcium

Cow's milk	300 mg. per 8 ounces (oz.)
Calcium-fortified orange juice	300 mg. per 8 oz.
Swiss cheese	272 mg. per oz.
Cheddar cheese	204 mg. per oz.
American cheese	174 mg. per oz.
Cottage cheese	77 mg. per half cup
Yogurt	345-415 mg. per cup

Mineral Water
    Gerolsteiner
    San Pellegrino
	
	80 mg. a cup
	50 mg. a cup

Canned oily fish with bones, such as salmon and sardines	200-300 mg. per 3-oz. serving
Tofu prepared with calcium chloride or sulfate	50-250 mg. per 3-oz. serving
Leafy greens such as kale, collards, or turnip greens	100-170 mg. per half cup

You need no more than 4,000 to 5,000 I.U. of vitamin A per day to promote healthy vision, ward off colds, and help your skin. Vitamin A deficiencies are extremely rare. If you take multivitamin supplements, avoid those that contain more than the recommended dose; large doses of straight vitamin A are associated with birth defects. However, supplements that contain vitamin A in the form of beta-carotene are safe.

B VITAMINS

Several B vitamins make up the B-complex family, including folic acid, B6, B12, niacin, thiamine, and riboflavin. They're found mainly in animal products such as meat, eggs, and dairy, although (with the exception of B12), they can also be found in certain vegetables. The B vita-

mins are water soluble, which means that they are not stored in the body for long-term use, so it's important to get enough every day. If you take a daily prenatal vitamin, it should contain a full B complex.

Thiamine (B1), 1.5 mgs a day

Thiamine, also known as vitamin B1, is used by your body to release energy from the carbohydrates in foods. Too little of it can make you feel listless. Pork is your best food source, with 0.7 mg. per 3 oz., but B1 is also found in watermelon (0.23 mg. per slice), avocados (0.2 mg. per avocado), and peas (0.41 mg. per cup).

Riboflavin (B2), 1.6 mg. a day

Riboflavin, aka vitamin B2, is also used in releasing energy from foods as well as for the growth and repair of tissues. Like B1, it's recommended that pregnant women get 1.6 mg. a day. If you drink two pints of milk a day, you should be getting plenty. It's also found in kiwifruit and avocados.

Niacin (B3), 18 mg. a day

Niacin, aka B3, also helps your cells convert food into energy and regulates the balance of fats in your bloodstream. It's recommended that pregnant women get 18 mg. a day. Salmon (14 mg. per 3 oz.), chicken (19 mg.), peanuts, and enriched cereal are good sources.

Vitamin B6 (Pyridoxine), 2.2 mg. a day

Vitamin B6 is especially important for protein metabolism, and helps your body build proteins, including hormones, blood components, and enzymes. Your body also uses it to help regulate your blood sugar levels. The FDA recommends that pregnant and lactating women get 2.2 mg. a day. Not getting enough can make you dizzy and cranky. Some research has shown that B6 may be helpful in reducing pregnancy-related carpal tunnel syndrome and other aches and pains because it helps nerve cells to communicate properly. For some women, B6 supplements can also reduce the symptoms of morning sickness.

Whole grain cereal, bananas (0.7 mg.), and chicken (0.8 mg. per 3 oz. serving) are good sources.

Vitamin B12, 2.2 mcg. a day

Vitamin B12 is found exclusively in animal products: milk, meat, shellfish, and eggs. Unless you're a vegan, you should have no problem getting the recommended 3 mcg. of B12 a day to maintain a healthy nervous system. If you are a vegan, talk to your care provider about supplement options. Symptoms of B12 deficiency, such as poor neurological development, can show up in children and breastfed infants of vegans.[10]

Folic acid (folate), 400 mcg. a day

All pregnant women and any woman planning on getting pregnant need an intake of 400 micrograms of folic acid daily. Folic acid, a B vitamin, has been shown to prevent neural tube defects in developing fetuses and, in some instances, it may help to prevent premature birth. For the vitamin to be effective, though, adequate amounts of it must be consumed pre-pregnancy, and followed through during the first six weeks of pregnancy, before most women know they are pregnant. Folate is fragile, and is easily destroyed by heat, light, and the decomposition of vegetables.

Most prenatal vitamins contain 400 mcg. Limit your folic acid intake to 1,000 mcg. per day to avoid overdose. A few cereals, such as *Total* and *Product 19*, contain 400 mcg. of folic acid, but most cereals do not contain those levels.

VITAMIN C (ASCORBIC ACID), 70 TO 300 MG. A DAY

Vitamin C is necessary for the proper function of your immune system. The FDA currently recommended daily allowance of vitamin

Sources of Folic Acid

Lentils, boiled	179 mcg. per half cup (4 oz.)
Oatmeal, instant	150 mcg. per packet
Asparagus, steamed	131 mcg. per 6 spear
Spinach, steamed	131 mcg. per half cup
Chickpeas, canned	80 mcg. per half cup
Lima beans	78 mcg. per half cup
Orange juice from concentrate	54 mcg. per half cup
Broccoli, steamed	52 mcg. per half cup

C for pregnant women is 70 mg., but recently the National Institutes of Health has recommended raising the recommended dose to 200 mg. Because vitamin C is water-soluble, it is almost impossible to overdose. Your body will just pass what you don't need through your urine. Generally, your body can't use more than 500 mg. a day. If you smoke cigarettes, be sure to get at least 300 mg. a day, because your body depletes its supply of vitamin C to fight the toxins in cigarette smoke, hindering your ability to fight illness.

IRON, 30 MG. A DAY

Most women don't get enough iron, and when you're pregnant, your need for this crucial mineral doubles because your body must produce extra blood to support your growing baby. During pregnancy, you'll need 30 mg. of iron a day. (Non-pregnant women need 15 mg., and a nursing mom needs 19 mg.)

The National Academy of Science recommends that expectant moms in their second and third trimesters take a daily iron supplement containing 30 mg. of iron.

It turns out that iron from plant-based foods is not as well absorbed as the iron from meat, chicken, and fish. The carbonates, oxalates, and phosphates in foods such as tea, cranberries, rhubarb, spinach, and soda actually block your absorption of iron to some degree. Consequently, a vegetarian needs to eat more iron to meet her needs. Consider drinking soy or cow's milk with three tablespoons of blackstrap molasses (found in health food stores) each morning and evening.

Vitamin C enhances iron absorption from plant sources. Drink orange juice with iron-rich foods, or try combinations like spinach with diced red peppers.

MAGNESIUM, 320 MG. A DAY

Magnesium is important to the function of the cells of your bones and tissues. Getting enough of it can spare you the pregnancy irritations

Iron Content of Common Foods

Cereal, ready to eat, fortified	1-16 mg. per cup
Clams, canned	11.2 mg. per 1/4 cup
Braunschweiger (liver sausage)	5.3 mg. per 2 oz.
Beef liver, fried	5.3 mg. per 3 oz.
Molasses, blackstrap	5 mg. per tablespoon
Baked beans	5 mg. per cup
Oysters, cooked	3.8 mg. per oz.
Sirloin steak	2.9 mg. per 3 oz.
Baked potato, with skin	2.8 mg. per medium potato
Soup, lentil and ham	2.6 mg. per cup
Burrito, bean	2.5 mg. each
Soup, beef noodle	2.4 mg. per cup
Rice, white, enriched	2.3 mg. per cup
Pop tart, fortified	2.2 mg. per pastry
Enriched pasta	2 mg. per cooked cup
Ground beef, lean	1.8 mg. per 3 oz.
Tofu, firm	1.8 mg. per 1/2 cup
Apricots, dried halves	1.7 mg. per 10
Cashews, roasted	1.7 mg. per oz.
Spinach, frozen	1.5 mg. per 1/2 cup
Bread, whole wheat	1.2 mg. per slice (varies with brand)
Broccoli, fresh cooked	0.7 mg. per 1/2 cup
Egg	0.7 mg. per egg

Magnesium Content of Common Foods

Avocado, Florida	206 mg. per medium avocado
Almonds	86 mg. per oz.
Mixed roasted nuts	66 mg. per oz.
Spinach	65 mg. per cooked 1/2 cup
Peanut butter	50 mg. per 2 tablespoons
Banana	30-45 mg. per medium banana
Chocolate bar	31 mg. per oz.
Kiwifruit	53 mg. a cup

of muscle cramps, mental disorientation, and even depression. Magnesium is needed for more than three hundred biochemical reactions in the body. It helps maintain normal muscle and nerve function, keeps heart rhythm steady, and bones strong. It's also thought to decrease your chances of preeclampsia and low birth weight. You need about 320 to 400 mg. of magnesium a day. Magnesium is found in all unprocessed plant foods to some degree. Many prenatal supplements also contain magnesium.

DOCOSAHEXAENOIC ACID (DHA), 200 TO 400 MG. A DAY

The FDA has not established a recommended daily amount for this variety of omega-3 fatty acid. However, recent studies have shown that pregnant women whose diets are rich in DHA have fewer instances of postnatal depression and give birth to babies with more developed brains.

Nutritionists currently recommend eating two or three weekly servings of coldwater marine fish (salmon, mackerel, sardines, tuna) to consume an average of 200 to 400 mg. of DHA a day. If you're concerned about pollutants such as mercury in fish, or you just don't like fish, you can take fish oil capsules, though this is thought to be less effective than acquiring your fatty acids through your diet. Omega-3 fatty acids are also found in soy foods, though there is suspicion currently that excessive amounts of soy can interfere with the hormones of male babies, causing birth defects to their reproductive organs.

If you're concerned about the birth difficulties that may arise from having a larger-headed baby, it is also an option to increase your omega-3 fatty acid intake during the first three months after birth, and supply your baby with DHA through your breast milk.

VEGETARIANISM AND VEGANISM

You can have a perfectly healthy vegetarian pregnancy, as long as you plan your menus well to include enough protein, calcium, iron, and vitamins D and B.

Protein is needed to build your and your baby's tissues, and to get the same amount of protein in two slices of cheese, you would have to eat two cups of beans.

If you're a vegetarian who eats dairy and egg products, you should have no problem as long as you carefully monitor your diet to make sure it's well balanced with a variety of vegetables, fruits, grains, legumes, and non-meat protein sources, such as beans, eggs, tofu, and cheese. Your body absorbs only three to

Microwaves

You may have heard some people express concern about microwave ovens leaking radiation that could harm a growing baby. Fortunately, this is just an urban legend—there's no evidence of any danger. Microwaves don't generate enough radiation for there to be a risk of exposure.

Is Organic Food Worth It?

Organic food is grown or raised by farmers who don't use synthetic pesticides or fertilizers made of synthetic ingredients or sludge from sewage treatment plants. Organic meat, poultry, eggs, and dairy products come from animals that are given no antibiotics or growth hormones. Herbicides, pesticides, and antibiotics consumed by cows can be passed along through their milk. Before a product can be labeled "organic," a government-approved certifier inspects the farm where the food is grown to make sure the farmer is following all the rules necessary to meet USDA organic standards. These higher standards mean that organic foods are more expensive for consumers.

Should you spend the extra money on organic foods? For fresh fruits, grains, vegetables, and dairy products, it's a good idea to pay a little more to lower the risk of your and your baby's exposure to unnecessary chemicals and pesticides. Chemicals such as dioxins are carcinogens considered to be potentially associated with cancer and with birth defects in animal studies. The foods most likely to be contaminated with pesticides are strawberries, rice, oats, milk, bell peppers, bananas, green beans, and spinach. Many of these crops come from overseas, where farmers are poorly monitored in their use of dangerous pesticides. Wash all fresh vegetables well, even organic ones.

eight percent of the iron in vegetables and grains, compared with about twenty percent of the iron in meat, poultry, and fish. You may want to take an iron supplement or a prenatal vitamin supplement. Be sure they contain at least 30 mg of iron. Also, eating foods rich in vitamin C and iron at the same time will greatly enhance the absorption of iron.

However, vegans who eat only plant foods may not consume enough B12, iron, calcium, and vitamin D. You need to take a supplement that contains 30 mg. of iron, along with 2 mcg. of B12 daily. In addition, diets with no animal products tend to be low in fat and high in fiber, so it can be difficult to get the

extra three hundred calories a day you need while you're pregnant.

Pregnant vegans should also be sure to get at least twenty to thirty minutes of sun on their hands and face two or three times a week, because vitamin D is produced by the body as a response to exposure to sunlight. Only take vitamin D supplements if your care provider approves; excess vitamin D is toxic and can produce fetal deformities. A vitamin D supplement of 10 mcg. (400 IU) daily should be taken by pregnant vegans who live at northern latitudes in the winter (due to reduced intensity of sunlight) and by those with minimal exposure to sunlight.

Managing Your Weight and Fitness

SHOULD YOU WORRY ABOUT GAINING TOO MUCH WEIGHT?

Pregnancy may be the first time in your adult life that people praise and encourage your weight gain. In fact, gaining is your duty! Can you eat whatever you want?

The answer is yes and no.

When you're pregnant, you should always eat when you're hungry. Now is not the time to go on a diet, go hungry, or deprive yourself of anything you're craving. But don't fully indulge every craving. Moderation and making every bite count can help you have an easier labor, give birth to a healthier baby, and recover more quickly from childbirth.

While the human body hasn't evolved much in the past five thousand years, the American diet is now full of more animal fat, processed sugars, and refined flours. Not all calories are equally satisfying; if you ate four apples, you'd feel full, but you probably wouldn't be satisfied by half a cup of ice cream. A cup of cooked brown rice has 90 calories, but a cup of pasta has 180. A diet high in high-calorie, high-sugar, and low-fiber foods will make both you and your baby large and undernourished at the same time.

HOW MUCH GAIN IS HEALTHY?

Most mothers of average weight gain between twenty-five and thirty-five pounds during pregnancy. Mothers who were underweight before they got pregnant are advised to gain twenty-eight to forty pounds, and mothers pregnant with twins may gain forty-five pounds or more.

The American College of Obstetricians and Gynecologists

recommends that pregnant women consume 300 to 500 extra calories a day beyond the standard 2,000. If you're carrying twins, you should consume about 2,700 to 2,800 calories. An extra 300 to 500 calories a day is not that many—an extra three to five tablespoons of butter or four tablespoons of olive oil. You won't need to make any effort whatsoever to get those calories unless your morning sickness is severe.

UNPLEASANT TRUTHS

1. Once you gain it, it's tough to get off.

Gaining weight in pregnancy can lead to a progressive weight problem for a lot of people. After you have your baby, you'll have a lot to deal with, and diet and exercise will probably not rank high on your list of concerns. Also, as you age, your metabolism slows down. You won't be able to drop extra pounds as easily as you could when you were younger. Pregnancy hormones may also play a role. Every pregnancy increases a woman's risk for obesity by seven percent, and her husband's by four percent.

The strategy of weight loss by breastfeeding may not work for you, either. While breastfeeding can burn five hundred calories a day, it also makes you really hungry. This may be why there's no link between how long a woman breastfeeds and how much she weighs in the long term.[11]

Exercise alone will not be enough to lose weight postpartum. Unless you make an effort to cut calories, your appetite will just increase to make up for the extra calories you're burning.

2. If you were overweight when you conceived, gaining even more excess weight can be harmful to you and your baby's health.

Recent studies have found that moms who are obese during pregnancy, defined as having a Body Mass Index (BMI) of more than thirty have double the risk of having babies with heart defects and double the risk of their babies having multiple birth defects. An obese mother can make it three and a half times as likely for her baby to be born with spina bifida, a neural-tube defect. Obese women are also more than three times as likely as other women to have babies with a defect known as omphalocele, which occurs in about one in five thousand births. The defect causes intestines or other abdominal organs to protrude through the navel. Researchers don't know exactly how obesity causes these various defects, but they suspect that women's diets that are high in empty calories may also be low in vitamins.[12]

The most accurate way to determine your BMI is to measure the thickness of the fat on your arm or abdomen with a caliper (or better yet, have your care provider do it). Calculators and equations that simply measure your ratio of height to weight won't take your muscle mass into consideration. Ask your care provider to measure your BMI and make dietary and lifestyle recommendations for you.

What Is Pregnancy Weight Made Of?

By the time you deliver, you will have added twenty or more pounds. Every pregnancy is different, but here is an estimated breakdown of what comprises your gain:

- Uterus: two pounds
- Extra blood volume: four pounds
- Breasts: one pound each
- Fluid retention: four pounds
- Extra fat, protein, and nutrients to support the pregnancy: seven pounds
- Placenta and membranes: one to one and one-half pounds
- Amniotic fluid: two pounds
- Baby: six to eight pounds

3. Extra pounds of fat can make you more uncomfortable and lead to health problems later.
The extra weight that pregnancy contributes also adds stress to your frame, and this can contribute to backaches and insomnia, making the later months of pregnancy more uncomfortable. Women who gain more than forty pregnancy pounds also increase their risk of post-menopausal breast cancer by sixty-three percent.[13]

4. The more junk you eat, the less room you have for healthy food.
Getting adequate protein, vitamins, and minerals—especially iron and calcium—is one of the most important things you can do for your baby's health. Consuming empty calories will leave less room for vegetables and protein.

OVERWEIGHT AND PREGNANT?

If you're like the majority of American women, you've got a little or a lot of extra poundage. Should you diet?

Actually, every pregnant woman should "diet"—that is, monitor her eating habits to make sure that the candy is not outpacing the vegetables. If you're overweight, though, you need to be particularly vigilant about portion sizes to keep your daily calorie intake at about 2,300 (or up to 2,500 if you're extra large or tall).

How important it is for you to make an effort to control your calories depends on how overweight you are. The risk of weight-related complications, such as birth defects and gestational diabetes, begins to increase in women who have a BMI of twenty-five, and it increases with every point. If your BMI is thirty or greater, consider getting help from your care provider or a dietitian.

Exercise

Unfortunately for couch-sitting types, the days of pregnant women being told to avoid physical activity are long gone. Thanks to researchers who have studied[14] thousands of exercising women in depth, we know that exercise has numerous benefits.

Exercising women, on average

- Gain less extra weight and are therefore less likely to suffer weight-related complications, like gestational diabetes.
- Have shorter labors.
- Are less likely to need medical interventions, including c-sections.
- Have fitter babies. Babies of moms who exercise are less stressed during labor and birth, and less likely to be overly large (in an unhealthy way), and recover from the stresses of birth more quickly.
- Retain less fluid.
- Are less likely to suffer depression and mood swings.
- Sleep better and have more energy when they're awake.
- Physically recover more quickly after childbirth—as much as twice as fast.
- Have bodies that regulate their temperature and utilize oxygen more effectively.
- Have increased body awareness and are less likely to suffer falls.
- Have a lower risk of injuries from accidents. Women who don't exercise are much more likely to

suffer from strains, sprains, and pain, even with exercise-related injuries taken into account.

When should you NOT exercise?

- If your care provider says not to.
- If you have an injury.
- If your membranes have ruptured.
- If the activity you've chosen causes you pain or exerts you to the point where you can't talk.
- If baby stays quiet and inactive for more than thirty minutes after you exercise. Make sure to discontinue exercise until you confer with your care provider to make sure that your baby is getting adequate oxygen.

STARTING FROM SCRATCH

If you've never exercised before, or it's been a long time since you were in the habit, it's not too late (unless your water just broke). You don't need to join a gym or sign up for a class, unless you want to. Exercise can be as simple as putting on your shoes and taking a walk. Here are some tips to get you going:

- Show up. Consistency is much more important than a spectacular performance. Some days you may be into your workout, other days you have to tell yourself, "I'm going to give it a try, and I'll stop if it's really not working." Most of the time, once you're out there, you'll be able to get into it. If not, you may need to find a new activity.

- Whichever exercise you choose, aim for at least half an hour three days a week, and work up to half an hour to an hour five or six days a week. Include five to ten minutes to warm up and stretch beforehand, and another five to ten to cool down.

- Pick something you like to do, and find something new if you get bored.

- Set time aside in your daily routine for exercise.

- Stop when your body tells you to. But don't be afraid to push yourself as long as it still feels like fun and nothing hurts. Your body's heightened sensitivity means that you can pretty well rely on it to tell you if you're doing something wrong.

- Drink lots of fluids before, during, and after. Not only is it good for you, but also it'll make your exercise much more enjoyable.

- Set time or distance goals so you'll notice when you start to make progress. If you're out of shape, you'll need to exercise for longer periods of time to gain benefits.

- Exercise to the point where afterward, you feel refreshed and energized—not tired or wiped out.

- For your comfort in late pregnancy, support yourself with a good sports bra and a belly bra.

The exercises traditionally recommended for pregnant women are walking, stretching or yoga, swimming, and stationary cycling. But if none of these inspire you, don't limit yourself. Before the effects of exercise on pregnant women began to be studied in detail in the late 1970s, doctors and pregnancy-book writers conservatively suggested that a host of activities be off-limits for normal and healthy women: horseback riding, hockey, racquetball, weight lifting, and so on. We now know that almost no exercises are off-limits, as long as you use common sense to avoid injuries.

The big things to avoid are

- Anything that risks trauma to your abdomen after your uterus has grown out of your pelvis (around week twenty).

- Strain to your abdominal muscles.

- Training, flying, or parachuting from an unpressurized aircraft at an altitude higher than 7,500 feet.

- Scuba diving (quick pressure changes can harm the fetus).

- Any activity that risks dehydration. Pay close attention if you're exercising in a hot, humid environment.

IF YOU'RE ALREADY EXERCISING

If you already have an exercise routine, keep it up! Discuss with your care provider if you'll need to make any safety modifications to your routine. Women who exercise and then stop in mid-pregnancy actually gain more weight (an average of five pounds and one to two percent more body fat) than women who never exercised at all![15] Researchers believe this is because the exercisers got into the habit of eating more to make up for the calories they were burning.

SOME EXERCISE IDEAS

Power walking

Walking is overwhelmingly the exercise of choice for pregnant women. You can do it almost anywhere at any time, you don't need to buy anything but a pair of comfortable shoes, it's safe, and you don't have to learn any new skills. It's also a great way to get fresh air and see what's going on in your neighborhood. Start by walking at least three times a week, if not daily. Set a goal to work up to walking for an hour, four or five times a week. If you've never exercised before, start slowly, listen to your body, and stop or slow your pace if anything hurts.

Running

There's no reason to avoid jogging or running during pregnancy, though you may need to make modifications to stay safe and comfortable. If you've never run before, though, take it easy. Use common sense—don't run on rough terrain you aren't familiar with or in a hot climate without access to water. In the later part of your pregnancy, you may need extra support in the form of multiple sports bras, worn one on top of the other, and a belly bra. Make sure that your shoes are in good condition; more weight will mean more wear. As with walking, exercise at least half an hour three times a week to get any benefit; work toward longer distances or more frequent runs. Be sure to rest at least one day a week.

Yoga

Yoga, which means union, was developed about five thousand years ago and consists of various poses and movements that reflect the natural world. Even if you think you've never done yoga before, you probably have: most childbirth classes, such as Bradley and Lamaze™, have incorporated yoga postures and breathing techniques into the curriculum. Yoga has been proven to reduce the amount of stress hormones in your body.[16]

Ideally, yoga tones muscles without straining them, promotes good circulation, reduces stress, helps clear mental fuzziness, eases nausea, and relieves some of the routine aches and pains of pregnancy. Learning yoga breathing techniques can also help you cope with contractions.

If you've never practiced yoga before, don't try to start from scratch on your own or with a video. Instead, sign up for a prenatal yoga class. (Almost all studios or health clubs that offer yoga offer a prenatal class.) That way, you'll be able to work with an instructor to make sure that you're doing the poses with proper alignment. A class is also a fun way to get out of the house and meet other moms-to-be.

If you're already an experienced yogi, then you'll need to modify your practice to avoid:

- Practicing in a room that's hotter than 100 degrees.
- Assuming or holding any pose that doesn't feel good for any reason.
- Poses that involve double leg lifts, such as the Boat, that strain your abdominal muscles.

- Back bends, which can increase pressure on your already stressed lower back.

- Positions that involve lying on your front, which put uncomfortable pressure on your uterus.

Yoga experts disagree about whether or not pregnant women should perform inverted poses, twists, and shoulder stands during pregnancy. We would recommend not attempting these postures unless a qualified instructor is present.

Certain poses are particularly helpful during pregnancy:

Mountain pose (tadasana), or standing with awareness, will help you maintain good posture as the distribution of weight in your body shifts.

Cobbler pose (Buddha Konasana) will help you learn to sit with proper alignment.

Cat pose (Marjaraiasana) is what your doctor would call a pelvic tilt. On your hands and knees, arch your back, and fold your pelvis, then release, sticking your chin up and your rump in the air. Repeat as many times as is comfortable.

Warrior poses (virabhadrasana) are modified lunges that can ease back and arm pain and strengthen your legs and ankles.

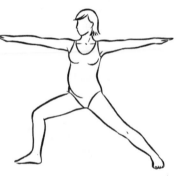

Warrior pose

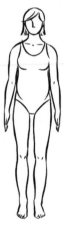

Mountain pose

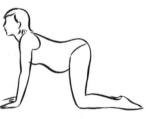

Cat pose

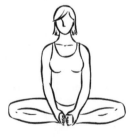

Cobbler pose

Swimming

Swimming is safe, low-impact, and in late pregnancy, a great way to relieve the pressure on your back. Even if you already know how to swim, you may consider taking a lesson to get your strokes into good form for maximum benefits. Kickboards, water aerobics, or water ballet can put variety into your swim routine.

Stationary biking

Stationary bikes can be a great solution if you're feeling bloated and don't want to jostle your breasts or stomach, or when the weather is bad. They're safe and don't bounce you around, and you can watch TV or read while you work out. Work up to five days a week, aim for half an hour of biking, and add time and intensity as you are able.

Even if you can't get outdoors or to a gym, you can still do exercises indoors instead of simply sitting in front of the television. Weighted wristbands and heavier ankle bands can help you work on muscle flexibility and tone while you're seated or lying on the floor. (But don't try to walk wearing the ankle weights; you could trip.) Moving around on a birthing ball while seated on it or leaning over it can help to improve your flexibility by stretching muscles. Try putting on the music and amplifying everyday household chores with extra range-of-motion movements. Scrubbing the kitchen floor on your hands and knees can help to strengthen and stretch muscles of your lower back; plus, it gives you practice for positioning during childbirth.

Managing Your Care

Only one person is going to be delivering your baby: you! The most anyone else can do is help. It's important to find the care provider who can give you the best assistance and to find a delivery environment that suits your needs. Because the location determines what kind of care provider is available to you (doctors don't do home births, lay midwives don't work in hospitals) you may want to first consider your birth environment.

Facilities

GIVING BIRTH AT A HOSPITAL

Currently, and since the 1960s, 96 percent of American births happen in a hospital setting. Though many studies disprove it, American women seem to be universally convinced that hospitals are the only safe place to give birth. This may not be true.

If you're trying to choose between one hospital and another, know that they can differ greatly in the extent of services and facilities available to birthing mothers. Because most insurance plans offer women a choice of hospitals, competition between facilities means that labor and delivery suites have evolved to be quite luxurious. In most hospitals, babies are delivered by obstetricians, but many also offer deliveries by *Certified Nurse-Midwives*. (See CNMs, below.) Some hospitals offer water birth facilities, which can be quite a perk.

It used to be that mothers would labor in one room and then be whisked off into an operating room for delivery. Now, everything almost always occurs in one room, which may look like a hotel room with lots of high-tech equipment (with the exception of c-sections, which are

still performed in operating rooms).
All hospitals offer regular tours of
their birth and labor floors (see
page 79, "Taking a Hospital Tour"),
which really is the only way to
assess your options.

Facilities can vary, and so can
standards to protect hospital staff
from making errors or being liable
to claims of malpractice. Just as
you may have created a birth plan
for what you'd like to have happen,
hospitals have their own standards
and procedures for dealing with
mothers and babies during labor,
birth, and recovery.

Labor and delivery policies
can determine such standards as
whether or not patients are hooked
up to continual monitoring equipment when in labor; whether or not
IVs are routinely given; how often
during labor patients are given
pelvic exams; and when providers
are to intervene in labors. If a hospital has adopted a philosophy for
the "active management of labor,"
then there may be a rigid timeline
on how quickly your cervix must
dilate and at what point interventions, such as an induction or a
cesarean, may be initiated.

The only way to know about
these policies is to ask your care
provider or to take a separate personal tour of the labor and delivery
area of the hospital you are considering. Take time to talk with the
supervisor of nursing or other personnel on the floor. Get a feel for
what the nursing staff's attitude is
toward birth plans (see "Some Ideas
of What to Include in Your Birth
Plan" on page 90); about staffing
ratios and how common inductions
and c-sections are on the floor.

(For details about the admission
process and how to manage your
hospital birth, see pages 272 and
277.)

Pros:

• If you turn out to be one of the
8 to 16 percent[17] of moms whose
births become complicated, then
you'll already be in the hospital.

• The hospital may be the safest
place to be if your pregnancy's
high-risk or you've had complications in the past.

• A variety of pain medications are
available, including epidurals,
narcotics, and opiates.

• Hospital stays are covered by
health insurance, if you have any.

• You get to stay for forty-eight to
seventy-two hours after delivery.

• Everything you may need is provided, from meals to nightgowns.

• Because of competition for
patients, many hospitals in larger
towns have very well-decorated
and homey birthing rooms.

• Some hospitals offer aftercare
services–a nurse or postpartum
doula who will visit you at home
in the days that follow birth to
answer your questions and make
sure you're doing all right.

Cons:

• If you don't have health insurance, a $6,000 to $15,000 hospital
birth can be extremely expensive.

• If your pregnancy is low-risk,
medical interventions may come
with risks. For example, the risk
of having operative interventions
(such as forceps or vacuum

extraction of the baby) for a healthy, normal delivery is much higher than at home or at a birthing center.[18]

- You may be more likely to have a cesarean.

- Women who give birth in hospitals are more likely to suffer postpartum depression[19] and post-traumatic stress disorder.

- The majority of your medical care will be administered by multiple labor and delivery nurses, whose shifts come and go.

- With a large, rotating staff, your birth plan wishes may not be known or honored.

- The environment can be intimidating.

- Many hospitals are not family-centered: you may only be allowed one or two family members with you while you give birth.

FREESTANDING BIRTHING CENTERS

If you want to try to avoid medical interventions and don't want a home birth, having your baby at a birth center may be a good option for you.

Freestanding birthing centers (those not physically connected to a hospital) can look like converted houses or may be more clinical in feel. Almost all of them have examining rooms used for checkups during the course of pregnancy and home-like amenities for families to use while birthing is going on, such as comfortable chairs and kitchen facilities. Unless the birth center has an anesthesiologist and obstetrician

on staff, you will not be able to have an epidural or a cesarean there. Complications may mean an ambulance ride to the hospital. Almost all birth centers discourage the use of any kind of painkilling medication and encourage you to take Lamaze™ or Bradley classes to learn natural pain management techniques. Most birth centers also don't provide aftercare—within hours of giving birth, you will likely return home with your baby to recuperate in your own bed. If you're at a low risk for pregnancy complications, delivering at a birth center is probably as safe as giving birth at a hospital. You are also much less likely to have your labor induced or to have an episiotomy.

Pros:

- Birthing centers tend to be family-oriented: Your partner, parents, kids, and friends can come and go.

- You'll be tended to by a midwife and labor assistants (doulas) who may stay with you through the whole experience.

- Birthing centers tend to have a homey atmosphere.

Cons:

- May or may not be covered by your health insurance plan.

- You may have to recuperate in your own home.

- If complications arise, you'll have to take an ambulance to the emergency room.

- Pharmaceutical pain relief options may not be offered.

GIVING BIRTH AT HOME

Women who choose home birth tend to believe that birth is a private, family affair and a natural process that requires as little intervention as possible. If you choose to have a home birth, then you'll be able to give birth wherever you feel the most comfortable, with total control over your environment. You'll be able to involve your family and friends at your own discretion and will be able to handpick any professional who will be assisting you. Many women feel that home birth is a spiritual experience.

Still, complications do happen, and with a home birth, you and the midwife you select will have total responsibility. While most births go without a hitch, they're never without some level of risk, and if an emergency arises at home, there may be a delay in how quickly it can be dealt with.

If you're considering a home birth, be sure to hire a competent and experienced midwife. The midwife you select may specialize only in home births; work out of a freestanding birthing center; be affiliated with an obstetrical practice that is hospital-connected; or have her own hospital affiliation that enables her to admit patients and attend births on an as-needed basis.

If giving birth at home appeals to you, there are plenty of worthwhile books on the subject, plus Internet sites with good information and chat rooms (see *Resource Guide*, page 538) that will help you begin your preparations. In addition, you may want to connect with other families experienced with home birth through local midwives and childbirth organizations (see page 176).

Pros:

• The baby is delivered in the comfort of your own house.

• You can choose who will attend.

• Depending on your insurance coverage, it may be the least expensive option.

• Statistically, it reduces your risk of injury from medical intervention.[20]

Cons:

• You may not be able to be fully equipped for emergency situations.

• You will probably need to prepare your own supplies.

• It's not a good idea if you've had a complicated birth or cesarean section in the past.

• Birth is a messy process—someone will need to clean up.

WEIGHING YOUR OPTIONS

If you're not sure if you want to give birth in a hospital, a birthing center, or in your own home, consider interviewing more than one healthcare practitioner, accompanied by your partner, until you find the one that feels the most comfortable to the two of you and who is the most aligned with your values and your communication style.

Most obstetricians and midwives welcome a preliminary appointment before you actually make up your mind about becoming a patient. It's important to inquire about the provider's hospital affiliations and their basic philosophy about handling labor and medical interventions. If you're serious about avoiding a cesarean section or an *episiotomy*, having a routine surgical incision in your vaginal opening, or aren't sure about whether you want to use pain relief measures, then bring up these topics for discussion. If you interview more than one provider, the contrast between the two will help you form a clearer picture of the kinds of services and support that are the most important to you.

If at any point during your pregnancy, you find yourself no longer comfortable with your practitioner or your plan—perhaps because of nagging doubts, poor communication, or inadequate attention to your concerns, or simply because there's a mismatch of personalities—it's okay to switch care providers. It's your body, your baby, and your money. However, many providers may be reluctant to accept new patients later in pregnancy for fear of being left "holding the bag" if a previous provider mismanaged your care. So if you have doubts, it's better to switch sooner, rather than later.

Care provider options

The medical professional who supervises your care during your pregnancy, birth, and postpartum period will be a part of your life for about a year. You'll see her at least eleven or twelve times, more if your pregnancy has been labeled high risk. You need to have great faith in this person's judgment, communication skills, and medical training.

OBSTETRICIAN/ GYNECOLOGIST

An OB/GYN has a medical degree specializing in the medical issues of pregnancy and childbirth. Though the field is changing, there are still more male OB/GYNs than female. OB/GYNs may have their offices in a hospital or arranged in a group practice with other doctors or with midwives. As babies can be born any time of the day or night, it's becoming less common to find an OB/GYN who works solo (unless you live in a very, very small town). If your OB/GYN works in a practice, consider making appointments for prenatal checkups with other members of the practice as your pregnancy progresses. This way, you'll be familiar with the partner who shows up at the hospital.

Pros:

- OB/GYNs all have advanced medical training and skills in dealing with special situations, including surgical skills for performing c-sections, forceps deliveries, and vacuum extraction.

Cons:

- Statistically, OB/GYNs are more likely to intervene medically in your delivery, and patients of obstetricians are more likely to experience episiotomies, labor augumentation, continual fetal monitoring, and the use of instruments such as vacuum extractors and forceps during delivery.

- OB/GYNs may spend less time with you when you are in labor than a midwife.

FAMILY PRACTITIONER

You can also opt to have your baby delivered by a family practitioner. Family practitioners are doctors who spent at least four years of their medical training in an OB/GYN residency program. They've been trained in pediatrics, adult medicine, and obstetrics.

All family practitioners (FPs) must be licensed as physicians and may be board certified in family medicine. Family doctors can preside over regular vaginal deliveries, and some with further training can do operative vaginal deliveries using forceps or vacuum extraction. You'll probably give birth in a hospital where your family practitioner will be able to consult with an obstetrician if the pregnancy or the labor becomes complicated. In addition to postpartum care, family doctors can also provide care to both you and your baby after birth.

Pros:

- A family practitioner can provide a continuum of care, treating you and baby together.

Cons:

- Unlike obstetricians, a family practitioner may not be trained in surgical interventions.

CERTIFIED NURSE-MIDWIFE

A CNM is a nurse who has also graduated from a nationally accredited midwifery program. CNMs are certified and periodically reviewed by the certification council of the American College of Nurse-Midwives. They can practice in hospitals and/or birth centers, and some may attend home births. In all but two states, CNMs can prescribe medications. CNMs usually practice in collaborative relationships with physicians. They provide care for normal pregnancies, provide support during pregnancy and labor, and manage labor and deliver babies with the backup of an obstetrician in case surgical intervention becomes necessary or other complications arise. Most CNMs do not perform cesareans and don't accept patients that they believe to be at high risk for needing surgical intervention.

CNMs also attend to patients after birth, conduct postpartum exams, and advise patients about proper aftercare at home. CNMs also attend to women's ongoing health needs, such as annual exams and birth control. Some CNMs provide a wide range of pain-relief options during birth, such as water birthing, massage, or TENS machines. (See page 298 in *Your Guide to Giving Birth* section for more on pain relief options.) If they do their deliveries in hospitals, most will have access to medically based labor pain management, such as epidurals. (Epidurals are discussed on pages 317–322.)

Be sure to ask your certified nurse-midwife about the types of pain medication and comfort measures available to you. You can find CNMs in your area on the ACNM Web site at www.acnm.org.

Pros:

- Many CNMs will stay with you from your arrival at the hospital until the baby's born.

- CNMs are more likely than physicians or OB/GYNs to have knowledge of alternative pain-relief measures.

- Some CNMs will also offer postpartum care, which may include house calls and lactation consulting.

- CNMs usually have obstetrical backup in case of complications.

Cons:

- CNMs are not trained or authorized to perform surgical interventions except episiotomies.

- CNMs may not accept certain high-risk patients.

CERTIFIED PROFESSIONAL MIDWIFE

A CPM, also known as a direct entry or lay midwife, has graduated from a nationally accredited midwifery program but does not have a nursing degree. They may not be accredited to work in all states. Certified midwives are less likely to work in hospitals and more likely to be found in birth centers or attending to home births. This means that they may not have direct access to a backup physician in case of complications, which may mean that you'll have to take an ambulance to a local emergency room if something goes wrong. CPMs tend to either work in communities underserved by physicians or with women who believe that technological interventions such as constant fetal monitoring, epidural pain relief, and surgical interventions should be avoided. The best feature of CPMs is the atmosphere they provide: an unhurried and family-centered environment.

Pros:

- Midwives can offer a more intimate atmosphere for delivery, such as a birth center or your home.

- If you don't have health insurance, a midwife is the least expensive option.

Cons:

- Without a nursing degree, midwives are not allowed to deliver in hospitals.

- Midwives are not trained or authorized to perform surgical interventions.
- Midwives may not accept certain high-risk patients.
- Depending on individual practices, it's possible that a midwife may not have medical backup other than the local emergency room.

Remember that it's not just the care provider who matters, but also the environment that they work in. You are less likely to be in continual contact with your doctor during your delivery, especially if your baby decided to be born at night or labor takes a long time. However, you will probably receive excellent support from labor and delivery nurses in the hospital. On the other hand, a midwife may be more likely to stay by your side.

Other professionals you may encounter

MATERNAL-FETAL MEDICINE SPECIALIST (PERINATOLOGIST)

A perinatologist is an obstetrician who, in addition to medical school, has also completed a three-year clinical and research fellowship to become a specialist in high-risk pregnancies, diagnostic prenatal tests, and fetal therapies. Perinatologists receive training in diagnosing fetal problems with ultrasound and can perform amniocentesis, CVS (chorionic villus sampling), and other procedures. If necessary, they can administer medications to the fetus, and some are even trained to perform surgery on fetuses in utero.

If your pregnancy has a higher-than-normal risk of complications (see *Managing High-Risk Conditions* on page 211) because you're carrying multiples, have a pre-existing condition, or have test results that show your baby has a higher-than-normal chance of a health problem, you may wish to consult with a perinatologist. Depending on your insurance company, you may also be able to select a perinatologist as the primary care provider for your pregnancy. A perinatologist can also help you locate other specialists, such as an appropriate neonatologist (doctor specializing in newborns) to care for the baby after she is born.

Perinatologists should be board certified through the American Board of Obstetrics and Gynecology, which is recognized by the American Board of Medical Specialties.

DOULA, LABOR ASSISTANT, OR MONTRICE

If you're opting for a hospital-based birth, and can afford it, it makes good sense to also think about hiring a labor coach, birthing assistant, or doula—a person dedicated to helping you during your entire labor experience. Hiring your own assistants saves you from depending on nurses who have other laboring women to monitor and who leave the hospital when their shifts change.

Studies have shown that the continuous presence of a support person at a birth reduces the likelihood of taking medication during labor for pain relief, requiring medical interventions, undergoing a cesarean delivery, or giving birth to a baby that is unresponsive, with a five-minute Apgar score of less than seven (see "Apgar Score" in *Your Guide to Giving Birth*). Continuous labor support has also been associated with a slight reduction in the length of labor.

Some hospitals offer labor assistant services, which may or may not be covered by insurance.

Labor assistance charges vary, but usually are between $250 and $800 per delivery. Some doulas-in-training may provide support for little or no fee.

LABOR AND DELIVERY NURSES

If you give birth in a hospital with an obstetrician, much of your care will be provided by labor and delivery nurses. These days, they do about everything: dole out the drugs, check your dilation by a pelvic exam, monitor your contractions and the baby's heart rate, bring you ice chips, and fluff your pillow. You won't have a choice about who they are, and there's no way to get to know them beforehand (unless your town or hospital is extremely small). As with any group of professionals, the majority are skilled and dedicated, but it's always possible to

---

Conditions That May Require a Hospital Birth

- If you have type 1 or gestational diabetes. (See *Managing High-Risk Conditions* on page 216.)

- If there is a significant risk that your baby will be born with a congenital disorder. (See "Testing: Risks and Benefits" on page 179.)

- If you have high blood pressure or pregnancy-induced hypertension. (See *Managing High-Risk Conditions* on page 214.)

- If you have a low blood count in the week prior to delivery. (See "Anemia" on page 367.)

- If you have a chronic illness such as lupus, heart disease, or kidney disease.

- If you have had a cesarean delivery before.

- If your baby is in **breech**, heads up, position.

catch someone on an off day. How much attention you get from the labor and delivery staff will depend very much on the size of the hospital and how busy the hospital is when you're delivering. A labor and delivery nurse should only have to care for one other patient while caring for you. While many hospitals may have this policy, only California mandates this ratio by law. On the hospital tour, ask about the hospital's policy for calling in extra nurses if the ward gets busy.

Childbirth classes

There are many good reasons to educate yourself about the process of labor and birth. Studies have shown that women who felt that childbirth was something being done to them, as opposed to feeling involved in the process, were far more vulnerable to postpartum emotional disorders, such as depression and **post-traumatic birth disorder**. Childbirth classes are also important for your partner. He also needs to know what to expect and how to be supportive. If he feels alienated from the process of pregnancy and birth, education can help him become more involved.

There's also the social aspect of childbirth classes. You'll get to meet other couples going through the same thing, a camaraderie that has forged many a lifelong friendship and/or toddler playgroup. Your un-pregnant friends may be tired of tales of your stretch marks, but not this group.

And finally, childbirth educators themselves are a great resource. After meeting hundreds of couples, they know the real lowdown on all kinds of topics: where to get a good prenatal massage, who the best pediatricians are in town, good lotions for an itchy belly, and sometimes even what other patients have had to say about your care provider.

How can you find these classes?

Although all courses should cover what to expect during labor and birth, pain management, common medical procedures, and newborn care, different courses have different philosophies. Your best bet is to get an idea of your own birth philosophy, and find a class whose approach you agree with. If you just want the basics, and you want them fast, consider a weekend hospital class. If you're dedicated to breastfeeding and want to focus on that, drop in on a free La Leche League meeting. If you want to avoid surgical interventions, try Bradley™ or Lamaze™.

Most preparation courses go for about six to twelve weeks and will be designed to end a week or two before your due date. Some groups, such as Bradley, may also offer classes during the first trimester, which can be quite helpful.

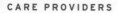

Care Providers for Pregnancy and Childbirth

TITLE	CREDENTIALS
PERINATOLOGIST	An obstetrician specializing in high-risk pregnancies. In addition to basic obstetrics and gynecology training, the perinatologist has completed a two- or three-year clinical and research fellowship. During this fellowship, he or she receives advanced training in comprehensive diagnostic ultrasound imaging of the fetus and in the management of medically complicated pregnancies.
OBSTETRICIAN/ GYNECOLOGIST (OB/GYN)	A licensed medical doctor who has completed three additional years of residency specializing in family medical care including obstetrics.
FAMILY PRACTITIONER (FP)	A licensed medical doctor who has completed three additional years of residency specializing in family medical care including obstetrics.
CERTIFIED NURSE-MIDWIFE (CNM), AND CERTIFIED MIDWIFE (CM)	A CNM is a registered nurse with a minimum of two years of advanced training in normal obstetrics and women's health care. A certified midwife (CM) is a professionally educated midwife who was not first educated as a nurse. Both certifications require a bachelor's, master's, or other advanced degree, and the midwife must pass a national exam.

ROLE	PROFESSIONAL ORGANIZATION
Usually hired on referral from an OB. They have advanced diagnostic skills and may perform invasive tests such as *amniocentesis* or chorionic villus sampling (CVS). May also deliver babies in certain high-risk circumstances, such as multiple births or when a mother suffers from a serious illness.	American Medical Association (AMA) American College of Obstetricians and Gynecologists (ACOG) www.acog.org Society of Maternal-Fetal Medicine (SMFM)
Usually work in group practices, perform deliveries in hospitals, and manage normal deliveries as well as deliveries that require medical intervention.	American Academy of Family Physicians (AAFP) www.aafp.org
May be a member of a group or individual practice. Do vaginal deliveries, but not all perform cesareans, but are likely to have collaborative agreements with obstetricians who do. They also can take care of your baby and family after birth.	American Academy of Family Physicians (AAFP) www.aafp.org www.familydoctor.org
Can be a member of a group of midwives, or a group of physicians and midwives, or individual practice, or employed by a hospital. Vaginal deliveries only. Will have collaborative agreements with obstetricians who provide backup in case of emergency. CMs and CNMs also offer postnatal health care and lactation support.	American College of Nurse-Midwives (ACNM) www.acnm.org

Care Providers for Pregnancy and Childbirth

TITLE	CREDENTIALS
CERTIFIED PROFESSIONAL MIDWIFE (CPM)	A Certified Professional Midwife is an independent practitioner who has met the standards for certification set by the North American Registry of Midwives (NARM). Requires successful completion of both a written exam and a skills assessment as well as training in birth centers or other out-of-hospital settings.
DOULA	A doula assists mothers and their partners during the process of birth. Most have special training, have read numerous books on birth and birth support, and are skilled in providing comfort measures for mothers. Postpartum doulas specialize in helping mothers and their newborns. A series of organizations train and/or certify doulas.

ROLE

PROFESSIONAL ORGANIZATION

Certified midwives are found in birth centers, attending to home births, and in hospitals. They perform vaginal deliveries only.

North American Registry of Midwives
www.narm.org

Doulas work in hospitals or birth centers, or attend home births. They're there for your comfort and to support you, but are not directly involved with assisting in delivery itself. Doulas can also be certified to assist mothers and their newborns.

Association of Labor Assistants and Childbirth Educators (ALACE)
www.alace.org

Doulas of North America
www.dona.org

MAJOR U.S. ORGANIZATIONS OFFERING PRENATAL EDUCATION

On a national level, the "big three" parent support organizations that train instructors to teach prenatal classes and oversee classes are the International Association for Childbirth Education (ICEA), the American Academy of Husband-Coached Childbirth (known as "The Bradley Method"), and Lamaze™ International.

La Leche League International also offers a free four-session course for pregnant and new mothers, which includes breastfeeding how-tos, birth topics, nutrition during pregnancy and after birth, and toddler nursing and weaning.

The Maternity Center Association is a national advocacy organization that also offers prenatal classes in the New York area and hosts an informative Web site to help families in making research-based, informed decisions regarding pregnancy and labor. The Centering Pregnancy and Parenting Association is an up-and-coming organization that provides prenatal care with education. (For more listings about pregnancy support organizations, see our *Resource Guide* starting on page 538.)

International Childbirth Education Association (ICEA)

Founded in 1960, this organization has more than twelve thousand members. The purpose of ICEA is to further the educational, physical, and emotional preparation of expectant parents for childbearing and breastfeeding. It also works to increase the public's awareness of current issues related to childbearing. The organization is committed to increasing parental participation in childbirth and to minimizing interventions in uncomplicated labors. It offers teacher certification programs for childbirth educators, conducts workshops, and operates a mail-order bookstore offering informative books on pregnancy, childbirth, breastfeeding, and parenting issues. ICEA-certified educators are usually found in hospitals, birth centers, churches, and community centers, or they may offer courses out of their own homes. ICEA also certifies doulas, and fitness and postnatal educators who can be located using its Web site.

Lamaze™ International

Lamaze International, formerly the American Society for Psychoprophylaxis in Obstetrics (ASPO), was founded in 1960 and currently has more than three thousand members, including physicians, nurses, nurse-midwives, parents who advocate for normal birth, and Lamaze Certified Childbirth Educators, who instruct parents in the Lamaze philosophy of childbirth and parenting. The organization is best known for its breathing and relaxation techniques; however, an array of labor skills and comfort measures are taught in Lamaze classes. Courses are based on the philosophy of supporting birth as normal, natural, and healthy and have the goal of empowering women to make informed decisions regarding their birthing options.

The organization's newly founded Lamaze Institute for Normal Birth sponsors mini-grants for the development of Birth Networks, which are local groups that provide support, education, and evidence-based information on interventions for parents and serve as a resource for caregivers who support normal birth. Lamaze also sponsors education workshops, forums, films, and written materials on childbirth, and it holds an annual international conference focusing on childbirth and topics of interest to professionals and parents. Its Web site includes a locator service for Lamaze childbirth educators and informative articles on pregnancy, childbirth, and breastfeeding and an online bookstore, which provides recommended resources that support normal birth and confident early parenting. Membership for parents is $40 a year and includes a subscription to *Genesis*, a quarterly newsletter.

The six care practices which support the Lamaze philosophy of normal birth are allowing labor to begin on its own without intervention (avoiding induction); non-supine positions for birth; allowing freedom of movement during childbirth; continuous support during labor; avoiding routine labor interventions; and keeping mother and baby together after birth.

American Academy of Husband-Coached Childbirth (The Bradley™ Method)

Founded in 1970 with more than 1,200 members, the organization advocates the Bradley Method of birth, named for obstetrician Robert A. Bradley, M.D. The Academy offers resources, information, film showings, lectures, workshops, and a national affiliation for Bradley Method teachers.

The method emphasizes the goal of an unmedicated, natural childbirth and teaches couples how to be effective consumers of medical services with the right to question medical intervention and to take responsibility for their own birth outcome.

Classes are based on a twelve-point list of endorsements: natural childbirth as the safest way to have a baby (in the absence of medical complications); active participation of husband as coach; excellent nutrition as the foundation for a healthy pregnancy; avoidance of drugs unless absolutely necessary; early classes starting in the sixth month; relaxation and natural breathing; tuning-in to one's body; immediate and continuous contact with newborn; breastfeeding; communicating with medical professionals; responsibility for the safety of the birth place; procedures based on education; and preparation for the unexpected.

La Leche League International (LLLI)

Founded in 1956, La Leche League has more than forty thousand members in three thousand–plus groups with more than 7,200 accredited leaders around the world. It sponsors 550 breastfeeding resource centers in forty-eight countries. The focus of the league is to help mothers to breastfeed through mother-to-mother support, encouragement, information, and education. Accredited leaders are volunteers who guide LLLI meetings, which are typically held once a month in homes in most communities. Most league groups list their numbers in the white pages of telephone directories and offer free, around-the-clock advice and counseling for breastfeeding mothers. The monthly topics of these meetings include breastfeeding, childbirth, nutrition during pregnancy, weaning, and toddler management. The national headquarters maintains a breastfeeding resource center, publishes brochures and articles of interest, and offers books, products, and brochures for sale. The $36 a year membership fee includes a subscription to *New Beginnings*, a bi-monthly journal. Most states have annual league conferences, and LLLI sponsors a semi-annual international conference as well as an annual conference for physicians.

Maternity Center Association (MCA)

Founded in 1918, the association is a coalition of laypersons and parents, physicians, nurses, nurse-midwives, childbirth educators, and public health workers interested in improving maternity care, maternal and infant health, and family life. The goals of MCA are to expand families' access to maternity care through collaboration, education, publications, consulting services, public policy initiatives, and demonstration projects, and it is involved in midwifery education. Its New York headquarters has a library of more than 2,500 volumes and additional reference materials on childbirth and maternity care. MCA publishes booklets and teaching aids and holds an annual meeting and periodic seminars on prenatal care topics.

The Centering Pregnancy and Parenting Association (CPPA)

Founded in 1994, CPPA is a new approach to prenatal care, merging routine prenatal care appointments with group childbirth education. After an initial obstetrical exam, women in a Centering Pregnancy program join with eight to twelve other expectant mothers or couples who have similar due dates. The groups meet monthly during the first six or seven months of pregnancy, then bi-weekly thereafter. With the group approach, mothers are responsible for their own self-care activities, including keeping their own charts for growth, weight, and blood pressure. Group members complete self-assessment sheets that stimulate group discussion about mutually shared pregnancy issues. At each meeting, a practitioner listens to babies' heartbeats, checks for uterine growth, and encourages women to talk about specific problems and concerns. Discussion topics, which are group-directed, include nutrition, exercise, relaxation, sexuality, domestic relations, pregnancy problems, infant care and feeding, postpartum issues, comfort measures, and parenting. A $50 membership fee to CPPA includes a subscription to *Circuit*, the organization's newsletter, as well as discounts for pamphlets, supplies, and workshops. CPPA's Web site offers connections to groups nationwide.

Online pregnancy classes

Thanks to the Internet, you can now take childbirth classes on your own time, which is good for working mothers with a busy schedule.

(See the *Resource Guide* for more information.) Many sites have been built to offer guided classes that you can read at your convenience. You'll miss out on the social aspects of birth classes, but do consider an online course as a supplement to your learning.

Genetic defects and testing

BIRTH DEFECTS: WHAT ARE THEY?

A birth defect is any type of mental or physical abnormality caused by either a genetic or environmental factor.

The good news is that thousands of genetic conditions have been identified so far, and many can be diagnosed by prenatal tests such as the Quad Screen blood tests, ultrasound, amniocentesis, and chorionic villus sampling (CVS). (Amniocentesis and choronic villus sampling are invasive procedures and carry a small risk of miscarriage.) These tests can identify more than ninety-five percent of disorders, including *Down syndrome*, trisomies, *hydrocephaly*, *anencephaly*, *spina bifida* (neural tube defects), *cleft lip* and *cleft palate*, pyloric stenosis, *omphalocele*, Huntington's Disease, muscular dystrophy, hip dislocation, and *clubfoot*.

Other blood screening tests can determine if one or both parents carry the gene for a specific disorder, such as screening tests for cystic fibrosis, most common in Caucasians; sickle-cell anemia, most common in African-Americans; *beta thalassemia*, most common in Greeks and Italians; *alpha thalassemia*, most common in Southeast Asians; and Tay-Sachs disease, most common in Ashkenazi Jews.

Non-genetic problems are those caused by environmental factors, such as alcohol consumption, obesity, or exposure to a *teratogen* (any substance that causes developmental malformations). As we mentioned on page 20 of *Your Pregnancy Week-by-Week*, if the fetus is damaged in the early weeks of pregnancy—in the time period before you knew you were pregnant—the pregnancy will most likely end in miscarriage. However, after the first few weeks, exposure to alcohol, drugs, or toxins can affect the development of a baby's organs and brain.

GENETIC DISORDERS

If you or your partner has a family history of genetic disease, your care provider will probably suggest that you take tests to show whether or not your baby has been affected. All of the genetic disorders below can be detected with CVS testing.

Genetic disorders are caused by abnormal genes or abnormal chromosomes, which can be the result of inheritance or mutation. Some disorders are passed by parent carriers that may affect only babies of a certain sex, such as disorders that are passed by mothers to their baby boys. For instance, Fragile-X is a condition that causes mental retardation and affects one in one thousand to one in two thousand babies, mostly males. If one parent has a dominant gene for a disease, or both parents carry the recessive gene for a disease, there is a chance that the child will inherit the gene.

Some ethnic groups and individuals from specific geographic areas are more at risk of certain genetic disorders. About four percent of Caucasians of Northern European descent carry the cystic fibrosis (CF) gene, and the disorder is rare in blacks and Asians. It is an inherited disorder of metabolism that affects the cells that line certain glands in a child's body. Children with CF have ongoing lung problems, digestive problems, and a shortened life expectancy. Complications may require medical interventions, and physical and respiratory therapy can help. Because CF results from as many as two hundred different alterations of the CF gene, it makes screening of parents as carriers a challenge, but it is currently possible to detect eighty-five percent of all carriers.

If there is an indication that your baby may have a birth defect, then you should seek genetic counseling for support and to discuss possible risks to your baby.

Chances of Having a Baby with a Birth Defect

Birth defects are any physical or mental abnormality present at birth. To put your baby's risk into perspective, your chance of having twins is 2.9 in 100[21] and of having triplets is 1 in 10,000.[22] (You'll find most of these conditions defined in more detail in the *Pregnancy Dictionary*, which begins on page 573.)

Heart defect. 1 out of 200 babies,[23] with 36 percent to mothers with diabetes.

Club foot (talipes). 1 out of 750 babies;[24] twice as common in boys than girls.

Cleft lip or palate. Cleft lip, 1 out of 800 babies; cleft palate, 1 out of 2,000 babies.

Down syndrome. About 1 in 1,250 for a woman at age 25; 1 in 1,000 at 30; 1 in 400 at 35; and 1 in 100 at age 40.[25]

Spina bifida. 1 out of 2,000 babies.

Down syndrome

Down syndrome, also commonly known as trisomy 21 (for the extra copy of the twenty-first chromosome), is the most frequently occurring genetic condition in the U.S. It affects approximately one out of every eight hundred to one thousand newborns. The risk of having a baby with Down syndrome increases with the mother's age. While a mother who is twenty years old has only a one in two thousand chance of giving birth to a baby with this condition, a mother who is forty-two has a one in seventy chance.

Children with Down syndrome often have distinctive physical characteristics, such as a flat facial profile (depressed nasal bridge and small nose) and an upward slant to the eye. Additionally, children with Down syndrome may have physical problems and other health concerns, as well as varying degrees of mental retardation.

Trisomy 18 and trisomy 13, other types of chromosomal disorders, are rarer disorders where extra chromosomes are involved. These disorders so severely affect babies that they rarely live more than two years.

Phenylketonuria

Phenylketonuria (PKU) is a genetic disorder that affects one out of every ten thousand babies. It disrupts normal metabolism and can result in mental retardation if a child's diet is not carefully regulated. Most newborns are tested for PKU at birth.

Thalassemia

Thalassemia is a group of related types of anemia caused by a mutation to the genes that produce hemoglo-

bin. The effects of the mutation can be minor and cause no symptoms, or they can be life-threatening. The two main types are called alpha and beta thalassemia, depending on which part of an oxygen-carrying protein (called hemoglobin) is lacking in the red blood cells.

Alpha thalassemia is found mainly in Africa, the Middle East, India, Southeast Asia, southern China, and sometimes the Mediterranean region. People whose hemoglobin does not produce enough alpha protein have alpha thalassemia. Most individuals with alpha thalassemia have mild forms of the disease.

Beta thalassemia is most commonly found in people of Greek and Italian descent and is also found in the Middle East. The most severe form of beta thalassemia is thalassemia major, or Cooley's anemia, which causes a life-threatening anemia that requires regular blood transfusions and extensive ongoing medical care.

Sickle-cell anemia

Sickle-cell anemia is a genetic blood condition that causes severe anemia. It mainly affects people of African, West Indian, and Mediterranean origin. In the U.S., approximately seven to eight percent of all African-Americans carry a gene for the disease. Carriers may not have symptoms of the trait. If both parents actually suffer from the condition, the baby will be affected. The implications of this should be discussed with your midwife or doctor.

A child with sickle-cell anemia will have blood cells that are limited in their ability to carry oxygen. Symptoms include anemia, fatigue,

Common Screening and Diagnostic Tests

NAME OF TEST	WHY IT'S PERFORMED	WHEN IT'S PERFORMED
URINALYSIS	To screen for sugar, indicating a diabetic condition; protein, which may indicate preeclampsia or a urinary tract infection (UTI); bacteria or blood cells, which would also indicate a UTI; or ketones, which would indicate dehydration or diabetes.	Sugar and protein screening at each prenatal visit, starting with the first; bacteria, blood cells, or ketones if your care provider suspects a problem.
BLOOD PRESSURE	To determine if you have unusually high or low blood pressure and to provide a baseline reading for later during pregnancy. High blood pressure (hypertension) can be a serious problem for both mother and baby.	At each visit to your healthcare provider.
VAGINAL SWAB	To check for the presence of certain bacteria, such as yeast and Group B Strep.	Usually performed at your first prenatal visit and between weeks thirty-five and thirty-seven LMP.
RH FACTOR SCREENING	To determine if you are Rh negative, which may cause your antibodies to attack your baby's blood if the baby is Rh positive.	During the first prenatal visit. If you are Rh negative, you should get a Rhogam injection around the twenty-eighth week of pregnancy or after any procedure with the potential to cause your and your baby's blood to come into contact.

HOW IT'S DONE

You urinate in a cup, then a nurse or technician inserts a paper dipstick that will instantly indicate the presence of sugar, protein, or ketones by changing color. For blood or bacteria, the sample is examined under a microscope.

ACCURACY & RISKS

Considered highly accurate. No risk to you or your baby.

An expanding cuff is fastened around your upper arm and inflated by squeezing a small bulb. Your pulse is monitored with a stethoscope with a dial indicating pressure readings. Considered to be accurate, although nervousness can affect blood pressure readings.

There is no known risk to you or your baby.

A swab is used to take a vaginal cell sample, which is then examined under a microscope.

No risks; one hundred percent accurate.

Blood is drawn and examined under a microscope to detect the presence of a protein called D Antigen on the surface of your red blood cells.

Highly accurate. No risk to you or your baby.

Common Screening and Diagnostic Tests

NAME OF TEST	WHY IT'S PERFORMED	WHEN IT'S PERFORMED
CHORIONIC VILLUS SAMPLING (CVS)	It is used to detect Down syndrome, cystic fibrosis, hemophilia, Huntington's disease, sickle-cell anemia, thalassemia, muscular dystrophy, and other genetic disorders.	Usually performed between eight and twelve weeks LMP.
ULTRASOUND (Sonogram)	May be used in the first trimester to detect a fetal heartbeat, to confirm your due date, or to rule out an ectopic pregnancy. Later, it may be used to find certain anomalies in the baby; to determine a baby's age; or to make sure the baby is positioned safely for invasive tests, such as CVS or amniocentesis.	At any stage of pregnancy, usually routinely during the eighteenth and twenty-second weeks.
AMNIOCENTESIS ("Amnio")	It is used to detect chromosomal defects, neural tube defects, certain diseases, chemical problems, and to assess a baby's lung maturity.	Fifteenth to sixteenth week of pregnancy (early amniocentesis is twelve to fourteen weeks).

HOW IT'S DONE

A small tube (catheter) is threaded into the cervix, or via a needle inserted through the abdomen to obtain a small sample of chorionic villi.

Ultrasound during the first trimester is usually done with a transvaginal probe. Later ultrasounds use an abdominal transducer to bounce high-frequency sound waves off your baby to produce an image on a screen.

A needle will be inserted through your abdomen into the amniotic sac to obtain a small amount of fluid.

ACCURACY & RISKS

About 98 percent accurate at detecting 95 percent of genetic disorders. Miscarriages occur in approximately one out of one hundred women.

It is accurate 25 to 75 percent of the time, depending upon what it is seeking, when it is done during pregnancy, and how skilled the technician (sonographer) is. The age of a fetus is best determined during the first trimester, screening for fetal anomalies between eighteen and twenty-two weeks. No specific risks have yet been identified for you or your baby.

Accuracy approaches 100 percent for 95 percent of genetic disorders. Although rare, the procedure can introduce infection into the womb, cause the rupture of the membranes, induce pre-term labor, or strike the baby with the needle. Miscarriages occur in approximately 1 in 250 women.

Common Screening and Diagnostic Tests

NAME OF TEST	WHY IT'S PERFORMED	WHEN IT'S PERFORMED
GLUCOSE TOLERANCE TEST	Detects the rate at which your body processes glucose (blood sugar). A high level of glucose indicates gestational diabetes.	Weeks twenty-five to twenty-eight if you have no history of gestational diabetes, earlier if you have risk factors or your care provider suspects a problem.
NONSTRESS TEST	Records uterine contractions over a period of time (usually twenty minutes) and judges the reaction of the baby's heart rate to contractions and movement.	Given in the third trimester, if the baby is past due, or if problems are suspected.
BIOPHYSICAL PROFILE	A test to assess the health of an unborn baby. Includes a nonstress test and also uses an ultrasound to look for breathing rate, movements, muscle tone, and the volume of amniotic fluid in the amniotic sac.	Given in the third trimester, if the baby is past due, or if problems are suspected.

HOW IT'S DONE

ACCURACY & RISKS

You drink a glucose-rich liquid, and an hour later, your blood is tested to detect levels of glucose.

No risks, other than possible nausea or vomiting after drinking the liquid.

Two belts, one with a uterine monitor and one with a fetal monitor, are placed around your abdomen and connected to a computer. Contractions and the baby's heart rate are printed out on graph paper. You may also be given a button to push when you feel the baby move. An increase in the baby's heart rate is a healthy response, called an acceleration.

No known risks. The test is not painful.

In addition to the nonstress test (above), ultrasound is used to observe a baby's body and breathing movements and measure the volume of amniotic fluid.

No risks.

delayed growth, and developmental problems. The clogging of blood vessels by abnormally shaped red blood cells can cause severe attacks of pain. Blood tests are used to determine carriers.

Tay-Sachs

People of Ashkenazi Jewish and French Canadian ancestry have the greatest chance of being carriers of Tay-Sachs disease, an enzymatic disorder. The chances of Ashkenazi Jews carrying this disorder are as high as one in thirty. Children with this condition die early in childhood. It's about eight times as common in these groups as with the general population. The disease results from a buildup of certain enzymes in the brain, and can be fatal in early childhood. There is presently no effective treatment for Tay-Sachs disease, so at-risk populations are urged to undergo genetic counseling and testing.

Testing: risks and benefits

RH-FACTOR SCREENING

During your first visit to your care provider, he ordered a blood test to check for the presence of a certain protein, called D Antigen, in your red blood cells. If your blood lacks this protein (is Rh negative), and your baby's blood has it (is Rh positive), then there's a chance that antibodies in your blood may attack the baby's blood. If this happens, the newborn can develop a condition called fetal erythroblastosis, a blood disease that causes anemia and jaundice.

If you're Rh negative, you'll need to get a Rhogam injection, usually around your twenty-eighth week of pregnancy, to stop your body from producing an antibody that may harm a future baby's blood.

The injection may be given earlier if you undergo an invasive test or procedure that has the potential to cause your and your baby's blood to come into contact. If you are Rh negative, you will also receive the injection if you miscarry.

The injection is usually given in your buttocks while you stand up. Your baby, if she turns out to be Rh positive, will also get an injection within seventy-two hours after birth.

GROUP B STREP

The American Academy of Pediatrics (AAP) and the Centers for Disease Control and Prevention (CDC) currently recommend that all pregnant women be screened for Group B Strep at thirty-five to thirty-seven weeks, with a simple swab test. Group B Strep (GBS) is an infection found in the genitals, rectum, and urinary tract of ten to thirty-five percent of pregnant women. It causes no symptoms and is not a sexually transmitted disease—streptococcal bacteria are naturally occurring in the human body. It's not the same as Group A Strep, which causes Strep throat. If you have a previous history of preterm labor, you may be tested earlier. If your care provider doesn't test you, you should ask to be tested. Only about one in two hundred babies exposed to the bacteria during birth will get a Group B Strep infection, but for those who do, it can be serious. Babies can contract meningitis, pneumonia, and blood infections (sepsis), and some can have brain, lung, or hearing damage, or more rarely, can die. If you're found to have Group B Strep, you'll be given a course of antibiotics and intravenous antibiotics during delivery. If you're allergic to antibiotics, make sure your healthcare provider is aware of this.

If your baby contracts Group B Strep, he will be given a ten-day course of antibiotics after birth.

CHORIONIC VILLUS SAMPLING (CVS)

CVS is a test which samples a fetus's genetic material to detect the presence of certain disorders, such as Tay-Sachs disease, thalassemia, cystic fibrosis, and Down syndrome. It should be considered if you have a family history of specific genetic disorders or if you are concerned that your age has put your baby at risk for a genetic disorder. Consider undergoing genetic counseling first to make the best possible assessment of your risk.

As opposed to amnio, CVS may involve a higher risk of causing you to miscarry a healthy baby. Approximately one pregnancy out of one hundred miscarries from the procedure (amnio is 1 in 250).[26] As with amnio, however, the so-called "loss rate" varies between doctors, and is lower with doctors who perform the procedure more frequently. Ask your doctor what his or her loss rate is. The test also may carry risks for limb defects as well. However, the test's main advantage is that it can be performed early on, between the eighth and twelfth weeks LMP, while amnio can't be performed for another month. If you're certain that you will terminate a pregnancy with major defects, knowing now as opposed to a month from now is obviously pretty important.

The CVS test involves extracting and analyzing a small piece of chorion from the placental tissue of the fetus. CVS can detect many of the same defects as amniocentesis except open neural tube defects.

If you have a CVS test, you'll have an ultrasound prior to and during the procedure. A CVS can be performed two ways, depending on the position of your placenta: transabdominally (through the abdomen) or transcervically (through the cervix).

If a transcervical CVS test is performed, a speculum will be inserted into the vagina to give the doctor access to the cervix, and the area will be cleansed with an antiseptic solution. Ultrasound will be used to help guide a thin plastic catheter (about the size of a toothpick) through the cervix to the placenta. The doctor will then withdraw a small piece of chorionic villi, the cells in the tissue along the edge of the developing placenta. The catheter does not enter the amniotic sac, and it does not touch the fetus. The sampling usually takes from two to five minutes and is not painful. If the collected sample is too small, another attempt may need to be performed. After the procedure, you may experience some spotting or mild cramping.

A transabdominal CVS test is very similar to an amniocentesis, except that villi are extracted instead of amniotic fluid. Ultrasound will be used to determine the position of the baby, and your abdomen may be numbed with an injection of local anesthetic. Then, ultrasound is used to guide a hollow needle to the chorion at the edge of the placenta. In a transabdominal test, the needle does enter the amniotic sac, but it should not touch the fetus. The test should take no longer than half an hour. After the procedure, you may experience cramping or bruising at the injection site.

If your blood is Rh negative, you will need to receive a Rhogam shot after the test, in case you and your baby's blood came into contact during the procedure.

After either test, the tissue sample will be sent to a laboratory, where the cells will be allowed to multiply. Then the cells will be stained with a special dye that binds to specific regions of the chromosomes. The cells will then be viewed under a strong microscope and photographed, and the chromosomes will be counted and examined for structural abnormalities.[27] The CVS test will also be able to tell you the baby's gender conclusively.

With either type of test, you will typically receive results within a

week, though some labs may be able to release results as soon as twenty-four hours. If you experience heavy bleeding, painful cramping, a fever, chills, or flu-like symptoms after the test, contact your care provider right away.

QUAD SCREEN (AFP)

The Quad Screen is a test that checks the levels of alpha-feto protein (AFP), human chorionic gonadotropin (hCG), and the hormones estriol and inhibin in your bloodstream. It's usually performed between weeks fifteen and eighteen. High levels of AFP may mean that the baby has a neural tube defect, and lower-than-normal levels may indicate Down syndrome. Elevated levels of hCG can indicate chromosomal abnormalities, as can lower-than-normal levels of estriol.

The Quad Screen has a fairly high detection rate. Abnormal chemical levels will reveal about 82 percent of cases of neural tube defects and about 74 percent of Down syndrome cases. But the Quad Screen also has a high false-positive rate—95 percent of women who receive a positive result are actually carrying healthy babies. Because this is a screening test, it can only alert you to the possibility of a problem, and a positive result will (with your consent, of course) lead to more testing procedures, such as an ultrasound or amniocentesis. You may want to ask your healthcare provider for a referral to a perinatologist who has extra training in testing procedure and interpretation.

ULTRASOUND

A detailed ultrasound between weeks eighteen and twenty-two LMP can detect approximately sixty to seventy percent of fetuses with anomalies.[28] If you're told that something on your ultrasound looks abnormal, don't panic—schedule another one, preferably with a perinatologist or a radiologist with a lot of experience. Technicians, who have varying degrees of ability, perform most ultrasounds. Because they aren't doctors or nurses, they are not authorized to make a diagnosis—this is done by a radiologist or perinatologist who will look at specific images and measurements collected by the technician. It may take a few days for your care provider to receive a report from the test, and you will probably only be notified if something appears abnormal.

If your pregnancy is high risk, or if screening tests have detected the possibility of a defect, your ultrasound may be performed by a perinatologist or radiologist instead of a technician.

The ultrasound test takes about fifteen to twenty minutes and is completely painless. You lie on a table with your belly exposed, and the technician or doctor covers your stomach with a cold gel. Then the technician or doctor moves a transducer painlessly up and down on your stomach, like a small Dustbuster. The transducer directs sound waves toward your uterus and fetus, and the sound waves bounce back at different frequencies to create a black-and-white image, with bones showing up as white, fluid as black, and tissues as gray. The technician can move in, out, and around the image, and take photos and measurements. These images can detect potential structural problems in a fetus as well as evaluate complications that you may have had, such as bleeding.

A nuchal translucency scan is an ultrasound that checks the thickness of the stem of the back of your baby's neck. If it is thicker than normal, your baby is at increased risk for chromosomal abnormalities such as Down syndrome. The test, combined with a blood test for two pregnancy-related proteins (free-beta hCG and PAPP-A), detects about eighty-five percent of abnormalities. This scan is usually offered at about ten to fourteen weeks. If this screening test is positive, it doesn't mean that your baby is abnormal—only that there is enough of an increased risk of a problem that you may wish to consider additional tests, such as chorionic villus sampling (CVS) or an amniocentesis.

An anomaly scan is carried out at about eighteen to twenty-two weeks and checks your baby's growth and development by measuring her head circumference, abdominal circumference, and thigh length. The doctor or technician will also check the amount of amniotic fluid in your womb, and examine your baby's organs and limbs. This scan detects about 60 to 70 percent of major defects and about 35 percent of minor ones. Again, if anything on the ultrasound makes the perinatologist or radiologist suspicious, your care provider may recommend that you consider additional testing, such as amniocentesis. Keep in mind that your chances of having a healthy baby are very, very good, even if you're over thirty-five and something looks abnormal.

If you want to know your baby's gender, an ultrasound may give you an answer. For a boy, the technician will look to see if there is a penis, and for a girl, she will try to identify the clitoris. If the technician can't see either one, she won't be able to tell you your baby's gender.

It's important to note that the ultrasound may not be without some level of risk. Researchers at the Karolinska Institute in Stockholm have discovered that male babies exposed to ultrasound are more than three times as likely to be left-handed, suggesting that ultrasound may have an effect on brain development. They theorize that the ultrasonic waves may cause bubbles in bodily fluids to vibrate, interfering with neuron distribution.[29] This is no reason to avoid a routine exam, but is a good reason to avoid unnecessary procedures.

4-D ULTRASOUNDS

In 2002, 4-D Ultrasound machines hit the market. These machines take regular ultrasound images, which are typically gray and grainy and then enhance them to create a real-time computer-generated image of a baby in utero. The "4-D" refers to the real-time aspect. They're often too expensive for your community-

---

Non-Medical 4-D Ultrasounds

Recently, some for-profit centers have opened to offer these advanced scans for non-medical reasons.

Some of these centers even offer comfy chairs and one-hundred-inch screens, so the whole family can come in to watch, and will burn a movie file onto a CD or DVD disk for you to take home.

• The centers suggest that you schedule your ultrasound between twenty-six and thirty-two weeks, and between twenty and twenty-six weeks for twins. That way you'll have plenty of amniotic fluid, and the baby's face will have filled out to maximum cuteness.

• The procedure is the same for a regular ultrasound, even though it is not a medical test. You'll just need to lie back, expose your belly, and be slathered with gel, and it's show time.

• Note that 4-D ultrasounds will also carry the same risks as regular ultrasounds—perhaps more, because recreational ultrasounds tend to last longer. If you're considering getting one, ask your doctor about the latest research on their safety.

• The whole experience costs about $75–$400, depending on when you go (sometimes weekdays are cheaper) and the package you buy. As of this writing, there aren't yet centers in all states. Search "4D Ultrasound" and your state's name online to locate a center in your area.

based OB's office but may be used if your care provider or a perinatologist needs to more closely examine the fetus.

GLUCOSE CHALLENGE TEST

You may be offered a test for gestational diabetes called the glucose challenge. The test is usually done between weeks twenty-four to twenty-eight if you have no family history of blood sugar issues and earlier in your pregnancy if you do. Gestational diabetes develops when a pregnant woman is not able to produce enough insulin to keep her blood sugar (glucose) within a safe range. The problem affects two to seven percent of pregnant women in America.

The one-hour tolerance test may or may not require that you fast for twelve hours. Either way, the test involves you being given a glucose-packed liquid to drink. You wait for an hour, then a blood sample is taken to check your levels of glucose. If you have blood sugar over 130–140 mg, then you'll be told to schedule another, longer, three-hour diagnostic test for a different day.

The procedure for the three-hour test is similar, except that your blood is checked before you drink the glucose cocktail and again once every three hours afterward. If you do have gestational diabetes, you'll be advised to adopt a low-carbohydrate diet, and, more rarely, you may need insulin. Gestational diabetes is a temporary condition that goes away after the baby's born, though you will need to be tested at your sixth-week postpartum

checkup to make sure that you don't have an underlying case of type 2 diabetes.

AMNIOCENTESIS

Amniocentesis (or amnio) is a genetic test that involves inserting a needle through your abdominal wall and into your uterus. It can reveal the chromosomal makeup of your baby, including the gender and whether or not she carries certain inherited diseases, such as Down syndrome or open neural tube defects. Other special non-routine tests can also be performed during the procedure if needed, such as tests for hemophilia, Tay-Sachs, or cystic fibrosis. If you're going to have amnio, it should be performed between the fourteenth and sixteenth weeks (LMP) of pregnancy. Later, if necessary, it can be performed to determine if there is an infection in the fluid surrounding the baby. If done at the end of pregnancy, it can show whether your baby's lungs are sufficiently developed to function after birth.

Your care provider will probably offer you the opportunity to take the test if:

• You're over the age of thirty-five. Amnio used to be routinely offered to every woman over thirty-five to test for chromosomal abnormalities (because as a woman gets older her chance of having a baby with a chromosomal problem like Down syndrome increases). Considering that the risk of a thirty-five-year old woman carrying a fetus with Down Syndrome (1 in 250) is about the same as the test causing a healthy baby to miscarry, the decision isn't so black-and-white.

- You already have a child with a genetic condition, such as Tay-Sachs disease, sickle-cell anemia, or cystic fibrosis.
- You and/or your partner are known carriers of an inherited genetic disorder.
- Your Quad Screen or ultrasound test reveals a possible risk for a chromosomal defect.
- You're certain you can't care for a special-needs child.

Amnio is administered by having a patient lie on her back. A doctor will then use ultrasound to locate the baby and make sure she's not in the way. Then the doctor or perinatologist will insert a long needle through the stomach skin and into the uterus and withdraw some fluid, which is sent to a lab for analysis. The needle is in the abdomen usually for less than sixty seconds. Naturally, this is uncomfortable. Some women report that they feel a menstrual-like cramp when the needle enters the uterus.

Good centers keep their statistics on their loss rate and will tell you what it is. It is unclear why these miscarriages occur—fortunately, they are rare. Some may be caused by bleeding from the placenta from a needle puncture (although the needle often goes through the placenta without causing any problem) or incurred by premature contractions set off by leakage of amniotic fluid. There is a small chance of the needle sticking the baby, although this doesn't appear to cause a problem.

Managing Your Medicine Cabinet

Common drugs

The blanket statement most pregnancy books and care providers issue is to not ingest any drug or herbal supplement while you're pregnant if you can avoid it. This is because so many drugs simply haven't been properly tested on pregnant women. The FDA does not require drug manufacturers to conduct proper long-term studies on pregnant women. The closest many drugs get to being tested for safe use during pregnancy is by being tested on pregnant lab animals during the routine approval process. While such testing could demonstrate major physical deformities, it's less able to show subtle defects, such as learning disabilities or long-term problems.

A 2003 study in the *American Journal of Obstetrics & Gynecology* showed that 91 percent of drugs put on the market since 1980 are still considered to have an "undetermined" risk of producing birth defects, because they have not been properly tested. The FDA requires extensive long-term testing in order to allow a company to label a drug as safe in pregnancy, which is why the label on everything from aspirin to Zyrtec instructs pregnant women to "consult a doctor."

For minor complaints such as headaches or congestion, non-drug remedies can often be effective.

But what if the natural remedy isn't enough?

ver-the-Counter Decongestants, Expectorants,

DRUG NAME	FDA PREGNANCY RISK CLASSIFICATION
Chlorpheniramine (Chlor-Trimeton®)	B Antihistamine
Pseudoephedrine hydrochloride (Sudafed®)	B Sympathomimetic decongestant
Guaifenesin (Robitussin®)	C Expectorant
Dextromethorphan hydrobromide (found in Nyquil®)	C Non-narcotic antitussive
Diphenhydramine (Benadryl®)	B Antihistamine antiemetic
Clemastine fumarate (Tavist®)	B Antihistamine

• For prescription drugs, make sure that your prescribing doctor knows that you're pregnant and is fully informed of any other medications that you're taking to protect you from harmful drug interactions.

• Remember that herbs are also drugs. Don't take any herbal medicines, dietary supplements, or therapeutic herbal teas unless your doctor or midwife has assured you of their safety.

• Also ask your doctor about any drug you apply to your skin— acne cream, for instance.

Take any drug in the smallest dose for the shortest time possible to be effective.

The FDA isn't completely silent on the issue of over-the-counter and prescription drugs during pregnancy. It does assign drugs to one of five categories:

and Nonselective Antihistamines[30]

DRUG CLASS CROSSES PLACENTA?	USE IN PREGNANCY
Not known	Antihistamine of choice
Not known	Oral decongestant of choice
Not known	May be unsafe in first trimester*
Yes	Appears to be safe in pregnancy
Yes	Will cause withdrawal symptoms in newborns if taken continually in pregnancy. Thought to cause still-birth when combined[31] with the sleeping medication temazepam (Restoril®)
Not known	Unknown safety profile

*Possible increased risk of neural tube defects.

Category A

Controlled studies in women show no risks to the fetus.

Category B

Either studies on pregnant animals have not shown a fetal risk, but no studies have been done with pregnant women, or animal studies have shown an adverse effect, but human studies have not.

Category C

The data is inconclusive. Drugs may have shown to cause harm in animals, but human studies have not yet been performed. Drugs should be given only if the potential benefit justifies the potential risk to the fetus.

Category D

There is positive evidence of human fetal risk, but the benefits from use

Over-the-Counter Antacids, Simethicone, and

DRUG NAME	FDA RISK CLASS	DRUG CLASS
Aluminum hydroxide, magnesium hydroxide (Maalox®)*	B	Antacid
Calcium carbonate (Tums®)	C	Antacid
Simethicone (Mylanta Gas®)	C	Antiflatulent
Cimetidine (Tagamet®)	B	Antihistamine
Ranitidine (Zantac)	B	Antihistamine
Nizatidine (Axid)	C	Antihistamine
Famotidine (Pepcid)	B	Antihistamine

*Contains magnesium sulfate.

in pregnant women may be acceptable despite the risk (e.g., if the drug is needed in a life-threatening situation or for a serious disease in which safer drugs cannot be used or are ineffective).

Category X

Studies in animals or human beings have demonstrated fetal abnormalities or there is evidence of fetal risk based on human experience, and the risk of the use of the drug in pregnant women clearly outweighs any possible benefit. The drug is contraindicated in women who are or may become pregnant.

Obviously no such categories exist for recreational drugs such as nicotine, alcohol, caffeine, and so on. Here as in elsewhere, we've tried to summarize the available research.

H 2-Receptor Selective Antihistamines

CROSSES PLACENTA?	USE IN PREGNANCY
Not known	Generally regarded as safe
Not known	Generally regarded as safe
No	Generally regarded as safe
Yes	Preferred after antacids; generally regarded as safe
Yes	Preferred after antacids; generally regarded as safe
Yes	Not recommended (adverse animal studies)
Yes	Probably safe, data needed

ALLERGY MEDICATIONS: DECONGESTANTS AND ANTIHISTAMINES

Allergy shots are thought to be safe during pregnancy. Most over-the-counter decongestants and antihistamines are also okay to use during pregnancy, though do ask your healthcare provider and/or a trained pharmacist about any drug you're considering taking. Pseudoephedrine (Sudafed®) or chlorpheniramine (Chlor-Trimeton®) is the decongestant many obstetricians recommend for congestion if natural remedies, such as avoiding allergens and humidifying the air, don't work.

As a side note, a study from Japan published in the *Journal of Agricultural and Food Chemistry* [32]

Over-the-Counter Antidiarrheal Medications[33]

DRUG NAME	FDA RISK CLASS BY TRIMESTER	DRUG CLASS
Kaolin and pectin (Kaopectate®)	B/B/B	Antidiarrheal
Bismuth subsalicylate (Pepto Bismol®)	C/C/D	Antidiarrheal
Loperamide (Imodium®)	B/B/B	Antidiarrheal
Atropine, diphenoxylate (Lomotil®)	C/C/C	Antidiarrheal

notes that certain compounds in green tea can also be helpful for treating allergies.

Antihistamines such as chlorpheniramine and triprolidine have a long history of use in pregnant women and are not associated with an increased risk to the mother or the fetus. If you need a decongestant, pseudoephedrine has the best safety record during pregnancy.

ANTACIDS

Antacids work by neutralizing excess stomach acid. They contain ingredients such as aluminum hydroxide, calcium carbonate, magnesium hydroxide, and sodium bicarbonate, alone or in various combinations.

Most antacids, such as Tums, Maalox®, and Rolaids®, are known to be safe to take during pregnancy. Still, you should discuss your antacid consumption with your doctor. If you're taking extra calcium, for instance, the additional calcium in antacids could cause side effects. Large doses of antacids may also keep your body from effectively absorbing iron.

You may want to choose a formula that contains both magnesium and aluminum, or calcium combined with magnesium (such as Rolaids®, Mylanta®, or Maalox®). A side effect of magnesium is diarrhea, and constipation is a side effect of calcium and aluminum—so combined they cancel each other out!

Do not take antacids within two hours of taking other medicines. The antacids can keep other medicines from working properly.

ANTIBIOTICS

According to a study in the *American Journal of Obstetrics*

CROSSES PLACENTA?	USE IN PREGNANCY
No	Antidiarrheal of choice
Yes	Not recommended—salicylates have caused birth defects in animal studies
Not known	Probably safe
Not known	Not recommended—shown to affect maternal weight gain and fertility in animal studies.[34]

and Gynecology, an astounding 46 percent of pregnant women receive some type of antibiotic during pregnancy or labor.

Many antibiotics, such as those in the penicillin and erythromycin families, are thought to be generally safe to take during pregnancy—safer than a bacterial infection, that is.

Certain antibiotics, however, are definitely not safe. Tetracyclines (including doxycycline) can cause permanent staining of a developing baby's teeth, and they may affect bone development. Cipro® can damage fetal joints. Sulfonamides are suspected of causing birth defects if taken in the first trimester.

Make sure that you really do have a bacterial infection that warrants the use of any antibiotic. Babies exposed to antibiotics during their mother's pregnancies may develop bacterial strains resistant to antibiotic use. This can lead to a decreased ability to fight off infections, which can be especially dangerous if your baby is premature.

Antibiotics taken by a mother can also cause drug-induced diarrhea in a newborn and place your baby at a higher risk for fungal and yeast infections.

Make sure that any doctor you see knows that you're pregnant, and avoid antibiotics unless you really need them. If you discover that you're pregnant while taking tetracycline, ciprofloxacin (Cipro®), or a sulfonamide, stop taking the drug immediately, and ask your doctor for a safer alternative.

ANTIDEPRESSANTS

About 20 percent of pregnant women suffer from depression,[35] which can have serious consequences. Depression is linked to a forty-five percent higher risk of miscarriage and to a higher risk of

Over-the Counter Topical Vaginal Antifungal

DRUG NAME	FDA RISK CLASS BY TRIMESTER	DRUG CLASS
Butoconazole (Femstat®)	C	Imidazole antifungal
Clotrimazole (Lotrimin®)	C	Imidazole antifungal
Miconazole (Monistat®)	C	Imidazole antifungal
Tioconazole (Vagistat-1®)	C	Imidazole antifungal

pre-term labor, premature delivery, and low birth weight. Infants born to depressed moms also have decreased cognitive skills and language development.

The selective serotonin reuptake inhibitors (SSRIs) paroxetine (Paxil®), fluoxetine (Prozac®), sertraline (Zoloft®), and fluvoxamine (Luvox®) are very effective at treating depression. However, these drugs have only been on the market for a relatively short period of time and have not yet been thoroughly studied. The FDA has given all four drugs a category B classification, meaning that they cause no harm in animal tests but that long-term human tests have yet to be performed. Fluoxetine is the oldest and most-prescribed SSRI; it ranks in the top twenty of all prescriptions written in the United States. Because the drug has been on the market since 1988, it has been the subject of the most longer-term SSRI studies.

However, the results of these studies have often been contradictory and inconclusive.

A 2003 study[36] in the *American Journal of Obstetrics and Gynecology* demonstrated that women who take SSRIs are at no higher risk for having babies with birth defects. A 1996 study in *The New England Journal of Medicine* reported that women taking fluoxetine during their pregnancies have no higher risk of miscarriage, or major fetal abnormalities, than women not taking the drug. However, this study found that women who took fluoxetine during the third trimester were at a higher risk of pregnancy complications such as premature birth.[37] Other studies have contradicted this finding and shown that women taking fluoxetine are no more likely to have complications than anyone else. One study published in *The Journal of Pediatrics* found an

Medications[38]

CROSSES PLACENTA?	USE IN PREGNANCY
Not known	Probably safe
Not known	Safe in second and third trimesters, based on human trials. First trimester studies are inconclusive
Not known	Probably safe
Not known	Unknown safety profile

increase in minor anomalies such as delays in fine motor skills and increased tremors in babies six to forty months old, but these findings did not show up in several other longer-term studies. Most notably, the longest-term study done so far, performed in 1997, followed up pre–school age children whose mothers had taken fluoxetine during pregnancy and found that these children did not experience any adverse effects on their neurological development.

As confusing as the body of evidence is, it does currently appear to indicate that the as-yet unproven risks on SSRIs make them a better choice than exposure to the very real risks associated with depression. Therefore, this is a decision only you and your doctor or psychiatrist can make, by weighing risks and benefits and the most current research.

ASPIRIN

Obstetricians generally recommend that you take acetaminophen (Tylenol®) instead of aspirin for routine pain relief. A small amount of aspirin, such as the eighty-one milligrams that may be prescribed by a cardiologist, has been shown to have no negative impact on your growing baby. In fact, some studies suggest that these low doses may actually help to prevent preeclampsia and premature delivery. But in very rare instances, large doses of aspirin taken during the last trimester can result in the failure of one of the baby's heart structures to close properly as well as cause jaundice after birth.

Vaccines

Vaccines that are made out of inactive viruses or proteins derived from viruses are safe during pregnancy and can be a good idea if you have a chronic illness or are at high risk because of your lifestyle. On the other hand, avoid any vaccine made from live viruses, such as those for measles, mumps, varicella (chicken pox), or rubella. Here's a breakdown on various immunization and vaccine options.

THE FLU SHOT

This is a very safe vaccine, made of inactive viruses and egg whites. The CDC recommends the flu shot for women in their pregnancy when it's flu season. If you have a chronic illness such as asthma or diabetes that makes the flu dangerous for you, you may especially want to consider taking the vaccine. Note that a flu shot will protect you only against the more serious strains of flu that tend to land people in the hospital, but not more familiar bugs, like the common cold.

TETANUS

You should make sure that you've had an immunization against tetanus in the past ten years. Though the virus is rare, if you contract it while pregnant, it can cause fetal death. If you get a dirty or deep wound, check with your care provider immediately to see if you need a tetanus shot.

HEPATITIS B

If you work in healthcare, with children, travel frequently to high-risk areas such as China and Southeast Asia, or live with someone infected with hepatitis B, you should seriously consider taking this harmless, genetically engineered vaccine. A pregnant woman with hepatitis B can pass the infection on to her baby during labor and delivery. If this happens, your baby will have to be treated at birth and again at one to six months with the vaccine and immunoglobulin, a serum made from the live virus.

HEPATITIS A

Hepatitis A usually does not affect an unborn baby. However, if you have a high-risk job (healthcare, child care, waste management), live in an area where this virus is common, or you travel frequently to developing countries, you may want to ask your physician about this vaccination.

PNEUMOCOCCUS

If you have a lung condition, such as asthma, your doctor may recommend the genetically engineered pneumococcal vaccine, which prevents some forms of pneumonia.

Recreational drugs

ALCOHOL

Drinking alcohol in any amount is not safe during pregnancy. It's more dangerous than almost any other drug known to science, because it affects the behavior of a protein necessary to the fetal brain, along with affecting a number of different neurotransmitters. Drinking alcohol in the first trimester can lead to facial malformations; in the second, it can interrupt nerve formation in the brain; and in the third trimester, it can kill existing neurons and interfere with nervous system development. Strangely, some fetuses seem unscathed by their mothers' drinking, while others are severely damaged by small amounts of alcohol. Just a drink and a half a week can lead to children being born with behavioral and learning disabilities. Avoid foods which contain alcohol (unless they've been cooked until the alcohol has evaporated), any medication which contains alcohol, and, of course, any alcoholic beverage.

BOTOX®

Even though you might be tempted to have Botox® treatments to remove those frown lines and little crow's feet that are creeping up on you, don't be tempted to do that while you're pregnant. Botox®, a facial muscle-relaxing agent, is derived from an ordinarily deadly botulism bacterium.

While there are no published studies of the effects of Botox on pregnant women, spontaneous abortions and fetal malformations have been observed in rabbits. If you plan to nurse your baby, you may want to postpone treatments until after your baby is weaned. Currently, it is not known whether Botox is secreted in breast milk.

CAFFEINE

Caffeine, a stimulant that increases your heart rate and metabolism, is the most commonly used drug in America. It can be found in coffee, tea, soda, chocolate, and even some pain relievers. During pregnancy, it is passed directly to the fetus through the placenta.

While your baby is able to handle occasional bouts of stimulant-induced stress, just as she would be able to handle it if you sprinted up a flight of stairs, exposing her to constant physiological stress from a drug is not a good idea.

In 1999, a review of studies on caffeine use in pregnancy found that there is no risk to babies whose moms consume less than 150 mg. a day, which is equivalent to one-and-one-half eight-ounce cups of home-brewed coffee, OR about thirty-six ounces (three cans) of regular or diet cola, OR two Excedrin.

Researchers disagree on the level of risk posed by moderate caffeine consumption, defined as between 150 to 300 milligrams a day (one

Over-the-Counter Pain Medications[39]

DRUG NAME	FDA RISK CLASS BY TRIMESTER	DRUG CLASS
Acetaminophen (Tylenol®)	B/B/B	Analgesic
Aspirin	D/D/D	NSAID analgesic
Ibuprofen (Advil, Motrin®)	B/B/D	NSAID analgesic
Ketoprofen (Orudis®)	B/B/D	NSAID analgesic
Naproxen (Aleve®)	B/B/D	NSAID analgesic

NSAID = nonsteroidal anti-inflammatory drug

*Associated with increased perinatal mortality, neonatal hemorrhage, decreased birth weight, prolonged gestation and labor, and possible teratogenicity.

†Large dosages are associated with oligohydramnios, premature closure of the fetal ductus arteriosus with subsequent persistent pulmonary hypertension of the newborn, fetal nephrotoxicity, and periventricular hemorrhage.

sixty-four-ounce 7-Eleven Big Gulp, three cups of home-brewed coffee, or four espressos).

However, studies agree that in amounts higher than 300 milligrams, caffeine becomes dangerous.

In 2003 researchers from Aarhus University in Denmark found that women who drink four to seven cups of coffee a day were 80 percent more likely to have stillbirths. The caffeine in coffee was presumed to be the culprit responsible for the increased risk, although the researchers noted that the increase in stillbirths might also be partly explained by other risky behaviors engaged in by pregnant women. Women who drank more than eight cups a day were found to be more than twice as likely to have stillbirths, according to the study.[40]

It's important to note that different brands of coffee can have very different amounts of caffeine. Starbucks drip coffee has 200 milligrams per eight ounces, while Maxwell House has 135, and instant coffee has just 95 milligrams. If you love your premium coffee beverages, try a cappuccino or latte that

CROSSES PLACENTA?	USE IN PREGNANCY
Yes	Pain reliever of choice
Yes	Not recommended except for specific indications*
Yes	Use with caution; avoid in third trimester†
Yes	Use with caution; avoid in third trimester†
Yes	Use with caution; avoid in third trimester†

dilutes the coffee with good-for-you milk.[41] And remember that serving sizes count: One cola means one can, not one Big Gulp.

Also note that caffeine dehydrates you, and dehydration causes headaches, muscle cramps, and even premature contractions. So be sure to match your caffeinated beverages with extra water.

The good news is that caffeine does not cause birth defects. Major studies over the past decade have shown no association between birth defects and caffeine consumption. Even offspring of the heaviest coffee drinkers were not found to be at higher risk of birth defects.[42]

ECSTASY

Ecstasy, also known as MDMA or methylenedioxymethamphetamine, has been shown to cause lasting damage in the areas of rats' brains that control planning, impulse control, and attention span. Rats exposed to ecstasy in utero have lasting learning and behavioral problems. If you've taken ecstasy during your pregnancy, inform your care provider.[43]

COCAINE

Because women who use cocaine tend to smoke and use other drugs, it's hard for researchers to isolate which drugs cause which side effects. Statistically, cocaine users have a much higher rate of spontaneous abortion, placental abruption, and *premature rupture of the membranes (PROM)*. Cocaine constricts the blood vessels that lead to the placenta, reducing the flow of oxygen. Cocaine also crosses the placenta, and because a fetus's liver is immature, it takes three times as long to pass through the body than an adult's. Babies exposed to cocaine in utero will test positive for the drug five to six days after the mother's use. Babies born to cocaine-addicted mothers also suffer painful withdrawal.

HEROIN, OXYCONTIN®, AND METHADONE

Maternal heroin use has been associated with low birth weight, prematurity, and nutritional deficiencies. Attempting detox during pregnancy is not recommended and can cause fetal death. Oxycontin, also an opiate, has the same effects. Opiate withdrawal is not recommended during pregnancy for addicts. The baby will also need to be kept in the hospital to undergo treatment for withdrawal.

MARIJUANA

Marijuana is the fourth most-used recreational drug in America (behind caffeine, nicotine, and alcohol) and has been studied fairly extensively. A link has not been found between moderate use

---

How to Break the Caffeine Habit

If you've ever tried to stop even a moderate caffeine habit, you know that withdrawal can be painful, causing headaches, fatigue, a spaced-out feeling, and bitchiness—a sure sign that the drug is powerful. Here are our suggestions:

- **Start slow.** Don't try to quit cold turkey all at once, but lower your intake gradually over one to two weeks.

- **Gradually make the shift.** Buy one tin of regular coffee and one of decaf, and then switch your "caf" to decaf ratio gradually until you're drinking all decaf.

- **Substitute.** After you've gotten yourself off the caffeine kick, start substituting your usual beverages and sodas with decaffeinated soda, seltzer water, and club soda or fruit juice.

2

(as in a few times a month) and pregnancy complications. Smoking anything deprives the fetus of oxygen, however. Daily smoking of marijuana has been linked to premature labor and low-birthweight babies. The drug definitely passes through the placenta to the baby—babies exposed to marijuana during pregnancy will test positive for the drug in their urine for two to three weeks after their mother's use.

TOBACCO

Smoking as few as six cigarettes a day, say researchers, is as toxic to your baby as cocaine or heroin addiction.[44] The damage to your and your baby's health associated with cigarette smoking are so well documented and are so numerous they could fill this book. But bottom line, smoking while you're pregnant can kill your baby. Nine percent of miscarriages and stillbirths are associated with smoking, and only 12 percent of pregnant women smoke. Statistically, smokers are two hundred times more likely to go into labor prematurely and three hundred times more likely to deliver a low-birthweight baby. Smoking just one cigarette a day increases your chance of giving birth to a low-birthweight baby by 70 percent. Smoking doubles your chances of placental complications such as placenta previa and abruption, the leading causes of newborn death. It keeps vital nutrients such as folate, calcium, and vitamin C from being absorbed by both you and your baby. It almost triples your baby's chance of dying of SIDS and is directly responsible for 10 percent

of all infant deaths in the first year. It doubles your child's risk of developing asthma. Kids of moms who smoke are shorter in height, smaller in size, and average three to five months behind in reading and math. Smoking has also been associated with Attention Deficit Disorder, hyperactivity, and poor social skills. Secondhand smoke also causes all of these effects, in different degrees, depending on the amount of exposure.

According to the American Lung Association, one in two smokers dies from causes directly related to the habit, and smokers die on average ten to twelve years sooner than nonsmokers. Quitting may be hard, but it's a day in the park compared to having something happen to your baby and forever having to wonder if it's your fault. Do whatever it takes to quit. If you gain 150 pounds, that's still healthier than smoking. If you have to drive one hundred miles to avoid certain places, friends, or situations, do it.

Talk to your care provider about getting help to quit. Plenty of resources are available. Also see our additional quitting suggestions on page 22.

NICOTINE REPLACEMENT DRUGS

What's worse for your baby—cigarettes or nicotine gum? Cigarettes. One of the main components of cigarette smoke is carbon monoxide, a known fetal toxin, and smoke also contains ammonia, hydrogen cyanide, benzene, and the poisonous gases of more than three thousand other potentially harmful chemicals. The safety of nicotine replacement products in pregnancy has not been adequately studied as of press time, but if gum or a patch can keep you from smoking even one cigarette, we'd wager that they're still a better choice. Talk to your healthcare provider if you think these products might help you.

Managing High-Risk Conditions

WHAT MAKES A PREGNANCY "HIGH RISK"?

To be told that you have a high-risk pregnancy can be quite alarming. It's a label that can be applied to a gamut of situations, from simply being thirty-five years old or older to having a life-threatening illness. Managing a high-risk pregnancy can involve any combination of remedies: more frequent checkups and testing, a special diet, drug treatments or lifestyle modifications, and limitations on where you can deliver. Most midwives and birth centers will not accept patients in certain high-risk categories. Here are some of the most common reasons why your pregnancy may earn the high-risk label:

- **If you're over thirty-five.** If you are in good health, your pregnancy isn't necessarily high risk, although there is a greater chance for some problems, including maternal diabetes and chromosomal (genetic) abnormalities.

- **You're carrying multiples—** twins, triplets, or more.

- **You have a serious medical condition,** such as cardiac disease, renal disease, hypertension, a thyroid condition, or diabetes.

- **Alcohol, heroin, cocaine, amphetamine, or prescription drug abuse.** These substances go directly to your baby and may have serious health consequences.

- **Viral infections, such as chickenpox, chlamydia, genital herpes, or HIV.** These infections can affect your baby, and some may cause miscarriage or prematurity. Prenatal screening for HIV is recommended for every mother, since the use of anti-retroviral therapy can potentially decrease the risk of transmission to the fetus from 25 percent to 88 percent.

- **You're at risk for pre-term labor.** Either you have a family or personal history, or you've been diagnosed with an incompetent cervix, or you're carrying multiples.
- **You have a family history of genetic disorders.** For example: if your baby's father has the sickle-cell trait; alpha thalassemia in Asian families; beta thalassemia in Mediterranean, North African, Indian, and Southeast Asian families; and Tay-Sachs disease in Jewish families.

MULTIPLES

Multiple births are on the rise. More women over thirty-five are becoming moms, and more women than ever are making use of fertility treatments. Overall, about 2.9 percent of women giving birth in the U.S. will have more than one baby. Twins occur naturally in about 1 in 90 births, triplets in 1 out of every 10,000, and quadruplets in 1 out of every 650,000 births. Conjoined twins (Siamese twins) occur in approximately 1 in 100,000 pregnancies.

Women between the ages of thirty-five and thirty-nine are more likely than any other age group to have multiples, because the body begins to produce higher levels of gonadotropin hormones. These hormones cause multiple eggs to mature and be released—kind of like the ovaries' version of a going-out-of-business sale.

As for fertility treatments, approximately one in five women undergoing treatments will have multiple babies. Women who take fertility drugs with gonadotropins, the egg-releasing hormones, are much more likely to have multiples than those who take fertility drugs which encourage estrogen production, such as clomiphene (Clomid®). Women who use *in vitro* technologies to conceive are also much more likely to have multiples, because fertility specialists performing the procedure will implant multiple embryos to increase the odds for success.

Multiples can also be hereditary. They're more common in African-American moms (occurring in about one in seventy births), and rarely in women of Asian descent (one in three hundred). And if you've been pregnant with multiples in the past, you're five times more likely to become so again.

Multiple pregnancies can result from two sperm fertilizing two eggs (*fraternal twins*, which are no more closely related than any other siblings and can be of either sex), or the separation of one fertilized egg into two embryos (identical twins, sharing genetic material). Triplets, quads, or quints can be a combination of either type of twins.

A multiple pregnancy is typically detected and confirmed by ultrasound. An abnormal result from an AFP screening test (see "Testing: Risks and Benefits," page 190), multiple heartbeats on the Doppler, extreme nausea, a larger-than-normal uterus and more severe pregnancy symptoms can also be a tip-off.

While being pregnant with multiples is certainly riskier than having just one, you still have more than a 90 percent chance of giving birth to healthy babies.

If you're pregnant with twins or more, you may experience these symptoms.

More intense pregnancy symptoms.

If you're pregnant with multiples, you can expect extreme tiredness, more nausea and vomiting, swollen and tender breasts, constipation, heartburn, and so on, because of the extra pregnancy hormones in your body. Later on, you'll experience more discomfort and side effects from the extra weight, such as backaches, hemorrhoids, and shortness of breath.

More, faster weight gain.

Women carrying multiples are advised to gain 1.5 pounds a week by consuming an extra three hundred calories a day per baby. Because of the additional nutritional needs of women carrying multiples, deficiencies such as anemia are more common.

A higher chance of delivering early.

Slightly less than half of multiple pregnancies end early. Preterm birth is the leading cause of neonatal death in multiples. Your doctor may advise you to take measures to lower your risk of preterm labor, such as beginning your maternity leave sooner, abstaining from exercise, or going on bed rest (see page 223). Fifty-three percent of twins and ninety-two percent of triplets are born early.

A greater risk of delivering low-birthweight babies.

The average birth weight for singletons is seven pounds, seven ounces; the average birth weight of twins is five pounds, five ounces. A difference of two to three pounds in birth weights between twins is not unusual.

A greater risk of complications.

Mothers of twins are more likely to be at risk of physical complications, such as pregnancy-induced hypertension (see page 214), preeclampsia (see page 215), and placenta problems. You can help reduce risks, though.

- **Get extra nutrition.** In addition to the extra three hundred calories per day per baby, take a prenatal vitamin supplement. Make every bite count. Try eating six small meals a day instead of fewer, large ones. A healthy gain is usually between thirty-five to forty-five pounds.

- **See your healthcare provider frequently.** Because of the high chance that you'll deliver early and/or need medical intervention, your pregnancy probably should not be overseen by a midwife. Typically, the first twin is born headfirst, and the second twin is in a different presentation, such as breech or transverse. It's not unheard of to deliver the first twin vaginally and then need to have the second delivered by c-section. Hire an obstetrician or perinatologist who has experience with multiples. Because of the risks, your pregnancy needs to be monitored much more closely, and you'll see your doctor much more often—usually twice a month instead of once, and once a week after gestational week thirty.

- **Get extra rest.** You'll be extra tired. Mentally and practically prepare yourself, your employer, and your family for bed rest should your doctor order it. Rest now to have the extra energy you'll need later.

You'll also have to prepare yourself and your family mentally and practically for the challenge of having two newborns. Prepare older siblings as well, because multiples will mean less attention for them, which may mean more jealousy. You will also need more help. In addition to enlisting more help from your family, consider hiring a helper, such as a retired nurse, for the first few months. Find a support group through the National Organization of Mothers of Twins Clubs (www.nomotc.com).

THYROID CONDITIONS

The thyroid is a gland at the base of the neck that regulates your metabolism and helps get oxygen to your cells. It produces several hormones, most notably triiodothyronine (T3) and thyroxine (T4). It knows how much hormone to produce from signals that come from the hypothalamus (a part of the brain). Conditions develop when something interferes with the signals or something interferes with the gland itself.

Thyroid conditions in women are fairly common—by age sixty about one in five women will experience some variety of condition. Postpartum thyroid conditions are also common and frequently misdiagnosed because the symptoms are often vague. Tell your doctor if, after birth, you have any or some of the following symptoms:

- You feel warm when others are cold, or vice versa.
- You have muscle weakness or cramping.
- You lose or gain weight rapidly.
- You are unusually nervous or irritable.
- You are extremely tired or have insomnia.
- You have heart palpitations.
- You feel swelling in your neck.
- You don't seem to have enough breast milk.

If your thyroid is underactive, it's called *hypothyroidism*. If it's overactive, it's *hyperthyroidism*.

If you already have a thyroid condition, you'll need to be in close contact with your doctor. You and your doctor and/or endocrinologist will need to evaluate the safety of the medications that you're taking (certain thyroid medications have been associated with minor birth defects). Your condition may make your pregnancy become classified as high risk. It almost certainly will be more difficult—women with thyroid conditions can also have far more severe pregnancy symptoms, such as heart palpitations and extreme *morning sickness* (hyperemesis gravidarium).

HYPERTENSION

Hypertension, in the form of chronic pre-existing or pregnancy-induced high blood pressure, is the leading cause of pregnancy complications. High blood pressure can cause preeclampsia, premature delivery, fetal growth retardation, abruptio placentae, and stillbirth. Your level of risk will depend on how high your blood pressure is. Blood pressure lower than 170 over 110 is considered mild to moderate and may be treated with lifestyle moderations. Higher blood pressure may require drug treatment, with medications such as methyldopa or hydralazine.

ABRUPTIO PLACENTAE

It literally means abruption, or the separating of the placenta from the uterus wall. It occurs in less than two percent of pregnancies, and usually later than the twenty-sixth week. It is often associated with hypertension-related problems in pregnancy and affects African-American women at least twice as often as women of other races. The mothers most at risk are older women and those who smoke.

Symptoms may vary depending on the severity of the abruption and generally include the following:

• Abdominal pain
• Bleeding (may vary from light to heavy, with or without clots)
• Abdominal cramping

If the abruption is so severe that a large part of the placenta has come away, the fetus is at risk of not getting enough oxygen to survive. Your risk is greatly reduced if only a small part of the placenta has been separated.

If the separation is small, the normal course of action is bed rest for the mother until the bleeding subsides, and you will probably need to be closely monitored for the rest of your pregnancy. If you start bleeding again, and your baby is near term, you may need to have a planned delivery. In cases of severe separation, you may require extra blood through a transfusion. Sometimes

babies who are endangered may need to be delivered right away by a cesarean section.

TOXEMIA (PREECLAMPSIA) AND ECLAMPSIA

Toxemia is a complication of pregnancy that usually shows up after the twentieth week, but is most common in the last month of pregnancy. The symptoms are swelling, vision disturbances, high blood pressure, and protein in the urine.

The causes of toxemia are not clear, although poor nutrition and genetic predisposition are thought to be contributors. One out of two hundred pregnant mothers who have toxemia will proceed to eclampsia, meaning toxemia with convulsions or coma. Preeclampsia can affect a mother's kidneys, liver, heart and blood.

Latter stage symptoms include abdominal pains, visual disturbances (seeing spots), severe headaches, and mental dullness caused by cerebral edema ("water on the brain").

If untreated, preeclampsia can lead to eclampsia and even death, but careful medical management can help to slow the progression of the disease, with total recovery once pregnancy is over.

DIABETES

Diabetes is a serious condition in which your pancreas can't produce enough insulin to control the level of glucose, or blood sugar, in your bloodstream. The unabsorbed glucose damages your organs, and without enough insulin fueling your cells, you may become tired, dizzy, and extremely thirsty, and you could even slip into a coma. High levels of glucose in your bloodstream in the first trimester can be toxic to your developing pregnancy and cause birth defects. If you were already diabetic when you became pregnant, your pregnancy is considered high risk, and you need to take and receive extra care to keep your blood sugar at safe levels.

GESTATIONAL DIABETES

Gestational diabetes is a special condition of pregnancy when a mother is unable to produce adequate insulin for herself during the latter months of pregnancy. Usually it will disappear after delivery, though it does mean you're more vulnerable to developing full-blown diabetes later in life.

Only about 3 percent of pregnant women have problems with their blood sugar during pregnancy. Still, the risks are significant enough that you'll be screened for the condition at least once during your pregnancy (see "Glucose Tolerance Test," page 186), early on if you have a family history of diabetes. If you have no risk factors, you may be asked to take the glucose tolerance test between the twenty-fourth and twenty-eighth weeks of your pregnancy.

If your care provider discovers that you have gestational diabetes, you may be advised to start a special diet and to take pills to stimulate your pancreas or injections to supply your body with insulin. With

adequate treatment, you have a good chance of delivering a healthy baby.

Untreated, your baby may grow too large, resulting in a difficult delivery. Your baby may also have difficulty keeping a normal blood sugar level after birth.

DES

It's important to know if your mother took DES (diethylstilbestrol) during her pregnancy. This drug is a hormone that was given to millions of women all over the world for more than thirty years, between 1938 and 1971, to prevent miscarriage. Not only did it not prevent miscarriages (demonstrated in research trials as early as 1953), but the drug caused structural abnormalities to the reproductive organs of female babies in utero, and rendered about twenty percent of exposed female babies sterile. DES has also been linked to a rare cancer. It's important to know if your mother took DES while she was pregnant, because malformations may put you at a higher risk for ectopic pregnancy, miscarriage, and preterm birth. Some researchers also believe that DES may cause reproductive problems for third-generation women (DES granddaughters), though the research is inconclusive so far. If you were exposed to DES, your pregnancy will be more closely monitored. For the latest research and information on DES, you can contact the Center for Disease Control's DES site (www. cdc.gov/DES /consumers) or DES Action USA (www.desaction.org).

CHLAMYDIA

Chlamydia trachomatis is the most common sexually transmitted bacterial disease in the United States, affecting about three million women a year, and is especially dangerous because 80 to 90 percent of infected women (and 50 percent of infected men) show no symptoms. Of women who do have symptoms, they can be hard to recognize, such as pain during intercourse, bleeding between periods, or abdominal pain. Untreated, it can lead to pelvic inflammatory disease (PID) which causes scar tissue to form in the fallopian tubes and can cause infertility or a higher risk of ectopic pregnancy. Untreated in pregnancy, chlamydia can result in eye infections or pneumonia in a newborn. The good news is that care providers routinely test for chlamydia with a painless cervical swab test at your first prenatal visit. If the test is positive, you'll be treated with antibiotics, probably erythromiacin, and you and the baby will be fine. If your test is positive, it's important that your partner is tested and treated also.

Pre-term labor: risk factors and prevention

Pre-term labor is labor that happens after twenty weeks of pregnancy, but before the end of the thirty-seventh week. Its symptoms include regular contractions occurring at intervals ten minutes apart or less for at least an hour accompanied by changes in the cervix.

No discernible cause is found for 38 to 50 percent of reported premature labor cases. In the remaining cases, however, many of the contributing factors are knowable, and in some cases, avoidable.

If you're over thirty-five or have delivered a baby prematurely in the past, consider working with a perinatologist in addition to your obstetrician (most midwives will not work with women in these high-risk categories). Being an older mother heightens your risk for pre-term labor, statistically speaking. Women who have had a previous premature birth are more likely to have another; their risk can be 2.5 times as great as that of women without this history.

If you are extremely high risk, your care provider may suggest that you be treated with progesterone, which has been shown to decrease the risk of a recurrent premature delivery.[45] Your doctor or perinatologist may also put you on bed rest for a large portion of your second and third trimesters.

If you're having multiples (twins, triplets, or beyond), you have a high chance of going into labor early. Close to 60 percent of twins, more than 90 percent of triplets, and virtually all quadruplets and higher multiples are born pre-term. The length of gestation decreases with each additional baby. On average, most singleton pregnancies last thirty-nine weeks; for twins, thirty-six weeks; for triplets, thirty-two weeks; for quadruplets, thirty weeks; and for quintuplets, twenty-nine weeks.

If you're having multiples, your doctor will want to schedule more prenatal visits than if you were having one baby. Even if you have no signs of pre-term labor, your doctor will probably recommend cutting back on your activities at around twenty weeks, and sooner if you're having more than two babies.

If you smoke: Women who smoke raise their risk of pre-term labor by 20 to 30 percent. As many as 15 percent of all pre-term births are attributable to smoking during pregnancy. (See our suggestions for quitting on page 22.)

If you're over- or underweight, your risk for pre-term labor rises if you are under- or overweight. Discuss with your doctor or midwife how much you should gain. Studies show that gaining enough weight in the first twenty to twenty-four weeks of pregnancy is especially important for women carrying multiples.

If you get a urinary tract infection during your pregnancy, have pain or burning when you urinate, or have any oral infections or problems with your teeth, let your doctor know. Early in your pregnancy, ask your doctor to test you for bacterial vaginosis, a common imbalance of organisms in the vagina. The condition often has no symptoms, and treating it may reduce your

chances of having a premature baby by about 20 percent. Other infections can have various short- and long-term health consequences, some of them quite serious.

If you have a vitamin deficiency: Iron-deficiency anemia is common, and it can increase the risk of pre-term delivery. Make sure that you get at least thirty milligrams of iron daily.

If you've been diagnosed with an *incompetent cervix*: An incompetent cervix is one that is prone to opening prematurely, when the weight of the uterus presses down upon it. This can lead to a miscarriage or premature delivery.

Miscarriages that result from an incompetent cervix generally occur four months into the pregnancy or later. This is when the fetus and amniotic fluid weigh enough to press down on the cervix and make it begin to dilate. About 25 percent of miscarriages that occur after the fourteenth week of pregnancy are attributed to cervical incompetence.

Usually, an incompetent cervix isn't diagnosed until it causes problems in your pregnancy, though sometimes an ultrasound or vaginal examination can reveal if your cervix is opening prematurely.

The exact cause of an incompetent or weakened cervix is unknown, though it is sometimes associated with a previous traumatic birth (during which the cervix was torn), a cone biopsy, or repeated or late-term abortion. It is also associated with an abnormally developed cervix, a finding in daughters of mothers who were exposed to the drug DES (diethylstilbestrol) during their pregnancy.

Standard practice for the treatment of an incompetent cervix in the past has been a procedure called *cerclage*, which involves basically stitching your uterus closed, and is usually done under general anesthesia. After having cerclage, a woman is usually prescribed medication to prevent a surgery-related miscarriage. The stitches are removed around the ninth month of pregnancy, or sooner if labor commences, to prepare for delivery.

Recent research appears to suggest that the risks of cerclage may outweigh its benefits, and that it may not be effective in preventing pre-term delivery.[46]

If you go into pre-term labor, your provider may recommend bed rest at home or in the hospital and, possibly, treatment with drugs that may postpone labor. If the provider does not believe labor will stop, and if the babies are likely to be born before thirty-four weeks' gestation, she will probably recommend that you be treated with drugs called corticosteroids. The corticosteroids help speed fetal lung development and reduce the likelihood and severity of breathing and other problems during the newborn period.[47]

Viral infections

HIV

During your pregnancy, you'll be offered a test for the Human Immunodeficiency Virus (HIV). Like every other test, you have a right to refuse it. However, knowing that you're positive means that you and your care provider can take preventive measures to keep your baby from also contracting the virus.

People catch HIV through the sharing of bodily fluids during unprotected sex, through blood that gets into wounds in the skin, or by dirty syringe needles. Individuals catch it when they have sex with an infected person, and more rarely, it can be passed through a blood transfusion that has been contaminated with the virus, or by sharing needles with other people when

doing drugs. Though HIV can be passed to unborn babies, amazingly, an unborn baby has only a one in seven chance of catching HIV if the mother is HIV positive, and as little as a one to two percent chance if mom receives drug therapy while pregnant. There's still a lot of research to be done, but it seems that women who contract HIV just before getting pregnant or while pregnant are the ones more likely to pass the virus on to their babies.

AIDS, which stands for acquired immune-deficiency syndrome, is the disease that results when HIV harms the immune system to the degree that the body is susceptible to a variety of infections. If a woman has AIDS, her baby is at much greater risk of being born with HIV. A cesarean delivery may be carried out if the doctors are of the opinion that normal vaginal delivery may increase the risk of the baby contracting the infection. Every baby whose mother has HIV is born with antibodies to the virus in her blood. However, these antibodies will disappear over time if the baby does not have HIV. Sometimes, it takes up to eighteen months for this to happen.

In developed countries, breast-feeding is not recommended to HIV-positive mothers because the virus can be passed to the baby during breastfeeding.

HEPATITIS B

Hepatitis B is a liver infection caused by a virus, easily transmitted from person to person through infected blood and also through sexual intercourse. Unlike hepatitis A (see page 204), which does not pass to the fetus or newborn, hepatitis B may be passed to the baby during birth or to the fetus during pregnancy if the mother is infected.

Up to 90 percent of pregnant women who are carriers of hepatitis B can pass it on to their newborns at delivery, and hepatitis B infection in pregnancy is associated with a 20 percent increase in preterm delivery.

A routine blood screening test will probably be performed during your first pregnancy exam to check for hepatitis B along with other infections.

If you're infected, you may be referred to a specialist. Your baby will be washed thoroughly after he is born to remove all traces of your blood, and he will be immediately injected with hepatitis B vaccine and hepatitis B immunoglobulin to help protect him.

Your baby will then need two more follow-up shots in the months after birth. You will not be separated from your baby or prevented from breastfeeding unless you have special circumstances.

HERPES

Did you know that more than 20 percent of American women have genital herpes? The virus can be transmitted when no symptoms are present, and 60 percent of people infected with the virus have never had an outbreak. Scientists estimate that up to 90 percent of people with herpes don't know it.

While most women with genital herpes have healthy babies, a small number pass the virus on to their babies during labor and delivery. The herpes virus can cause neonatal herpes, a rare but life-threatening disease. Neonatal herpes can cause eye or throat infections, damage to the central nervous system, mental retardation, and even death. The good news is that a dose of acyclovir (an antiviral medication) taken in the month of delivery, is very effective (though not foolproof) in preventing an outbreak.[48] So it is especially important for you to recognize the symptoms of the disease, and to seek immediate medical treatment if you think that you could be infected. If you've ever had an episode where the skin in your genital area became unusually red and sensitive (painful, itchy, or tingly), with one or more blisters or bumps appearing at the area afterward, be sure to mention this to your care provider.

The biggest herpes-related threat that your pregnancy faces is to have a first outbreak close to delivery. Acquiring the disease during pregnancy has been associated with spontaneous abortion, prematurity, and congenital and neonatal herpes. So if your partner is infected but you're not—even if you've managed to avoid getting the disease in the past—the risk is high enough that you should consider abstaining from oral or digital genital contact for the duration of your pregnancy.

It is currently standard practice in the United States to perform cesarean delivery on pregnant women with recurrent herpes outbreaks to reduce the risk of transmission of the virus to newborns. Still, 20 to 30 percent of all infants born with herpes simplex virus (HSV) are delivered via cesarean, which may indicate that the practice isn't very effective. If you have herpes, shop around for an obstetrician who has specific experience with herpes patients and follows the latest research.

GENITAL WARTS

Genital warts are one of the most common sexually transmitted diseases in the world, affecting about 1 percent of the U.S. population. They're caused by one of at least one hundred strains of the human papilloma virus (HPV). In the majority of cases, the virus is dormant and shows no symptoms. Because of hormonal changes during pregnancy, the dormant virus may wake up, and warts may appear for the first time or may grow larger. The warts can vary from almost invisible little bumps to larger growths. Sometimes larger growths can cause problems, such as obstructing the urinary tract or the vagina during delivery.

The good news is that HPV and genital warts are only very rarely transmitted to the baby.[49] The bad news is that if they are, very rarely they can grow in the baby's throat, obstructing breathing. To be safe, if you have visible genital warts, your care provider may prescribe a topical cream called imiquimod to treat them. There is little known about the effects of this medication on an unborn baby. You should not be prescribed podophyllin, 5-fluorouracil cream, or podofilox because they are absorbed by the skin and may cause birth defects in your baby. Large warts can be removed with laser surgery or by freezing with liquid nitrogen.

SYPHILIS

While syphilis seems like a disease from another era, it remains quite common in the U.S., and some researchers even believe that it's on the rise. Your healthcare provider will test your blood for syphilis at your first prenatal visit. If your test is positive, you'll be treated with antibiotics, in the form of injections or oral doses of penicillin. Your healthcare provider may prescribe erythromycin if you are allergic to penicillin. Your partner also needs to be tested and treated. Prevent syphilis and other STDs by using condoms if either you or your partner are not monogamous. Being treated for syphilis before the sixteenth to eighteenth week of pregnancy will usually prevent the fetus from getting the disease. Treatment is very important, because without it the chances of your baby being stillborn, deformed, or very unhealthy is high. Later treatment may lessen your baby's infection, but the baby may be born with some problems caused by syphilis.

A baby born with syphilis will be treated with penicillin given as a shot or intravenously (IV).

GONORRHEA

Gonorrhea, another common STD, affects about a million women a year. Healthcare providers routinely test for it during your first prenatal visit with either a cervical swab or a urine test. If the test is positive, you'll be given a round of antibiotics. Effectively treated, you and your baby should have nothing to worry about. Like chlamydia, untreated it can cause pelvic inflammatory disease, and can cause an eye infection in your newborn if you're infected at the time of delivery. Healthcare providers routinely apply erthyromycin ointment to babies' eyes after birth to prevent this, even if your test was negative. Like any other STD, if your test is positive, it's important that your partner is tested and treated also.

Vaginal birth after a cesarean (VBAC)

"Once a cesarean, always a cesarean," is the typical medical stance about mothers giving birth vaginally after having undergone a cesarean section in the past. Giving birth vaginally was thought to be risky because labor would put stress on the previous incision site and possibly cause a uterine rupture. Only 12 percent of women with a previous cesarean opt to attempt to deliver vaginally.

However, a study published in 2003 in the *American Journal of Obstetrics* that pooled studies covering nearly 48,000 births found that women who had undergone previous cesarean births, but were allowed to go into labor (sometimes called a trial of labor) experienced signifi-

cant benefits over those who underwent a repeat cesarean section.

While the strain of labor and vaginal delivery on the uterus did cause a small increase in the rate of uterine rupture and complications for babies when compared with elective repeat cesareans, the women who gave birth vaginally had fewer fevers, less need for blood transfusions, and their risks of life-threatening bleeding, hysterectomies, and fatal injuries were reduced.

VBAC should not be attempted if you have had a vertical or T-shaped incision, which makes you more vulnerable to having your uterus rupture or if you're pregnant with twins after having had a prior c-section.

It is also not advised if your baby is estimated to be larger than normal, if your baby isn't positioned head downward, or if there are inadequate facilities at your hospital for performing an emergency c-section should you need one.

You and your healthcare provider will need to carefully review your medical records to study what caused your prior c-section. If it was the result of having a breech baby, having your placenta misplaced or coming loose (abruption), your baby having a cord accident, or because a previous baby went into fetal distress, you still have a 74 to 94 percent chance of a successful vaginal delivery. Your chances of successful vaginal delivery are lowered to between 35 and 77 percent if you had *cephalo-pelvic disproportion (CPD)*—a mismatch in size between your pelvis and your baby, or if you had an induction that failed.

Because of the small increased chance of rupture if you attempt a VBAC, you'll have to be more closely monitored during labor. Induction is not recommended, and you should not attempt to have your baby at home or in a birth center unless a blood supply has been set aside for you and there is a nearby hospital that has been notified in advance that can offer immediate help. Otherwise, labor and birth can proceed normally.

Coping with bed rest

Many pregnant women are sent to bed by their doctors at some point in their pregnancy, for conditions such as pre-term labor, pregnancy-related hypertension, slow fetal growth, carrying twins, placenta previa, and incompetent cervix. Bed rest is believed to increase blood flow to the uterus and placenta, help kidney function, take pressure off your cervix, and possibly lower high blood pressure.

These complications, or the fear of possible complications, may provoke your healthcare provider to instruct you to hit the bed for days, weeks, or even months. However, lately, many doctors and researchers are beginning to rethink bed rest as a solution. The side effects can be severe, and there's no medical evidence to guarantee it works.

While lying in bed seems like a harmless activity, side effects can include headaches, blood clots in the legs, muscle atrophy, weight loss, depression, and anxiety. Often, even after delivery, the effects of passive immobility can continue, such as difficulty walking up and down stairs and deep soreness in your back and leg muscles.

The bed rest prescription also means you have to stop work, certainly a shock to your employer or anyone else who relies on you.

Currently, there is no standard protocol for prescribing bed rest. Being put on bed rest, and the extent to which your activities may be restricted, may depend more on your care provider's style than on your physical symptoms.

Many healthcare providers prescribe bed rest for problem pregnancies because they want you to feel like you're doing everything you can—even if the complications are out of your control.

Ask your healthcare provider the following questions if you've been prescribed bed rest:

- **Predicted outcome.** How and why will bed rest help my condition?

- **Side effects.** Are you aware of the side effects of bed rest, and do

you think that the benefits will outweigh them?

- **The details.** Make sure you know what he means by the concept of bed rest. Are you going to be allowed to sit up? Or, should you lie on your left side all the time? Can you get up to go to the kitchen or bathroom? Can you hook up a laptop and work from home? Should you limit your sexual activities?

- **Second opinion.** Get a second opinion, particularly if you begin to experience the side effects listed above.

Managing Other Risks

IF YOU GET SICK

Catching a cold while you're pregnant is more miserable than at almost any other point in life—not only did you already feel heavy and congested before, now you're scared for the baby and don't know if you should feel guilty about taking medicine.

Here's a quick guide of what you should know:

Colds and flu won't hurt your baby, even if they make you miserable. The exception is if you have a high temperature (102°F or above) for more than a day, especially during the first trimester, or if you become dehydrated, which may cause premature labor.

Treat your cold as soon as you begin to feel ill.
Go home, drink plenty of liquid so your body can wash out the germs, take a zinc lozenge, and get under the covers.

Monitor your temperature, and control a fever.
If your temperature is above 101°F, take a dose of acetaminophen (Tylenol), and call your care provider.

Avoid echinacea.
Some researchers believe that echinacea can stimulate uterine contractions and cause premature labor. Other researchers say that because no definitive studies have been conducted, it's too soon to tell. Either way, major studies have shown that echinacea has no benefit in shortening the duration or severity of a cold—placebos are apparently just as effective.

Read labels of all herbal products.
If you drink herbal tea, check the label, and avoid any teas which contain echinacea, ma huang, pennyroyal, mugwort, and/or any type of cohosh. All of these are suspected of causing premature labor. If your tea of choice has ingredients you haven't heard of, ask your care provider if they're safe.

Stay hydrated.
Chicken soup, water, juice, sports drinks, and green tea are good choices. Calcium-fortified orange, tomato, and carrot juice are nutritious choices while juice-drink combinations loaded with sugar, sucrose or high fructose corn syrup are carb-heavy. (Read the label.)

Take something if you're miserable.
It is a good idea to avoid unnecessary medications while you're pregnant, but most cold and flu medications are safe to take during pregnancy, so there's no need to suffer. Call your care provider, and ask her to recommend an over-the-counter medication for your symptoms.

Be cautious with antibiotics.
Antibiotics are useless against any illness caused by a virus. They only cure bacterial infections. Taking unneeded antibiotics will make you (and your baby) more likely to be plagued with infections caused by drug-resistant bacteria in the future. Don't take them unless you and your care provider are sure that a bacterial infection is the cause of your ills.

If you're vomiting, it won't hurt the baby unless you reach the point of becoming dehydrated. Drink water, Pedialyte®, or sports drinks, even if most of it just comes back up. If you're sick and can't keep anything down for twelve hours or more, call your care provider.

Try steam from a humidifier, shower, facial steamer, or a washcloth soaked in hot water over your face.

Elevate your head if your sinuses are congested. Use pillows to keep your head and neck up so your sinuses can drain.

IF YOU HAVE AN ACCIDENT

If you fall or are hit on the abdomen, it's terrifying—but probably okay. Your baby is in liquid, in a membrane, surrounded by the muscles of your uterus, with your abdominal muscles on top. To harm the baby, the impact would have to be hard enough so that if you weren't pregnant, it would cause damage to your internal organs. One author of this book was hit by a car, in the stomach, while eight months pregnant, and the baby was fine. Since occasionally hitting your stomach or falling can cause serious problems for the pregnancy, do inform your care provider of any falls, accidents, or incidents of domestic violence. He can order a sonogram to make sure the baby's okay.

HIGH ALTITUDES

If you live above seven thousand feet, your body is already used to functioning with less oxygen. If you don't, then it makes sense to avoid traveling anywhere with an altitude of higher than seven thousand feet or flying in an unpressurized cabin above this level. The decreased oxygen will put a strain on your system and may even cause altitude sickness: nausea, headaches, and vomiting.

INSECTS

Pregnancy makes you more appealing to mosquitoes and other biting insects, because your blood vessels are more dilated, and you're giving off more body heat. Mosquitoes also are attracted to carbon dioxide, and pregnant women take larger and more frequent breaths. Use insect repellants that are labeled as being okay for children, and avoid products containing DEET—they've been associated with neurological and dermal reactions in humans. Also avoid natural repellants that contain oil of pennyroyal—though you probably won't absorb enough through the skin to make a difference, pennyroyal is known to induce abortion.

If you're unlucky enough to get an ant, roach, termite, or flea infestation while you're pregnant, investigate what measures you can take to avoid bombing the house. No one knows whether the bug sprays used by exterminators are safe for pregnant women or not, but the lists of warnings are certainly scary and extensive. If you must bomb, we suggest staying somewhere else for a week, and letting someone else go in and air out the house and wipe down the surfaces before you move back in.

If your neighborhood is being sprayed, stay inside with your windows closed. Again, no one knows whether the sprays are safe for pregnant women or not, but if they can kill all those bugs, it makes sense to avoid them.

CORD BLOOD BANKING

Along with the coupons for diapers and formula most pregnant women find in your mailboxes, you may also find some literature from for-profit "Cord Blood Banks," urging you to spend thousands of dollars to have your child's umbilical cord blood cryogenically frozen. What's the deal?

Blood from the umbilical cord contains stem cells, truly amazing unspecialized cells that can divide and renew themselves, and also differentiate—that is, develop into specialized cells. Because many diseases are the result of problems with certain cell types (leukemia, for instance, is a blood cell dysfunction), stem cells have the potential to help cure a huge variety of diseases. But emphasis is on potential. At this point, the only application for cord blood stem cells is to treat certain very rare life-threatening leukemias and rare blood disorders such as Fanconi's Anemia in siblings—essentially the same afflictions that would be treated with a bone marrow donation.

It's important to know that doctors can only rarely use a child's own cord blood to treat disease, because that blood would most likely carry the disease too. The chance of any child developing a disease that can be treated with their own stem cells has been estimated at less than one in ten thousand; some experts put the figure as much smaller.

Therefore, storing your child's own cord blood is really only worthwhile when there is a child in the family who already has, or has had, leukemia or some other specific disease. Under these circumstances, there is a one in four chance that the new baby will be a perfect match for her sick sibling.

Another option is to donate the cord blood to a stem cell bank through the National Marrow Donor Program. To join, you must fill out a questionnaire, give a blood sample to determine your tissue type, and sign forms consenting to being listed on the registry. You also must give birth in a participating hospital. If you choose to donate cord blood, then after you deliver the baby, cord, and placenta, the cord blood stem cells will be collected by a trained nurse, then rushed to a collection facility, where they're registered in a computer system, then cryogenically frozen until or if they're needed. And should your family need it, the donation will be available to you too.

For more information, visit the National Marrow Donor Program at www.marrow.org.

IF YOU BECAME PREGNANT WHILE USING BIRTH CONTROL

If you became pregnant while using some method of birth control, you have a lot of company. One-fourth of all pregnancies in America are due to contraceptive failure—that's more than a million pregnancies every year! If your pregnancy is one of the "lucky" ones, you may have extra concerns about birth defects or pregnancy problems. Most often, there's nothing to worry about in terms of the baby's safety.

Birth control pills and contraceptive patches

Birth control pills can fail if a dose is skipped, when there's a chemical interaction with certain antibiotics or antacids that block their absorption, or if anything prevents them from getting digested, like a stomach virus or food poisoning. Birth control patches and rings, which eliminate these problems, are therefore theoretically more reliable. All three methods, even when used absolutely correctly, do fail on rare occasions.

If you became pregnant while taking the pill or while wearing a contraceptive patch, there's no need to worry. There appears to be no increased risk of problems with the pregnancy or fetus. Just stop taking the pills or remove the patch as soon as you know you're pregnant.

Spermicides

The majority of birth-control-failure pregnancies are from the failure of spermicidal methods, such as a diaphragm with spermicide, contraceptive foam, the sponge, or contraceptive film. The failures of these methods result in more babies every year than there are residents of the city of Baltimore. Fortunately, studies have found no link between spermicides and birth defects or pregnancy problems.

An IUD (intrauterine device)

The IUD is very effective, with an average annual failure rate of less than one percent. Still, failures do occur, usually if the IUD has fallen out unnoticed. If you become pregnant with an IUD, call your gynecologist right away, and check to see if you can still feel the IUD string. If you can't find the string, the device has either fallen out or has gotten out of position. Your care provider will probably order an ultrasound to see which is the case. If it's still in there, your pregnancy will be left to progress as usual, because the device is off to one side and unlikely to get in the way. Your care provider will just deliver it with the baby.

However, if you can still feel the IUD string when you discover you're pregnant, your care provider will carefully remove the device.

Though no one knows for sure, researchers believe that an IUD works by causing a chain reaction of chemical messages that disorient sperm. You're about five percent more likely to miscarry if you become pregnant with an IUD.

Becoming pregnant with an IUD also increases your risk for an ectopic pregnancy—be alert and notify your provider immediately if you experience bleeding, cramps, or fever.

Depo-Provera®

Depo-Provera is a contraceptive shot which contains a medication similar to the hormones in birth control pills, but in doses high enough to prevent pregnancy for three months. It's extremely effective: You're as likely to get pregnant in the three months after getting a Depo-Provera injection as you would be if you had an operation to be sterilized.

Before you got the shot, your care provider should have tested you for pregnancy or administered the shot during your period, because some studies have shown the drug to be statistically associated with an increase in the incidences of low birth weight, stillbirth, and infant death,[50] particularly in women who become pregnant in the one to two months after the shot. If this happens to you, discuss the risks with your care provider.

If you've decided to stop taking the shots and want to conceive, many practitioners recommend using a non-hormonal birth control method (such as condoms) for at least six months before you start trying.

Tubal sterilization (tubal ligation)

Hard to believe, but women do sometimes become pregnant even after their fallopian tubes are "tied," sometimes many years after the operation. Almost always, these are ectopic pregnancies—meaning that a sperm has somehow managed to cross the divide and fertilize the egg, but the zygote can't descend into the uterus and implant and instead grows in the tube and must be removed surgically or treated medically. If your pregnancy is the one in vast myriads that implants normally, discuss it with your care provider.

On the other hand, it's quite possible to get pregnant after you or your partner has had the sterilization operation reversed. How likely and easy it is to get pregnant afterward depends on the type of sterilization procedure. The pregnancy rate after a male vasectomy is reversed can be as high as ninety percent. For reversed female sterilization, the rate can vary between fifty-five and eighty-five percent, depending on individual circumstances like which sterilization procedure was employed, and how well the reversal operation went. If you do become pregnant after a reversal, however, there's no reason why your pregnancy shouldn't proceed as usual.

PREVIOUS ABORTION

If you're worried about whether a previous abortion may affect your ability to give birth now, you needn't be.

If you've had one or more abortions in the past which were uncomplicated and performed in a modern, medically adequate facility, you have no greater risk of fertility problems, ectopic pregnancy, premature birth, low birth weight, deformities, or miscarriage than any other woman.

If you did suffer from complications after an abortion, such as infection or perforation, make sure that your care provider is aware of the details, so you can be monitored.

TIPPED UTERUS

If you've been told you have a tipped uterus (also known as a retroverted uterus), there's no need to be concerned about your pregnancy. This simply means that your uterus points towards your back instead of your front (called anteverted). While the condition is associated with higher incidences of *endometriosis* and painful intercourse, it has not been associated with any pregnancy problems or complications.

HOT TUBS, BATHS, SAUNAS, AND ELECTRIC BLANKETS

Experts advise against exposing your body to temperatures higher than 102°F during the first trimester. Studies have linked early fetal heat exposure to neural tube defects and to a higher risk of first-trimester miscarriage. So for the first months of your pregnancy, don't soak in water that's uncomfortably hot. Avoid water temperatures that feel painfully warm when you stick your toe in, or tubs, saunas, or steam rooms that make you feel flushed and sweaty. If you decide to soak and sweat after the first trimester, be wary of lightheadedness and dehydration.

If you use an electric blanket, avoid higher settings during the first trimester.

UTERINE FIBROIDS

Fibroids are non-malignant growths that can develop in the muscle tissue of the uterus. It's possible to have one or several. The growths are made up of muscle and fibrous tissue, and the hormone estrogen encourages them, making them more common in women who use birth-control pills or are pregnant. About fifteen percent of women have uterine fibroids[51] at some point in their life (most commonly after age thirty-five), and about 4 percent of pregnant women have them,[52] a number that's gone up as the pregnant population has aged. For reasons unknown, African-American women are more susceptible to developing them at an earlier age.

Most often, uterine fibroids pose no problem, and women don't even know that they're there. They don't appear to have any effect on fertility. Sometimes, though, large fibroids can cause issues such as lower-back or abdominal pain, feelings of pressure, or abnormal bleeding. Because of the risk of miscarriage, fibroids shouldn't be removed while you're pregnant.

If you had fibroids removed at some point before you became pregnant, this shouldn't affect your ability to carry a baby to term unless the fibroids were extremely large and removing them was complicated. In this case, your uterus may be weaker than normal, and your care provider may recommend a cesarean delivery.

If you're pregnant and have fibroids, ultrasound should be able to detect their size and position. Your care provider should then be able to discuss with you how they may affect your pregnancy. In some cases, they can increase your risk of ectopic pregnancy, miscarriage, placenta previa (when the placenta blocks the baby's way out), abruptio placentae (when the placenta prematurely separates from the uterine wall), premature labor, and/or a baby in a difficult-to-deliver position. So if you have fibroids, be attentive to signs of trouble: pink discharge for several days, bloody show, bleeding, or cramping.

TRAVELING

You don't need to avoid air travel (other than in unpressurized craft above 7,000 feet) unless you're at risk for premature delivery or have a condition that may need constant monitoring by a physician, such as high blood pressure.

Airlines usually have no restrictions on pregnant passengers up to eight months, and most will take your word for it when you tell them how far along you are. Still, always call and check with the airline you're flying with to verify their policy, because some airlines may require a doctor's note stating that you're okay to travel, signed within the past seventy-two hours. Others may require a doctor's note if you're at all visibly pregnant. Their main concern is that you won't go into labor on board, forcing an emergency landing.

Tips for Flying When You're Pregnant

- Avoid lifting heavy bags.
- Make your seat request as soon as the airline will let you. Being close to the front of the plane will make it easier for you to get on and off, and the air is fresher there.
- Ask for a bulkhead seat. Bulkhead seats at the very front of the cabin nearest first-class seats allow the most legroom, and you can take off your shoes and put your feet up on the carpeted cabin divider if your back starts to ache or your legs feel swollen.

- Choose an aisle seat. You can get to the bathroom without having to disturb fellow passengers. It's also a good idea to walk around and stretch your legs every hour or so to reduce swelling.
- Get up and walk around the plane once an hour. This will help prevent you from getting blood clots in your legs, to which pregnant women are slightly more prone than non-pregnant women.

WORRYING OBSESSIVELY ABOUT THE BABY

Every mom wants to know if her baby will be healthy and normal. It's terrifying, after all, to know that you are responsible for this little person. The world is full of mysterious chemicals, and tests seem to only give you the barest information. The odds are overwhelmingly in your favor that your baby will be fine, but you can't stop thinking, "What if I am that one in 250? Somebody has to be that one." If your worry seems out of control, here are some things to do:

- **Don't try to push thoughts out of your head.** It doesn't work. Spend serious time with your worry instead. Say it out loud, even write it down. When you can hear it and see it, it'll carry less weight.
- **Don't worry about your dreams**. Almost every pregnant woman has a dream of giving birth to a deformed baby or some kind of animal. Dreams indicate your current emotional state, not what's going to happen in the future.

- **Carry your thoughts out to the finish.** If you have a vague fear that "something" is wrong with the baby, try to pinpoint exactly what it is you worry about the most. Deformities? Disorders? Then address those worries one at a time, by talking to your healthcare provider about them specifically and doing research.
- **Step up your classes.** If you're only planning to take a short childbirth class, consider switching to one that meets weekly for several weeks. You can use class time to get your worrying out of the way for the week.
- **If you have had a test that shows that something might be wrong,** know that the odds are still in your favor that the baby will be healthy. Ask your healthcare provider what the test's false-positive rate is, and don't hesitate to get a second opinion.
- **If it's clear that something specific is wrong** with the baby, do as much research from as many different types of sources as you can. Try to meet adults with the condition, and locate and talk to parents of kids with the condition. Ask your care provider to refer you to specialists, and find online bulletin boards.

Managing Family and Emotional Issues

Your dreams are full of talking babies and animals. Your family has something to say about every bite you eat. Your drinking buddies are acting like you've joined a weird cult, and your husband is brooding around the house with a pint of ice cream—or is downright freaking out. Welcome to your pregnant emotional life! We can't remedy all of the craziness in your life, but here are some common emotional and relationship issues pregnant women face, some information about what's going on, and some suggestions to help you cope.

THE STRANGE DREAMS OF PREGNANCY

As the third trimester progresses, your sleep becomes lighter, and your dreams may seem more intense.

More often than not, a pregnant woman's dreams are more vivid, more emotional, and more memorable than ordinary dreams. During your pregnancy, you'll probably have at least one or two dreams that you remember for a long time, because they were so strange, scary, marvelous, or symbolic. Why?

There are countless theories about the causes and meanings of dreams, many thousands of years old: that they are the way the dead communicate with you, that they bring omens or symbols that predict the future, that they bring messages from the almighty.

One of the newer theories about dreaming is that it helps your subconscious mind sort the information it received during the day, kind of like a secretary filing a pile of the boss' random message slips. Information from the recent past is being added in with older memories, and the mingling of the old and new information creates a strange story, a sort of mental Mad Lib. Add to this mix all of the extra hormonal messages and physical changes your body and brain are going through, and all of the new sensations and worries, and your dreams may be very unusual, indeed.

Right now, your whole body and brain is in a state of high alert. It's critical to your baby's survival that your subconscious mind, the part that has you swerve before your car hits a tree, is ready to react to new potential threats and surprises. Perhaps this is why pregnant women often report having dreams about things like giving birth to a litter of kittens, or dreams where their babies are demonic. It doesn't mean that your baby will actually have a tail, of course. More likely, your brain is just rehearsing, so that if your baby is born, and he doesn't look like you expected, or there are surprises while you're giving birth, you'll be able to react appropriately to keep you and your baby safe.

DEPRESSION

Do you spend more than half of your life being tired and sleeping, crying, feeling annoyed and irritated, or feeling overwhelmed and out of control? Do you not want to do the same things you used to do, and feel isolated? Then you're not just pregnant, you're probably depressed too. Some women become depressed for the first time during pregnancy, while women who have a history of depression are at risk for a recur-

rence of their depressive symptoms. Some studies of premature birth and low birth weight have appeared to link stress and depression.

Medical research appears to show that serious depression can be caused by biochemical imbalances in the brain and can be triggered by stressful circumstances. Considering what a stress pregnancy is on your body, lifestyle, and body chemistry, it comes as no surprise that some of the milder symptoms of depression are the same as pregnancy symptoms that are almost universal in pregnant women.

The most common treatment for depression in America today comes in pill form, and modern drug therapy is thought to be safe for you and your baby, although long-term research results aren't in yet. Should your symptoms persist for more than a week, or they get worse, or if you have feelings of wanting to hurt yourself, your baby, or your partner, it's important that you contact your healthcare provider and tell her about your symptoms. If your doctor or midwife brushes off your symptoms as normal, seek the guidance of a psychiatrist.

Since depression and stress are associated with low birth weight, you and your doctor or psychiatrist must weigh the risks and benefits of medication. Unlike therapists, social workers, psychologists, or counselors, psychiatrists—who are also medical doctors—can prescribe the appropriate medications for you.

If you feel like you want to hurt yourself, get to your care provider as quickly as possible to get help. Depression is a disease, like diabetes, and can be treated and controlled.

Non-Drug Options for Depression

There are also non-drug treatments that may work just as well for you or even better for minor symptoms of depression, and if you're on medication for depression, they can help your medication work better:

- **Magnesium.** Make sure you get enough depression-fighting magnesium (found in fruits, nuts and vegetables) and omega-3 (DHA) fatty acids (found in olive oil and fish).

- **Low carbs.** Avoid sugar and processed flours.

- **Balanced blood sugar.** Keep food in your stomach at all times, and drink water: low blood sugar can increase feelings of depression and irritability.

- **Moderate exercise.** Exercise has been shown to help alter feelings of depression. Try moderate exercise such as walking, swimming, or yoga forty minutes a day to make your body release more endorphins, which elevate your mood.

- **Control stress.** Avoid stressful situations if you can. Now is not a good time to take on new responsibilities if you can avoid them.

- **Avoid self-medicating.** Any antidepressant in the world will likely be better for you and your baby than alcohol, smoking, or recreational drugs. Seek safer alternatives.

The most common medical solution is a prescription for a selective serotonin reuptake inhibiting drug (SSRIs), such as fluoxetine (Prozac®) (see "Antidepressants" in the drug guide), sertraline (Zoloft®), or fluvoxamine (Luvox®). None of these drugs have currently been linked to birth defects or developmental delays in babies.

PREGNANT AGAIN

Second and successive pregnancies have their perks: you're used to the symptoms, you've scouted out the good maternity shops, you probably already have a healthcare provider that you know and trust, and you may even still have baby supplies left over from last time. You know what supplies you need and what's a waste of money. Your partner is probably a little calmer too, and may already be in the habit of doing chores—you both know what you're getting yourselves into, more or less. And you can take comfort in knowing that labor gets shorter with every successive pregnancy, sometimes by a lot. If you had a thirty-hour labor of misery the first time, you'll almost certainly not have to suffer that the second time.

On the other hand, you may find that you get a lot less attention this time around. Of course, ladies in the grocery store will still ask you personal questions, but at home, your partner may have to be prodded a little bit harder to make you a sandwich.

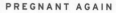

Ways to Prepare a Sibling

If your child is two or younger:

- Let Dad take responsibility for more of your child's daily routine, so it won't be a big shock after baby arrives.

- Talk up the concept. Even very young children model their attitudes on what you say and do, and understand things before they can speak. Use this to your advantage by pointing out babies in books, on TV, and in the shopping mall with great delight, saying things like, "Babies are great! What a cute baby! I love babies!"

- And avoid using the word "baby" in a negative context in front of your child. No "Ow, this baby is killing me!" or "Stop acting like a baby!"

- Visit as many babies as you can, and talk over the rules of babies with your child. "We have to be very gentle and not poke or scare the baby."

- Get your child in the habit of walking instead of being carried. Get him in the habit of walking from the car to the house and back and up and down stairs while holding your or Dad's hand as soon as possible.

- Prepare to stay in a while. If you have a babe-in-arms and an older child in the middle of the terrible twos, going out to eat, shopping, or taking a stroll anywhere but an open field is going to be nearly impossible if you don't have extra hands to help hold the baby or get your toddler out of trouble. Collect phone numbers, e-mail addresses, and information from anywhere that delivers, such as grocery stores, dry cleaners, and pharmacies. Consider ordering bulky items such as pet food, diapers, and baby wipes online, and see what bills you can pay online.

If your child is between two and six:

- Let your child feel the baby kick.

- Bring out the baby pictures of your child, and tell him about what it was like when he came home for the first time.

- Play house with your child and a baby doll, and talk about what babies are like.

With successive pregnancies, you'll feel symptoms sooner and begin to show almost as soon as you get a positive test result. Even if you've worked hard to get your *rectus abdominus* muscles (abs) rock-hard since your last pregnancy, they "remember" the drill from last time and quickly get into the outward uterus-supporting position. Looser abs also means you get to feel fetal movement sooner.

It's worthwhile to get a copy of your medical records from your last pregnancy and look them over. There may be things you've forgotten, and if there were any complications in your past deliveries, talk to your care provider about how

- Visit a baby, or invite one over. If baby's mom lets you, sit the child on your lap, and hold the baby together.

- When you've run out of lap, tell your child that a new baby sister or brother is on the way.

- Prepare them for your time in the hospital. If you're planning to have a relative or neighbor to your house to babysit, encourage your babysitter-to-be to drop in during the weeks before your due date. Ideally, have her over for dinner, a few hours of playtime, and the going-to-bed ritual, so she'll have some idea of your house routines. If your child will be staying somewhere else, like with grandparents, consider a sleepover beforehand.

- Emphasize what's great about not being a baby anymore: "You get to use the potty, and drink out of a cup, walk around in galoshes, turn the faucet on and off..."

- Don't leave a child younger than the age of four alone with the baby. They don't yet understand cause and effect.

If your child is older:

- Think of some age-appropriate chores that your child could learn to help you with: sorting laundry, folding clothes, picking up toys, emptying wastebaskets, and so on. Consider offering rewards for jobs well done.

- Bring your family to a prenatal appointment, and have your partner bring your child into the exam room when it's time to listen to the baby's heartbeat.

- Let your child and partner plan the "welcome baby" party and help open gifts. Few kids can resist the allure of an extra birthday party being added to the family calendar!

- Ask your child what baby names he likes.

likely they are to recur and if there are ways to prevent them from happening again.

Particularly if you suffered from depression during or after your last pregnancy, be alert for symptoms this time around. Also know that it's possible to be depressed even if you weren't during your previous pregnancies.

Even if you didn't get **stretch marks** or **hemorrhoids** or **spider veins** the first time around, you still might this time. Sorry.

You're older this time around, obviously, and if you're like most American women, you're a bit heavier. Remember that you need a good balance of exercise and rest during this pregnancy too.

YOU AND YOUR CHILD-FREE FRIENDS

Being pregnant is a whole-life makeover. You're expected to go cold turkey with your every vice, make every bite count, prepare everyone at work for your absence, exercise, get plenty of sleep, solidify your relationship with your partner, save money for the future, and get on waiting lists for preschools. When you're pregnant, suddenly it gets virtually impossible to think about anything but being pregnant. You will never lack for pregnancy, birth, and baby-related things to think and talk about. If this is your first pregnancy, you may have plenty of friends who see your condition as a kind of debilitating disease that keeps you from having any fun, and they wonder why you've gone and done this to yourself. To your childless friends who want kids, you're going to a party where they haven't been invited, which may make you want to tone down your joy.

And a part of you might be jealous of those who are kid-free. Wouldn't it be nice to just worry about your car or your hairdo for a while? No matter what you may be gaining by having this child, there will always be the path you didn't take, as a freewheeling single who's not responsible for anything but a bar tab and who can leave the country on a whim.

It could be that you and your childless friends will cross paths less often in the future, but it doesn't have to be that way. Remember that everything about pregnancy but the baby is temporary. While the next year or two might make you want to keep closer to home, there really isn't anything that you can't do once you become a parent; activities just require more advance planning. Either by bringing your baby along or by using family, babysitters, and the support of your partner, you'll be able to go on vacations, write your novel, socialize, and do just about everything you could do before. You'll still have the same sense of humor and taste that you've always had. If you can't identify with your single friends' lives right now, you may reconnect in the future as you get more free time.

In the meantime, seek out activities that you and your friends can enjoy without drinking, eating sushi, or participating in body-contact sports. You don't have to avoid bars or parties while you're pregnant, but you may find that sitting for hours and sipping a club soda while your friends get sloppy is not much fun. Rather than making plans to just sit at a bar, try planning activity dates. Shop, sew, swim, see a movie, and get out in the world. It's as good for them as it is for you!

UNSOLICITED ADVICE

Are you sure you need to eat that? Have you thought about preschools? Are you sure it's safe to go skiing? Are you going to breastfeed? Are you going back to work? Perhaps the most annoying of all pregnancy complaints is that everyone—friends, family, and people on the street—has an opinion on your every move. You may spend much of your mental energy devising snappy comebacks and arguments to defend your choices. Unfortunately, this is one pregnancy complaint that doesn't go away after the baby is born. Why is pregnancy and parenthood an invitation to the world to comment on your decisions? Here are a few theories:

- **They really want to help.** It's always possible that whoever is dispensing advice wants to impart information to make things easier for you.

- **They feel a kinship with you.** Every woman who's ever been pregnant remembers the experience.

- **They feel insecure about their own choices.** Sometimes, and not even consciously, people can see the choices that you make as a criticism of their own decisions. Of course it's silly; opting to buy a different brand of stroller than your best friend did doesn't mean that you think her choice is inferior, and she's an inferior parent for buying it. But there's so little reassurance in parenting, and so few clear right or wrong answers, it makes people desperate for affirmation.

- **Nagging is a hard habit to break.** Your family has plenty of experience in giving you their opinion, and for some parents, their daughters' pregnancy is the Olympic nagging event they've been training for their whole lives. And sometimes just an expression of doubt can make you question your decisions, which will make you even more resentful. Pregnancy may remind you of high school again—you feel the need to assert your authority and independence.

What can you do about unsolicited advice? Our advice is, if smiling and nodding isn't enough, kindly thank the nags for their opinion, and change the subject in a hurry. If the nagging extends to your partner, or makes you feel negative or helpless, it's time to take a stand. While you may need your family's loving support, you also need to keep your stress level low.

Taking a stand is good practice for mothering. You have a right to decide what you want you and your baby exposed to, and if you offend anyone, you can blame it on pregnancy hormones.

SCARY MEDICAL STORIES

If you have a lot of older, female relatives, they may have some scary hospital stories to tell. Hospitals of twenty and thirty years ago were very different places, and the whole childbirth experience has changed a lot since then.

Back in their day, hospitals hadn't embraced the concept of informed consent, and patients were not expected to be involved in their own care. Having a *doula* or labor support person was unheard of, dads were not in the delivery room, and women were subjected to a lot of unnecessary and uncomfortable procedures that aren't done anymore, like pubic shaving and enemas. So don't let your older relatives or your mom scare you. Also feel free to interrupt the beginning of a story to say, "Is this story positive? If not, I'd rather not hear it right now."

FORGIVING YOUR PARENTS

All of your life, your parents have held more sway over your opinions and perspective about the world than any other human beings. Now that you're about to have a child of your own, you can see the man (and woman) behind the curtain—your parents are just people. They probably weren't any more prepared to become parents than you are right

now. Like you, they already had personalities before they had children. They kept secrets from you, just like you're going to keep your diaries from Junior, and they did the best they could. When you have a child of your own, your relationship to your parents changes and almost always for the better. You'll never be their equal, but you will become more of a peer. You'll have new respect for their efforts and successes and are in a position to improve on their mistakes.

You and your partner

FATHERHOOD: WHO'S A MODERN DAD?

A hundred years ago, a man with a pregnant wife was considered actively involved in his wife's pregnancy if he took her on walks after dark (to disguise her unbecoming condition). As recently as thirty years ago, a husband in the delivery room was unheard of. A family was structured as a hierarchy of power, not a camaraderie of companions, and roles were well defined. A Victorian dad would be quite happy to never have to hear word one about any female trouble.

A modern expectant dad, on the other hand, can be found in childbirth classes taking notes and assuming undignified positions, driving through the snow for pork chops and doughnuts at midnight, or scooping the cat box and arguing the merits of

perineal massage. When the time comes, modern Dad is expected to be right there in the delivery room, able to weigh and argue the risks and benefits of any possible intervention with the doctor while applying acupressure points during contractions, before catching the baby, cutting the cord, and gifting his wife with a nice piece of jewelry.

Modern Dad is expected to be a bastion of emotional stability, a best friend and virile breadwinner, playing the roles that servants or extended family would have provided in times past, unless he has servants or family to fulfill them. Although most men still do less housework than their wives, that gap has been halved since the 1960s. Today, forty-nine percent of couples say they share child care equally, compared with twenty-five percent in 1985. And dads spend more time with their kids today than they have at any point in history.

This is all time well spent—kids benefit emotionally, financially, and educationally from having involved dads, even dads who don't seem to know what they're doing. And dads find that fatherhood makes their lives more emotionally rewarding, rich, and meaningful. Hands-on fathers make better parents than men who let their wives do all the nurturing and child care. They raise sons who are more expressive and daughters who are more likely to do well in school—especially in math and science.

So how can you help your partner go from dude to Dad?

Help him vocalize his fears.

If he's normal, your partner has a laundry list of fears. Will he pass out in the delivery room? Is he doomed to be the kind of dad his own father was? Your husband may be reluctant to talk about his fears because he doesn't want to burden you, but it's now more important than ever that you keep the lines of communication open and listen, even if you don't like what he has to say.

Reassure him that he's more to you than earning power.

The first thing many, many men say when they find out that they're going to be dads is, "Can we afford it?" It's still our cultural expectation that Dad will carry the primary financial responsibility for the family. That's not sexism—somebody has to bring home most of the bacon, and somebody has to be baby's caregiver. But emotional contributions are at least equally as important.

Promote active involvement.

If Dad's game, prepare him to be your eyes, ears, and voice while you're in labor and giving birth. Offer to let him come along to prenatal appointments if he's interested, and make sure he can make it to any ultrasounds. But also understand that he may not feel able to leave work for portions of the day very frequently.

Don't spare him.

If something goes wrong, don't think that you're doing him a favor by withholding information.

Know that distance is normal.

You may have heard of couples who decide to have kids to bring them closer together; that's a misguided notion, to say the least. The physical and emotional changes of pregnancy can make you feel worlds away from your husband, especially in the first half of your pregnancy when you certainly feel pregnant but aren't yet showing. And as much empathy as he has, he won't be able to understand what you're going through, and vice versa. Developing sympathy and empathy even when you don't quite understand is an important skill for both of you.

Don't make him cut the cord.

Let your husband know that he doesn't have to do anything he doesn't want to do. Most dads these days want to be where the action is and like being a part of it, but if your husband is more comfortable passing out cigars in the waiting room, there's nothing wrong with

Notes for Dad

If she asks you to do something, do it. If you can't do it, make an effort. If you can't make an effort, pretend.

Don't tell "funny pregnant wife" stories at parties, unless she starts telling them first. There's a fine line between laughing "with" and "at," and the fog of hormones can blur the line.

Take her to and from any ultrasound or glucose tolerance tests. Ultrasound because you get to see the baby together. Glucose tolerance because it can make women nauseated and dizzy.

Careful with the breasts. They look great, but they can also be achy and sore. Be gentle unless otherwise instructed.

Remember that moods are fleeting. Pregnant women are going through a hormonal hailstorm—a certain level of neurotic behavior should be forgiven, even expected. Try to be the voice of reason and stability, and try not to take it personally. Your real wife is in there somewhere, and she'll be back someday. If she seems depressed (crying a lot, sleeping too much or too little, acting listless) for more than a week or so, though, that's not healthy. Use your influence to get her help, for both of your sakes.

Say "I love you" with chores and errands. It's been scientifically proven by marital researchers that guys who do more chores have more sex! Dishwashing, laundry, and straightening up are to women what revealing lingerie is to men.

---

that. Also tell him that it's fine and good if he stands at your head during delivery. It's important that he's there, not that he see every graphic detail.

Talk about both of your expectations for life after birth.

Some people say that the key to happiness is managing your expectations. In other words, if you don't expect your partner to throw his socks in the hamper, you're not going to be angry if he doesn't. Think about what you do and don't expect from your partner, now and after the baby arrives.

- To stay in a job he hates to provide financial support for the family?
- To pitch in with chores?
- To let you sleep late sometimes?
- To clean up a spill completely instead of just throwing towels on top of it?
- To come home from work promptly so you can take a break?

It's better to be up-front about what you expect, rather than quiet, or worse, constantly nagging or remarking on his perceived shortfalls.

After baby arrives...

Learn to cook a few things. If you're confused in the kitchen, learn to make a few dishes that you both like. If you've never cooked before, use a cookbook, and follow recipes. Or better yet, have a member of her family show you how to make some of her favorite things. Just don't improvise and dare her to eat what you come up with.

Talk through her fears. Every woman worries about the health of her baby. You may have the "what if something's wrong with the baby?" conversation several times a week. Try to get her to narrow down her concerns as specifically as possible and vocalize them.

Ask about appointments. Call her after prenatal appointments, and take time to talk about them.

Don't drink in front of her if she misses drinking. And don't smoke in her presence—quit with her. If you can't, do your smoking on the other side of town.

Exercise with her. Get into the habit of taking walks, going for a swim, or stretching together.

Be familiar with her birth plan. Know what she wants and why, so that if she's too busy during labor to voice her preferences, you can reinforce them to the medical staff.

Play the protector. Open car doors, walk on the side of the street closest to the curb, and offer your arm. Take phone messages while she naps, or if she doesn't feel like talking.

Pump breast milk.

Many men feel left out by the bond that breastfeeding creates. The solution is not to deny your baby nutrients by adding formula feedings, but to express milk so that your husband gets to feed the baby sometimes too.

Trust him with the baby.

Don't interfere with dad's baby bonding by having a "you're doing it wrong" attitude. Unless he really is endangering the baby, let him figure out his own methods for getting things done.

Plan a vacation.

Formulate a plan now to get away together after the baby's weaned, even if it's only for a weekend or a night. Your baby needs you around, but he also needs his parents to have a strong relationship. And it's much easier to handle the stress of parenting when you have a break to look forward to.

Separate but equal?

Is it possible to have separate but equal roles? Pregnancy and childbirth can come as a surprise to couples who are used to feeling like equal companions, because there's simply no male equivalent for the pregnancy, birth, and breast-feeding experience. And having a baby does make you dependent on your partner to an extent you may not be used to. It's not always possible to avoid playing traditional roles, with Dad doing most of the earning, hunting, and gathering, and Mom covering the nurturing, at least until the child is weaned. And until she is old enough for school or full-time day care, somebody has to play the role of primary parent. It's possible, but rarely cost-effective, to put a child under the age of two into full-time day care. And naturally, the home duties fall to the person at home.

And the next thing you know, you're a stay-at-home mom, in a strange new universe. It's a role that you may cherish or chafe at (or both at different times). If you think that the easiest day at home with an infant is ten times harder than any office job, and he thinks you just sit around all day, you're going to have issues. If you both feel that you and your partner are doing your best to support the team, then you'll be in good shape.

Finding that balance, though, is a whole other book.

COUVADE SYNDROME

You're not the only one who may be experiencing the discomforts of pregnancy. Your partner may be affected, too. *Couvade syndrome* is the medical term for when your partner starts showing pregnancy symptoms along with you. The term comes from the French word *couvée*, meaning to hatch. The concept has

long been a subject of jokes ("Hey, your belly's getting bigger than mine!"), but now researchers are taking men's symptoms more seriously.

According to a Canadian study, men who live with their pregnant partners show a decline in the aggression-producing male hormone testosterone by more than a third and an increase in their levels of the hormones prolactin, cortisol, and estradiol. Prolactin, a hormone that stimulates lactation, also acts as a mild sedative. Cortisol is known to help people focus during stressful situations, and estradiol is a female sex hormone.

His hormonal shifts are in no way as dramatic as the ones you undergo, but your partner may indeed experience some nausea, indigestion, heartburn, change in appetite for food, weight gain, and, notably, a loss of interest in sex.

The universal nature of Couvade syndrome has long suggested to scientists that more is going on than a psychological experience. Reports of sympathetic pregnancy symptoms and rituals have been found in many diverse cultures around the world, from North and South America to Africa, India, Spain, France, and China.

So now there's proof that your partner's connection to your pregnancy is more than mental. These hormonal changes are thought to help your partner be a better father—more relaxed, nurturing, and less aggressive.

Some form of Couvade syndrome may also continue after birth. For every child a couple has, a man's risk of obesity goes up by four percent.[53]

ABUSE

At the opposite end of the spectrum from the broody husband is a violent partner. The American College of Obstetricians and Gynecologists estimates that as many as twenty-five percent of women are abused while pregnant. Abuse happens at all income levels and in all ethnic groups.

Some abusers say that they're jealous of the bond between the mother and unborn baby. Other men may be angry at their partners for becoming pregnant. Controlling men may also take advantage of what they perceive as their partners' vulnerability. The emotional stress of a baby on the way can create conditions in which violence can explode.

Abuse isn't just hitting. It can also take the form of psychological intimidation, sexual force, or social isolation. Women who are physically and/or emotionally abused have a greater chance of many complications, including miscarriage, low birth weight, and *premature rupture of the membranes*. Living under constant stress can retard fetal growth. Abdominal blows can cause fetal death.

If you're in an abusive relationship, your first step is to acknowledge it for what it is. Many abused women see each event as an isolated one, and convince themselves it won't happen again or that a partner who hits is better than none

at all. Unfortunately, one abusive incident almost always leads to another, and the level of violence and damage often goes up with each incident.

If your partner hits or intimidates you, he certainly will do the same to your children. In some cases, anger management classes or therapy may help—but only if your partner genuinely wants to stop. He's the only one that can make that decision.

Are you in an abusive relationship? If your partner has ever struck you on purpose, yes. But also ask yourself these questions:

- Do you ever feel afraid of your partner?
- Has your partner ever destroyed your belongings?
- Has your partner ever forced you to have sex against your will or forced you to engage in acts that made you feel uncomfortable?
- Has your partner ever prevented you from leaving the house, seeing friends or family, getting a job, or going to school?
- Has your partner ever threatened to hurt you or your children?

If you answered "yes" to any of these questions, talk over your concerns with someone whom you trust to give you an objective point of view. Talk to your care provider, childbirth educator, or the National Domestic Violence Hotline at (800) 799-7233. Don't be ashamed. Violence isn't your fault, and it's much more common than you think.

Single motherhood

In 2002, thirty-four percent of babies were born to parents who weren't married.[54] The label of single covers a lot of different situations: cohabiting parents, gay parents, and mothers who are single by choice.

The good news for single moms-to-be is that studies have shown that Mom's marital status (or sexual orientation) is not by itself an indicator of a child's well-being. Parental attention, access to social support, education, and financial resources are much more important to a child's overall mental and emotional health than a ring on Mom's finger. Kids from amicably divorced couples actually do better than kids from high-conflict married couples, and financially stable, well-educated single moms have healthier children overall than impoverished married couples.

The bad news is that single motherhood can make it difficult to become financially stable, or to become educated if you weren't before you became a mom. It's a high-stress situation, akin to working in an emergency room 24/7. Parenting an infant just can't be done by one person.

Also, for far too many women, single motherhood equals poverty—forty percent of single mothers have incomes of less than $10,000 a year. But don't let statistics make you feel doomed. Just realize that because you can't be in more than one place at one time, you're going to need extra practical help until your child reaches school age.

Consider what options you have that can give you and your baby maximum stability: perhaps moving in with relatives or moving a relative or good friend in to your home to help. Take advantage of any social programs, scholarships, or food programs that you can.

And also important, try to avoid burnout. Schedule social time for yourself, and use child care help even to just get extra sleep. Your baby needs a mother who isn't a basket case.

What about the name?

Married or not, you can give your child any last name you want to on his or her birth certificate, including none at all, à la Cher. As far as the law is concerned, the bestowing of a name doesn't establish paternity. You'll still have to go to court for that, or have the father sign an affidavit of parentage. Dad can still deny paternity of a baby with his last name if he wants to.

Think long and hard about giving your child his dad's last name if you aren't married to him and aren't sure that you ever will be. Giving your child a last name that's different than yours, while it may seem like a way to keep Dad involved, can become stigmatizing when you realize that it exposes your situation to the world. And if Dad is less than involved, you'll resent that he gets the legacy while you get the work. Consider hyphenation, or tell the father that you'll change your child's when and if you get married.

What about custody?

One in two kids born since the 1970s has had to deal with custody and visitation issues at some point in their life. In a best-case scenario, exes can agree to a custody, visitation, and child support arrangement that works for everyone involved and keeps working if someone moves away or gets remarried. If not, you may enter the world of family court.

If you and your baby's father have a good relationship, consider a session with a mediator (usually a family-law attorney) who can help you come to an agreement about rights and responsibilities, which a judge makes official by signing. If you can't agree, or if your ex already has a lawyer, then it's important to contact a family lawyer or legal aid in your area to establish custody, visitation, and child support. You need someone who understands the laws of your state, because every state is slightly different. But in any state, without a court order to establish parentage, custody, and support, your child's father has no rights to visitation, nor is he obligated to pay any share of your child's expenses.

Religious matters

If you're in a mixed-faith relationship, or have family members and in-laws who are vehement about their chosen religion, the disagreements about how your child will be raised will probably crop up as birth nears.

If religion has or will ever matter to you, it will matter more than ever during your pregnancy, as you and your partner consider what values and moral principles you want to raise your child with. You're making sure that the emotional and spiritual environment that your baby will be born into is the healthiest one you can create. If you and your partner share a faith, then you may be closer to agreement on what your parenting mission statement and your guiding principles will be. Issues such as where to attend services, whether or not to send your child to a religiously affiliated school, or whether or not you want to participate in rites such as baptism or circumcision probably won't be major points of conflict.

But even if you nominally share a faith, you may still have profound differences about how to put principles into practice. Not all Jews choose to circumcise their sons, and not all Christians believe in baptism. Not all Catholics want their children to attend Catholic schools. Some Muslims even put up Christmas trees.

Now that you're pregnant, what were once casual dinner conversations between you and your partner can become major philosophical showdowns. Add your parents and in-laws and their respective beliefs into the mix, and there's a high chance of faith-based conflict in your pregnancy forecast.

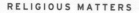

How to Handle Family Religious Conflict

Focus on what you have in common.
Even an atheist, an Imam, and a rabbi would agree that children should be raised with some kind of guiding ethical principles and a value system. When you have disagreements with your friends or family, try to put them into perspective and focus on what you do agree on.

Identify the real deal breakers.
There may be some things where you just have to say, "I will never, ever raise my child that way!" Put your foot down if you must; it's your right. But see if there are some things that you can compromise on in return. Many a mixed-faith family decorates a Hanukkah bush.

Remember that faith is a lifelong practice.
One compromise won't make or break your child's religious and/or ethical development. Your child will learn by watching and copying what you do and say on a daily basis.

Remember that religion is also about community.
Religion is not just about what you want your child to believe, it's about what kind of community you want your child to feel affiliated with.

Find where you belong.
As much as a faith can be a matter of conflict, it can also be an infallible source of support.

If you and your partner have religious leanings but aren't practicing, you might consider auditioning various religious establishments in town to find a place where you share beliefs and feel at home. Even if you're an atheist, it's worthwhile to find a group of like-minded people who can serve as a consistent point of reference during the often-disorienting years ahead.

Managing Your Finances

At work

When should you tell your boss you're pregnant? Conventional wisdom is that you should refrain from telling your employer and co-workers until you've been pregnant for three months. If something goes wrong with your pregnancy, you don't want to be in the position of explaining that to Barb in accounting. There are, however, some good reasons to consider telling your employer about your pregnancy sooner rather than later:

- Your work environment exposes you to toxins, radiation, or other dangerous conditions, or involves moderate or heavy physical labor.
- Your co-workers might figure it out and tell the boss before you get the chance.
- You believe it may protect your job (at least in the short term) if your boss fears a discrimination lawsuit or doesn't want the bad PR of firing a pregnant woman.
- You're close to your boss and co-workers and are not comfortable being deceptive or evasive about your physical symptoms or medical appointments.

While your family and friends may be thrilled for you, your employer's response may be a bit more lukewarm. You may be gaining a baby, but they see it as losing an employee. They fear that you'll take your leave and then leave them high and dry. Considering how much your life is going to change between now and then, it's entirely possible that your boss's worst fears will come true. But then again, it's possible you'll be ready to come back with more commitment than ever.

With bosses, it can be a fine line between pregnancy discrimination and making practical decisions to avoid a loss of productivity.

BOSS-TELLING TIPS

Wait, if you can, until your first trimester is over. Depending on your age, you have a risk of miscarriage during the first trimester. You don't want to have to "untell" your news.

Pick your moment.

Definitely wait until your boss is in a good mood. Set up a time to talk with your employer privately, and break the news then.

Prepare in advance.

Find out how your company has dealt with pregnant co-workers in the past. Someone who's just returned from maternity leave can be your best ally and give you tips on how to negotiate your leave and return.

Offer solutions.

Inform your employer how you plan to deal with issues, such as identifying someone to cover for you while you take time off for doctor's appointments, or how to modify your work routine to avoid your exposure to toxins.

When it gets to be closer to time for your maternity leave, consider drawing up a written proposal for your employers for any alternate arrangement you'd like them to consider for your return, such as part-time hours, job sharing, or working at home. Make sure your proposal addresses salary, hours, and responsibilities. Don't be afraid to ask for the arrangement you want: It's in your company's interest to keep you if you're good at what you do.

Keep it professional.

Your boss is interested in making sure the work gets done. Don't try to promote your cause by trying to appeal to her emotions or by sharing personal information that's irrelevant.

Review your rights before your meeting.

Make sure you're aware of federal, state, and your company's work leave policies in advance. If you suspect discrimination, save e-mails, notes, and anything that might support your case.

Postpone questions you aren't prepared to answer.

Avoid making promises you may not be able keep, such as planning to take on a huge project the first day you return from maternity leave.

Keep in mind that as much as you want to say what your employer wants to hear, it's better for you (and for other pregnant employees who come after you) to be on the level. Don't be afraid to say, "I'm not ready to discuss that now," or, "I don't know the answer to that, but I promise you that I'll always be honest with you about my intentions."

Ask about savings options. Some companies may match savings for college plans or child care. Also consider raising contributions you may be making to life insurance or 401(k) plans.

Secretly consider the possibility that you really won't come back. If you think a career change may be in order, quietly make sure your résumé is up to date, collect contact information for anyone who could serve as a reference, and take home samples of your work that you can add to your portfolio.

WHAT LAWS APPLY TO YOU?

The Pregnancy Discrimination Act

Prior to the Pregnancy Discrimination Act of 1978, female employees could be fired just for becoming pregnant. This act made it illegal for workers to be discriminated against just because of pregnancy, and requires employers who have fifteen or more employees to treat pregnancy as they would any other medical condition. In addition:

- You can't be fired, denied a job, or denied a promotion simply because you are or may become pregnant.

- You cannot be forced to take pregnancy leave if you are still willing and able to work.

- You must be provided the same level of medical benefits, disability insurance, and leave as are offered for other medical conditions or disabilities. Vacations, raises, and other fringe benefits cannot be denied to you because you're pregnant.

- Your husband's insurance must cover pregnancy-related conditions if he has comprehensive health insurance coverage.

If you can't perform your job (you're a supermodel or perform heavy lifting), your employer must treat you just as any other temporarily disabled employee—modify your tasks, find you alternative assignments, or provide disability or unpaid leave.

If you feel that you're being discriminated against, make sure to keep detailed notes (including times and dates) about everything that happens. Make copies of performance reviews, correspondence, and anything that might support your claim. Then contact your local office of the Equal Employment Opportunity Commission (EEOC), which is listed in the local or state government section of your telephone directory, for advice on how to proceed.

The Family Medical Leave Act (FMLA)

The Family Medical Leave Act of 1993, or FMLA, allows both you and your husband to take up to twelve weeks of unpaid leave during a twelve-month period for pregnancy, birth, or child care.

It applies to workers with companies that have more than fifty employees, who have been employed for 1,250 hours in the twelve months prior to leave. If your workplace isn't covered, your employer may not owe you any considerations by federal law. It does not apply to you if you're a part-time employee or you've worked at your company for less than a year.

If you are covered by FMLA or similar state or company policies, you should be able to choose to take your leave in a single block, or use some for the baby's birth and save other time to use in case of health complications or family issues, as long as you give thirty days' notice to your employer about your foreseeable plans.

If your job permits it, you can use the act to allow you to return to work part-time for a period of time. But while you're not on the job, you may be required to pay your own health insurance premiums.

Consider using your accrued personal or vacation time as paid leave for a time. However, your boss may be able to require you use your paid vacation time during your twelve-week leave. The act and your employer may not allow you to roll over personal or vacation time between calendar years.

At home

WHO'S GOING TO STAY HOME?

At some point, you and your partner are going to have to discuss the modern American dilemma—who's going to watch the baby for the first years of his life? If you're a dual-income family, and you aren't lucky enough to have Grandma living next door, willing and able to watch the baby for forty hours a week, a baby will most likely mean some major financial sacrifice. There are as many child care arrangements as there are couples in the world, but here are some of the most common:

Traditional

Whoever makes the most money, has the best benefit package, or hates their job the least stays at work.

Family help

Grandma, grandpa, aunt, or uncle are on duty while you both work.

Live-in help

You find a live-in nanny or *au pair*.

Care outside of your home

You and your husband work, and baby goes to an infant day care center.

Mutual compromise

You both change your work hours to take turns staying at home or find ways to work from home.

Wills and Life Insurance

"What would happen if one of us died?" It's not the most romantic way to start out a date with your spouse, but it's a conversation you need to have while you're pregnant or soon after the baby's born.

WILLS

It's a good idea for both you and your spouse to draw up wills to name a guardian for your child in case something happens to you. You can hire a lawyer to draft the document, or simply write down your intentions and date and sign the document with a witness. Store your wills in a safe place where the surviving spouse or other family members will be able to find them easily.

LIFE INSURANCE

How much life insurance should you have?

The consensus among financial planners is that you need at least enough life insurance to replace the income and job benefits (such as health insurance) of the deceased parent until your child moves out or graduates college. If it's the stay-at-home spouse who dies, the newly single parent will need enough support to hire people to replace the labor that will be lost. You may also wish to assume that the living parent will want to limit their work hours.

These calculations can get complex, especially if you try to project expenses adjusted for inflation. Insurance expert Timothy Pitcher, author of *Making Sense of Group and Medical Insurance*, suggests using a formula called "Cash + One + Half."

The cash is the amount of debt carried by the family: mortgage, car payments, credit card debt, the balance of student loans, and so on. One is one year of the highest-paid spouse's salary after taxes. This would provide for the surviving spouse during a one-year transitional period. Add to that the half—half the annual salary of the deceased spouse until the youngest child reaches age eighteen or until they graduate college. This will give you a minimal amount. If you want to be sure your child can afford expensive schools, you may want to consider more.

If you're single, you'll want to name a beneficiary for the policy whom you trust to make good financial decisions. Insurance benefits are usually paid in a lump sum. Ideally, the sum should be invested, allowing your child's expenses to be paid from the interest payments, not the principal.

Also remember that Social Security will pay a monthly death benefit (currently $255) to a surviving spouse. A surviving spouse may also be entitled to a monthly benefit based on the full retirement benefits of the deceased.

Your
Guide
to Giving
Birth

3

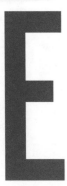

very woman's labor has its own rhythm and flow, and giving birth is a healthy, natural, and dynamic process. As you will discover when you go into labor, your body is already equipped with its own built-in program for getting your baby from the inside to the outside. Hopefully, the more you understand about what your body is doing, the more at ease you will feel about letting go and allowing nature to take control. A woman's most basic requirements during birth are to feel safe and supported and to have her body needs met with as few interruptions or interventions as possible. The ultimate reward is the birth of a healthy, wonderful baby.

This section gives you an easy-to-follow road map as you prepare for your huge, one-day, baby-birthing marathon. It describes the body mechanics of labor and birth and your options for managing discomforts and making informed decisions about medical interventions. In addition, you'll find lots of practical, mother-centered ideas for getting through.

How Birth Starts will give you the signs of true labor and tips for coping with practice contractions and "false alarms." You'll also find strategies on how to deal with being overdue; information about being admitted into the hospital; and the importance of taking an active role in your labor decisions.

All about Labor takes you step-by-step through the four stages of labor, the actual birth, and your recovery. Each stage is described in detail: how long it is likely to last, how it will feel, and numerous tips for managing the whole process.

Coping with Labor Pain explains the natural sources of labor discomfort and gives you descriptions of many drug and nondrug options for making yourself more comfortable during labor. You'll also find the benefits of adopting a pain-coping mindset to help you get through.

During and after Labor discusses your baby's post-birth experience, including how babies are evaluated once they're born, and it also covers your own recovery in the hours after giving birth. (For more about your recovery at home, see page 361.)

The Non-Hospital Birth Experience presents what it's like to give birth in a freestanding birthing center or at home and offers basic "first aid" for giving birth by yourself should you find yourself in an emergency situation with no one to help.

Special Situations describes the guidelines used by hospitals to measure the progress of labor and common medical interventions. Artificial induction and augmentation are discussed along with their risks. The experience of having a ***cesarean section (c-section)***, the surgical delivery of a baby by cutting through the mother's abdomen and uterus, is described in detail along with the issues surrounding vaginal birth after a cesarean section (VBAC).

As with other sections of this book, terms defined in the pregnancy dictionary at the end of this book starting on page 574 are set in ***italics*** and ***bold*** the first time they appear in this section. You'll also find numerous page designations that refer you to other parts of the book so you can navigate quickly from one section to another when you discover a topic you want to explore in more detail.

The information presented in this section has been carefully collected from hundreds of medical studies, from the wealth of birth wisdom and knowledge in the field of obstetrics, family practice, midwifery, and nursing, and from the experiences of childbirth educators and ***doulas***. We have also incorporated wisdom from mothers who have shared their experiences with us and from our own vivid experiences of labor and birth.

Remember, though, that this section cannot duplicate the knowledge and judgment of a seasoned healthcare provider. An experienced, well-informed obstetrician, physician in family practice, or midwife can play an important role in supporting you and guiding you through your birth and delivery. She will also assist you in weighing a wide range of options; will keep your preferred strategies for pain relief and your birth in the forefront; and will refrain from recommending any medical interventions that are not in the best interest of you and your baby.

SOME TYPICAL QUESTIONS

During the final stage of pregnancy, most mothers carry a mental list of gnawing, unanswered questions: "When will I finally go into labor?" "How long will my labor last?" "How big will my baby be?" "Will my baby and I get through it okay?"

Unfortunately, not even the wisest and most experienced healthcare providers can answer these questions with much precision. If you ask them, you'll typically get a shrug and be told "it depends," or a hazarded guess. That's because every woman's labor and birth is unique.

Even though it is impossible to exactly predict what will happen during your own birthing experience, we can offer a general picture to help you prepare in advance.

When will I go into labor?

Calculations of a woman's due date and her baby's weight are famous for being wrong. The length of an average pregnancy is about 266 days from the date of conception until delivery. In the normal model, conception happens 14 days after a woman's last period. Rather than trying to guess the actual date of conception, healthcare providers simply add 280 days (or forty weeks) to the first day of a mother's last period. But, a pregnancy can last three weeks longer or shorter (thirty-seven to forty-two weeks) and still be on course.

A wrong due date is more likely to happen when a woman's periods have been irregular or her menstrual cycles closer together or further apart than the average 28 days. In any event, it's quite likely that your baby will choose to arrive on a different day than your official "due date"—the one you've been quoting to everyone for the past nine months.

First-time moms typically go into labor a few days to a week later than their estimated due dates, while mothers who have previously given birth generally come closer to their due dates or go even a little earlier than expected. Again, we're talking averages, and your baby may surprise you by arriving before his crib does or aggravate you by being tardy.

Having your baby's age estimated by a sonogram before you're twenty weeks pregnant is considered the most accurate way to tell how many weeks along your baby really is. However, ultrasound gets less and less accurate in predicting a baby's age as pregnancy progresses. (Being overdue is discussed on page 269.)

How long will my labor take?

First-time moms take an average of fifteen hours to give birth from start to finish—approximately three hundred contractions after their waters break. Some labors take hours longer, others hours shorter. While some labors proceed in a straight line from start to finish, others lose steam and come to a halt, only to start up again. Either way can still result in a perfectly healthy birth and baby.

If you've had a baby before, it may be comforting to know that giving birth the next time around can be approximately four hours shorter and two hundred contractions less.

Whether this is your first or your fifth baby, during labor, you'll probably be too preoccupied to keep checking the clock or to carve contraction marks on your headboard. Time will seem to speed up or slow down, depending upon your sensations at the moment.

How much will my baby weigh?

So you've gotten really huge, and you're worried that you're cultivating a gigantic monster that could be the death of you when it's time to get from the inside to the outside. Not to worry: Most of your weight gain during pregnancy isn't your baby, but his life support system.

Your extra stores of fat will account for 7 pounds or more. Add 4 pounds for your extra fluid supplies, and 2 pounds (or more) for your breasts. Your uterus now weighs 22 pounds or more, and the placenta and umbilical cord weigh about one to 1½ pounds. Then factor in a mere 7½ pounds for the little creature floating around inside of you.

Your baby's weight isn't going to affect birth as much as you might suppose. Your baby's head is the largest part to be delivered, and it's adapted for birth. Unlike the hard and well-formed skull of a child or an adult, a newborn's skull is made up of soft, moveable plates of bone that are joined together by membrane-covered spaces. This allows the plates to slide over one another, making the baby's head more compact for birth, called *molding*. This could mean your newborn will have an oddly shaped skull, but it won't hurt his brain. It will round out and start looking normal in a week or so.

During the last weeks of pregnancy, your hormones soften the connective tissues between your pelvic bones so they can stretch apart during birth. The lower rim of your pelvis will expand by as much as one-third for your baby's descent down and out. Positioning yourself in an upright or side-lying position will take pressure off your tailbone area and enhance the natural expansion process during birth. Both your pelvis and vagina will return to normal shape once birth is over, although some mothers continue to experience pelvic aches and pains for a while afterward.[1]

Will my baby and I survive birth?

Most mothers secretly fear that their babies may have something wrong or that they won't survive the trauma of birth. It's important to know that even if you're over thirty-five, overweight, or a smoker, or have been put on bed rest, the odds are still incredibly good that both you and your baby will sail through this experience unscathed—tired, sore, and groggy, yes, but healthy, alive, and well.

In centuries past, many mothers *did* die during birth. In 1900, the complications of pregnancy cost the lives of approximately 850 mothers out of every 100,000 live births. Today the U.S. pregnancy-related mortality ratio stands at about 11.3 deaths per 100,000 births, or 0.000113 percent according to the Centers for Disease Control and Prevention. Your drive to the hospital will be four hundred times more dangerous, so wear your seat belt, and tell your driver not to speed!

In spite of medical advances, the maternal mortality ratio has remained relatively constant over the past twenty-five years and isn't improving. There is no single answer as to why the rate has stopped improving, but the rising proportion of pregnancies among older women is thought to play a part.

Although the overall risk of pregnancy-related death is small for all mothers, it is two to three times higher for women over thirty-five than for those in their twenties, and even higher for women older than forty. It can't be ignored that the maternal mortality ratio for African-American women is estimated to be three to four times higher than that for women of other races—a glaring disparity that deserves more research.

Studies have estimated that more than half of mothers' deaths could have been prevented with attentive prenatal care that intervened at the early sign of problems, and also if mothers changed their lifestyles, such as getting better nutrition, letting go of harmful habits (no drinking, drugs, or smoking), and being better informed about early signs of impending trouble. It's worth noting that mothers who have no apparent risk factors may have the same (and many studies say, even better) outcomes regardless of whether they give birth in a freestanding birth center, at home, or in a hospital.[2]

When it comes to baby survival, the U.S. infant mortality ratio is currently 7 infant deaths per 1,000 live births. The majority of infant deaths are from unpreventable, congenital defects. The rate is lower for Asian and Pacific Island babies, at 5.2 per 1,000, and highest for African-American women: 14.1 per 1,000 for live births. There are regional differences: the infant death ratio for San Francisco is 2.6 per 1,000, but for Washington, D.C., it is 14.9 per 1,000.[3] Given even the highest ratios, the chances are only 1 percent or less that your baby will die during birth or his first year of life.

What if I'm labeled high risk?

Approximately 70 to 80 percent of all pregnancies are considered low risk. The remaining pregnancies are labeled high risk, meaning that a mother or baby have physical problems that are sometimes associated with something wrong.

As we pointed out in the "Managing Your Pregnancy" section, prenatal tests make mistakes. Being labeled high risk doesn't mean you will develop a complication. Most likely you won't. It only means your risk is higher than for other women. On the other hand, sometimes mothers develop complications during labor that couldn't be predicted ahead of time.

Even if you fall into the 20 to 30 percent of pregnant women at risk for pregnancy complications (perhaps because you're over thirty-five or you or your baby are thought to have potential health problems), the chances are still excellent that both you and your baby will beat the odds and survive beautifully.

Age or lifestyle factors, such as drinking, smoking, and exposure to toxic chemicals increase your statistical risk of problems such as your baby's being born prematurely, being low birthweight, or having mental retardation or deformities, but how these things may affect you or your particular baby can't always be predicted in advance. Giving birth, just like parenting, sometimes calls for submitting and accepting what is out of your control.

Hopefully, whatever complications you face will be surmountable.

How Birth Starts

By the final weeks of pregnancy, you'll probably be visiting your healthcare provider more frequently. He will want to measure your rising "bump" to confirm your baby's growth and watch for signs of change in your *cervix*—the neck and mouth of your uterus. He will also monitor your blood pressure and urine to ensure that there are no signs of preeclampsia, a serious condition unique to pregnancy. (Preeclampsia is discussed in *Managing Your Pregnancy*, on page 215.)

Some mother's bodies undergo changes in the weeks prior to birth. You may be told that the mouth of your cervix has started to soften, thin, and widen, and the tip end of it has moved forward and down. Palpating (see *palpation* in the *Pregnancy Dictionary*) your abdomen will help your healthcare provider figure out your baby's position.

Your baby's back will feel smooth and hard, while the front area will be soft with hard bumps that move when pressed. Your baby's head will feel hard and round and will move in response to a gentle nudge. The baby's forehead and brow will also feel hard, and your care provider will try to tell if his head is in a normal chin-down position or extended upward. The rump will feel larger and bulkier than the head and won't move as readily as other body parts.

Most babies rotate themselves around from being head-up to being head-down sometime during the last weeks before birth. When that happens, you'll be told your baby has engaged, and it will feel as though he has settled deep and low into your body. (See "lightening" on page 263.)

Other babies wait until the last possible minute to get into proper position. This is especially true if their mothers have previously given birth. Should your baby continue to stay head-up after your labor has started, then he will be born rear-end first, which is called a **breech birth**. This is a matter of concern for healthcare providers because it tends to make labor last longer and can be hard on both mother and baby. Delivering a baby presenting as a breech vaginally may be riskier for the baby, and now most obstetric care providers are recommending cesarean delivery for women carrying breech presenting babies when they go into labor.

If your baby stays breech by thirty-six weeks or later, your healthcare provider may suggest **external cephalic version (ECV)**, manually turning your baby by manipulating your abdomen. You will be asked to empty your bladder and to lie on your back with your knees bent. Your practitioner will use a sonogram to determine the baby's position and will listen to the baby's heart rate before and after ECV has been done. An **epidural** may be used to help your uterus relax. (Epidurals are discussed on pages 317–322.)

Since there is a small risk of the placenta being pulled off the wall of the uterus, this procedure requires skill and should only be done by someone with special training and lots of experience. It's important to ask about the person's training in the procedure and how many times she has performed it.

Sometimes ECV works, but other times the baby may revert to being right side up. If ECV is successful, and your baby remains head downward, you may be asked to walk around for an hour or so after the procedure to encourage the baby to fix into the head-downward position.

Your baby's "I'm ready!" signal

Most moms honestly can't answer the question "What time did your labor start?"

For many women, the body's process of preparing for going into labor can last a week or more. It's not unusual to have labor build up slowly and gradually for days with starts and stops along the way. Getting started could be compared to a snowball gaining momentum as it rolls down a hill instead of, say, a horse leaping out of the gate when a pistol fires.

While your uterus had the job of keeping tightly closed to hold your baby securely inside and keeping germs out, when it's time for labor, the mouth of the uterus will drop lower and will begin to soften and stretch. If labor starts, and these things haven't happened yet, a mother will be said to have an unripe cervix.

Most of what we know about the hormones and mechanics of how labor gets underway comes from research conducted on animals, so it's still not totally clear what actually signals labor to start. But, there appears to be scientific grounding for the old saying, "Only the baby knows when it's time to be born."

Researchers believe that a hormone secreted by the baby's pituitary gland in the base of her brain initiates a complex cascade of hormonal interactions—a chemical conversation, if you will—between baby and mother that signals when it's time.

When your baby's body gives the go-ahead, a cascade of hormones will be released that instruct the cervix to soften (ripen), and the muscle fibers in the uterus will begin the process of contracting up and around the baby. Then they will help to push her down and out, ejecting her from her comfortable water world into the cold, gravity-heavy place we call home.

WHEN BIRTH IS JUST AROUND THE CORNER

Signals that labor is on the way

These signs don't mean you'll be racing off to the hospital any minute now, only that you'll be having your baby in a few days, a week, or maybe a week and a half. Not much help, but better than having a couple of months to go!

Lightening

A week or so before labor begins, your baby will probably settle more deeply into your pelvic area. The official words are **engagement**, lightening, or dropping because your bump will appear to be lower.

When the baby moves down, it will feel as though you've got more room at the top of your abdomen with less pressure around your rib cage. Breathing will be easier and deeper. If you've suffered from nagging **heartburn**, especially at night, the release of pressure off your stomach could cool that down too.

The relief from dropping brings a whole new set of discomforts: twinges and pains in your lower half, like lower-back aches, cramping in your buttocks, or shooting pains down your inner thighs. If you have hemorrhoids or **varicose veins**, they may become even more enlarged from the pressure of the baby's body on your veins. (Hemorrhoids and varicose veins are described in more detail on pages 133 and 143.)

Sometimes, a baby doesn't engage in his mother's pelvis until labor actually starts. Your baby may wait until show time, particularly if this isn't your first baby. Your care provider may recommend frequent walking and/or pelvic tilts (curling your pelvis while you're on your hands and knees) to encourage your baby to get into position. It's worth a try—it can't hurt. (See the discussion of "lie" on page 88.)

Show

When your care provider examines your cervix, he will see a blue-tinged ring the size of a mini-doughnut with a dimple in the center. As labor nears, the cervix will start to thin (efface) and the hole in the center will widen (dilate).

As that happens, you may discharge a jelly-like mucus plug, called **show**, or bloody show. The plug serves to keep germs from traveling up into your cervix. Some mothers lose only part of the plug before birth, and others don't ever see it. It can be white, clear, or pink, and appear chunky or stringy. A pink or reddish tinge is from tiny blood vessels rupturing during the thinning and opening process. Show is not to be confused with the thicker, light brown discharge that sometimes follows intercourse, or the bright red discharge that

"When we got to the hospital, the nurse asked me when my labor began. I felt dumb, but I couldn't give her a specific day or time. I was tired and bleary-eyed, and it had taken a couple of sleepless nights before things started to really heat up."

may come after an internal exam. Anything more than that should be reported to your healthcare provider right away.

Unfortunately, show isn't a very good predictor for when labor is going to start. It can appear days or even weeks earlier, or happen while you're actively laboring. As long as you are thirty-seven weeks along in your pregnancy, there's probably no need to worry about it. If you have heavy mucus discharge earlier than your thirty-seventh week, especially accompanied by bleeding, then contact your care provider immediately: it could mean that you're going into labor prematurely.

Breaking of the waters

All during pregnancy, your baby has floated inside a tough, watery balloon called the **amniotic sac.** Usually the amniotic sac breaks sometime during labor. That is called **rupture of the membranes (ROM)**. It is painless, you may hear a pop, and you'll simply feel gushing, warm fluid coming out. Most likely your contractions will get stronger soon afterward. In about one out of ten labors, the sac ruptures on its own before labor starts, and when that happens, the majority of women go into labor within twelve to twenty-four hours.

It's not clear what makes some sacs break before labor, but recent research appears to show that one out of three mothers whose waters break before labor have mild infections. Typically, it will break while a woman is at home in bed, or while she's sitting on the toilet. Nothing special about these places, they're just where third-trimester moms spend most of their time.

If your membranes rupture, you may see the mucus plug and white flecks of vernix, the sloughed-off waxy covering for your baby's skin. If you're walking around, the fluid may dribble out and dampen your underpants, or it could gush out and run down your leg, which some witty care providers call a sock soaker. There are a couple of ways to tell a simple urine leak from amniotic fluid: urine is yellow and has its own familiar, ammonia-like smell. Amniotic fluid is clear or slightly milky and sticky with a briny, sea-like aroma.

If the fluid is greenish or foul smelling, it could be caused by **meconium** (baby stool), a sign that your baby could be in trouble. Call your care provider immediately, regardless of what time it is. Sometimes a baby's umbilical cord can get pulled out into the birth canal when the waters break. That's called a **prolapsed cord,** and it's very rare, but can be life-threatening to the baby.

Write down the time your water broke. Should your labor fail to start within twenty-four to forty-eight hours, you may be given antibiotics to protect you and your baby from infection, and your healthcare provider may suggest that your labor be artificially induced using drugs that make your uterus contract to protect you and your baby from infection. (Induction is discussed on pages 335–344.) In the meantime, avoid anything that could contaminate your vagina or birth canal such as tampons, sexual intercourse, or soaking in a bathtub, and don't allow anything except a care provider's sterile glove inside your vagina.

Contractions

Some women who have never given birth mistakenly believe that labor is just one long pain. Actually, the uterus contracts in rhythmical waves of hardening and softening throughout labor with time to rest in between. The pain of a contraction builds and then peaks for a few seconds in the middle of the wave, and then it slowly disappears. No contraction lasts more than ninety seconds, and the time between contractions can be ten minutes, five minutes, or one and a half minutes, depending upon what stage of labor you are in.

By now, you've experienced plenty of contractions during your pregnancy, but most of them were so painless and mild, you probably weren't aware of them. A simple test for whether you're having a contraction or not is to press down on the top of your uterus—the ridge at the top of your belly below your rib cage. If the ridge feels soft like the tip of

Signs That Birth Is Nearing

Here's a quick checklist to help you decide where your body is in preparation for going into labor.

"Labor day" is nearing, but not here yet
Backache. A nagging backache and an overall feeling of restlessness.
Cramps. Menstrual-like cramps that come and go.
Diarrhea. Stools that are softer and more liquid.
Nesting urges. A sudden, uncharacteristic surge of energy that makes you want to clean house and actively get things in order.

Starting to change, but labor's not completely established yet
Passing blood-tinged mucus. Mention it to your care provider, but don't page her in the middle of the night. You may have a week or two yet to go.
Your water breaks. It can be a trickle that seems like lots of watery discharge or an unmistakable gush. Still there's no need to panic. You'll probably have a good six to twenty-four hours to go before labor starts. If it's flecked with brown or green spots or smells bad, page your care provider no matter what time it is.
Prodromal labor. Your contractions may last about the same amount of time, but they don't seem to be getting any stronger or closer together. Try recording them for an hour—when each contraction starts, when it ends, and when the next one begins. If they're more than five minutes apart and lasting less than thirty seconds, just rest and wait.

Pack your bags
Any two of these signs usually mean that labor is truly getting underway.
Stronger contractions. You can say without a doubt that they're getting more intense.
Closer contractions. You are having more in the same amount of time.
Longer contractions. Contractions are lasting longer than, say, an hour ago.

Understanding Your Contractions

STRENGTH OF CONTRACTIONS	HOW LONG THEY LAST	HOW OFTEN THEY HAPPEN
Mild (the beginning of labor)	Less than 30 seconds	Six minutes apart
Strong (labor getting established)	35 to 45 seconds each	Four to five minutes apart
Very strong (the middle to the end of labor)	45 to 60 seconds each	Two to three minutes apart

your nose, then you're not having a contraction. If the ridge feels hard like your forehead, then you are.

Unless your contractions are getting stronger, longer, and closer together, then you're probably not in labor, but having Braxton-Hicks contractions, the painless tensing of the smooth muscle fibers of your uterus as it stretches and adapts to your baby. You can usually make these practice contractions go away by drinking water, changing positions, or lying down for a while.

Prodromal labor involves contractions that lead up to labor, but start and stop in the weeks and days before active labor gets underway. Prodromal labor helps the mouth of your cervix start to soften, thin, and stretch open.

If you aren't certain whether your contractions are prodromal or real, get a watch with a second hand, a pen, and a piece of paper, and write down the time when each contraction starts, when it ends, and when the next one begins for about an hour.

Contractions that end in the birth of a baby usually get stronger and closer together over time. They also tend to become progressively more painful. Typically, the discomfort of these contractions starts as a low backache or a band of pain that begins in the back and radiates toward the front. The pain crests

HOW YOUR BELLY FEELS	HOW THE CONTRACTIONS FEEL
Partially soft	Crampy, like menstrual cramps, but regular and undeniable. Like an elastic band tightening under your belly and around to the small of your back that pulls and then lets go.
Slightly firm	Bearable. Gripping, hurting more in the middle of a contraction wave than at the beginning or the end.
Very hard	"Wow! Mamma never told me it would hurt like this!" Each powerful contraction wave seems more unbearable than the one before, but then it releases. Sometimes, you barely have time to catch your breath before the next one comes, and you may feel as though you are losing control. You may begin to feel exhausted and dispirited thinking this torture will never end, and your baby will never arrive. Then, the urge to bear down announces itself with a groan followed by the quite bearable pushing stage and the birth of your baby.

in the middle of the contraction. Abdominal pain that hurts all the time and doesn't come and go is a danger sign and should be reported to your healthcare provider.

A mother who is moving into active labor will have trouble talking during a contraction. So if you can keep chatting without skipping a beat, then you're probably still in the latent, early part of labor. If you find yourself having to stop talking, sucking in your breath, and whimpering, then it's probably getting time to pack your bag, and contact your healthcare provider for instructions. With contractions, if you have to ask if it's the real thing, it probably isn't.

Vaginal secretions and diarrhea

Birth may be womanly, but it isn't ladylike! Most mothers' bodies do some housekeeping in the twenty-four to forty-eight hours before labor begins. Your vaginal secretions may increase, you may experience diarrhea, and you may also discover that you're peeing more often than usual from the pressure of your baby's descent.

The nesting instinct

Even if you've been obsessively arranging your house since your first pregnancy test turned positive, when birth nears, you may find

Pre-Labor Versus Real Labor Contractions

CONTRACTION CHARACTERISTICS	PRE-LABOR	LABOR
Frequency	More random than regular.	Getting closer together over time.
Duration	Variable: contractions sometimes brief, sometimes longer.	Steadier and lasting longer as time goes on. (Different than an hour ago.)
Effects of movement	Moving around can sometimes make them go away.	You feel restless, but walking or moving doesn't seem to make much difference.
Pain and uterus	No relationship between pain and your uterus feeling hard.	The intensity of discomfort is related to how hard the uterus is.
Strength	Stay mostly the same without getting stronger.	Steadily get stronger over time.
Your reaction	You can chat or eat while they're happening.	You have trouble completing a sentence or eating while you're in the grips of one.
Location on body	Nagging, lower-back ache, or mainly in the front of the abdomen.	Pain usually starts in the back and moves around to the front with each contraction like a tightening band.

your organizational activities kicking up a notch. There are no scientific studies on this, but the rule appears to be that if you stay up way past bedtime indulging the urge to cook, clean, or organize, labor will start in the next twelve hours.

The benefits of getting started at home

Unless you have pregnancy complications, and your labor has been labeled at-risk, it makes sense not to rush off to the hospital at the first signs of labor. Consider staying at home while your labor patterns are getting firmly established. Rest as much as you can, drink plenty of water, and eat nutritious snacks to fortify your body for the heavy workload ahead. Waiting to go to the hospital might translate into having fewer exams too, and it could protect you from extra interventions.

When your baby is overdue

It's normal to feel worried and discouraged when your due date comes and goes without going into labor. Before you start thinking your baby will never get born, remember your due date is simply an estimate. And even though your baby may appear to be overdue, there's also a good chance that your estimated due date was inaccurate, especially if you didn't have a sonogram, or waited until after the twentieth week to have one.

Sonograms have been proven to be increasingly less accurate as pregnancy progresses. Their measurements of a baby's age conducted during the first twenty weeks of pregnancy are considered accurate within one week, but during weeks twenty to twenty-eight, they're only considered accurate within two weeks. Past the twenty-eighth week of pregnancy, measurements could be off by as much as four weeks. Unfortunately, artificially inducing labor because a baby is thought to be overdue can have serious repercussions, especially if a baby's lungs are still immature.

Some researchers have estimated that nine out of ten babies are considered overdue as the result of human error, not because the baby is running late. Usually, the problem is a miscalculation about when con-

ception actually happened since many women don't keep accurate records about their periods. A baby may appear to be abnormally late even though he's right on schedule according to his mother's cycles.

About eighteen out of every one hundred pregnancies go beyond forty-one weeks; and approximately one out of every six mothers—seven out of one hundred pregnancies (about one out of fourteen)—has a pregnancy that lasts beyond forty-two weeks.

In rare instances, an overdue pregnancy can signal a medical problem. A mother's **placenta** may lose efficiency in supporting the baby. Her amniotic fluid may begin to dry up; a baby's growth may be halted; or he may keep on growing larger, making his trip through a narrow pelvis more challenging. Babies who are seriously overdue are more vulnerable to **asphyxia**—not getting enough oxygen during labor and birth—and being **stillborn**.

> *"With my three babies, false labor and true labor felt exactly the same. It's just that the false kind kept me awake all night and wore me out, while the true kind ended up with my babies' births."*

Coping with Nighttime Contractions

Sometimes Braxton-Hicks contractions feel more intense and bothersome at night, especially as they begin to shift into prodromal labor. If you're awakened by discomfort in the middle of the night and are having trouble sleeping, try to conserve your energy for the big work ahead. Drink water, eat something, and try to relax around your contractions as best you can. Here's a handy list of coping strategies:

Stop watching the clock. While you do want to check your contractions once in a while to see if they're changing, you don't need to record every contraction over the many long hours of early labor—you could wind up staring at the clock for days. Trust your contractions to let you know in no uncertain terms when it's time to take them more seriously.

Take a shower or bath. Nothing soothes like warm water. Dunk a full-size bath towel in warm water, and use it as a blanket for your back or belly, or roll it up to make a warm compress to drape across your neck and shoulders. (Not too hot, it will make your baby's heart rate speed up.)

Drink a soothing beverage. Try non-caffeinated liquids, such as warm milk with honey, or an instant breakfast beverage to make you sleepy.

Urinate frequently. It will make you more comfortable, and an empty bladder will make more room for your baby to move down in preparation for birth.

Eat a snack. Try eating cereal, a banana, or a turkey sandwich. Turkey contains an amino acid called tryptophane that may make you drowsy.

Turn on some music. Listen to a relaxing CD of surf or nature sounds, or pull out your self-hypnosis birthing tapes. (See hypnosis for birth on page 307.)

Change beds. Try sleeping on the couch wrapped in a cozy comforter and propped up with piles of pillows.

Ask about medication. Take Tylenol PM® or Benadryl® if your health-care provider has already given you the go ahead. Carefully follow his instructions for what dose to take, how often, and for what span of time.

If you've gotten to forty-one weeks of pregnancy with no signs of going into labor, you may be asked to take tests to evaluate your baby's activity levels and heart rate and to measure the volume of fluid in your amniotic sac to make sure it is adequate to support your baby. (See *nonstress test* in the pregnancy dictionary on page 624.) The size of your baby's head will be compared with the size of its body to ensure that his growth is normal.

You care provider may also suggest inducing your labor with a synthetic hormone that makes the uterus contract. If you're concerned about whether it's time to have your labor induced, consider getting a second opinion from a specialist in maternal-fetal medicine and the pediatrician you've chosen for your baby.

Nonmedical ways to encourage labor to start

Throughout human history, women have tried to jump-start labor, but usually without much success. Here are some of their strategies:

Oral or vaginal sex. A man's *semen* contains *prostaglandins*, hormones known to start labor that, in their synthetic form, are sometimes used for medical inductions. Intercourse delivers these hormones to the cervix, but in some circles, it is thought that oral sex involving swallowing the ejaculate is more effective. (Avoid intercourse if your water has broken.)

Nipple stimulation. *Oxytocin*, also used in a synthetic form for medical induction of labor, is released naturally when a mother's nipples are stimulated, either manually or with a breast pump. The strategy may not be very effective. Studies have failed to show it works.

Herbs. There is a long history of midwives using tinctures, teas, and infused oils of herbs to assist with bringing on labor to help with weak contractions, and to help mothers heal after giving birth. There is little solid research to show whether using plant infusions is beneficial or harmful. Black cohosh and blue cohosh have long been suggested as ways to induce labor, but one study found that blue cohosh increased the rate of meconium staining for babies, fetal heart rate problems, and inconsolable baby crying after birth.

Other herbs that have been used historically are raspberry leaf and

FLASH FACTS

The risks of getting admitted to the hospital too early

Recent research appears to show that mothers are more likely to have a normal vaginal birth when they complete the early part of their labors at home, rather than in the hospital. The early-stage labor is thought to be especially sensitive to stress and interruptions, which can affect the rhythm and effectiveness of contractions. Stress hormones can also interfere with labor.

A 1998 study found that admitting women too early during labor, before they had reached three centimeters dilation, was associated with longer labor, more obstetric complications, more technical interventions, and it exposed them to a greater risk of undergoing a cesarean section.

In spite of the recommendations of the American College of Obstetricians and Gynecologists against augmenting labor with drugs during its early stage (before three to four centimeters of dilation), or performing cesareans for lack of progress during labor during the early stage, the practice of intervening too soon is still happening.[4] (Dilation is discussed on page 281-284, and cesareans for lack of progress on page 337.)

nettle, which are thought to promote easier labor and better postpartum recuperation, and shepherd's purse infusion to control bleeding after the placenta has been delivered. There is inadequate scientific research to demonstrate their effectiveness. If you do use any herbal preparation, it's important to inform your healthcare provider, since some herbs may potentially interact with drugs you may be given.

Getting admitted to the hospital

Admission procedures vary among hospitals, so it's important to discuss the process in advance with your healthcare provider during one of your office visits. It's also an excellent idea to take a tour of the hospital prior to going into labor to get a general lay of the land. You may want to converse with a nurse in labor and delivery, and if you have any questions about your health insurance coverage, this would be a good time to talk with the hospital's billing office.

When you're admitted to the hospital, you'll be asked to submit your insurance card, your birth date, your social security number, and other identifying information. You may be given waivers and other paperwork to sign, where you agree not to sue the hospital in case something goes wrong; that you'll allow them to perform emergency surgery; and you'll pay your medical bills if your insurance company won't.

You will then be rolled in a wheelchair with your patient record to the labor and delivery area of your hospital. A labor and delivery (L&D) nurse will assess your general health, and she will try to determine how far along you are in labor.

Here are some questions you may be asked: "What is your due date?" "How many times have you been pregnant?" "Have you previously had a cesarean section?" "When did your contractions start?" "How often they are coming?" "How strong are they?" "Has your water broken yet?" "If so, when did that happen, and what color was the fluid?" "Is your baby moving as much as usual?" "Have you had any problems during your pregnancy?" "Do you have any ongoing medical problems, such as diabetes or heart problems?"

You'll also be asked about any medications you may be taking (bring along your bottles); if you have any allergies, your diet preferences, and whether you plan to breast- or

Castor Oil and Contractions

Some people swear it works, others say it doesn't—but either way, what you go through just may end up being worse than labor itself. Basically, castor oil causes your digestive system to spasm, causing diarrhea and/or vomiting, possibly bringing on labor as the result of your body becoming dehydrated. Even if it does work, you'll have a sore, red bottom, making the whole ordeal even more painful than just letting nature do it her way. Don't do it!

bottle feed your baby, which will determine if you get breastfeeding help, or baby is automatically fed formula.

If you have a birth plan or a list of your birthing goals that you've discussed with your healthcare provider, this would be a good time for you, or your partner, to present a copy to be inserted in your medical folder. (Birth plans are discussed on page 90.)

Keep in mind that even though you have strong wishes about how you would like to have your labor and birth handled, decision-making in labor is an ongoing process that depends a lot upon how your labor progresses and your baby's signals about his condition. Your healthcare provider may have ongoing standing orders at the hospital about how the labors of her patients are to be managed that will be followed by labor and delivery nurses in addition to the recommendations of professional guidelines and hospital protocols about how every labor is to be handled.

Your vital signs, including your temperature, pulse, respiration, and blood pressure will be taken. Your baby's heart rate will also be listened to using a *fetoscope*, a special, handheld stethoscope, or using a Doppler that uses ultrasound technology. You may have a belt strapped around your abdomen to take twenty- to thirty-minute readings of your contractions and your baby's heart rate using a small sensor box connected to an *electronic fetal monitor (EFM)*. The monitor provides a continuous printout of your baby's heart rate in relationship to your contractions. Small wires with sensors on the

> *"Hospitals frighten me and make me anxious. If anxiety can contribute to a longer labor, messed-up contractions, and a more difficult labor, then I'm setting myself up. I've decided to use a midwife, and I'm hiring a doula to help me get through."*

ends may be inserted inside your birth canal and into your baby's scalp after your waters have broken to track your baby's heart rate and the strength and timing of your contractions. These actions are represented as separate lines, which appear on a strip of paper printed out by the monitor.

As part of your labor evaluation, you will probably be given an internal exam to determine if your cervix has started to thin (efface) and begun to stretch open (dilate). If your amniotic sac has ruptured, the nurse or practitioner will don sterile gloves and collect a sample of the fluid with a cotton swab. It will be examined on a slide under a microscope to determine if it is just vaginal secretions or amniotic fluid.

After your initial assessment, she will notify your care provider and provide information needed to determine how far along you are in your labor, and how well you and your baby appear to be doing.

If you are dilated four or more centimeters (about 1 1/2 inches), you will likely be labeled as being in *active labor*. On the other hand, if you are having regular contractions, but are not dilated to that magic mark, you may be given the option of strolling around the hospital for an hour or two (or may even be told to go home) and return to labor and delivery to be reexamined to see if you have reached four centimeters. (See our discussion about the "active management of labor" on page 279.)

After you're officially admitted, you may be given a routine blood test to check if you're anemic, to confirm your blood type, and possibly to determine if you have blood clotting problems. At this point, the hospital may place a catheter (tiny tube) with an anticoagulant in it (to

> *"With your health-care provider's help, create a great birth plan well in advance of going into labor. Then, keep flexible about last-minute changes. Plan to make one decision at a time according to how things unfold."*

prevent blood clotting) on the back of your hand, which gives caregivers constant access to your veins in case they want to give you an IV of intravenous fluids. You may want to request not having a routine IV to allow yourself freedom to move around during labor unless it is medically necessary.

Once you're in active labor, you and your baby will be monitored, either continually, every fifteen to thirty minutes, once an hour, or less regularly depending upon the policies of your care provider and the hospital. The timing and strength of your contractions may be measured, and how your baby's heart rate responds to your contractions. The opening of your cervix will also be monitored through periodic pelvic exams.

How often you'll be given exams depends upon the policies of your care provider and hospital. If your care provider suspects problems, he may place you on an electronic fetal monitor and attach a wire lead to your baby's scalp, or a blood sample may be taken from your baby's scalp to ensure he is getting sufficient oxygen and is not under stress.

Your rights as a patient

Informed consent refers to an important ethical and legal principle of medicine designed to empower patients to actively participate in their medical planning and care and to protect them from unwanted procedures or treatments. The American College of Obstetricians and Gynecologists, the leading professional organization of obstetricians, states that every patient has the right to have information disclosed by obstetricians in such a

FLASH FACTS: EFM Benefits vs. Risks

Multiple research studies have failed to prove the superiority of electronic fetal monitoring (EFM) over the use of a traditional stethoscope or fetoscope for monitoring normal, non-risk births. One major drawback of the EFM machine is that its tracings are not always easy to interpret, and care providers differ in what they see when they view the tracings on the printout.

This sensitive, high-tech device sometimes fails to detect the difference between mothers' and babies' heartbeats, and sometimes this can lead to diagnosing a baby as being in trouble, when, instead, it's the mother's heart rate that has speeded up. In rare instances, EFM has missed a baby's death because it continued to record the mother's, rather than the baby's heartbeat.[5]

Numerous scientific studies have concluded that EFM conveys virtually no proven benefit to the mother, and mothers placed on EFM machines are more at risk of having needless cesarean sections. The American College of Obstetricians and Gynecologists has deemed EFM unnecessary for low-risk mothers. Nonetheless, monitors are in widespread use in contemporary hospitals as a tool for managing normal labors, and it is also felt to be useful for providing a printed record of a woman's labor should there be a lawsuit.[6]

From a mother's point of view, the biggest downside to being on continuous EFM monitoring is that she will be tied down to the machine, which interferes with her freedom to walk about and seek comfortable and effective positions for labor that might help her with pain and the aligning of the baby's body for birth.

way that enables her to understand her situation and her options.[7] Patients are also given the freedom to agree to interventions and other options presented to them, or to refuse them. Similar ethical guidelines also exist for physicians in family practice, midwives, and labor and delivery nurses.

In simple terms, you have the right to know how your healthcare provider wants to care for your birth; to have a thorough description of the treatment being proposed, including why it's being suggested for you; and to be fully informed about the potential risks and complications associated with the treatment.

Your healthcare provider should discuss these options with you in a forthright, honest manner, rather than just presenting all the "good" reasons for doing it. You should be fully informed of all your options, the merits of not having the treatment at all, and an accurate estimate of how likely it is that the treatment will succeed or fail.

If you're in doubt about whether to have a procedure, you have the right to request a second opinion from another healthcare provider. This may be important for those that could affect your and your baby's health and well-being, such as having an artificial induction, having your labor augmented with drugs, having an epidural, or being given a cesarean section.

If you don't have an expert in mind, and you're in the hospital, you can request to confer with the on-duty head of obstetrics or medicine for the hospital, or you can seek the opinion of another, more specialized practitioner, such as a *perinatologist* (maternal-fetal specialist). If the procedure poses a potential risk to your baby, consider putting in a call to your baby's pediatrician. The supervisor of

nursing for your floor may be helpful in offering guidance about where to turn, but keep in mind that she may have biases for or against certain procedures or feel duty bound to support your healthcare provider.

Serious medical emergencies sometimes unexpectedly arise during labor. In that case, postponing an important medical decision could mean the difference between life and death for you or your baby. Examples are when your baby's heart rate becomes dangerously slow, signaling serious oxygen

Percentage of Mothers Having Interventions During Labor[8]

(Based on a report published in 2000)

Electronic fetal monitoring (EFM)—a monitoring machine attached to a mother's body	85%
Epidural—pain medication injected into a space in the spine	66.6%
Episiotomy—cutting of the perineum to widen the vaginal opening	32.7%
Cesarean section—surgical delivery of a baby through an incision in the uterus	22.9%
Amniotomy—artificial rupturing of the amniotic sac	22.3%
Artificial induction of labor—labor initiated with drugs to make the uterus contract	19.9%
Augmentation of labor—using drugs to make contractions stronger	17.5%
Vacuum delivery—using a suction device to pull a baby out of its mother	8.4%
Forceps delivery—using metal tongs to pull a baby out of its mother	4.0%

deficiency; when labor goes too long with no progress; or if you're having serious bleeding.

Should any of these emergencies happen to you, your care provider will discuss the risks of delaying your decision. You, or your partner, will probably be presented with a special informed consent form to sign that details the seriousness of the situation and potential risks involved in intervening (or not intervening). (The most life-threatening emergencies are described on pages 355–357.)

Your partner's role in childbirth

In the old days, numerous cartoons were drawn of anxious husbands pacing in the "waiting room" while their wives gave birth behind closed doors. Now, husbands, lovers, or other chosen birth partners are playing an active role in helping moms get through birth. Fathers-to-be are much more likely now to be actively involved from the first minute a woman finds out she's pregnant, through the final cutting of the umbilical cord, or escorting newborns to the nursery for observation.

It's up to you to decide how involved you'd like the man of your life to be in your birth experience. It's critical to have support from at least one other familiar person during your labor to help you stay relaxed and to assist you with important decisions, but there's no hard-and-fast rule that says the person you choose has to be your husband or boyfriend.

Many of today's fathers-to-be want to play an active role in the birth process. Most fathers who have been able to be present during birth report afterwards that it was an important and unforgettable transition for them, too. But, if your baby's dad is skittish about blood or medical procedures, there are other ways he can still help, such as transporting you to the hospital, alerting family members, and making sure your other children and pets are taken care of while you are hospitalized.

Your healthcare provider and the labor and delivery nurses that care for you during your birth will handle the medical details; and, hopefully, they will make certain that you and your partner are allowed to weigh in on critical decisions about the way your birth is handled, which is your right as a patient.

The primary role for your chosen birth partner is to stay at your side as much as possible; to talk with you and reassure you; to bring you water and food as allowed; to alert the medical staff when you have needs; and to provide TLC and touch to help you to relax, such as massaging your feet, or reminding you to breathe deeply. Even before you begin labor, your partner should be reminded that there may be times when could become unpleasant or irritable, especially during "transition," but he shouldn't take it personally.

Tips for managing your hospital birth

Trust that your body knows what it's doing. Your body has a very sophisticated, built-in program for laboring and giving birth. Relax, and allow your body to do its work.

Select a secure setting. Familiarize yourself with the hospital in advance, so you can rehearse how it will look and feel to give birth there. If you're not comfortable there, take steps to

Questions to Ask about Procedures

Here is a list of possible questions to ask before agreeing to an intervention or medication during labor and birth.

Why is this needed?

What are the realistic risks to me, or my baby, if I declined this intervention? (Keep in mind that risk and safe are general terms. For instance, a cesarean section may be safe in that it is unlikely to result in death, but it also results in risks and a painful recovery period.)

What are the risks or side effects, even rare ones, to me, or my baby, if I agree to have this done?

What will my recovery be like afterward?

What are my other options?

What might happen if I choose to wait (thirty minutes? an hour?) to make this decision?

May I have some time alone to talk with my partner about this?

How might I get a second opinion?

find the birthing option that feels the safest and most comfortable for you. Anxiety, stress, and a sense of estrangement can lead to the secretion of catecholamines that can increase tension and pain.

Check in late, rather than early. Studies have shown that mothers who arrive at the hospital in the early stages of labor are much more likely to undergo serious interventions than those who wait to arrive until strong, active labor has gotten underway. (See "Flash Facts" on page 271.)

Surround yourself with supportive people. Handpick the people who will be with you during this most intimate of events, and keep the group small. Choose a clinician with excellent training and lots of experience, who will respect your preferences. A supportive caregiver at your side, such as a

partner or another experienced mother, can help to protect you from unwanted interventions. We recommend that in addition to your partner, you consider hiring a doula or personal labor assistant to accompany you through your birth process. She will bring a wonderful bag of tricks to make labor more comfortable. (See "Flash Facts" about support on page 304.)

Conserve energy. When labor is just getting started, it may be tempting to pull out all of the positions, movements, and breathing techniques you learned during childbirth classes. If they help, go for it—just don't exhaust yourself too soon.

Post a sign on your door. Ask for quiet, if that's what you want. If you don't want pain medications, indicate that, and respectfully request to not be offered those options unless you specifically ask for them.

Who Will Oversee Your Labor in the Hospital?

If you elect to give birth in a hospital, the person who will have responsibility for your care during labor and birth depends upon whether the hospital is affiliated with a medical school and whether you have chosen to use the services of an obstetrician, a physician in family practice, or a midwife. In a teaching hospital, a resident (a physician-in-training for obstetrics) may be responsible for managing your labor until your healthcare provider arrives for delivery.

If you give birth in a community hospital, where most babies in the U.S. are born, your labor will be overseen by your private healthcare provider, and if she is not physically present, it will likely be managed by a labor and delivery nurse using your caregiver's standing orders and telephone instructions for procedures, monitoring, and interventions to be used with you, such as performing an amniotomy or starting **artificial induction** or **augmentation of labor**.

Most labor and delivery areas in hospitals are also guided by a set of written protocols based on current practice guidelines established by national professional organizations in medical specialties, including obstetricians, family practice physicians, midwives, pediatricians, and labor and delivery nurses. Some guidelines have to do with monitoring and recordkeeping rules designed to protect the hospital and its staff from being vulnerable to malpractice suits.

Some hospitals and healthcare providers adhere to an approach called the **active management of labor**, designed for use on first-time mothers (**nulliparas**), which calls for continuous nursing support; continuous monitoring; routinely performing amniotomies on mothers when they are admitted into labor and have reached three to four centimeters dilation; and augmenting labors when the progress of dilation and the descent of the baby fail to occur within certain time limits. Current research demonstrates that although this approach may shorten labors for first-time mothers, it has not consistently resulted in a reduction in cesarean sections, the original justification for using this approach.

While midwives generally remain with their patients throughout labor, it is not uncommon for obstetricians to be physically absent for their patients with normal labors until the time of birth nears. If your healthcare provider is seeing patients or is busy with another patient or out of town, your labor may be mostly managed by telephone or turned over to another medical professional.

A 2002 survey sponsored by the Maternity Center Association of more than fifteen hundred U.S. women who had recently given birth found that 19 percent of the mothers (nearly one out of five) said they were delivered by healthcare providers they hardly knew or were strangers. (The entire survey can be accessed at www.maternitywise.org.)

Ease into the pain. When you're in the middle of a contraction, try to relax as best you can, moving toward, rather than bracing against the discomfort.

Keep things in perspective. Labor is tricky: you can feel utterly exhausted and think you can't go on another moment, then comes the pushing stage and wellsprings of energy you didn't know you had. Keep focusing on the fact that your labor will soon be over, you'll have your wonderful baby in your arms. Be bold about demanding pain medication when things become truly unbearable. (See our discussion of pain relief measures on page 315.)

Use comfort measures. A mildly warm bath or shower can help you relax. Bring along your favorite CDs to listen to. Consider bringing something familiar from home, such as your favorite pillow, teddy bear, or religious object that says home to you. (See other pain relief measures on pages 303–315.)

Think of creative ways to use your bed. If you find yourself confined to a hospital bed because of monitoring devices or the wires and tubes of an epidural, crank up the back support, and try to stay as upright as you can. Don't be shy about squatting in the bed or putting up the sidebars and using them to help you get comfortable or to push. If you've had an epidural, ask the nurses to help you change positions at least once every thirty minutes, which will help labor to move along. When it comes time for delivery, you can request that the bottom portion of the bed be left in place rather than removed for your healthcare provider's convenience, if doing so makes you feel more comfortable and secure.

Coach others about how you wish to be treated. Be positive and polite, but let others know how you would like to be treated. If you're in the middle of a contraction, and your caregiver wants to examine you, ask him, or her, to wait until you signal you're ready. If you don't want your baby's amniotic sac artificially ruptured, say so before your first in-hospital exam. (See our discussion of *amniotomy* on page 341.) The same goes for whether you want to be touched, massaged, coached, or simply left alone.

Go with the flow. The most intense part of labor will be directed by a different part of your brain than the part that thinks. Trying to keep control can make things slow down. At some point, you just have to surrender.

Claim your baby. You'll always remember those first precious moments: Don't let others steal it away from you. Ask to be given first dibs on your baby before all the cleaning, testing, weighing, and assessing get underway. Lay your naked newborn on your bare chest under a warm blanket over the two of you, and wait to see if your baby tries to crawl to your nipple or makes mouthing motions for nursing.

Plan ahead for privacy. Consider paying extra for a private room in the hospital. That will give you the space you need to recoup, have undisturbed bonding and breastfeeding time with your baby, and have quiet time with your partner.

All about Labor

In medical circles, labor is usually described having four distinct stages. From your point of view as a patient, the stages will probably pass through in a blur, since you'll simply be engrossed in the strong sensations and signals your body is sending you. But being aware of the stages of labor and its complexities can help you feel more in control of what is happening to you and less anxious.

The first stage of labor defines the process of the uterus drawing up to make the cervix open up so the baby can be born. The second stage is the pushing, or bearing down stage when the uterus and its owner push the baby through the birth canal to the outside. The third stage is when the placenta and membranes, known as the afterbirth, are expelled, and the uterus starts to shrink back to its regular size. The fourth stage covers a mother's recovery immediately after giving birth. Here is a detailed description of each stage with practical suggestions to help you get through each one.

STAGE 1

What's happening

Picture your uterus as a large, upside-down pear. The neck of the uterus (stem of the pear) faces downward toward your vagina. The neck and tip end of the uterus are called the cervix, the Latin word for neck. During this stage, the cervix softens and becomes thinner and wider. The thinning process is called *effacement*, and it is described as a percentage, with 50 percent effaced meaning the cervix is halfway through its thinning process, and one hundred percent, or fully effaced, meaning the cervix has become paper-thin and has almost disappeared. It can happen over the process of hours, or even days, of mild, irregular contractions.

Dilation (or dilatation) refers to the widening of the mouth of the cervix. During this stage of labor, contractions draw the side walls of the uterus upward causing the diameter of the cervix to widen. Dilation

The Phases of Stage 1

Some clinicians divide labor into two phases: latent and active. The latent phase refers to the time before a mother's cervix reaches three to four centimeters dilation. The active phase is dilation from four to seven centimeters. "Transition" is an informal division within the active phase that refers to the last, intense part of labor before a mother reaches full dilation. Some women find the contractions in the latent stage quite

STAGE 1 PHASES	HOW LONG THE STAGE LASTS (first time mothers)	WHAT'S HAPPENING
Latent (beginning)	5 hours or longer	The cervix is slowly effacing and dilating at the rate of 0.6 centimeters (about one-quarter of an inch) an hour until it reaches 3 to 4 centimeters ($1^1/_4$ to a little over $1^1/_2$ inches).
Active (middle)	Approximately 3 hours	Cervix dilates to about seven centimeters ($2^3/_4$ inches).
Transition (end)	2 hours or less	Final stretching of the cervix over the baby's head and contraction of the uterus before the baby moves down into the birth canal. It dilates from 8 to 10 centimeters (a little more than 3 inches to nearly 4 inches).

is expressed in centimeters as the diameter of the hole, or more casually, as fingers. (A centimeter is equal to a little more than a third of an inch.) A mother is considered to be in active labor when her dilation reaches three to four centimeters (two to three fingers), and fully dilated when it reaches ten centimeters (five fingers). Once that happens, the mother enters the second stage of labor.

As with effacement, it can take hours, or days, for the cervix of a first-time mother to make it to three or four centimeters (approximately uncomfortable, others find that walking or other techniques make them tolerable, and still other women barely notice any discomfort at all. Some healthcare providers and anesthesiologists prefer to wait to administer an epidural until a mother has passed the latent stage, while others allow mothers to have epidurals whenever they request it. (More about epidurals on pages 317–322.)

LENGTH OF CONTRACTIONS	HOW CONTRACTIONS FEEL
Last 30 to 40 seconds, start at about 10 minutes apart, and slowly move to 5 minutes apart	Crampy. May start in the lower back and migrate toward the front in the lower abdomen, or feel like a sharp squeeze.
Last about 60 seconds and go from 5 to 3 minutes apart	More intense and regular.
Last 60 to 90 seconds and are 2 to 3 minutes apart	Intense with little time to rest in between. Some mothers experience trembling, nausea, and vomiting, or hot and cold flashes.

one to two inches). That's because it takes the uterus two to three times more effort to dilate the cervix one centimeter during early labor than it does later on. The dilation process will probably move slowly at first and get much faster as you near ten centimeters.

During first births, effacing and dilating are usually two separate processes, with effacement (effacing) happening first before dilation begins in earnest. For mothers who have previously given birth, effacement and dilation often happen simultaneously, which is why labor

Quick Guide to Dilation

Dilation is the width of the opening of the cervix as the baby's head descends.

One centimeter = width of a Cheerio®
Three centimeters = slice of banana
Four centimeters = Oreo® cookie
Five centimeters = lid of a small orange juice can
Seven centimeters = lid of a soda can
Ten centimeters = width of a bagel

1 2 3 4 5 6 7 8 10

is generally shorter the second time around. Don't be discouraged at the news that you're not dilating if this is your first time around. Ask about how well you're effacing instead.

How long the first stage lasts: How long the entire first stage lasts varies widely among mothers. It'll probably be longer if this is your first baby. This stage is estimated to take approximately six to eighteen hours from the time labor starts for first-time mothers, and between two to ten hours for mothers who have given birth before.

How the first stage feels: At first, contractions may resemble waves of menstrual cramps, except that they come and go. Labor pain generally starts in the back and moves around to the front, and sometimes it radiates into the upper thighs. There are regular pauses between each contraction. Contractions usually become stronger and more uncomfortable as labor goes on, with discomfort peaking for a few seconds halfway through each contraction. Contractions never last longer than a minute and a half, while the breaks in between contractions go from five minutes at the start of labor to less than thirty seconds toward the end.

How this stage will feel to you will depend upon how you've elected to deal with labor pain. If you've decided to forego painkilling drugs, you'll probably be walking around, breathing, and assuming various positions for comfort. If you've decided to have an epidural and it took properly, you'll be lying down and probably won't be feeling pain, though you may be aware of pressure and experience nausea, itching, or other side effects from the drugs. If you've chosen to have narcotics, you'll probably feel groggy and a bit out of it. Some mothers experience temporary waves of nausea, regardless of their pain management method. (We discuss pain management on pages 302–322.)

Active phase

During the latent stage of labor, you may feel stuck at three to four centimeters for hours, while the dilation of your cervix will start to pick up speed during the active phase. It can be a great feeling to know you're finally making progress. The downside is that contractions become more uncomfortable to the point of being annoying or almost unbearable. Pain management techniques that worked earlier, such as massage or warm water, may no longer distract your brain from the pain.

> *"The magic words all mothers need to hear during transition are: "You can do this!" And, "We can do this together."*

Transition phase

The final part of the first stage is called *transition*, or the transition phase, when the cervix progresses from about seven to ten centimeters dilation, which is considered fully dilated, or complete. This phase can feel very challenging and exhausting. Contractions descend one after another with little rest in between. And sometimes they're out of rhythm, with two peaks cresting into one continuous, long contraction.

The intensity and length of these contractions will demand everything you've got just to ride through them. You may have hot flashes and get red-faced, only to feel cold a few minutes later. You may tremble, have hiccups, burp, feel nauseated, and even vomit.

During transition, many mothers feel unusually irritable and demand that people not touch them, or they become hypersensitive to the things people are saying around them. And you may have the urge to yell, curse, or make sounds to express what's going on inside. Low tones from the bottom of your lungs work better than high-pitched sounds that strain your body and make it harder to breathe.

Psychologically, most mothers at this stage come to the point of being ready to throw in the towel. They think they're going to die and wish they could, just to get out of the incredible intensity of this rapidly progressing, brief storm.

This is the time during labor when you most need the encouragement and support of your partner and doula, or your labor and delivery nurse. The words you need to hear are that you're doing a fantastic job and that it won't be long until you're holding your baby in your arms.

If you've resisted having an epidural up to this point, you may beg for one just to get relief, not realizing that you're almost over the hump.

Sometimes mothers get the urge to push before they're fully dilated. Some healthcare providers will allow the mother to push whenever she gets the urge, while others may tell you that you're pushing too soon and warn you that doing so will make your cervix swell and become puffy, making birthing harder. Your healthcare provider will suggest how to handle the situation.

What to do during the first stage

- **Relax through early contractions.** There's no need to go crazy with labor positions or breathing exercises you learned in childbirth class unless they really help. Try to not wear yourself out too early in the process.

- **Breathe.** Inhale through your nose and out your pursed lips with deep breaths during contractions, but don't pant or hyperventilate. Try to breathe deeply to the bottom of your lungs. Making low-pitched noises may help.

- **Relax, and trust your body.** Try to maintain a positive outlook. Stress and anxiety can cause the body to produce chemicals that increase muscle tension and pain. Ask for a foot massage or other comfort measures if you find yourself tensing up.

- **Move around.** Moving around can help to stimulate nature's own painkillers, endorphins. If you're not connected to monitoring lines, change positions frequently, especially if your contractions appear to be getting weaker or further apart.

- **Try out some gadgets.** Patient rooms in progressive hospital birth centers and freestanding birth centers often are equipped with laborsaving devices to help mothers. If you aren't offered labor "toys," ask, because they may well be sitting in a closet somewhere. An exercise ball, or birth ball, can be great for sitting on, rolling your hips around, draping your body over, or for a footstool. Many newer hospital beds come equipped with a squat bar that pops out to transform the bed into something that looks like a luggage rack. You use the bar to pull up and stretch.

- **Sit on the toilet.** Staying on the toilet for a while can help to open the pelvis and rotate the baby. Use a footstool if one is available.

- **Try temperature and pressure changes.** Warm or cold compresses to your back or lower abdomen may help in the middle of a contraction. Getting a shoulder massage or having pressure applied to your back or hips may be temporarily soothing. A soft

The Benefits of an Upright Labor

Many hospitals and care providers once routinely placed mothers in bed for labor and on their backs for delivery. Old-fashioned doctors were not too keen on the idea of laboring women wandering around and getting underfoot, and women who could afford it were knocked out with "twilight sleep" anyway. Keeping the mother to the bed made it easier and more comfortable for the doctor to deliver the baby.

Fortunately, these are more enlightened times, and we know that lying on your back is an inefficient position for both labor and giving birth. As long as it feels comfortable, walk around, squat, sit up straight on a birth ball, and otherwise keep yourself as upright as you can and still feel comfortable.

If you've had an epidural and are confined to bed, having the top of the bed raised can help. Here are some of the advantages to staying upright and moving around, especially during the first stage of labor:

Better circulation. Being upright takes pressure off your main arteries and keeps them from being compressed.

Better use of gravity. An upright position uses the force of gravity to naturally pull the head-heavy baby downward and realigns your pelvis to make a straighter outlet for birth.

Improved alignment of baby's body. Walking and standing improves the alignment of your baby's body from head to toe during his descent and distributes the pressures of birth more evenly on his body.

Better contractions. Being upright makes contractions stronger and more efficient. It can also help to shorten the second (pushing) stage of labor.

Wider outlet. Your pelvis has the capacity to expand up to one-third more and an upright, squatting, or lunging position can help, but most modern-day mothers can't squat comfortably for very long.

Less awareness of pain. If you don't have an epidural, women who continue to walk, stand, and squat during labor report that they experience less discomfort and that their pain is more tolerable than mothers who passively lie down or sit during labor.

Fewer interventions and less tearing. A systematic research review found that in the second stage, being upright is associated with less risk of forceps delivery, vacuum extraction, or cesarean sections, and that translates into less blood loss and quicker healing.[9]

paint roller or a rolling pin is sometimes used by doulas to help lower back pain.

- **Make the most of your hospital bed.** If you're stuck close to bed because of monitor wires, an IV, or an epidural connection, try to sit as upright as is comfortable and request extra pillows for support. You can also lie on your left side if that feels comfortable to you, but avoid lying flat on your back (being supine). Doing so can affect your blood pressure and could deprive your baby of needed blood circulation and oxygen, and it may dislodge the catheter inserted in your back for your epidural.

- **Urinate frequently.** Drink sips of water between contractions to make up for your sweating and panting. Make sure to urinate frequently to keep your bladder empty so there's more room for your baby to move down. If you've had an epidural, you may have a catheter inserted, a tube inside your urinary tract that drains to a waterproof pouch clipped to the side of your bed.

- **Be kind to your partner.** Arrange for a labor assistant or family member to keep you company, so your birth partner can take a break once in a while to rest or eat.

- **Ask for help.** If pain becomes overwhelming, discuss the benefits and risks of various medication options with your care provider.

- **Don't give up.** Although transition may feel awful, it means you're getting closer and closer to having your baby.

"What can I eat?"

The process of labor makes heavy energy demands on a mother's body. Just as for performers in athletic events, if a laboring body isn't being supplied adequate carbohydrates and energy supplies, body stores can become depleted, forcing the body to metabolize its own fat and muscle tissue. That's great if you're trying to lose weight, but not so great if you're expending a huge physical effort over a long period of time to give birth.

For decades, laboring mothers were automatically put on standing orders for NPO, the initials for the Latin *nil per oram*, meaning nothing by mouth. The order was based on the threat of mothers' suffering lung damage from breathing vomit and stomach contents into their lungs when they were rendered unconscious by *general anesthesia*. The orders meant that a mother would not be permitted to eat or drink during labor, even when labor dragged on for eighteen hours or more. The wisdom of restricting mothers' food and beverages is now being debated in medical circles.

General anesthesia is rarely used during deliveries and c-sections now, primarily because it has a profound effect on the baby, and it has caused maternal deaths. Instead, regional anesthesia, such as epidurals or spinal anesthesia, or a combination of these two is being used for cesareans. In addition, inhaling the contents of the stomach into the lungs during general anesthesia is now thought to be more of a result of the lack of an anesthetist's skill, rather than anesthesia itself. Newer devices are designed to shield the airway to prevent the problem.[10]

FLASH FACTS: Is It Okay to Wait to Push?

Often mothers are coached to start pushing as soon as it is determined that they are fully dilated (ten centimeters). Waiting to push until your baby has moved down into your pelvis (between a +1 and +3 station) and his head has begun to rotate can save you a lot of energy and make your pushing efforts more efficient in moving your baby down for birth.

Pausing for an hour, relaxing, and waiting for your baby to descend rather than spending that hour trying to push your baby down has recently been shown to delay pushing only by an average of fourteen minutes during the second stage of labor (one hundred six minutes versus one hundred twenty minutes). In addition, waiting to push also may help protect your pelvic floor from damage.[11]

Although some hospitals continue to rigidly hold to the NPO rule, or only allow mothers to drink clear liquids, many facilities are now in the process of liberalizing their policies regarding mothers' freedom to eat and drink during labor. Typical foods being allowed: water and fruit juices; low-residue, low-fat foods, such as light meals; clear soup broths; gelatin and jelly candies; ice cream; toast and jelly; packaged crackers; boiled or scrambled eggs; cooked fruit; and light cereals.

STAGE 2 (THE PUSHING STAGE)

What's happening during the second stage

During the process of labor, the muscle fibers of your uterus draw it up and then thicken at the top in order to expel your baby. During this stage, your baby's head and body descend downward and rotate to find the best way to negotiate the zigzag path down through your pelvis.

Even though your cervix is fully dilated (five fingers or ten centimeters), there typically will be a pause before the urge to push sets in. Meanwhile, you'll feel the pressure of your baby's head and body as it gradually moves downward in a two-steps forward, one-step backward fashion with each contraction. This pressure will initiate the *Ferguson's reflex* in your body, causing the secretion of oxytocin, which will stimulate your pushing urge.

Unless your lower body is numbed by your epidural, the arrival of this urge will probably evoke a groan, and you will find yourself tightening your abdominal muscles and pressing down using the muscles of your chest to exert pressure on the top of your uterus. Contractions may spread further apart, giving you more time in between to rest and catch your breath.

As your baby comes closer to being born, your *perineum* will bulge with each contraction, and your baby's head will become increasingly more visible. His scalp may appear folded, wrinkled, lumpy, shiny, or maybe even mushy. If your baby has hair, it will probably be announced, along with its color.

The Phases of Stage 2

STAGE 2 PHASES	HOW LONG THE STAGE LASTS	WHAT'S HAPPENING
Passive stage	Approximately 15 to 20 minutes	Your cervix has dilated between 8 1/2 and 10 centimeters. Your baby is in the process of descending downward and is getting aligned for birth.
Expulsive (active or bearing down) **stage**	20 to 30 minutes (an uncomplicated active stage can last an hour, or longer, and still be normal)	Your baby has moved deeply into your pelvis and is putting pressure on your lower body and vaginal area.

Crowning is when the skin of the vagina surrounds your baby's head like a halo, and it's a sure signal that delivery is at hand. Your care provider may ask you if you want to reach down and touch your baby's head, or you might be provided with a hand mirror so you can see for yourself. Your vagina will appear stretched, expanded, and thinned out so that the tissue is almost white. Contractions will be quite intense, but the pressure of your baby's head will make your vagina tingly and then numb.

Some healthcare providers give advance orders that a mother's epidural medication be reduced (backed down) at this stage to make her more aware of her pushing urges and to shorten the second stage of labor. Backing down on an epidural can cause a mother to experience more pain than if she were not on powerful numbing drugs. Their effect will have altered her body's response to pain so that it produced fewer natural endorphins, nature's potent painkillers that are much stronger than commercial morphine.

Laboring down describes a recent medical practice that allows a mother with an epidural to hold back from pushing until she has the urge to do so or until certain signs of readiness appear. When the time for pushing is ripe, the baby will have begun his descent down into his mother's pelvis (at least one centimeter below the ischial spines, two bony knobs inside the pelvis); his head will start to rotate to facing rearward; and the mother's softened cervix will begin to pull back over the baby's head with each contraction. If you would like to have the chance to labor down rather than having to push from the time you are fully dilated, you should discuss this with your healthcare provider.

CONTRACTIONS	WHAT TO DO
Contractions slow down.	Rest, and collect yourself. Don't attempt pushing unless you have a strong urge to do so.
Contractions are accompanied by a sudden, strong urge to push, and you may find yourself making loud groaning sounds.	Go with your instincts. There's no need to hold your breath and push to a count of ten. Light pushes three to five times per contraction are more natural.

If your baby has descended, but you still feel no pushing urge because of your epidural or other medication, your care provider, nurse, or doula may place her hand on your abdomen to sense when your contraction starts to help coach you when to push.

How long the second stage lasts: This stage can last between thirty minutes to three hours for a first-time mother. It can be less than thirty minutes and up to two hours for a mother who has given birth before. Some mothers take much longer and still have healthy babies.

How the second stage feels: It may take a few contractions for you to figure out what your body is doing. The urge to push will become very compelling on its own, and when it does, it will be difficult to do anything but push when the contractions hit.

Most of the discomfort you'll feel at this point will be from the pressure of your baby's head on your stretching lower body and vagina. You'll feel the sensation of pressure even with an epidural. Although this stage seems challenging, many mothers say they also find it deeply satisfying. Others report that the sensation of pressure from the baby's head while they're pushing can be scary, intense, or painful. Even though your body is designed to stretch and accommodate the baby, most women have a momentary fear of tearing or splitting open.

"A ring of fire" is what midwives use to describe how a woman's vagina may burn, tingle, and then go numb from the pressure of the baby's head as it presses forward and recedes backward near the end of the second stage. Most non-medicated mothers find this part of birth quite bearable, but if you find

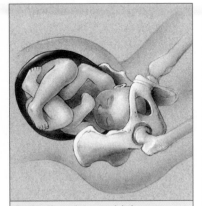

Getting through your pelvis is your baby's hardest job.

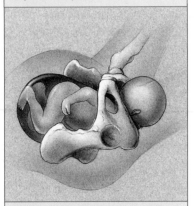

His whole body will rotate to make it through.

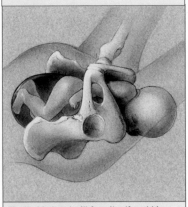

Finally his head will free itself and his shoulders will emerge one at a time.

yourself in pain, you can request that your healthcare provider give you medication for relief.

During this stage, the bones at the base of your pelvis, including your tailbone will need to be free to flex outward instead of being pressed inward toward the front of your body, as they are when you lie down or sit.[12]

A variety of positions can help your pelvis to efficiently expand. Sitting up works well for some mothers, as does a temporary squat or semi-squat. If you're experiencing *back labor*, continuous pain in your lower back, pushing while you're down on all fours may be the most comfortable for a while. If you're exhausted from long hours of contractions, lying on your left side for this stage will allow you rest between contractions without hampering your stretching.

What to do during the second stage

- **Request time to rest and regroup.** Even though you're fully dilated, if you haven't felt the urge to push yet, you're probably in passive stage, as your baby is aligning and descending downward. Simply rest for a while.

- **Push effectively.** While you're pushing, relax your perineum, and try to direct your bearing down toward your lower pelvis, rather than concentrating all your pushing forces in your chest area.

- **Breathe deeply in between.** Take deep breaths between your contractions to help maintain good oxygen levels for your baby.

If You're Instructed to Hold Back

Once you begin to bear down during the second stage of labor, it's next to impossible to stop yourself; however, your care provider may ask you to hold back for a number of reasons, including your cervix isn't yet fully dilated and pushing could cause swelling; your vagina may need a little more time to relax and stretch; or your baby is about to emerge and his shoulders need to be gently freed. Here are some tips about how to hold back from pushing:

Blow. It's impossible to blow and push at the same time. Purse your lips and blow as though you're blowing out birthday candles. Be careful not to hyperventilate. Stop blowing if you start to feel lightheaded or dizzy.

Lean back and go limp. Keep your eyes open during the contraction. Find something in the room on which to focus.

Relax down below. Try to relax the muscles you aren't using for pushing.

Let your body do the work. Just let your contractions do all the work without your adding additional pressure.

Push, but differently. Give in to the urge to push, but respond to it differently: push in brief, light pulses while keeping your throat open.

• **Don't worry about soiling the bed.** Your baby's head will be exerting pressure on your rectal area. Even if it feels like you're about to go, you probably won't, since your body has probably already cleaned everything out.

• **Try to stay upright.** You will be able to bear down more effectively if you are in an upright position, a forty-five degree angle, rather than lying flat or semi-reclined. Have the back of the bed raised, and use the sidearm of the bed, or towels tied to the sides to pull yourself up. If tubes and wires from your epidural have tied you down, sit in as upright a position as you can, or lie on your left side with a pillow between your knees while your back is supported by pillows.

• **Get off your tail(bone).** Having your tailbone (coccyx) compressed by the weight of your body can prevent your pelvis from expanding as your baby descends. If you are able to move about, there are

"Just because your baby is taking her own sweet time about getting herself born doesn't automatically mean your doctor should suggest you have surgery."

FLASH FACTS: Research vs. "Purple Pushing"

In hospital rooms across the nation (and on reality birth shows), nurses can be seen commanding mothers in the second stage to push: "Ready, take a deep breath, now hold it and push, push, push!" Then, the count begins: "1-2-3-4-5-" until the number ten is reached and the purple-faced mother is allowed to gasp for air before the push command and the counting begin all over again.

In 2000, the Association of Women's Health, Obstetric, and Neonatal Nurses (AWHONN) issued an evidence-based guideline recommending that breath-holding or forced pushing be avoided during this stage. It suggests that mothers be free to rest and not push in the early part of this stage, even if they are fully dilated; that they be allowed to rest through some contractions if they wish; and that they be allowed to push in any way they feel comfortable, such as pushing only for four to six seconds with only a slight exhale. (AWHONN's guidelines can be found on www.awohnn.org. by searching "second stage.")[13]

numerous positions that will free up your pelvis. Try leaning forward while standing or squatting with support from your partner, the bed, or a chair. Swaying your hips can feel good. Or you may feel the urge to get down on all fours or even to climb stairs. Let your body do the talking.

- **Make working sounds.** Your facial expression will change as the urge to push starts. You are likely to grimace and frown. Don't be shy about grunting, groaning, or making other noises during this phase if that feels natural to you.

- **Ask for support.** Ask others to help you get into positions, to fetch pillows and blankets, to give you something to drink, or anything else that will help you stay comfortable. There should be a nurse or midwife with you during your entire second stage.

- **Sip on water, and urinate.** Remember to keep yourself hydrated, but don't overdo. Try to keep your bladder empty. That will cause less discomfort and make room for the baby to move through.

- **Ask unwanted onlookers to leave.** If your room becomes overly crowded with idle viewers, including extra hospital interns and relatives, select the two to four people you want to have with you for birth, and request that the others leave, or ask your nurse or midwife to do that for you.

- **Reach for your baby's head.** If your care provider gives you the option, you can reach down and feel your baby's head with both of your hands as your baby starts to crown. It may be a sensation you'll remember for a long time.

- **Protect yourself from injury.** If you've had an epidural, don't try to turn in the bed by yourself unless someone is supporting you at your feet, your back, and your shoulders. The temptation for caregivers and support people is to pull your legs far apart when you're pushing to help get the baby out, but that could tear muscles and ligaments and cause you a great deal of pain afterward. Don't allow staff members or your support person to stretch your legs farther apart during pushing than you would ordinarily position them.

Your baby's birth

Usually, babies' heads come out facing their mother's tailbone, so only the top rear of your baby's head will appear first. With his head facing toward the floor, your baby's forehead, brows, eyes, nose, and cheeks, then the mouth and chin will slide free of the band that holds them. The baby's head will then rotate sideways and will gently move to face the inside of your thigh. Your healthcare provider will be helping to support your baby's head to prevent putting too much pressure on your perineum.

Once the head, the largest and hardest part, is out, then the shoulders will be birthed, one shoulder at a time, with the top shoulder first and the bottom one second. Then, your baby's slippery body will slide out with no pain or effort on your part.

When your baby's face emerges, he may take his first breath, and start mewing and gasping for air even before his body gets birthed. If your baby is being delivered by cesarean, his crying may start before he is completely lifted out of your body.

Your care provider will quickly work to suction out the mucus and amniotic fluid from the baby's mouth and nostrils so he can breathe. All the while, your baby's body is rotating inside so the shoulders can get out. Until then, your baby has been tunneling out on his side or belly, butting his head against your bony pelvis.

FLASH FACTS: Do Healthy Babies Need Suctioning?

Although suctioning the baby's nose and throat and even stomach is routine in many hospitals, research shows that this procedure isn't necessary for a normal baby who isn't having problems. Sometimes suctioning is important for helping a baby to clear his nostrils and lungs, but a healthy, full-term baby who is breathing without problems doesn't need the annoyance of being suctioned.

In some instances, there is concern that suctioning too forcefully may actually make some babies stop breathing. Also, evidence indicates that suctioning of the stomach may impede a baby's suckling and nursing later. Harsh suctioning may cause irritation to the baby's mouth and throat. A gentler alternative is to simply place the baby face down on your chest.[14]

STAGE 3

What's happening during the third stage

This stage of labor begins immediately after the birth of your baby and ends with the delivery of your placenta. All during your pregnancy, the placenta has been anchored to the wall of your uterus by hundreds of capillaries and supportive connectors. These anchoring threads are bathed in a pool of blood. After the sudden decompression caused by your baby's evacuation, several contractions will quickly close off the placenta's attaching fibers to help stop bleeding.

You may be asked to push when your care provider sees the first signs of the placenta detaching. Expelling it usually takes less than fifteen minutes.

Once the placenta arrives, it, and the part of the umbilical cord still attached, will be examined to make sure there are no parts still remaining inside, which could cause infection. When that happens, your uterus will begin shrinking and hardening. You'll be able to feel the top of it near your navel. Nursing your baby will encourage your body to release oxytocin, which will help your uterus remain firm, or you may be given an IV of Pitocin or an injection to help it contract.

How long the third stage lasts
Five to thirty minutes.

How the third stage feels
In your eagerness to see and hold your baby, you may be mostly oblivious to this stage of delivery. That is, unless your care provider presses the top of your uterus as your placenta comes out, or massages your uterus immediately after the placenta is born, in an effort to help close off open blood vessels. That can be painful.

What to do

- **Get hold of your baby.** While your placenta is being delivered, ask to have your baby's cleaning, rubdown, and other procedures delayed so you can hold and greet him. Gently massage the white, waxy substance, the *vernix* into his skin. It has protective antibacterial properties.

- **Place your baby on your abdomen so you can see his face.** Let him rest on your bare front, with a blanket covering both of you. See if your baby begins crawling motions to move himself up to your nipples. If he nuzzles, offer your breast for nursing. Some babies are very alert and eager to nurse right away, while others need more time to get acclimated.

STAGE 4

What's happening during the fourth stage

Your uterus is starting to firm up and shrink. Open blood vessels and capillaries in the uterus are closing off. Your hormones are beginning to shift. Your milk-making glands start to activate, which stimulates your breasts to produce high-protein colostrum. Your milk will come in in a couple of days. Your body starts processing all of the fluids and tissues of pregnancy so it can return to its non-pregnant state.

How long the fourth stage lasts: The official dimensions of this stage are twenty-four to thirty-six hours during the immediate postpartum. Actual recovery takes about six weeks for your body to become completely functional and up to six months to feel like your normal self again.

How the fourth stage feels
After your elation and adrenalin rush wears off, you may begin to feel deeply tired and achy. Your perineum may be sore and swollen, and you may experience aches and pains. If you've had an epidural, you may start to have a pins-and-needles feeling in your legs and hips as the painkillers wear off. (If you've had a c-section, see pages 343–350.) You will have heavy bleeding from your vagina and require maxi-pads for a while. Your breasts may become swollen and hard after about a day, called **engorgement**. Walking may make you feel weak and dizzy, but you will be encouraged to get up and walk within hours of birth to discourage blood clots. Your body

will stay in its pregnant size for quite a while, and your belly will probably stay mushy for months. Tiredness and temporary baby blues are typical. (You can find more about recovering from birth beginning on page 329, and in "You and Your Baby," starting on page 361.)

"This was my first baby, and I was truly terrified that I might die during childbirth, or something awful would go wrong with my baby. During my last months, I just kept reminding myself how badly I wanted to see her and hold her in my arms. Actually, the experience of giving birth was pretty calm, like doing heavy work. Others were very kind, and I really didn't need to be so afraid. We both cried when she was handed over to us. She was so beautiful!"

Coping with Labor Pain

It's only human to shy away from pain. Most of us would do anything to not have to endure it. And, yes: childbirth hurts. For most mothers, it's more than the discomfort that birth instructors once labeled the sensations of labor in order to minimize mothers' fears. Pain has a utility in birth. It's a powerful signal for a mother to find a safe place and to encircle herself with caregivers.

What hurts about labor? Two words: contractions and pressure. By the time you're ready to give birth, your uterus has grown into the largest muscle in your body. During labor, it will be undergoing profound change. It will thin at the bottom and get denser at the top by progressively pulling itself upward. Basically, it's moving itself out of your baby's way, shaping him into a compact ball, and pressing him downward using waves of muscular action that start at the top and radiate downward.

Surprisingly, pain isn't necessarily related to the strength of contractions. Braxton-Hicks contractions that occur throughout pregnancy are usually painless, but are identical in strength and intensity to the real contractions of labor. Contractions following birth that close down and shrink the uterus are even stronger than labor contractions, but the pain is much milder.[15]

Some mothers find their labor surprisingly easy and bearable, while others find it verging on unbearable or at least exhausting. Words mothers use to describe labor pain are "achy," "sharp," "cramping," "intense, "throbbing," "stabbing," "shooting," and "heavy."[16]

The type of pain you feel depends upon what stage of labor you're in and where in your body your baby is. Pain is usually unfocused and diffuse during the first part of labor. Most mothers feel it in their lower back and rectal area and radiating around to their lower bellies. As the baby begins to move downward and the cervix stretches around his head, contractions can be intense.

Even though most women dread the final part of birth, the pushing stage, it doesn't usually hurt as much as the stage that immediately precedes it. The stretching of the vagina sometimes evokes a temporary burning sensation, sometimes called the "ring of fire," but it's usually followed by numbness. Often, knowing the baby is about to be born, the intense work of pushing him out comes as a relief that almost feels good.

While it's useful to not worry about labor in advance, it's important to have some idea of how you plan to manage the pain of labor before it actually starts. You'll need a "Plan B" in the event that things go differently than you pictured.

For instance, even though you plan to have an epidural, you may find your labor more bearable than you imagined, or you may move into the pushing stage before there's time to get one.

Or, you could be adamant about remaining drug-free, only have your labor drag on for so many hours that an epidural seems like a godsend. No matter what, the decision about how you handle labor pain is yours, and yours alone, to make. And you should never feel coerced by anyone else into making choices you don't want.

Factors that affect labor pain

The intensity of pain you'll be feeling during your personal baby-bearing marathon depends upon a series of factors:

- **Your comfort level.** Your experience of pain is apt to be milder when you feel relaxed, secure, comfortable, and supported by others. Your body is more likely to tighten up and cry out with more pain if your birthing environment makes you feel anxious, scared, or threatened. Studies show that mothers who give birth at home surrounded by their families report substantially less pain in childbirth than those who give birth in impersonal hospital settings surrounded by strangers.

- **How far along you are in your birthing process.** Contractions are generally less painful as they're getting underway and more painful once they become more established.

- **Your baby's position.** Contractions are apt to be less painful if your baby's faced head downward and toward your back, and more painful if the baby is facing forward, positioned sideways, or rump downward, called breech (discussed in detail on page 261.)

- **How many times you've given birth before.** Your first experience with labor is apt to feel more painful, while experienced moms generally report less discomfort.

- **Hunger and thirst.** Being dehydrated or hungry could amplify your experience of pain. The old dictum that a laboring mother shouldn't eat or drink during labor is giving way to newer research showing that mothers with adequate hydration and nutrition fare better during labor. The uterus is a muscle that needs adequate hydration and energy supply to contract effectively. (See our discussion of this topic on page 288.)

- **Movement.** Being active and moving around can help make your contractions more effective and help your body to work with, rather than against, gravity. Upright positions help, such as sitting, using a lunge with one foot on a chair seat, standing upright, standing while leaning forward, or getting down on all fours. Lying on your back doesn't help labor and can affect your blood pressure, while lying on your left side causes contractions to spread further apart, but become stronger. Side lying is a good position to use during the pushing stage if you're tired. (The left because it takes pressure off your arteries). If your labor has been augmented or you have an epidural, you may find yourself wobbly on your feet and confined within two feet of your bed by monitoring wires and your IV line, which will limit your freedom of movement.

- **Nausea.** Getting nauseated and throwing up can intensify feelings of pain. Some women don't experience nausea at all, some experience it as a natural part of labor, and others have it brought on by the mix of drugs used in their epidurals and spinals. On the other hand, vomiting often strengthens contractions. To ease waves of nausea, some mothers find that applying pressure on the acupressure point on the wrist approximately two finger widths below their thumbs can help. You may want to consider bringing your own "Sea Bands®," elastic wristbands with a small, smooth knob to press into that specific seasick and nausea acupressure point.

Adopt a pain-coping mindset

Today's obstetrical mindset is that labor is pure anguish, and no mother should have to suffer through it. It is true that no mother should have to suffer pain if she doesn't wish to, but there are also a number of solid reasons for not choosing to have heavy medication during your one-day labor marathon. Here are some of the reasons to consider going drug-free:

Dread is the worst part. While you're actually in labor, you'll be too busy to be afraid. Just as with any other extreme situation—driving on an icy road, for instance—you'll do what it takes to get through. Because you know what's happening to you, it's not frightening at the time, especially if you've taken time to prepare yourself in advance for the nature of the birthing experience.

Pain comes in waves. Labor pain isn't the same thing as passing a kidney stone, having a broken leg, or an inflamed appendix. The on-and-off nature of contractions means that you get mini-breaks in between. With every contraction, the sense of pressure starts and then builds, peaking in intensity after about thirty seconds. The strongest sensations come at the pinnacle of each contraction and last only for seconds before they start to ease off.

Contractions change. Some contractions are more (or less) painful than others. You could have three bad ones in a row, then a milder one, or vice versa, with each one being different. It's perfectly normal to have times when you feel overwhelmed by weariness and exhaustion and get ready to throw in the towel, only to have your labor shift on a dime into a different dimension.

It's not going to kill you. Unlike injury or illness, you can be confident you'll survive this—no matter how uncomfortable it may temporarily be. Your body produces endorphins, nature's own pain relievers that are far more powerful than morphine. These substances belong to a family of proteins that interact with specific parts of your brain to affect your perception of pain. They soothe your central nervous system, reduce your sensation of pain, and help you feel calmer, more at ease, and relaxed. Although your endorphin rush won't be sufficient to get rid of your labor pain, it will make it more bearable. If you have pain-killing drugs in your system, or your epidural wears off, your pain may feel more acute and unbearable than if you hadn't been given the medications. That's because your endorphin production slows when pain signals are chemically dulled. There are specific things you can do to help your body with its job, like eating snacks so you're not starved, drinking liquids so you're hydrated, changing positions to help your pelvis stretch, and urinating frequently so your bladder stays empty to leave more room for your baby to move down.

Just when you think you can't stand it any longer, it's nearly over. Many a woman has given in to an epidural at the very moment when the first stage of labor is coming to a close, only to be too numb to push effectively. Just before giving birth, it's not uncommon for a woman to utter something like, "I think I'm going to die," or "Please give me a c-section," at which point everyone in the room smiles knowingly, because that means the baby will be born very soon.

When it's over, it's over. When your baby is born, you'll have some post-birth contractions to expel the afterbirth and shrink the uterus, but other than that and vague afterpains, you'll be done. Unless you've lost a lot of blood, you'll be able to get up, get in the bed on your own, eat a big meal, whatever you choose to do.

Baby safety and easier recovery. Although medications may appear to be benign for babies, virtually every drug that enters a mother's body is also transferred through her bloodstream to her baby. Babies have very poor resources for processing and eliminating chemicals. Research is lacking on the potential long-term effects of epidurals or narcotics on a baby's delicate brain and nervous system, particularly if the effects don't show up until later, although there is currently no evidence of harm to babies.

Using medications sparingly during labor, or not at all, can protect your baby and help to maintain efficient contractions. That, in turn will help to protect your baby from being oxygen-deprived, particularly when medications lower your blood pressure or speed up or slow down your contraction. Plus, you'll have more freedom of movement and avoid unpleasant drug-related side effects, such as drug-induced nausea and vomiting, itching, or having a hangover afterward.

No worries about side effects. Even though most epidurals succeed in removing the pain of labor, they are still far from ideal. An epidural can cause you to have problems urinating; numb your lower body to the extent that your balance and ability to walk safely are affected; mute your natural urge to push during the second stage of labor; and change your sensations and awareness of giving birth. Sometimes epidurals work unevenly or not well for some women, and the drug mix can cause nausea and itching, or more rarely, serious side effects, such as drastically lowering your blood pressure; affecting your sense of being able to breathe; or leaving you with a severe, prolonged headache. (Newer techniques are helping to combat that.) Some opiate-derived narcotics can cause constipation, making your first bowel movement after having your baby a truly painful ordeal.

NONDRUG APPROACHES

There are a host of nondrug alternatives available to help you in dealing with the pain of labor. Most nondrug approaches rely on the fact that the body's pain signal system can only allow one signal to be processed at a time. So giving the body alternative sensations during contractions can help to interfere with the delivery of the pain signal to the brain.

With the exception of acupuncture and water injections, most nondrug strategies only serve to distract you from pain signals, but they don't have the power to completely erase the pain in the same way that drugs can. And frankly, during the transition phase, that period between active labor and the time for pushing your baby out, nothing's going to distract you enough, but that's only a short phase of labor.

During transition, most mothers are cranky and have a compelling need to be left alone and untouched by others. In that case, any effort to do things to you, mechanical or human, may only serve to raise your level of irritation. But once you know that's where you are and that you'll soon be pushing your baby out, even transition can become bearable.

Some strategies are practical and easy to apply, such as the use of aromatherapy, applying warm compresses or ice packs, standing in a warm shower, or sitting in a tub of warm water. (See hydrotherapy and water birthing.) Others require practice or the help of an expert.

Biofeedback and *TENS* require electronic devices for mastery. Massage during labor, especially for your lower back, and foot reflexology are best learned from a skilled practitioner, your doula, or your midwife. Having acupuncture, and the administering of homeopathic

> *"Since I spent my whole pregnancy avoiding drugs, even simple over-the-counter stuff, it seemed so illogical to request the world's strongest painkillers and narcotics at the very moment when my baby's life was most in danger. I figured I could stand anything for one day."*

remedies may require expert help during labor and delivery.

We suggest learning all you can about nondrug pain management techniques before you go into labor. Enroll in a series or two of childbirth classes with your partner months ahead of your due date to familiarize yourself with the best strategies. Also consider hiring extra around-the-clock labor support, such as a trained doula who will stay by your side and present you with a variety of nondrug comfort options to help you through contractions if you choose to go unmedicated, or if your drugs fail to completely eradicate your pain.

Even if you plan to take the epidural or use other drug options for pain, it makes sense to have some effective nondrug pain management strategies up your sleeve. They will come in handy when you're at home and in early labor. Plus, an epidural or other medical interventions can be delayed when there are staffing shortages, or when it's a full moon and the middle of the night, and every pregnant woman in town has gone into labor too. Also, drugs sometimes don't work well for some people, and often the painkilling strength of drugs fades over time. (See our pain management strategies on pages 302–322.)

Most remedies for nondrug pain relief during labor are fairly straightforward and familiar to hospital personnel, while others, such as TENS, biofeedback, acupuncture, or self-hypnosis, may not be. Be prepared for raised eyebrows and pressure from medical personnel to have an epidural or other pain medication strategies that are more familiar and routine to them.

> *"Even though I love him dearly, my husband is not much of a nurturer. I chose my best friend, Beth, a very motherly and caring person, to serve as my birth partner. I knew it was futile to try to morph my husband into a nurse. It's just not in his genes."*

Continuous support

The gold standard for coping with the discomforts of birth and for celebrating its joys is to have someone accompany you through your experience who will be there for you, encourage you, acknowledge your progress, and make you feel protected and nurtured. That person could be your life partner, your sister, or someone else of your choosing, such as a calm and reassuring friend. Bear in mind that many obstetricians don't appear until you get closer to time for delivery unless you or your baby is thought to be having problems. Realistically, for most of your labor in a hospital, your support will come from labor and delivery nurses. In most hospitals, nurses may have other patients to assist too, particularly when there are staffing shortages.

FLASH FACT: Support During Labor

Having continuous support during labor can make a big difference. Support can be from a partner, a chosen friend, a midwife, a doula, or others. An extensive research review on the effects of support on labor published in 2003 found that mothers having continuous support

Need less medication. Mothers with adequate human support are less likely to require an epidural or need other pain medication.

Have more effective labors. Supported mothers are less likely to need a forceps or vacuum extraction during birth.

Are less likely to have surgical deliveries. Supported mothers are less likely to need cesarean sections.

Have a better birth experience. Supported mothers give higher ratings for overall satisfaction with their births and had a feeling of having more personal control over their labors.

Have the best outcomes. Starting support early in labor, relying on someone other than hospital staff members, and not having an epidural promise the best outcomes for both mother and baby.[17]

Acupuncture and acupressure

The skill of acupuncture has been used in China for many centuries to help women move painlessly through labor. This ancient art involves the insertion and small movements of extremely thin needles in different parts of the body. This stimulating of specific points in the body's energy meridians is thought to help balance the body's energy flows and to soothe pain. Acupuncture points most commonly stimulated to reduce pain during labor are located on the hands, feet, and ears.

There are various Western theories as to how acupuncture works. One is that pain impulses are blocked from reaching the spinal cord or brain at various points. Another is that acupuncture stimulates the body to produce endorphins, the body's natural painkillers.

Acupressure (the application of pressure on acupuncture points) is an alternative to using acupuncture needles. Applying pressure to certain points along the palm of the hand and on the big toe can sometimes help to reduce the sensation of pain during contractions. Electronic devices are also available that are designed to use the same points on the body without piercing the skin.

If you decide to use these approaches in labor, it makes sense to become familiar with them well in advance of giving birth. You may also require the skills of a trained practitioner during your labor.

Aromatherapy

Aromatherapy is the use of natural fragrances to aid in relaxation and healing. Aromatherapy has long been used as an aid to laboring mothers, and essential oils are thought to increase the output of the body's own relaxing, sedating, and stimulating chemicals. Typically, the oils are massaged into the skin or inhaled by using a steam infusion or burner.

If you decide to use aromatherapy during your labor, you may need to check in advance with the labor and delivery area of your hospital about whether you will be permitted to use a burner or electrical device for spreading the aroma in your room.

Most facilities will not allow an open flame in patients' rooms and may not accept the concept of having the air infused with a scent that could linger on the furniture, bedding, and walls long after you've checked out. In addition, using the strong-scented oils to massage your body during labor might interfere with your baby's bonding to your own body aroma immediately after birth, since newborns quickly learn to identify their mothers by their scent.

An alternative is to place small amounts of the scents on your hands and feet, or to put droplets of the essence on a large bandage that can be pulled off your gown after your baby is born. You can also put the fragrance droplets on a handkerchief that you store in a zippered plastic bag.

Seek the advice of an aromatherapist prior to labor to select the right oils for your needs. Jasmine and sage are thought to help contractions and ease muscular pain; lavender is thought to be antiseptic and to also help with pain; frankincense is thought to calm and to deepen breathing.

Biofeedback

Biofeedback uses a computerized monitoring device to help you learn to control and manage your body's stress responses. The device will give you immediate feedback about your biological functions such as muscle tension, skin temperature, brainwave activity, skin resistance, and heart rate.

During your training sessions, sensitive instruments will be used to measure your physical processes and offer feedback to help you learn how to control fear and stress responses.

Training can take four to six weekly sessions to help you become aware of your body's reactions and to help you alter and control your responses through relaxation, deep breathing, imagery, or meditation. The more you practice, the more adept you will become, since the biofeedback method uses as much skill as medical therapy.

Biofeedback is the technique for learning the relaxation skills. Once you've mastered them, you will no longer need the feedback devices. An extra plus is that you will be able to apply those skills not only during labor and birth, but also to other stressful situations that arise in your life.

Having an empty bladder

Sometimes pain during labor, including pain that breaks through an epidural, is caused by an overfull bladder. The bladder is a balloon-like structure that can cause crowding and congestion in a woman's lower body. Ask your partner to remind you to void every hour, particularly if you are being given extra fluids through your IV or do not have a catheter up your urinary tract.

Conscious relaxation

Being able to relax during labor is vital. If you are stressed and uptight, you will exhaust yourself, and the hormones secreted in response to stress can affect the efficiency of your uterus. It can produce contractions that are uncoordinated and painful. When stress and tension last for a long time, it can reduce the oxygen supply to your baby in the same way that stress can affect your digestion, or it can speed up your heart rate, alter your circulation, or give you a headache. Learning how to consciously relax can help you monitor your own tension levels.

Good relaxation techniques will help keep you centered and focused so you feel more in control of your labor.

One relaxation system has been widely used in Europe for decades. It is called the autogenic method, or Schulz method, named after Dr. Johannes Schulz, who was the first to describe this technique. Schulz discovered that focusing on specific body sensations, such as imagining feelings of heaviness and warmth, can help the body to relax.

To apply the Schulz system, the student must master a series of relaxation techniques that are applied to various parts of the body. The client is guided to focus on feeling a sense of heaviness in the arms and

legs, starting with the dominant side, followed by sensing a feeling of warmth in the arms and legs, then warmth and heaviness in the heart area, in the breathing, in the abdomen, and ending with coolness in the forehead.

Slow breathing accompanies each step in this progression, and a silent phrase is repeated five to seven times with each formula, such as "my arm feels heavy," "my heart feels warm," before you open your eyes and stretch. It is recommended that each focus area be mastered individually before moving on to the next by using twice daily repetitions. The concept is to be an alert but passive observer of body sensations. Some mothers have active imaginations that easily can picture what is being asked and respond to it, but others may not be able to operate very well in that visualized realm.[18]

Most childbirth education courses offer parents helpful relaxation strategies. For example, the Bradley Method® teaches a series of relaxation techniques coupled with deep breathing exercises to encourage physical, emotional, and mental relaxation during the stress of labor. Bradley® classes are offered in many locations throughout the U.S. There are a number of other forms of meditation and relaxation including Transcendental Meditation (TM), Buddhist practices, and yoga breathing techniques that can be applied not only to labor and giving birth, but also to the everyday stresses of life.

Homeopathy

Homoeopathy is taking extracts of natural substances internally, such as herbs and minerals, to help with stress, pain, and healing. Homeopathic remedies are highly diluted amounts of substances applied in varying potencies.

The homeopathic approach to pain and stress was discovered by a German physician named Samuel Hahnemann, who discovered that remedies for some illnesses could arouse the same symptoms as the illnesses themselves. He reasoned that if a healthy person suffers from certain symptoms after taking a particular substance, then a sick person who naturally has similar symptoms could be cured by that same substance. He found that only minuscule amounts were needed to effect the desired result.

During labor, homeopathic remedies are administered according to the type of pain and emotional reactions a mother is experiencing. The remedies are thought to stimulate the mother's innate body processes to enable her to function well and stay strong so she is better able to cope with labor. Certain remedies are used to help soothe and relax and others to reduce the sense of pain.

Homeopathic remedies have not been embraced by the wider scientific community as being effective, however some families routinely rely on homeopathy to help them through times of illness and crisis. If homeopathy is of interest to you, confer with a homeopathic practitioner. Practitioners can generally be located through nutrition centers, health food stores, and local publications featuring advertising from practitioners in alternative medicine.

Hypnotherapy

Being able to enter a hypnotic state is thought to help you remove the fear and anxiety that sometimes surrounds pain. Hypnosis can help your body relax, so your muscles and your uterus can work at peak efficiency. You can be taught self-hypnosis techniques in advance of going into labor that you can then employ during contractions.

Hypnosis techniques are actually very simple and rely on focused concentration. You will learn with practice how to put yourself into a very relaxed state of mind in which your attention is deeply focused; yet you can remain highly aware. With proper training, you can learn to come in and out of your hypnotic state at will.

Hypnosis bypasses the active, critical part of the mind and gives suggestions for eliminating fear and pain. Through instruction or tapes, you can learn how to use an hypnotic cue, sometimes called an anchor, to help you enter the hypnotic state.

Cues can also be used to help you feel anesthetized and numb to help in relaxation and comfort. Since fear and tension increase the sensation of pain during labor, you will be shown ways to release fears so that you can enter into birth positively with visualizations of birthing comfort and breastfeeding success.

Mothers give hypnosis in birth a high rating for satisfaction, and current research suggests that hypnosis may be effective in reducing pain during labor. Studies show that mothers who use hypnosis are less likely to require drug-related pain relief; less likely to have their labors augmented; and more likely to have vaginal, rather than cesarean, deliveries.[19] (See hypnosis sources in the *Resource Guide*, page 538.)

Massage, effleurage, and reflexology

Massage involves using hands, elbows, and sometimes the feet or rollers to help stimulate and relax the muscles and tissues of the body. During all stages of labor, massage can bring welcome relief from the tension and intensity of contractions.

You are the best guide for the type of massage strokes that feel best to you. Some mothers prefer *effleurage*, lightly tracing in circling motions on their abdomen or wherever they are feeling discomfort. Although effleurage is useful in the early stages of labor, it may not be as helpful when contractions become more intense.

Having someone massage your shoulders, neck, lower back, legs, or feet using cream or oil as a lubricant can help to release tense muscles, improve circulation, and leave you feeling more soothed and calm.

> *"My labor wasn't unbearable. I thought it was going to get worse, but it didn't. Honestly, getting a tattoo hurt more than my contractions!"*

A woman who is experiencing lower back pain during labor may find deep massage of her lower back between and just above the buttocks using the heels of the hand or pressing of the pelvis on both sides during a contraction can bring relaxation and temporary relief.

Firm massage of the hands or feet can also be very soothing and help a mother stay relaxed. Rolling pins and small paint rollers are sometimes handy for helping with back pain. Having someone stand behind you and press your hipbones firmly from both sides can also help ease discomfort.

Reflexology relies upon reflex points on the feet that correspond to organs and structures of the body. By gentle manipulation and pressing certain parts of the foot, the sensation of pain during labor can be reduced.

Movement and positioning

Movement and frequent position changes are age-old (and instinctive) comfort measures for labor. Mothers-to-be have historically used standing, swaying, and leaning forward or backward with support from others as a means for getting their babies out.

During late pregnancy, changes in hormones help to relax the ligaments and connective tissues of the pelvis so that the joints and bones that support the pubic area can stretch to accommodate your baby.

Moving a lot—rocking your pelvis, swaying, walking, squatting, or raising one leg and supporting it on a chair, and bending forward while being supported in the front or the back—can all help the bones and cartilage of your pelvis to realign

Labor Positions

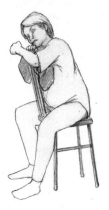

Leaning against a chair's back

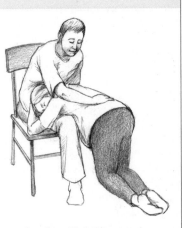

Kneeling with loving support

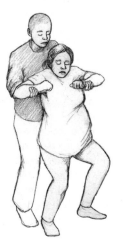

Semi-squat supported from behind

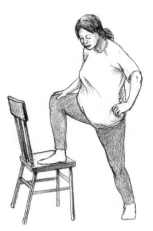

One-legged lunge

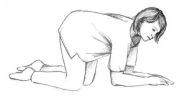

Hands and knees

positions and stretch. In addition, being upright helps work with the force of gravity, rather than against it, which happens when you're lying down, and your pelvis is reclined.

Upright positioning and movement also make contractions more efficient. When a mother lies on her back, the baby must negotiate an angled exit, but when a mother stands, sits upright, or bends forward, a straight pathway is formed.[20] Mothers often report that being in an upright position and being free to move around also makes their contractions stronger, but less painful.

There are numerous positioning strategies you can use, even if you're in a cramped space. You can position yourself leaning over an adjustable hospital table with a pillow for support, sit on the toilet backward while using a pillow to support you under your arms and head, use a birth ball to posture yourself, lean back on your partner while being supported under the arms, rock in a rocking chair, or use modern-day birthing aids such as a suspended strap or labor bars.

Prayer

Many mothers report that prayer was one of the most powerful tools they had to get through labor. If faith and prayer can move mountains, it could very well move babies too. Certainly, if prayer is an important part of your religious faith, then it also belongs in your hospital room.

Relaxation breathing

The way you breathe can affect your baby, and it can also help you make it through contractions by altering your awareness of pain. Think of breathing as bringing in oxygen to send to your baby. Breathing too rapidly and shallowly, either on purpose, or because you're fearful and anxious, will change your body chemistry and contract the blood vessels that feed your brain, which in turn, will affect the flow of oxygen to your body and to your baby.

Breathing too fast can also increase a feeling of anxiety during labor, which then leads to increased tension in the body, heightening the sense of pain. In turn, a chain reaction gets started: fast breathing, more anxiety, and more pain sensations.

Slow, deep breathing using the muscles of your abdomen delivers air into your lungs and oxygen into your body and to your baby. Here's how it works: As you breathe in, move your diaphragm, the muscle deep at the bottom of your lungs, downward while pushing out your belly. This increases the volume of air flowing into your lungs by creating a partial vacuum to suck air in. Then, when you breathe out, your diaphragm muscle should rise back up into your chest while your abdomen sinks down to push out air.

It's easiest if you take air in through your nose and then breathe it out through pursed lips, although you can do both inhaling and exhaling through your nose or both through your mouth if your nose is congested. Take five to six seconds for each inhalation, and slow down from fifteen to seventeen breaths per minute to five to seven breaths, exhaling gently for the same amount of time after each breath.

Your chest should be relaxed, rather than tense. Most of the movement during breathing should be in your abdomen as it expands first, followed by your chest as it contracts to let out air. Air exchange should be flowing and relaxed with no pausing or holding your breath at any point.

Mastering the art of deep breathing will come in handy in the midst of labor. Try practice sessions three or four times a day where you change from shallow chest motions into the deeper breathing pattern that engages both your chest and your abdomen. Try to make your breathing slow, steady, and regular.

Again, if done correctly, your abdomen will rise when you breathe in, and contract and fall as you breathe out. Gradually, your everyday breathing habits will start to change. For help and support in getting your breathing straightened out, take a prenatal yoga class; attend a meditation group; listen to tapes on breathing; join groups practicing chi-kung (qigong) or tai chi, both of which emphasize breathing skills.

Making sounds

A birthing mother's throat and voice can be useful tools for encouraging the progress of labor. Many believe a woman's vaginal area appears to have a connection with her throat and the use of her voice.

One way to experiment with that connection while pregnant is to consciously relax and "open" your throat when you are having sex, rather than focusing only on your genital area. Speak the words "open," or "I will fully open now," out loud, followed by a deep breath while continuing to maintain an open and relaxed throat. The effects on the musculature of the vaginal region are usually immediate.

Speaking your intentions out loud can help to change the state of your body too. Consider yielding to the urge to make moaning or groaning sounds during contractions to give vocal expression to your body's work. Speak out loud your intent for your birth: "I let my body go so my uterus can do her work." "I am going to fully relax now and allow my baby to come out." "I love you, baby, very much, and I surround you with warmth and comfort."

If you are in the bearing down mode, instead of closing your throat to push downward, try keeping your throat relaxed and slightly open with only brief stops ("tuh…tuh…tuh"), or pulling your attention away from your vaginal area to your neck, your jaws, and your forehead to simply experience the sensations of pushing without forcing. (See our discussion on pushing strategies on pages 289–294.)

Sterile water injections

Injecting sterile water directly under the surface of the skin has been used to eliminate lower back pain for mothers experiencing back labor with no known side effects and excellent results. The injections are done at specific points below the base of the spine (the sacrum) and are followed by the formation of a small, temporary swelling (weal) where the injection was done. Pain relief follows within two to three minutes and lasts up to two hours or longer.

If hospital policies permit it, nurses can administer the injections. First, the back is wiped with antiseptic, and then a small amount of sterile water is injected in four places. Ideally, the procedure is done with two people administering the injections on both sides simultaneously. The injections cause an intense burning and sensation of pain that lasts thirty to ninety seconds. Relief from the procedure follows within two to three minutes.

It's not clear exactly why the injections are so effective, but it is thought to do with the way nerves can act as gates, closing off the transmission of pain to the brain when there is more than one competing signal.[21] Although effective for lower back pain, the injections don't appear to have any effect on front labor—the discomfort of contractions.

If you'd like to have the technique available as a part of your pain relief arsenal, discuss it with your care provider beforehand. Request that written instructions and doses be included in your hospital record along with your birth plan.

TENS

TENS stands for Transcutaneous Electric Nerve Stimulation. By stimulating one set of nerves a person can competitively block the perception of impulses from another set of nerves—a form of distracting the body from the pain.

A small, handheld TENS unit delivers mild electrical shocks to specific areas on your back through small adhesive pads that are applied at specific points. The unit produces a pins-and-needles feeling in the back and legs that is thought to block contraction pains and to stimulate the body to release endorphins, the body's version of morphine. Most models have dials that allow you to adjust the intensity of the stimulation, since your body may slowly adapt to the sensations as time passes.

TENS appears to work best with chronic low-level pain and can be reasonably effective in early labor. It is thought to be the most useful in the first three or four hours of labor, or until about five or six centimeters dilation, but research does not appear to show that it is very beneficial during advanced labor.

Water Birthing the British Way

Deluxe versions of British water birthing pools offer a semi-inclined, supportive seat for the mother, bars for grasping during pushing, built-in thermostats, and underwater lights. Some models come with throwaway liners to prevent mother-to-mother infections. These well-designed birthing environments provide an entirely different laboring experience for British mothers than for U.S. mothers who find themselves trying to squeeze into Jacuzzi-style bathtubs installed in the tiny bathrooms in some hospital birthing centers. In fact, tubs with pulsing water vents are not thought to be optimal, since the vents and pipes may harbor infection.[22]

You may be able to rent a TENS unit for labor (ask your childbirth preparation instructor), or you can purchase one online.

Water birth and hydrotherapy

Women who have used warm water bathing and showering during labor report it to be more effective for pain relief than drugs that alter a mother's awareness of pain (*analgesia*). Studies show that as many as ninety percent of mothers who gave birth in water rate their birth experiences extremely positive.

Water birth is extremely popular in the United Kingdom, where thousands of mothers have given birth underwater in spacious, portable pools available in most hospitals. The tubs enable them get down on all fours, to move freely about, float on their backs, or do whatever else makes them comfortable during contractions.

Laboring in water and water birth also appear to give mothers a private space where they feel less vulnerable. It can also help to reduce a mother's need for drugs and other interventions, including an epidural.

The ideal time for entering the tub or pool is when a mother is dilated between five and six centimeters. Entering the pool earlier than that can cause labor to slow down.

The perfect depth of the water in the tub is up to the mother's breasts prior to birth and below the mother's breasts once the baby is born to allow him to nurse. Water levels that are too high can impede the mother's sweating, which is important in helping her body to control its temperature.

A floating thermometer is usually used to carefully monitor water temperature. Warm or cold water may need to be added from time to time to maintain body temperature in the tub.

The water exerts an even pressure on the mother's body and vaginal area, which is thought to discourage tearing during birth, and it gives the mother's body buoyancy, which makes it easier to find comfortable positions than on land. It is also useful for mothers with conditions such as physical disabilities or asthma.

Water birth requires careful monitoring of the baby's heart rate and the mother's condition and should only be used by mothers with normal labors that are progressing as expected. The baby must be full term, and not pre-term or post-term, and in a normal, head-down (cephalic) position.

Water birth should not be used if there are signs of fetal distress, such as irregular or slow heart rate or when your baby is passing meconium (stools). Mothers who have been given painkilling drugs should not attempt to labor or birth in water, nor should it be used if there are any complications for either mother or baby during the process of birth, such as a baby with insufficient oxygen during the second stage of labor, or for babies known to have cleft palates or other anomalies. Mothers having breech births and those whose waters have been broken for more than twenty-four hours also shouldn't attempt water birth.

Although parents are concerned that their babies could drown during a water birth, babies have a dive reflex that enables them to hold

Questions to Ask Your Provider about Pain Relief Alternatives

If you hope to have a minimally medicated birth, it's useful to explore your healthcare practitioner's concepts and practices about that. Here are some questions to ask:

- **What are your standing orders for your patients regarding pain relief measures?**

- **What are your thoughts about my not having a routine IV so I am free to move around?**

- **What proportion of your patients gives birth without pain medication?**

- **What is your opinion of nondrug pain relief options such as self-hypnosis for birth, relaxation and breathing techniques, water injections, or other remedies instead of using analgesia or anesthesia?**

- **Is water birth an option for me? What is your opinion about giving birth in water?**

their breaths until their noses and faces are exposed to air; plus, they're still being supplied oxygen from their umbilical cords.

Within seconds after a baby is born under water, he will be immediately lifted up and out of the water so that he can take his first breaths. First breaths are different for water babies than land babies. A water baby's breathing will start slowly with almost invisible breaths, whereas land born babies are more likely to gasp.

The birthing room should be kept warm, and dim lights used to help create a secure and inviting atmosphere. Water temperature is very important. The pool should be body temperature and no hotter. If the pool becomes too warm and the mother's temperature goes up, the baby, who is normally two degrees warmer than his mother will be in danger of becoming overheated.

If the mother gets too cold, her endorphin production will go down, and her muscles will become tenser. Drinking a lot of water is important for everyone in the room, since the humidity and heat of the environment can lead to dehydration.

Ventilation and an extra heat supply will help in maintaining a comfortable room temperature. A mother should be able to stay in the tub or pool without having to sit on the side or get out completely in order to have her baby's heart rate monitored. Waterproof fetal heart monitors are now available to do that job.

The room where the tub is should be equipped with nonslip mats, a soft, warm robe for the mother, towels, and if possible, a mat so that the mother can continue her delivery should she need to get out of the tub. An extra attendant may be needed to help maintain careful records during labor and birth. Normally, the birth attendant is kneeling beside the tub, and wearing long, waterproof gloves to assist the mother and baby during birth.

MEDICATIONS FOR PAIN RELIEF

There are a variety of pain relief options that use medications to help mothers with the pain of labor and birth. Analgesia is the term used for drugs that mask pain or change a mother's mental state so that pain becomes less anxiety producing. Analgesia is usually administered through an injection or fed into your veins through an IV line. Besides making you drowsy, analgesia can affect the baby and cause him to be sluggish or have trouble breathing after birth.

Anesthesia refers to a category of drugs that completely numb pain by altering the transmission of pain signals from the mother's nerves to her brain. Regional anesthesia injects painkilling medications into a mother's spinal column, cervix, or area surrounding her vagina and rectum to produce a complete loss of sensation in that specific area. General anesthesia administered through a face mask renders a mother completely unconscious and is usually reserved only for emergency cesareans where speed is of the essence due to the drugging effect the anesthesia has on the baby.

Local anesthesia (a local) is directly injected into a specific part of a mother's body to provide specific numbing to that body area. An epidural, which allows for a continuous flow of numbing medication into the epidural area of the spinal column, is by far the most popular painkilling method for labor. It can provide almost total relief from labor pain while allowing a mother to remain awake and aware. (Epidurals are discussed in detail on pages 317–322.)

Spinal anesthesia (getting a spinal) is similar to an epidural but uses a different kind of medication injected in the space under the membrane that covers the spinal cord. It is often used for cesarean sections when rapid painkilling effects are needed. More recently, spinals and epidurals are being combined, which is called a CSE (combined spinal epidural).

Regardless of the pain relief options you choose for labor, it's important to weigh the side effects on both you and your baby. Some medications can cause nausea and vomiting; others make a baby sluggish and may interfere with breathing immediately after birth. Some have been shown to place the

> *"Avoid birthing shows on television, particularly the crisis-oriented ones. They will only raise your level of anxiety, and you might have flashbacks during birth."*

FLASH FACTS: Drugs During Labor

Most mothers presume that the drugs used during labor are known to be safe for both themselves and their babies and have been tested and approved by the U.S. Food and Drug Administration (FDA). In reality, the decision to approve a drug for use by pregnant women is based on the FDA's opinion that the benefits of the drug outweigh its risks. If you want to learn more about any labor-related drug and its precautions for use, consult the Physicians Desk Reference, available in most libraries, and also request a copy of the package insert for the drug from its manufacturer. A pharmacist can help you locate the information you need.[23]

mother at greater risk for having her labor augmented or having to have forceps or vacuum extraction used to deliver your baby, or they're more likely to put you at risk for a cesarean section.

There are a variety of ways to learn about pain-relief options. Your healthcare provider should be your number one source, but many childbirth preparation courses discuss these options.

How to talk with your healthcare provider about pain

Openly discuss your fears. If you have an overriding fear of hospitals, procedures, or needles, discuss these in advance with your healthcare provider. Should you not feel heard or supported, consider changing providers or moving to an alternative healthcare system, such as a non–hospital-based birth center, which may feel less threatening.

Learn about drug benefits and risks. Ask your healthcare provider for written materials about the drugs she commonly uses for pain relief during labor. The information should detail the benefits and risks, including short-term and long-term

side effects of drugs for labor and birth on you and your baby. Ask when these drugs are most likely to be advised.

Tailor your use of drugs to your own philosophy. If you have scrupulously avoided alcohol, caffeine, and cigarettes during pregnancy to protect your baby, or seldom choose to use medication for your own aches and pains out of a strong belief in the healing power of your own body—then consider preparing for a non-medicated delivery. (See our list of alternatives on pages 302–315.) If this path feels best to you, explore your healthcare provider's approach to natural, non-medicated labor and birth.

Ask about labor induction and augmentation. Having your labor started or made stronger by chemicals can increase the intensity and sometimes the pain of your labor. Ask your provider under what circumstances he uses *Pitocin*® or other induction medications, and what percentage of his patients is given inductions and augmentation of labor. Find out if any of the pain-relief medications recommended by your healthcare provider could potentially increase your risk of requiring augmentation. Ask how he feels about elective inductions, or a patient's right to refuse an induction. (See our discussion of induction on page 335.) If you do have an induction, the contractions will probably be more bearable with pain relief.

Epidural precautions. Check to see whether your hospital provides twenty-four-hour anesthesiology services for labor and delivery. Schedule an appointment with the anesthesiologist in charge to learn about the procedure and any potential risks. This is particularly important if you are overweight, extremely short, have a chronic skin infection, are allergic to any medications, or have serious medical, neurological, or spine problems that could have an impact on your epidural experience.

Having an epidural

Epidurals are by far the most effective painkilling method for labor and birth. In fact, it has been estimated that as many as ninety percent of laboring mothers in community hospitals are opting for epidurals or spinal blocks.

Some medical situations may require an epidural. For example, an epidural, spinal, or CSE will be used in place of general anesthesia for cesarean sections, except during dire emergencies when speed is of the essence. The type of medication and dosages may be different for these situations than during labor.

A healthcare provider may also recommend a mother have an epidural if she appears to be in extreme pain, or if her labor has lasted for many hours, she seems to need time to rest, or if she has been

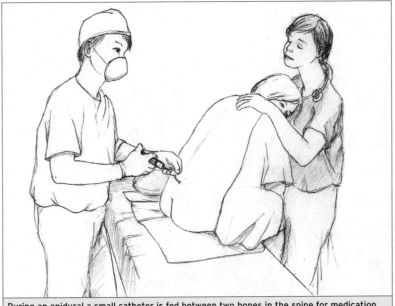

During an epidural a small catheter is fed between two bones in the spine for medication that numbs labor pain.

Medical Reasons for NOT Having an Epidural

If you have any of these problems, make an appointment with the anesthesiologist or nurse-anesthetist who will be handling your epidural prior to going into labor to discuss potential complications. Here are some medical reasons for avoiding an epidural:

- **You're taking blood thinners.** If you have been taking anticoagulants because of heart or stroke problems, it could affect the healing of your epidural wound.

- **You have a skin condition or infection.** An infection on your lower back near the injection site could cause problems.

- **Blood-clotting problems.** If you have blood-clotting problems, your epidural may have problems healing.

- **Spinal deformities.** Abnormalities in your spine could affect the ability of your anesthesiologist to administer the epidural in your spinal column and could affect the spread of the medication.

- **Nervous system disorders.** Since an epidural affects the way your nerves transmit pain signals, a CNS (central nervous system) disorder may make having an epidural unwise.

given a labor-inducing drug such as Pitocin that has caused her contractions to intensify.

How an epidural feels

Hospitals and healthcare providers have different policies about the best time during labor to administer an epidural. Some prefer to postpone it until a mother's dilation is four centimeters or more, so there is no possibility it will interfere with the delicate balance of labor becoming established.

Prior to getting an epidural, a catheter will be inserted into the back of your hand, or in your arm, and taped down to keep it in place. A blood sample will be taken from your arm into a tube to test the clotting speed and to obtain your blood count. An IV bag will be attached to a hanger beside your

bed and connected to the neck of the catheter taped to your hand to administer fluids to prevent a fall in blood pressure.

An anesthesiologist or a nurse anesthetist will perform the actual epidural, and getting one usually takes between ten and twenty minutes, sometimes longer if he has a problem finding a workable location for inserting the needle between the vertebrae of your lower back. If you are petite, be sure to remind the anesthesiologist of your height, since being less than 5'4" may affect the strength of your dosage.

The anesthesiologist will wear gloves, a mask, and sterile gown to help prevent infection. You will be asked to sit upright and then to lean forward with your legs dangling from the bed or supported by a stool, or you may be instructed to

The "Wiring" of an Epidural

As a safety precaution, when you have an epidural, you are likely to be connected to a series of tubes and wires that supply your medication, drain your urine, and provide a continuous, electronic printout for comparing your baby's heart rate to the pattern of your contractions. (See electronic fetal monitor on page 275 and in the dictionary.) Below is a list of the wires and tubes that may be connected to you:

1. Epidural catheter—the tube in the back to flow medication into the epidural space of your spinal column.

2. Urinary catheter—a tube inserted into the urinary tract and attached to a collection bag to ensure a mother's bladder remains empty.

3. Blood pressure cuff—to keep tabs on the mother's blood pressure since epidurals can cause sudden drops in blood pressure.

4. IV—intravenous tubes to send fluids and medications to your body should your blood pressure drop unexpectedly.

5. Pitocin drip—medication to strengthen your contractions if they are weakened by the epidural, particularly during the second bearing-down stage of labor.

6. Oxygen mask—used when there is concern that you or your baby are not getting enough oxygen.

7. Electronic fetal monitor (EFM)—belted onto a mother's abdomen. A sensor may also be fastened to the baby's scalp inside the mother's body and connected to the EFM to monitor the variations in the baby's heart rate. (EFM is discussed on page 275.)

8. Pulse oximeter—fastens like a clothespin to a mother's finger or toe to keep tabs on her oxygen levels.

9. Intrauterine Pressure Catheter (IUPC)—in some cases, a long, slender probe with a sensor on the end will be hooked up to the electronic fetal monitor (EFM) and the other end inserted through the cervix into the uterus to monitor the frequency, length, and strength of contractions.[24]

10. EKG leads (four or five)—used in some hospitals to monitor a mother's heart rhythms.

Symptoms of an Epidural Headache

- Stiff neck. Pain that radiates to your neck. Pain in your forehead and back part of your head that increases when you're sitting up or standing, but decreases when you're lying flat.

- Pain that lessens when pressure is applied to your abdomen.

- Nausea and vomiting accompanying the headache.

- Vision problems, such as sensitivity to light, seeing double, or difficulty focusing.

- Auditory symptoms such as a loss of hearing, ringing in the ears, or extreme sensitivity to noise.

fold your legs in front of you on the bed Indian-style. Some mothers are instructed to lie on their sides in a curled-up fetal position. All of these positions round your back and help to enlarge the space between the small bones of your lower back.

Your back will be wiped with an antibacterial liquid, after which you will receive a numbing injection near the insertion site a little lower than halfway down your back. You may momentarily feel a stinging or burning sensation. After the area becomes numb, a long, thin needle will be inserted between spaces in the vertebrae of your lower back until the epidural space that surrounds the spinal cord is located.

An extremely thin tube (catheter) will be threaded through the needle, and the needle removed. The tube will be secured on your back with tape to keep it from moving. A syringe will be fastened onto the other end of the tube to administer a drug, or a combination of drugs, such as bupivacaine, a numbing anesthetic, and possibly a narcotic (such as fetanyl) used to strengthen and lengthen the effects of the drugs. After it's inserted, you probably won't be aware that the tube is there.

The length of time your first dose of epidural medication lasts depends upon the type of medication used, and how big a dose you received. There are individual differences, too, in how medications act and are absorbed by women's bodies.

As your epidural takes over, your legs will begin to feel heavy, warm, or tingly. Then your belly and hips will also start to become numb, but you will still continue to feel pressure signals for your lower body.

Once the epidural is in full effect, you may feel euphoria from having the pain taken away, and want to simply converse or nap. When your dose begins to wears off, the pain will slowly edge back in again. That will signal the time for more medication to be fed into the catheter fastened on your back.

Potential epidural side effects

Itching and nausea. Approximately one out of five mothers experiences itching and nausea caused by synthetic opiods related to the morphine/heroin family used to strengthen the epidural and make it last longer. Symptoms for most mothers are mild and temporary, but more rarely, symptoms can be extreme. Medications are available to treat them.

Fever. Epidurals can cause epidural fever, a rise in a mother's temperature not related to infection. First-time mothers are five times more likely to have a fever higher than 100.4 than mothers who have previously given birth, and it is estimated that 24 percent of first-time mothers will experience fever. A baby's body generally remains two degrees warmer than the mothers', so when the mother's body heats up, the baby's will too, which in turn, speeds up the baby's heartbeat.

Fever could also signal an infection, which is of serious concern and could be treatable. Both mother and baby may be treated with antibiotics as a precaution against infection, and the baby may be shipped off to the nursery for a septic workup, which could translate into several days of observation in the nursery. The baby may be given blood tests and possibly a spinal tap. One study of newborns whose mothers had epidural fevers were almost twice as likely to undergo sepsis evaluations than mothers who didn't and had to stay in the hospital a day longer than babies whose mothers did not have a fever.[25]

Sudden drop in blood pressure. Epidurals can cause *hypotension*, a sudden drop in a mother's blood pressure, which can affect the baby's oxygen supply. Treatment includes administering extra fluids and drugs known as vasopressors, such as ephedrine or phenylephrine, through an IV, which constrict small blood vessels to restore blood pressure to normal.

Longer labor. Unless epidural medications are reduced during the second stage of labor when it's time to bear down, mothers having epidurals may not feel the urge to push. Mothers having epidurals will generally take longer to push the baby out than those who haven't. They are also more likely to be given oxytocin (Pitocin®) or other drugs that make contractions stronger and closer together.

Increased rate of instrumental and cesarean deliveries. There is an increase in the number of deliveries with forceps or vacuum extractions during the bearing down stage. Some believe that epidurals are associated with an increase in cesarean section for dysfunctional labor (dystocia), but it is not clear from current research whether epidurals actually lead to more cesarean sections, or mothers with longer, poorly progressing labors are more likely to use epidurals and require cesareans.

An out-of-position baby. Studies of epidurals have reported a 20- to 26-percent incidence of babies being out of position or failing to rotate normally during birth. *Malpresentation* can prolong labor, and lead to instrumental delivery using forceps, vacuum extraction, or cesarean section.

Headache. Spinal headache, post dural puncture headache (PDPH), affects approximately one out of one hundred mothers who have epidurals. Symptoms can last from two to ten days or longer. It is caused by the leaking of spinal fluid from the sac that surrounds the spinal column. (See "Symptoms of an Epidural Headache" on page 320.)

Rarer complications. Some mothers experience prolonged tingling and weakness in their legs; and very rarely, temporary or permanent paralysis in the legs that affects walking. Some patients having epidurals have convulsions (seizures). While epidural-related deaths are extremely rare, potentially life-threatening complications are estimated to occur in about one out of four thousand cases. When major neurological and brain damage has occurred in patients, it has been associated with oxygen deprivation caused by profound drops in maternal blood pressure. There are also rare reports of enduring spinal nerve damage.[26]

Other Forms of Regional Anesthesia

The following additional medications are given by injection during labor to numb you, but not put you to sleep:

Paracervical block. Local anesthesia is injected into the tissues around the cervix to numb the pain caused by cervical dilation. The effect lasts an hour or two, and additional injections can be given if needed. It is often used in a forceps delivery or vacuum extraction, and for episiotomies. This form of anesthesia can slow down a baby's heart rate, and should be avoided if your baby is showing abnormal heart rate patterns.

Pudendal block. Two injections are used to numb the nerves of the vaginal area and the area between the vagina and rectum. It is usually used during the second ("bearing down") stage of labor. It delivers rapid relief, is simple to perform, and has no ill effects on the baby, but can't be done if the baby's head is too far down into the birth canal. Risks include patchy, incomplete numbness, or, more rarely, accidental injection of the medication into blood vessels, affecting a mother's breathing, heart rate, blood pressure or resulting in seizures or convulsions.

Caudal block. Sometimes called a "saddle block," anesthetic is injected into the spinal fluid at the lower back to produce numbing in the vaginal area that would come into contact with the saddle of a horse. It works rapidly, but can lower a mother's blood pressure affecting the delivery of oxygen to her baby, and, as with an epidural, it can result in a post-delivery headache, temporary impairment of bladder function, and, very rarely can cause convulsions (seizures) or infection. It is not recommended for mothers with *preeclampsia* or *eclampsia*.

During and after Birth

Your baby's position and other vital signs will be monitored throughout your labor to ensure that he is doing well. One way that a baby's progress during labor is tracked is through noting the baby's position in his mother's body.

Station describes where the top of the baby's head is as he descends through the center of a mother's pelvis. A baby's station can be measured by examining your pelvis. Your care provider will track where your baby is in relation to two bony knobs on either side of the interior of your pelvis called **ischial spines**.

A baby is said to be at zero station when the head (or with a breech baby, the rump) is level with the ischial spines. If the lowest part of the baby is above the spines, it is said to be at a minus station, "minus five" being five centimeters above the spines, and "minus one" being a centimeter above the spines. Positive numbers (+1, +2, +3, etc.) mean the baby's presenting part has passed the spines and is on the way down through the pelvis, expressed as 1, 2, or 3 centimeters below the ischial spines, with +5 the closest to being born.

Your baby's heartbeat

The speeding up (accelerations) and slowing down (decelerations) of your baby's heart rate in relation to your contractions are thought to be indicators of how well your baby is doing during labor. Normally, a baby's heart rate is between 120 and 160 beats per minute (bpm), or about twice as fast as an adult's. The rate naturally speeds up at times during and in between your contractions.

Abnormal changes in the speed of a baby's heart rate are thought to be a survival response in a baby

> "*I have given birth to three children. Every time I got to hold my new baby, it was as though I had just accomplished the greatest deed in the entire universe. It felt like falling in love over and over.*"

Your Baby's Apgar Score

Soon after your baby is born, your healthcare provider may tell you that your baby was given a seven, a nine, or a ten Apgar score. The score will be written down in your baby's record. It is used to help birth attendants assess how well a newborn is doing right after birth in order to make a decision about rescue operations, such as helping the baby to breathe. The word Apgar is derived from the name of Dr. Virginia Apgar, an anesthesiologist in obstetrics who developed the scoring system more than fifty years ago.

Each letter of Apgar's last name—A-P-G-A-R—stands for things birth attendants observe in the baby immediately after birth—Activity, Pulse, Grimace, Appearance, and Respiration. Your baby's score will be calculated twice—one minute and five minutes after he's born. More recently, the score refers to a baby's color, respiration, heart rate, reflex irritability, and tone.

Experienced practitioners make the calculations in their heads. The score at the five-minute point is the most telling. If the baby's score is seven to ten, everything is progressing normally. A score of four to seven says the baby may require some extra measures to help him breathe. Babies with scores of three or less are in serious trouble and need emergency care, such as CPR or deeper suctioning to clear their lungs of fluid. In some cases, babies with very low Apgars may be showing the first signs of lasting problems, such as damage from oxygen deprivation, but many babies with very low scores at first turn out to be perfectly normal over time.

who is getting into trouble during labor. A prolonged, slower-than-normal heart rate could be caused by a mother's blood pressure dipping too low, or a baby not getting enough oxygen for other reasons. It can also signal that a mother's uterus is contracting too quickly, or freezing up from too large a dose of the drugs used to make the mother's contractions stronger. A slow heart rate can also signal that the baby's umbilical cord is being squeezed. An extremely slow heart rate may be a serious sign that the baby's life is in danger.

When a baby's heart rate, or other signs, gives signals that he is potentially in trouble, it is called *nonreassuring fetal status,*

fetal distress, or fetal compromise. How rapidly a baby's heart rate returns to normal after a contraction is a good indicator of the baby's general well-being.

Tachycardia, the speeding up of the baby's heart rate to faster than 160 bpm without slowing down during contractions may signal the baby isn't getting enough oxygen *(hypoxia)*, or it may be caused by his mother's fever from an epidural or an infection. A mother's overactive thyroid (hyperthyroidism) or certain drugs she is taking can also cause a faster-than-normal heart rate. *Bradycardia,* or brady spells, is the medical term for when a baby's heartbeat remains less than 120 bpm.

The Points of the Apgar Score

WHAT'S BEING MEASURED	ZERO POINTS	ONE POINT	TWO POINTS
[A] Activity	Limp	Arms and legs tight and pulled up close	Active motion
[P] Pulse	No pulse	Less than one hundred beats per minute (bpm)	More than one hundred bpm
[G] Grimace (baby's reaction to having his nose and throat suctioned) (Can also be measured as reflex irritability by flicking the soles of the baby's feet)	No response at all	Baby grimaces	Baby sneezes, coughs, or pulls away
[A] Appearance	Blue-gray or pale all over	Body pink, arms and legs blue	Entire body completely pink
[R] Respiration	Not breathing at all	Weak, irregular breathing	Regular breathing, strong cry

A fetoscope is a specially adapted stethoscope for listening to a baby's heartbeat. How fast or slow the heart is beating in relation to a mother's contractions is an important measure of how the baby is bearing up during labor. A fetoscope is noninvasive and provides all the information needed to monitor heart rate changes.

Your baby after birth

Once your baby arrives, there will probably be a deafening silence in the room. Everyone will be waiting for your baby to breathe: the most important, first step of surviving in this world. After what may seem like an eternity, at last you will hear sputtering, gasping, and then the lusty, high-pitched screams of new life. As long as it seems to take,

Things That Happen Right after Birth

Your baby will be weighed and measured, evaluated (see Apgar score), given an ID bracelet or anklet (or both), given a shot of vitamin K, have antibiotic ointment applied to his eyes to ward off infection, and have his or her footprints recorded. A sample of blood from his umbilical cord will be sent for tests. Ask the hospital staff for a copy of the footprints as a memento.

If you're in a hospital, you may be given an IV of Pitocin to stop post-partum bleeding and help your uterus contract. If you had an episiotomy and/or tearing, you'll be given a shot of a local anesthetic and stitched up, usually with dissolving stitches that won't need to be removed but will need to be kept clean. (The pros and cons of episiotomies are discussed on page 344.)

Soon after giving birth, you'll be wheeled to a recovery room to be attended to by a new staff of nurses. You may remain in the delivery room for recovery, or wheeled into a separate room from where you labored and gave birth. A postpartum nurse will help you pack your pants with a large sanitary napkin and cold packs for your perineum. And she may wake you up if you're napping to change the pads and cold packs.

You'll be transferred from the labor and delivery room area to your own room. If your baby is "rooming in," he will be given a bassinet in your room. If the baby is in the nursery, he should be brought to you at least every three hours for feeding. If he is in your room, doctors and nurses will come in a few times a day to check the baby's vital signs.

most babies will breathe within a minute after birth. Then, everyone heaves a collective sigh of relief. The baby's breathing! The baby's okay! It's a girl! (or) It's a boy! You'll find yourself elated by that news, even though a sonogram may have told you that months ago.

Your newborn will be gently suctioned with a rubber bulb with a pointed end to remove blood and fluid from the mouth and nose. Your baby's chest will be watched to see that the breathing is normal and regular, and his heart rate monitored to see if it speeds up to about 100 bpm or more. His color will be assessed from blue to pink, and he will be checked for how well his muscles flex by looking at how tight his fists are.

He will be dried off quickly to reduce heat loss and chilling from evaporation. Then, your baby will be wrapped in a warm, dry towel and presented to you, a tiny pink head wrapped in a white cocoon. At last you get to meet this little person who has been squirming around inside for so long.

First breaths

While your baby was still in the womb, he floated inside a warm balloon of amniotic fluid with his lungs filled with a mildly salty liquid. Babies swallow the liquid and take practice breaths from time to time, but that's a far cry from inhaling the icy cold air of planet Earth for the first time. Those first breaths are critical and sometimes can make the difference between life and death.

During your baby's trip down the birth canal, up to one-third of the fluid filling his lungs will be expelled from the pressure exerted on his small chest. Lung tissues will absorb the remainder of the fluid.

As your newborn gasps in air with every scream, his skin coloring will rapidly change from a rich, purplish blue into a bright, cherry red as his circulatory system changes from getting oxygen through his placenta and umbilical cord to getting it through his lungs. Sometimes whether a baby needs extra help or not can't be determined until after he is born.

At other times, certain signs are used to tell if a baby might need help right after birth. These include the baby being born before thirty-four weeks of pregnancy; too slow or irregular baby heartbeats during labor; fresh stooling from the baby (meconium) that arrives before the baby does; a baby's having retarded growth during pregnancy; twins

and multiples; abnormal presentations, such as feet first; a birth that requires a forceps delivery or vacuum extraction because she gets stuck; a baby born by cesarean section; when a baby and mother have blood incompatibility; and when a mother's been put to sleep with general anesthesia.

If a baby needs help, he will be laid on a special padded cart with the bed tilted so his head is slightly lower than the feet to help fluids to drain out. The equipment on the cart includes a heater, an oxygen supply, suctioning devices, a stop watch, a resuscitation bag to pump air into the baby's lungs, a baby-size face mask, a laryngoscope for peering down the baby's throat, special tubes for suctioning and draining, and drugs for stimulating the baby's system if needed.

Clamping and cutting the cord

Within a few minutes of birth, your baby's umbilical cord will be squeezed together by a plastic clamp, and then painlessly cut off, leaving a stump. Usually the stump and the umbilical area will have medication put on it to help protect it from infection. It may make the stump a different color, such as purple.

It will take two to three weeks for the cord to dry and wither before it falls off on its own, leaving the belly button behind. As it dries, it's likely to stink, but don't try to manipulate it into coming off early—that can cause bleeding and make your baby more vulnerable to infection.

In the meantime, newborn diapers with a "U" shaped belly cutout will help keep the diaper from irritating the cord. If you're using cloth diapers, you can simply

> *"Three years later, I don't remember who sent me flowers, but I'm still grateful to my co-worker who sent a basket of fruit, crackers, cheese, and chocolate. My visitors and I ate the whole thing in a day."*

Sensations after Birth

Once the initial adrenaline rush and the excitement of finally giving birth is over, the hormones will die down, and you may begin to feel some of these other sensations:

- **Exhausted.** As if you just ran a marathon or went a round in the boxing ring.

- **Sore and swollen.** Your vaginal and perineal area has undergone a lot of stretching and trauma, and if you got stitches from an episiotomy, they may hurt. The pain is worse when you sneeze or cough, and at first when you sit down or walk. ("Please, don't make me laugh!")

- **Crampy.** You'll have contractions or after-pains as your uterus shrinks back to its pre-pregnancy size.

- **Woozy and trembly.** If you've lost a lot of blood, you may feel woozy and shaky.

- **Headache-y.** Tell your nurse right away if you have a headache. If it's severe, it could be a side effect of your epidural, or it could be a sign of eclampsia, especially if it's accompanied by swelling in your face, your fingers, and your ankles.

- **Uncomfortable going to the bathroom.** Urinating the first time may be difficult if you had a catheter inserted during a cesarean or epidural. Most women are also constipated for a few days after birth. Drinking a lot of water may help. Note that opiate-derived painkillers, such as Demerol® and codeine, may make constipation worse. If you're too shaky to get out of bed, you'll be given a bedpan.

- **Sweaty.** Much of the fluid you retained in the weeks before birth will be sweated out in the days after birth. You may wake up with the sheets soaking wet. You may be too unstable to shower for a little while too. Many new moms report that the first postpartum shower was the best of their life.

- **Achy.** Your muscles may be strained from the exertion of labor and pushing. Your tailbone area (coccyx) may hurt.

- **Bruised.** It's not uncommon to have bruises on your body that you don't remember getting. If you had an IV, epidural, and/or injections, you could have bruises from them too.

make a fold to be sure the stump is exposed to air. Some healthcare practitioners suggest gently cleaning the stump with a cotton ball dipped in plain water, or they may suggest rubbing alcohol, which could cause your baby discomfort because it burns. Be sure to contact your baby's healthcare provider if there is any bleeding, pus, or swelling that suggests an infection. The way your baby's cord is cut has nothing to do with whether your baby will have an "inny" or an "outy" belly button. That's determined by the muscular structure of your baby's abdomen.

YOUR RECOVERY AFTER GIVING BIRTH

Most hospitals have a policy of getting new birth moms up as quickly as possible to help speed recovery and to protect them from forming blood clots in the legs. Don't be surprised if you're weaker than you imagined. You may be terrified of having your first bowel movement after birth. If you had a c-section, you won't be released from the hospital until you've passed gas. You'll probably be supplied with a small, plastic squeeze bottle to fill with warm water for rinsing off your sore perineum every time you go to the bathroom.

If you had a vaginal birth, you can at least wait until you're in private and familiar surroundings. And it may not be as bad as you think—but still, take your time, and try to relax and take it easy.

It's okay to ask your nurse to take your baby to the nursery when you need a rest. Also, call the nurse to take the baby to the nursery if you need to take a shower or leave the room for any reason.

If your hospital has *lactation consultants* on staff, take advantage of their skills. You'd think that like most bodily functions, breastfeeding would be self-explanatory, but if you've never done it before, it can be tricky and frustrating. Trust the advice of the lactation consultant above all others—even postpartum nurses have been known to give conflicting or erroneous advice. Ask if the hospital has a number that you can call later if you have breastfeeding questions or problems. (Also see our discussion about breastfeeding on pages 408–418.)

If your baby is being observed or treated in the NICU, you and your family members should be allowed to don sterilized scrubs and visit.

Your care provider, or a partner in the same practice, will check on you. She will feel your uterus to make sure it's contracting properly, check your stitches or incision site, and startlingly, may "honk" your breast to make sure you're making milk. Your care provider should also instruct you on how to care for any stitches or incisions, and give you a Sitz bath, a small shallow basin that fits under the toilet seat, to use and take home to keep stitches clean. She should also check to see if you have hemorrhoids, and give you cream to use for them, if necessary.

Make sure that your partner has installed a car seat in time for the ride home. Hospitals won't let you drive off without one.

What to do during the first hours after birth

Rest. Hospitals are noisy, interruptive places, and each new change in staff means a visit and a check of your signs, and for filling out the information for your baby's birth certificate, so be prepared for being awakened over and over.

Drink water. Keep yourself hydrated, especially if you lost a lot of blood.

Page a nurse or ask your partner to help out. You'll need help lifting your baby in and out of your bed for nursing and diapering.

Use painkillers. Ask for medication if you are in pain.

Get coaching on breastfeeding. Get a nurse, or ask for your hospital's lactation consultant to show you how to position your baby on your breast so you won't have sore nipples. Consider using lubrication to protect them. (See breastfeeding advice on pages 408–418.)

Watch for symptoms. Report any of the following symptoms immediately: a fever; a headache; a gush of blood; feeling faint; sharp pain, and swelling or heaviness in one leg; unusual pain in your chest.

Babies who need help

All expectant parents look forward to bringing their new babies home with them from the hospital. But if you have a baby or babies who are premature, or if your baby is fullterm but has problems with breathing, an infection, or a condition that requires surgery, he may be transferred to the neonatal intensive care unit (NICU, pronounced "nik-ewe"), a specialized baby-care facility found in larger medical facilities.

Walking into the NICU after your baby has been whisked away can feel like a scary and surreal experience. You will be instructed how to wash your hands and arms, and you may be expected to wear a special gown inside. Your baby may be hooked to wires and tubes and a respirator to assist with breathing. You may be encouraged to pump and freeze breast milk to feed your baby and to help in the feeding process.

The NICU's staff is made up of specially trained nurses, doctors, doctors-in-training, and other health care professionals to take care of your baby. The list may include a clinical nurse specialist who is an RN with a master's degree in nursing; a neonatologist, a pediatrician with special skills and training in caring for premature and sick newborn; a

neonatal nurse practitioner (NNP; and special dietitians and therapists to help manage your baby's needs. There will likely be a social worker assigned to you too, who is trained to counsel you and your partner through the experience, including managing health care arrangements and financial issues. He may also oversee a parent support group for parents of babies in NICU.

The NICU is a noisy, hot place. Each baby is connected to a pulse oximeter and a respiratory and heart rate monitor. These monitors go off frequently and are constantly attended to by the staff. A beeping monitor is usually nothing to panic about. It usually signifies a false alarm, a warning that something needed to be adjusted, or a warning that the baby needed some brief attention. And if your baby is extremely tiny, there may be a series of crises that happen during his growth and recovery that he will have to overcome. You will be coached about how to show your love to your baby through gentle, careful touching.

The emotional experience of having things go awry for your baby can be incredibly stressful. You will want to be with your baby, and you may find yourself being unable to eat or sleep out of concern for him. You'll likely have trouble concentrating on everyday activities and taking care of routine things, including tending your other children. You can expect to go through strong emotional ups and downs, from feeling angry to confused or depressed, to numbness, and back again. It helps that the NICU staff really care and that there are other parents there who are going through similar experiences.

The Non-Hospital Birth Experience

If you've chosen to give birth in a freestanding birth center (not to be confused with the "birth center" name given to the labor and delivery areas inside hospitals), your birth will likely be managed by a trained midwife or healthcare professional who has expertise in assisting women through the normal child-bearing process. (For information to help in deciding whether to use a freestanding center, see pages 162 to 165 in *Managing Your Pregnancy*.)

Research has shown that for healthy mothers, midwife-attended births, whether in birth centers or at home, turn out equally as well as physician-attended births. In 1999, the *Journal of Obstetric and Gynecology Research* reported a survey that compared midwife-attended births with obstetrician-attended births. The researchers concluded that midwife-managed care was equally as safe as obstetrician-managed care for low-risk pregnancies and births.[27] (For more information on freestanding birth centers, contact the National Association of Childbirth Centers, www.birthcenters.com.)

Your birth center's healthcare provider will not only be concerned about your and your baby's physical health during labor, but will also try to support your emotional and psychological well-being. The central focus of your care will likely be on honoring your birth wishes, and the natural progress and timetable of your labor.

Only medically necessary interventions will be used, and most centers are stocked with essential safety and emergency equipment should serious problems arise. If your labor has complications requiring obstetrical intervention, you will be transported to an appropriate medical facility for delivery.

The center also will also be equipped with innovative birthing aids designed to encourage your labor and improve your comfort. Included on the list might be a large tub for waterbirth; a suspended birth sling; birth stools, squatting bars, birth balls; an abundance of pillows and blankets; hot and cold packs; and tools for massaging your back. All are on hand to help your labor be as effective and comfortable as possible.

Preparing for a home birth

If you are expected to have a healthy, uncomplicated labor, having your baby at home may also be an acceptable alternative to a hospital or birth-center birth. Home birth is not as safe an option if you have a preexisting physical condition that could negatively affect your labor, such as a history of stillbirths; bleeding problems; a prior cesarean section; or other preexisting physical problems associated with complications. Should complications arise that could not have been anticipated in advance, you may be transported to the hospital for specialized care.

Using the services of a trained, certified midwife is essential. One overview of the outcomes of six studies of 24,092 planned home births found home birth to be an acceptable alternative to hospital care for selected, low-risk pregnant women. Mothers who had a home birth had fewer medical interventions.[28]

Having a home birth is also your least expensive option and will provide you with uninterrupted privacy in the comfort of familiar surroundings. If you elect to have a home birth, you can find excellent sources online to help you in preparing for your big event, including the equipment you should have on hand and what your midwife will probably supply. (See the *Resource Guide* on page 538.)

EMERGENCY CHILDBIRTH

When most mothers think about emergency childbirth, they usually picture giving birth in an elevator, on the side of a highway, or in a cab caught in rush-hour traffic. We've all watched television scenarios of a small child being talked through the birth of his little sister by the 911 operator.

Sometimes mothers have what is called a *precipitous birth* when their babies are born very quickly, which can't always be anticipated in advance. This can be hard on the baby and cause tearing and damage to a mother's insides. Most babies give their moms and dads more than enough time to get to the hospital with lots of hours to spare.

Discuss your fears about giving birth unexpectedly with your care provider. But, just to reassure you that you can get through a birth on your own, we're offering some simple instructions about how it's done.

Instructions for an emergency childbirth

If you go into labor, and giving birth seems imminent, you will probably have someone there to help you. The surest sign that birth is about to happen is an enormous sense of pressure between your legs and a compelling desire to push. Reach down, and feel between your legs. If your baby is about to come, you'll be able to feel his hard skull pushing down into your vagina. Here's what to do if delivery is imminent, and you know you're not going to make it to a hospital or birthing center in time:

- **Keep calm.** Just focus on your body sensations, and rest between contractions.

- **Don't try to drive yourself.** Stay where you are, and try to conserve your energy. If you're already in the car, pull over, and put on your blinkers. If you have to, you can give birth in the backseat of the car. That's better than having a wreck racing to the hospital.

- **Contact your doctor or midwife.** Let the office know this is an emergency call and that you are about to give birth. If you can't get through to the office, call 911. Mentally prepare yourself for the sounds of sirens, rushing personnel, lots of commotion, and a possible ride to the hospital.

- **Unlock your front door.** That will speed up getting emergency help to you.

- **Use your hands to guide you.** You will be able to feel your baby's head moving forward and backward during your contractions.

- **Find a comfortable position.** Some mothers naturally gravitate toward a squatting position, others prefer to be propped up semi-upright in the bed, to sit on the toilet, or lie in a tub of warm water unless you're all by yourself. Birth is messy, so protect the bed or floor with extra sheets or towels if you can manage it.

- **Take your time.** Don't feel you've got to hurry to get the baby out. Just relax, and let nature do its work.

- **Soften your pushing.** You can help protect yourself from tearing by keeping your throat open during the pushing urges so the baby has adequate time to ease his way out of you.

- **Don't try to pull on the baby or his head.** Simply guide the baby out. You may need to press on his shoulders to help them through.

- **Help the baby breathe.** Stroke downward on the baby's nose to help expel excess mucus and fluid from his nose and throat.

- **Leave the umbilical cord alone.** It's okay for the baby to remain connected to the cord. Don't pull on it or allow it to stretch tight.

- **Put the baby next to your skin.** Lay the baby across your belly or near your breasts with his head slightly lower than his body for mucus draining. Cover both of you with towels or a blanket.

- **Allow the baby to nurse.** If the baby is willing, let him begin suckling at your breast. That will help your uterus contract, push out the placenta, and then slow down any bleeding you have. The placenta's birth can take up to twenty minutes or more. Make sure your breast doesn't cover your baby's nose so your baby can breathe while nursing.

- **Save your placenta.** Put it in a plastic bag if you have one. Keep it next to the baby, and don't try to cut the umbilical cord yourself. Leave everything intact until help arrives.

Special Situations

A mother's labor is considered normal when her contractions are efficient in causing her cervix to efface and dilate. It's considered abnormal if it isn't happening in a reasonable amount of time. Some of the reasons that labor gets stalled are a baby being out of position; when contractions don't appear to be effective in moving the baby down; and if a mother has a pelvis shaped in such a way that it hinders the baby being born. In some cases, ineffective labor can be the result of painkillers given a mother during early labor.

Healthcare providers use certain time limits and milestones for labor progress to help discern whether labor is moving along as it should. It has been estimated that 8 to 11 percent of births when babies are in a normal, head-downward position have complications during the first stage of labor.

Clinical guidelines are printed statements used to determine when labors are normal and at what point in a labor that intervention will be called for. Just as many mothers enter the hospital with their birth plans in hand, healthcare providers and hospitals rely on preset guidelines and their own education and

experiences regarding birth to determine when to apply technology and medical interventions to their laboring patients.

Labor guidelines are often based on the Friedman Curve created more than fifty years ago by Dr. Emanuel Friedman, an obstetrician and Harvard Medical School professor who sought the best way to measure the progress of women's labors in order to help physicians judge when to intervene. He found that the dilation of a mother's cervix and the progress of a baby downward through the mother's pelvis, called fetal descent, were the two most useful tools to measure labor progress.

When Friedman published his study, he included a graph, the ***Friedman Curve***, that graphed out labor for first-time mothers based on how their cervix dilated and their baby progressed through the pelvis. The curve has since become the standard for judging whether a mother's labor is on schedule or not. The curve has been widely published in obstetrical textbooks for use as a decision-making tool.

The latent phase of labor on the curve shows the line slowly rising from two to three centimeters as a woman begins labor and during her first 8 hours. The active phase of labor finds the line taking a sharp upward slant as dilation and the baby's descent become faster. The active phase of dilation from three to four centimeters to full dilation of ten centimeters is depicted as lasting approximately 5.8 hours for first-time mothers and approximately 2.5 hours for mothers who have previously given birth.

Friedman found that approximately one centimeter of dilation per hour during the active phase represented the labor progress of the slowest 10 percent of women.[29]

Most hospitals have adopted the one centimeter rule as their guideline for mothers' speed for labor once she moves into active labor. That is, a mother's cervix will be expected to dilate by one centimeter per hour from the time it reaches four centimeters until ten, or she may be labeled as having a labor that is taking too long *(protracted labor)*. If your labor is ineffective or lags behind, it may be suggested that your labor should be augmented with drugs that cause your uterus to contract, or a cesarean may be recommended.

Artificial induction and augmentation of labor

Induction, sometimes called *induction of labor (IOL)*, is using medical means such as drugs or mechanical stretching devices to make a mother go into labor. *Elective induction* is the term for a patient's decision to have labor induced for any reason other than medical indication. Some women seek the security of being able to schedule the exact date their babies

will be born. Others are just ready to get the whole thing over with. Many women also fear the pain of labor, preferring controlled circumstances to the seemingly capricious whims of nature.

Instead of going into spontaneous, active labor anytime day or night, inductions are run on a schedule that brings mothers in the night before so that they can be induced in the morning and give birth by the end of the day.

Elective induction is not without potential risks. A baby may be delivered before he has completely matured, which can result in serious lung and physical problems. Induction has also been associated with the uterus contracting too frequently and too hard *(uterine hyperstimulation)*. When the uterus overworks without stopping, a baby is deprived of much-needed oxygen. That can affect the baby's heart rate and result in the diagnosis of non-reassuring status.

Mothers who undergo elective inductions are more at risk for having cesarean sections and to experience *postpartum hemorrhage*.

These complications are rarer in mothers who have previously given birth, but are significantly higher for first-time mothers. This group of women is also more likely to require instrumented delivery using vacuum extraction or forceps; and to have their babies admitted to neonatal intensive care units (NICU).[30]

Augmentation of labor is the strengthening of labor with contraction-inducing drugs once it has already started, although the word induction is popularly used to refer to both induction and augmentation. If a mother's cervix is hard and closed tightly, medications may be used to soften it before induction is done.

According to the National Center for Health Statistics, the national induction rate has more than tripled since 1989. The American College of Obstetricians and Gynecologists has issued a guideline that, whenever possible, induction should not be performed until a mother is at least thirty-nine weeks along in her pregnancy, and only then, when it is clear the benefits of being induced outweigh its risks.

Medical reasons for induction include a failing placenta; a baby in trouble or not thriving; a mother who is seriously ill with preeclampsia; a mother's high blood pressure; uncontrolled *diabetes mellitus* or lung disease; an infection of the uterus *(chorioamnionitis); isoimmunization* (Rh factor); stillbirth (a baby's having died inside his mother); or, the signs of infection after a mother's waters having broken too early (rupture of the membranes).

If your baby is overdue, induction may be suggested as an option, particularly if your care provider determines that your placenta is beginning to fail in supporting your baby. Placentas work most efficiently up to forty weeks, and forty-two weeks is about the longest most clinicians will let a pregnancy go on without suggesting to mothers that their labor be augmented with drugs or other interventions to make them start.

Drugs used for forcing the uterus to contract are given to a mother to take by mouth, or inserted inside her cervix as a tablet, gel, or suppository. Amniotomy, purposely rupturing a mother's amniotic sac; *sweeping the membranes*; and using a *Foley catheter*, a balloon-like mechanical device are ways of trying to speed up labor.

The *Bishop's score* is a forty-year-old scoring system used to determine if a mother is ready to have her labor augmented. The score is derived from counting points for five signs of labor's progress: the effacement and dilation of the cervix; how far down the baby is inside; the consistency of the cervix (firm, medium, or soft); and where the cervix is positioned inside the mother (to the back, to the center, or to the front).[31]

Each of these conditions is assigned ratings from zero to three with three being the most favorable. If the mother's score is zero, then it is thought to be too soon to augment her labor. But if her score is greater than eight, then the conditions for augmentation are thought to be favorable. The mother's and baby's status will be taken into account as well as the strength of her contractions.[32]

DRUGS COMMONLY USED FOR INDUCTION AND AUGMENTATION OF LABOR

Prostaglandin-like drugs

Misoprostol® (PGE1, or cytotec), and prostaglandin E2 (Prepidil®, Cervidil®), also called dinoprostone, are synthetic forms of prostaglandins, a hormone naturally present in the uterus. These drugs are used to help a woman's cervix to soften

FLASH FACTS: Cesareans for Lack of Progress in Early Labor

Cesarean sections can be lifesaving when there is a serious obstetrical emergency, but sometimes they are performed for reasons other than emergencies. Cesarean sections are now done on more than a million U.S. mothers a year (twenty-six percent), and lack of progress—*dystocia*—is the most commonly cited reason for doing them.

A 2000 study of more than two thousand U.S. births found that 68 percent of unplanned cesareans were performed for lack of progress, and 16 percent of these were performed during the early (latent) stage of labor, prior to the cervix reaching three to four centimeters, the indicator used to show that a mother is in active labor.

According to the American College of Obstetricians and Gynecologists, risk factors for dystocia include having an epidural; the baby being faced to the front; a first-time birth; a very short mother; a large baby; and a baby who is not descending well inside his mother even though she is fully dilated.

A cesarean section is serious surgery that carries the risk of hemorrhage (sudden, uncontrollable bleeding), infection, life-threatening blood clots, placenta problems in subsequent pregnancies, and other complications including a three times greater risk of stillbirth in subsequent pregnancies.

Giving a mother a cesarean for lack of progress in the early stages of labor goes against the current practice guidelines issued by the American College of Obstetricians and Gynecologists (ACOG) and most major medical organizations worldwide. And once you've had a cesarean the first time, it is highly likely you will have a cesarean for all of your future babies.

If there are no signs that your baby's life is endangered or your well-being is at stake, yet the "C" word is being used with you, as in "if you're not dilated by 'X' centimeters in the next 'X' minutes, you're going to need a c-section," we suggest moving around as much as feels comfortable; drinking water, and urinating often (sitting on the toilet can sometimes help); and simply waiting for your labor to develop on its own.

If you are feeling as though the staff is putting undue pressure upon you regarding having a cesarean section without a solid medical reason for doing so, request a second opinion from the head of obstetrics for the hospital or a specialist in maternal-fetal medicine. In the meantime, post a sign on your door asking not to be disturbed; try to postpone internal examinations for a while; turn down the lights; breathe deeply; relax; decide to trust your body; and if it's in your faith—pray.

and ripen so induction works better. In some cases, the drugs are administered by mouth as a tablet, or a dose can be placed inside a mother's cervix.

Numerous studies have shown that misoprostol works well for cervical ripening for full-term pregnancies, but it should not be given more often than every four to six hours.

Misoprostol's biggest risk is uterine hyperstimulation, which is estimated to occur in eight out of one hundred women and can be damaging to the baby. While Pitocin® is given through an IV, and the dose can quickly be backed down, misoprostal is not as easily controlled, and if it is not carefully administered, it can cause a mother's uterus to overcontract, endangering the baby's oxygen supply. Muscle relaxants may be required.

Misoprostol has also been associated with increased meconium staining, a sign of fetal distress and life-threatening *uterine rupture*, particularly if the mother has previously undergone a cesarean section. Women with prior cesareans who have their labors augmented with prostaglandin-based drugs were found to be fifteen times more vulnerable to experiencing uterine rupture than women who had prior cesareans but did not receive the drug. Its use also remains controversial for women who are expecting multiples or who are suspected of having fetal macrosomia. As of this writing, this drug has not been approved for use during pregnancy by the U.S. Food and Drug Administration (the FDA),[34] but is commonly used "off label."[35]

Oxytocin (Pitocin®). A mother's body naturally produces a hormone called oxytocin to stimulate contractions. Oxytocin, or Pitocin®, as the synthetic version of oxytocin is called, is one of the most commonly used drugs for making a mother's uterus contract or to

---

FLASH FACTS

Should you be induced if your baby is thought to be too large?

Macrosomia is when a mother is carrying a baby that weighs more than four thousand grams (nearly nine pounds). An extra large baby is thought to have trouble fitting through a mother's pelvis and to cause a mother's contractions to be ineffective.

Even though healthy pregnancies are sometimes induced because the babies are thought to be growing too large, current studies show that macrosomia by itself is not a valid reason for undergoing an induction.

A 2002 review of eleven research studies covering 3,751 women given inductions for macrosomia found that 16.5 percent ended up having cesarean sections. On the other hand, only 8.4 percent of mothers with macrosomia who were allowed to undergo a normal, non-induced labor required c-sections.[33]

cause weak contractions to become stronger. Pitocin® is usually administered with an IV. It can be used to start a labor that may not have started on its own, or to speed up a labor that has slowed down or stopped.

The dose of Pitocin® you receive will gradually be increased over time until contractions become strong. There is a danger of over-stimulating a mother's uterus when cervical ripening agents, such as Misoprostol®, are used, and for that reason, it is recommended that a Pitocin® IV not be started until six hours after you've had cervical ripening. Pitocin® should also be stopped after five hours if it does not succeed in getting labor started. Sometimes when labor does not start after induction, a mother may be encouraged to eat and rest with induction resumed again in the morning. Rarely, an induction may be stopped and the woman sent home to wait for labor to start on its own or for her body to show more signs of being ready to go into labor.

Sometimes Pitocin® can cause contractions to become too intense—uterine hyperstimulation—which can affect the baby's circulation of blood and oxygen through the umbilical cord. If that happens, your medication dose may be reduced or stopped completely. If there are signs of nonreassuring fetal status that don't improve after the Pitocin® is stopped, it may mean that you'll be given a c-section. Pitocin® should be used cautiously if a mother is at risk for having her uterus tear (uterine rupture) along the scar of prior surgery to her uterus, such as a prior c-section.

MECHANICAL FORMS OF INDUCTION AND AUGMENTATION

The following are nondrug ways to stimulate the uterus to contract.

Sweeping the membranes

If you are more than a week overdue, your healthcare provider may suggest sweeping, or stripping, your membranes during your routine physical exam. The procedure involves inserting a gloved finger up into the rim of your cervix and rotating it between your baby's amniotic sac and the rim of the cervix. This detaches the amniotic membranes from the lower part of the uterine cavity in order to encourage the start of labor.

The sweeping is used to help stimulate the hormones that start labor, but this can be painful, and lead to minor bleeding afterward. In some cases, the procedure can't be performed because the mother's cervix is still too tightly closed to allow the insertion of a finger.

A series of studies have found that sweeping the membranes increases the chances of going into labor within a week. Women who've had sweeping done are less likely to have their labor artificially induced. There appears to be no increased incidence in adverse outcomes for mothers who had the procedure or higher levels of infection, although the procedure may cause temporary bleeding and discomfort.

The Risks of Artificially Inducing Labor (IOL)

Heightened cesarean risk. An induction nearly doubles your risk of having a c-section. A retrospective study of the induction experiences of more than 14,409 women found that having an induction was associated with an 11 percent higher risk of having a cesarean section for first-time mothers. Being older than thirty-five and carrying a baby longer than forty weeks were contributors to the mothers' c-section risk. For mothers who had given birth to more than one baby, having an induction nearly doubled the risk of a cesarean. For these mothers, the risk was heightened by being over forty and carrying a baby beyond forty-one weeks.[36] (See our list of c-section risks on page 346.)

Uterine hyperstimulation. Uterine hyperstimulation is defined as having contractions lasting longer than ninety seconds or having more than five contractions in ten minutes. Hyperstimulation can affect the delivery of oxygen and blood to your baby, which can affect your baby's well-being. Sometimes hyperstimulation is caused by having too strong a dose of an induction medication. Some drugs are associated with presenting a higher risk for uterine hyperstimulation than others. If it happens to you during an induction, your drugs may be reduced or discontinued, or you may be given a drug to counteract the effects of the induction medication. You will probably be placed on your side for half an hour, and both you and your baby will be monitored continuously until the rhythms of your contractions return to normal.

Uterine rupture. Having an induction after you've previously had a cesarean section is associated with having uterine rupture, which is a tear in the uterus and bleeding inside that can be dangerous for both mother and baby. The risk of rupturing is higher if your previous cesarean used an incision down the center of your uterus. A scar down the middle of your abdomen does not necessarily mean your uterus was opened in the middle. The only way your obstetrician can know for sure is from your past hospital records that detail the kind of incision made in your uterus. Other mothers at risk for rupture during induction are older mothers, women who have given birth to a large number of children, women carrying larger-than-normal babies, and women with an enlarged uterus. Approximately 25 to 30 percent of babies die when their mothers have uterine rupture. (Uterine rupture is also discussed on page 222.)

Immature baby with lung problems. Sometimes healthcare providers miscalculate an unborn baby's age and maturity, which can result in the baby being born with severe lung problems. Inductions have also been associated with babies having a poor measurement of functioning immediately after birth (lower Apgar scores). (We describe the Apgar system for rating newborns on page 324.)

Amniotomy (Artificial rupture of the membranes, ARM, or AROM)

If you've started labor and your sac still hasn't broken, some practitioners may decide to rupture it for you. The procedure is called an amniotomy, *artificial rupture of the membranes (ARM or AROM)*. It consists of using a long device that resembles a crochet hook to painlessly puncture a hole in the sac. You have a right to refuse this procedure, and you should consider doing so unless your care provider has an obvious and compelling reason for using it.

Although ARM is simple and easy to do, it is a form of labor augmentation that causes labor to speed up, sometimes by one to two hours. Because of the danger of infection, breaking the waters also commits a mother to giving birth on a schedule. (Our discussion of induction procedures starts on page 335.)

If you have no signs that your baby is in trouble, such as heart rate abnormalities, consider requesting that the sac be left intact to break on its own. Temporarily preserving your baby's water cushion will help to provide him with a buffer zone during the squeezing of contractions and as his head moves down through the hard ring of the pelvis. The fluid will provide lubrication and make shifting positions easier for him.

Medical reasons for performing an amniotomy are to see if your baby is passing meconium, a nonreassuring sign that the baby may be in trouble; to take a blood sample from your baby's scalp; or to attach a monitor to the baby's scalp because of concerns for his well-being.

Mechanical dilation devices

Mechanical dilation devices can be inserted in the mouth of the cervix to help stretch it. Some dilators use small balloons to apply pressure to the cervix. The balloon is inflated with water, which causes the cervix to soften and dilate. The device is sometimes used when labor goes on for many hours with the cervix showing little or no change. It can only be used if a mother's cervix is adequately open enough to allow the catheter to be inserted. Oxytocin is usually administered in the following six to twenty-four hours. In some cases, the dilator can cause the amniotic sac to rupture, or it may introduce infection into the cervical area. Another way to dilate the cervix, *laminaria* are small reeds placed inside the cervix that swell from moisture, which causes it to stretch open.

Operative vaginal delivery

Instruments, including forceps or a large suction cup are sometimes used to help a baby be delivered during the second stage of labor. They may be employed if the pushing stage is taking a long time, or when the baby needs to be removed for the safety of either the mother or the baby. It is important that your care provider be very experienced with using these instruments to ensure that you and your baby are not injured in the process.

Forceps delivery

Forceps are a two-piece, spoon-shaped metal instrument with two blades and interlocking handles. One of the blades is first placed around the baby's head, and then the other blade is secured to enable the baby to be grasped in front of his ears. Gentle pulling is applied from outside. A mother's cervix must be fully dilated before forceps can be used.

Forceps are more likely to be used during the second stage when a first-time mother who has been given an epidural doesn't succeed in pushing the baby out within three hours, or within two hours if she has no anesthesia. Those time limits are shortened by an hour for mothers who have previously given birth. In some instances, forceps may be used to assist a baby in rotating or to help a breech baby get born.

Forceps may result in injury and lacerations to the muscles surrounding a mother's birth canal and may require that the mother have an episiotomy, the cutting and stitching of the region between the vagina and rectum, which may increase bleeding, be painful during recovery, and make her more vulnerable to infection. In rare instances, forceps can result in temporary or permanent nerve damage to an infant's face. (See episiotomy "Flash Facts" on page 344.)

Vacuum extraction

Recent evidence suggests that vacuum extraction is another alternative to the use of forceps for delivering a baby whose head is engaged in the birth canal but is not making progress toward being born.

A vacuum extractor has a plastic cup on one end that is placed on the top of a baby's head and is attached to a suction device on the other end. The baby is then pulled along the birth canal as the mother bears down.

Vacuum extraction is normally used when a mother's cervix is fully

FLASH FACTS

Amniotomy and c-sections

An overview of research on the artificial breaking of mothers' amniotic sacs found the procedure carries both benefits and risks. While rupturing membranes shortened the average length of mothers' labors by one to two hours, it also markedly increased the risk of their having to undergo cesarean sections because of nonreassuring status for the baby (fetal distress). On the plus side, mothers who had amniotomy had a reduced risk of having their labors augmented and their babies generally had higher Apgar scores than mothers who did not have amniotomies. Because of the increased risk of injury that cesarean sections pose, the researchers concluded that amniotomy should be reserved only for women with abnormal labors. (Apgar scores are discussed on page 324, and cesarean sections on pages 343–350.)[37]

dilated, and the baby's head is positioned for birth. This intervention is only recommended for use with a full-term baby who is arriving in the head-down (*vertex*) position. It is not recommended for use with a baby who has had a blood sample taken from his scalp to minimize the risk of injury.

The baby's head will be wiped clean. The cup that will be attached to his scalp and the suctioning part of the device will then be compressed and inserted. Your care provider will sweep his, or her, finger around the cup to make sure none of your own tissue is trapped inside. Your care provider will then apply pressure in an inward and downward pull.

When you have a good contraction, the suction pressure will be raised, and traction will be applied to gently help pull your baby out. Once your contraction goes away, your provider will stop pulling, and the suction will be reduced.

As your baby's head gets closer to coming out, you will probably be given an episiotomy, and the direction of traction will be changed to an upward, forty-five-degree angle to help your baby's head navigate your pelvic bones and the curve of the birth canal. Once the baby's head is delivered, the cup will be removed.

Your caregiver will likely stop the procedure if it fails to achieve the birth of your baby's head within a reasonable amount of time or if it is suspected that your baby's scalp has been injured.

The benefit of vacuum extraction over forceps is that it is easier to use; there is less room for error when applying the suction cup; less

anesthesia may be needed for the mother; and there may be less damage to the mother's soft tissues.

Vacuum extraction has some disadvantages over forceps. If proper technique is not used, the extractor may lose its vacuum. Delivery may take longer than with forceps, and babies are more likely to have bleeding, bruising, and swelling of the scalp called *cephalohematoma*.

Cesarean section

The medical term for surgically delivering your baby by cutting open your abdomen and uterus is a cesarean section (or c-section). Cesarean sections can be a life-saving option for a mother or baby. Most frequently, c-sections are performed at short notice during labor when complications arise that might be risky for mother or baby. This is usually called an emergency section.

Giving birth to a baby through the vaginal route is generally safer for both mother and baby, and recovery is much less painful and quicker than with cesarean sections. Nonetheless, c-sections have now become the most commonly performed surgical procedure in the U.S. Approximately 825,000 c-sections are performed every year in the U.S., or approximately one out of every four pregnancies.[38]

There are different types of c-sections. A section may be performed through the upper part of the uterus when a baby is lying sideways, when the baby is very small and premature, or when there is insufficient amniotic fluid. But the lower segment of the uterus is the most common place where the incision is done

FLASH FACTS

Will you need an episiotomy?

An episiotomy is a surgical procedure. It is the cutting into the connective tissues and muscles in the area between the vagina and the anus to widen the birth canal in order to ease the baby out.

For a long time, episiotomies were a routine procedure for childbirth. Healthcare providers thought that giving a woman a surgical incision would ease her delivery and avoid the deep, jagged tears that might happen. It was also thought to prevent **urinary incontinence**, to keep the muscles of a woman's pelvic floor from becoming too lax, or to prevent a prolapsed (dropped) uterus, but research has failed to prove that having an episiotomy can prevent any of these things from happening.

In fact, recent research now shows that having an episiotomy actually increases a woman's chances of severe tearing, excessive bleeding, infection, and swelling. It can cause severe discomfort after birth and make sex painful.

Episiotomies today are most often performed when forceps or vacuum extraction are used. And having an epidural increases a woman's risk for needing to have these instruments used to help pull her baby out. There are times when babies are in dire trouble and may need to be delivered quickly. In that case, an episiotomy may be important.

Ask your healthcare provider to discuss the pros and cons of having an episiotomy. Let her know your preferences, and ask what strategies might help you to avoid the surgery. Your caregiver may perform massage of your perineum, use care in supporting your baby's head, or apply warm compresses to help your vaginal area relax and stretch in order to reduce the risk of tearing. You can also master breathing techniques that will help you hold back should your baby be arriving too quickly, which could reduce your risk for tearing.

because the scar holds up better there for future pregnancies.

Full anesthesia is seldom used for cesareans nowadays. Instead, you will likely have a stronger-than-normal dose of numbing drugs through a spinal or an epidural or a combination of both. (See the discussion of these procedures on pages 315–322.)

An elective caesarean section is one that is chosen for reasons other than an emergency. It is usually performed one to two weeks prior to a baby's official due date with special care being taken to make sure the baby's lungs and body are mature enough for survival.

Suggestions for avoiding a c-section

Here are some suggestions of ways to help protect yourself from having an unnecessary cesarean section:

Choose a healthcare provider and hospital with a low cesarean rate. Midwives and family practitioners generally do not perform cesareans. Some obstetricians and hospitals have inordinately high percentage rates for performing cesarean sections. In 2002, the national cesarean rate was 26.1 percent for all birthing women, while the ideal rate set by Healthy People 2000 is 15 percent or lower. In some cases, a high rate may be due to the high-risk patient loads that certain hospitals and physicians carry. Most obstetricians will furnish the percentage of their births that are c-sections upon request. (One place to search for your hospital's c-section rate is on www.healthgrades.com.)

Give your labor time to get established. Early medical interventions can start a cascade of problems that cause labor to stall and may lead to a cesarean. Rest at home until your labor is clearly established. (See our discussion about when to check into the hospital on pages 271–277.)

Adopt baby-friendly positions during late pregnancy. During the latter part of pregnancy, try not to sit for long periods of time. Practice standing and leaning forward in a moderate jackknife position using a desk, chest, or other piece of furniture for support. Frequently getting on your hands and knees during late pregnancy can help to strengthen your back, and it might help to move your baby into more favorable position for labor.

Have your baby turned. Many obstetricians choose not to deliver breech babies vaginally, but a few obstetricians and midwives still practice the art of vaginal breech delivery in selected patients, but doing so presents risks to your baby.

If your baby is breech or in another unfavorable position for labor, and your due date is getting close, consider having the baby turned by external cephalic version (ECV). (Breech birth is discussed on page 261, and ECV on page 262.)

Avoid having your labor induced. Sometimes having an induction is medically important for saving the life of your baby, but if it's not, don't agree to it. Induction can increase your risk of a c-section anywhere from 11 to 50 percent.

Move during labor. Keep upright, and if you can, change positions frequently to help your labor progress. (We list position possibilities on pages 287 and 309.)

Ask for a different kind of monitoring. Unless your baby is clearly endangered, request that he be monitored intermittently, rather than continuously by an electronic fetal monitor. (We discuss electronic fetal monitoring on page 275.)

Use an alternative birth setting. If your pregnancy is low-risk, consider a freestanding birth center or having your baby at home. (We discuss these centers on pages 164–165.)

Will a cesarean save your lower body from damage?

Sometimes cesareans are offered to healthy mothers with the promise of protecting the deep tissues of her lower body from the stretching and damage caused by the baby's descent and birth; to prevent urinary and fecal incontinence that is sometimes associated with vaginal birth; and to keep the uterus from slipping down into her vagina.

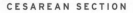

The Risks of a Cesarean

Dying. The risk of a mother dying as a result of having a cesarean is small, but the risk is considered four times greater (four per ten thousand) than for a vaginal birth (one per ten thousand births).

Problems for the baby. Babies born by cesarean section are four times more likely to suffer from respiratory distress than babies born vaginally.

Higher post-birth complications. Rates of infection, hemorrhage, thrombosis, and pulmonary embolism are higher for mothers who have had cesarean sections than mothers who have had vaginal deliveries.

Slower recovery. Recovery from a caesarean birth takes longer than for a vaginal birth. Women who have cesareans require more support at home and suffer more psychological after-effects from cesarean births.

Stillbirth. A survey of 120,633 second births to women who had previously given birth vaginally or by cesarean section published in 2003 found that having previous cesarean sections made mothers three times more at risk for their next babies dying. Women who had c-sections for their first births were twice as likely to have stillborn babies with their second pregnancies. After thirty-nine weeks of pregnancy, the risk of unexplained stillbirth was and 0.5 per one thousand in women with previous vaginal delivery, but 1.1 per one thousand women with a previous cesarean delivery. The causes for baby death are still not clearly understood.[39]

Infection. In spite of the routine administration of antibiotics to mothers undergoing c-sections, it is estimated that each year in the U.S. between 41,000 and 206,000 women develop an infection of the uterus or their surgical incisions after undergoing a cesarean section.[40]

However, research appears to show that it isn't vaginal birth itself that leads to these problems, but pregnancy itself. These problems are also associated with the use of forceps and vacuum extraction to deliver a baby; episiotomies; birthing an abnormally large baby; a prolonged second (pushing) stage of labor; and with mothers whose bodies are changed over time from giving birth over and over.[42]

You can have a vaginal birth and still take active measures to help protect your pelvic area. Avoid forced pushing during the second stage of labor. (See our pushing suggestions on pages 289–295.) Change your position frequently, and try to stay in an upright position during the second stage of labor and during birth, rather than lying flat. Don't agree to have an episiotomy or forceps unless there are clear medical indications for it. (Epidurals are associated with a slower second stage of birth, and a higher rate of forceps deliveries; in turn, forceps are associated with an increased risk of serious tears in the vaginal area.)

Placenta problems. Complications of the placenta such as abruption and placenta previa are more common in women who have previously undergone cesarean section, and the risk of those problems increases with each cesarean.

Hemorrhage. Cesarean sections are associated with heavier blood loss and a higher risk of hemorrhage—severe, difficult-to-control bleeding.

Uterine rupture with next birth. Tearing of the uterus is serious and rapid and can be deadly. It is associated with neurological injury to the baby. A study of the second births of more than twenty thousand women over a nine-year period who had had cesarean sections with their first babies found that eleven women out of twenty thousand had a rupture while undergoing a second cesarean without labor, and fifty-six had rupture after spontaneous onset of labor. Uterine rupture increases the possibility that a woman will have to have her uterus removed (*hysterectomy*). (See our discussion of vaginal birth after a cesarean section [VBAC] on page 350.)[41]

Placenta problems with the next birth. A repeat cesarean delivery carries significantly higher risk of having placenta previa (a misplaced placenta that interferes with birth) and *placenta accreta* (a placenta buried deeply into the uterus that does not detach normally). The risk of placenta previa and placenta accreta increases with each subsequent cesarean delivery, reaching a risk of greater than sixty percent in women who have undergone four or more cesarean deliveries.

Pain and discomfort after birth. Pain in the incision area can interfere with a mother's picking up and holding her baby, and that can make routine baby management and breastfeeding during the early, vulnerable stage of bonding more of a challenge.

How a c-section feels

In preparation for surgery, your pubic hair will be shaved for the area where the incision will be done, and you'll be wiped down with antiseptic. You will have a catheter, a small tube, placed into your urethra to make sure your bladder stays empty. If you haven't had an epidural yet, the insertion can be uncomfortable, and you can ask that it not be done until your epidural goes into effect. (See our description of epidurals on pages 315–322.)

If you have sufficient pain relief, you should not feel the incision. If you do feel the doctor cutting, or any pain, inform your anesthesiologist immediately. Some medications used in epidurals can temporarily cause you to experience nausea or itching.

The table you are on will be tilted to the left or a pillow placed under your right lower back to keep the pressure of the weight of your womb and your baby from pressing down on important arteries inside your body, which could cause your blood pressure to decrease.

Your hands will be fastened down on each side of you to prevent them from contaminating the sterile operating area. A sheet about eighteen inches high will be draped like a tent in front of you at about chest level to serve as a shield so you won't be able to see the surgery. But your partner may be allowed to take pictures or a video of your baby when she emerges from your belly.

Your abdomen will be opened with an incision through your skin and abdominal tissues using a scalpel. The incision will likely be done along the lower abdominal crease a little above your pubic bone, called a bikini cut. The scalpel will cut through fat, and the opening will be pulled apart, with some of the muscles being cut with scissors. Tissues will be separated either with tools or with the surgeon's fingertips.

Once an adequate opening has been made, your obstetrician will reach inside your uterus, and place a hand under your baby's head. Your baby's head will be exposed first, and then the doctor will gently ease out the rest of the baby's body, which will feel like a sense of pressure followed by a strong tug as your baby's body emerges through your incision.

Some hospitals offer to hold a mirror so a mother can see the baby being pulled out, but you can elect not to use it if the thought of watching makes you queasy. It's normal to have temporary feelings of vulnerability or fear. Having your partner or labor assistant telling you what's going on can help.

Your baby's mouth and nose will be suctioned while pressure is being placed on your uterus from the outside. The baby will finally begin to cry, and your baby will be given an Apgar rating. (See "Apgar" on page 324.) Your baby's weight, length, and time of birth will be recorded.

You may then be aware of the pushing and pulling of tissues and organs as they are being handled after delivery. You will likely be given oxytocin intravenously to help your uterus contract after your baby is removed. The placenta will be delivered while the surgeon feels inside to make sure that the entire placenta has been removed, so no pieces of tissue are left inside to cause infection.

The next step will be to place your intestines, your bladder, and your uterus back into their proper place and sewing together the layers of abdominal tissue cut during the surgery. Your incision will be closed with stitches, usually in two layers. The interior stitches will dissolve on their own. You may have a drainage tube left in to help the wound drain. Staples may be used along the outside of the cut; they will be almost painlessly removed later. Sometimes surgical tape is used instead to seal the wound. It will dissolve on its own.

It will take five to ten minutes to remove your baby; after that, it will probably take between thirty to forty-five minutes to remove your placenta, replace your organs, and stitch the inside layers of your abdomen.

Once your surgery is complete, you will be rolled into a recovery room, and in some cases, you may be transferred onto another bed by nurses or orderlies who will pick up your sheets and slide you effort-lessly across from one surface to another.

You'll be covered with a warm blanket and are likely to stay in the recovery room for an hour or more, while your blood pressure and other vital signs are being closely monitored. You may continue to be hooked up to an IV solution hanging from a pole on wheels. While you're there, the hospital staff will be checking your blood pressure and temperature repeatedly to make sure you're not experiencing any complications from your surgery.

If you were given general anes-thesia because of the emergency nature of your c-section, you will probably feel groggy after surgery and just want to nap. Some mothers also feel waves of nausea, and a sore throat from being intubated (having a tube placed down the throat to protect the lungs from inhaling stomach juices).

If you elect to breastfeed, you'll need help in putting your baby to your breast. You may be able to breastfeed in a side-lying position. Ask the nurse who is there for you, or your partner to help you arrange pillows to make you feel more com-fortable. Soon after delivery, you may be asked to do simple foot exercises to help prevent blood clots from forming in your legs, and deep breathing exercises to help clear your lungs.

Recovery from your cesarean section

Immediately after the birth, you'll be given pain medications that may make you woozy but will help to reduce swelling and speed up your recovery. The first sign that your epidural is wearing off will probably be a pins-and-needles feeling in your legs and pain at your incision site. How quickly you start to get your sensations back will depend on the type of analgesia you had, how strong a dose was used, when you received your last dose, and your own body's response to medication.

Don't be shy about asking for more pain medication if you need it. Studies show that painkillers work best when you take them before pain gets unbearable. Make sure your nurse knows that you plan to breastfeed, since some medications aren't recommended for nursing mothers.

You may also begin to feel stom-ach cramps from trapped gas, which is common after any sort of abdomi-nal surgery. Pulling in your abdomen and grunting as you exhale helps expel the gas. Just as with mothers who have given birth vaginally, you may become aware of your uterus cramping as it squeezes shut and shrinks as it recovers from birth.

You may be encouraged to suck on ice chips or be offered clear liquid or juice to drink. Later, you may be offered regular foods. The purpose is to stimulate your intestines and colon so your bowels will start acting again. Avoid carbonated beverages, though, because they may lead to more gas pain.

You'll also be encouraged to get up and walk within hours after your surgery, unless your legs are too wobbly to support you. Within twelve hours, you'll be encouraged to sit in a chair or to go to the bathroom to take care of your stitches. Until then, you'll be offered a bedpan.

Although catheters can be painful going in, you may also have momentary, mild discomfort and a burning sensation while it is being removed. A nurse will remove it upon the orders of your care provider. You may have difficulty urinating for a while. Drink plenty of water, because urinating is important to flush germs out of your urinary tract.

You are going to need help for the first weeks after your surgery. If your partner is unable to stay with you to help you around the clock, consider enlisting the support of other family members or hiring a nurse or postpartum doula. You should never be left alone in the house with the baby until you've recovered enough to get out of bed on your own and pick up and carry your baby.

The surface of your cesarean incision will heal around six weeks after your surgery. You may initially have numbness at the scar site, and some mothers develop scar tissue, called keloids. A cesarean is major abdominal surgery. It will take at least six weeks for you to recover, and some mothers experience pain or numbness at the incision site much longer.

VBAC–Vaginal Birth after a Cesarean

It has often been said that "once a cesarean, always a cesarean," but that isn't necessarily true. Going into labor in hopes of giving birth to your baby vaginally after having had a cesarean section in the past is called having a *trial of labor*.

The advantages to trying to give birth vaginally after a cesarean (called VBAC—vee-bak) are that your chances of dying or having things go wrong is less with a vaginal delivery than with a cesarean section, plus vaginal deliveries are far less expensive.

The disadvantages of trying to give birth vaginally after having had a c-section from a prior birth are that you will require very close monitoring during the procedure and afterward, and you will have a higher risk of having the scar on your uterus separate, or more seriously, your uterus rupture, which is very rare, but can be life-threatening.

A mother whose uterus is rupturing may go into catastrophic shock with internal bleeding. When that happens, she will feel acute pain. It is sometimes hard for medical personnel to detect if a rupture is going on, even though there is considerable bleeding inside. A mother's blood count may go down slowly, but an ultrasound may show the baby in an abnormal position. The extreme nature of the problem may not give enough time for a sonogram.

A study of the second births of more than twenty thousand women who had cesareans for their first babies over a nine-year period compared their relative risks for uterine rupture depending upon their deliveries. Eleven women out of twenty thousand had a rupture while undergoing a second cesarean with no labor; fifty-six had a rupture after spontaneous onset of labor.

Whether to allow women who have had prior cesarean sections to give birth vaginally is a hotly debated topic in the medical world right now. Some healthcare providers and hospitals are flatly refusing women the right to have vaginal births, while other settings and providers may be more open to allowing it.

The prime consideration about whether you are a good candidate for VBAC depends upon the type of incision made on your uterus during the previous cesarean section, how many cesareans you've had in the past, and how old you are.

We suggest obtaining your prior hospital records for your last cesarean section; becoming fully informed on VBAC issues from books, research, and reliable Web sites; and then discussing the risks and benefits of VBAC with your healthcare provider.

Giving birth to twins and multiples

Twins occur in about 2.9 pregnancies out of 100, triplets about 1 in 10,000, and quadruplets in 1 out of every 512,000. The use of *in vitro fertilization (IVF)* and fertility drugs are increasing the chances of mothers having multiples. Women ages thirty to forty are also more likely to give birth to twins, as are African-American mothers.

Identical *(monozygotic)* twins come from the same egg splitting in two, while fraternal *(dizygotic)* twins come from two eggs fertilized by two different sperm, but other than having genetic testing, or discovering your babies are different sexes during a sonogram, there's no way to know which type of twins your babies are until childhood.

Twins may share one placenta, but have two different amniotic sacs, or each of your babies may have its own placenta. Twins and multiples bring a number of risks. They may be *low birthweight*; they may

suffer from twin-twin transfusion in which one twin steals blood from the other; they may have a greater risk of preeclampsia (toxemia), placental problems, or cord accidents; and they may be out of position for birth. The greatest risk is that your twins will set off the labor process early and be born prematurely before their body systems have had adequate time to mature.

If both babies are positioned head downward, which happens with 45 percent of twin pregnancies, and your babies are full term and a good size, you will probably be able to deliver them normally. Twins often weigh less than normal because they've had to vie for space inside, and they typically arrive between the thirty-sixth and thirty-seventh week of pregnancy, and between 10 and 15 percent of twins are born by twenty-eight weeks.

You have a 45 to 50 percent chance of needing a cesarean if you have any risk factors, such as placenta previa or *intrauterine growth retardation* (IUGR), if your babies are out of position for birth, or if you start labor early, rather than making it to full term. If you're carrying three or more babies, then it's almost certain you will be delivered by cesarean section.

Even if both of your babies are in the right position, your labor and delivery may be more difficult than normal. For example, your second baby may have trouble getting down the birth canal. An epidural may be suggested for you, which will enable you to have a quicker transition into a c-section if something goes wrong. It will also allow your healthcare provider to manage a breech birth or to massage your uterus should there be excess bleeding.

Vaginal delivery for your first twin has been shown to be safe for both mother and baby, and for your second baby, if he is large enough to make it through safely. But if your babies are both breech (bottoms down) or are in other odd positions, then your healthcare provider may feel that it's wisest to allow you to carry your babies as long as possible, and then to schedule a cesarean section.

Your birth experience with twins is likely to be very similar to mothers giving birth to singletons, except things may take a little longer. Whether you give birth vaginally or your babies are delivered by c-section, they will be temporarily named "Baby A," and "Baby B," depending upon which baby comes out first.

Carrying multiple babies will cause your pregnancy to be considered high risk because multiples raise the potential for complications during labor, including premature delivery. As with other conditions, careful monitoring will help to ensure that your pregnancy and labor progress normally and that you and your babies aren't endangered in the process.

Rarer medical concerns

Dystocia is a general term for a difficult labor that can be caused by the position or size of the baby or by problems with the mother's contractions or her having a pelvis that is too small. A mother may be said to have dystocia if her cervix dilates less than half a centimeter per hour during active labor, which happens after three centimeters of dilation.

Obstructed labor is when a baby gets stuck inside a mother during labor so it can't get out. The cause may be ineffective contractions by the uterus. Macrosomia, discussed earlier, is when a mother has an unusually large baby that may make labor harder. *Cephalopelvic disproportion (CPD)* is when a mother's pelvis is too small, or a baby's head is too large, making birth difficult or impossible. An out-of-position baby who is facing forward instead of rearward, or lying sideways can also impede birth. A cesarean delivery may be the best answer for these problems.

Shoulder dystocia happens when a baby's shoulders are too large to fit through the mother's pelvis so his body doesn't rotate normally during the last part of birth. It happens in less than two out of one hundred births and doesn't become apparent until after the baby's head has already come out. Sometimes a mother's position can help to release the baby's shoulders. A mother may be asked to bend her knees and bring her legs up while her provider presses down on the baby's shoulder from the outside, and then gently rotates the baby's body. In rare instances, a baby's collarbone may be deliberately fractured to save the baby's life.

Uterine inversion is when a mother's uterus gets turned inside out after the baby is born. This causes the tissues of the uterus to become starved for oxygen, and it is considered a serious crisis. Inversion is most often caused by a healthcare provider pulling on the part of the umbilical cord that is attached to the uterus after the baby has been born in an attempt to speed up the delivery of the placenta. It is estimated to occur in one out of two thousand mothers.[43]

Polyhydramnios refers to a mother's carrying too much fluid in her baby's amniotic sac so that it becomes distended and swollen. In one out of five cases, this condition is associated with a baby's having congenital anomalies (birth defects), and it can result in premature birth, the baby being out of position during birth, and the mother's placenta pulling away from the side of her uterus (placental abruption), and premature rupture of the amniotic sac. It also increases the risk of a mother needing a cesarean section or having excess bleeding (hemorrhaging). Mothers with diabetes mellitus are more likely to have the condition. Amniocentesis may be used to remove the excess fluid. (The risks of amniocentesis are discussed on page 184.)

Oligohydramnios is not having enough amniotic fluid for the baby, and it is most frequently associated with the premature rupture of membranes (PROM), a mother's amniotic sac breaking too early so the fluid drains out. If the condition goes on for long, it can affect a baby's lung development and lead to severe respiratory problems after birth, and sometimes deformities and death. Sometimes the condition happens when a pregnancy is long overdue, and the placenta begins to shut down. Your healthcare provider may recommend bed rest and drinking plenty of water, which can increase amniotic fluid by as much as 30 percent.

Oligohydramnios is frequently associated with chorioamnionitis (amnionitis), an infection of the membranes that surround the baby (see below). *Amnioinfusion*, adding fluid to the amniotic sac through the cervix at the time of delivery, may be used to ease delivery and keep the baby's umbilical cord from being squeezed shut.

Serious infections

Fever during labor can be associated with an epidural, but it can also be a serious sign of infection that could harm the baby and is associated with baby death. Mothers who have sexually transmitted diseases, those whose amniotic sacs have broken early, and those who have had cesareans are the most at risk for infection. In these situations, usually antibiotics will be given in advance of birth as a protective measure.

When a mother has a fever during labor, it is usually a sign of inflammation of the fetal membranes due to infection. This fever is strongly associated with infection-related neonatal and infant deaths among both preterm and term infants. Approximately 1.6 percent of mothers come down with *intrapartum fever*, and mothers who have previously had babies have a 30 percent greater chance of the fever. Untreated, it can be deadly, tripling the risk of a baby dying soon after birth.

Chorioamnionitis (amnionitis) is an infection of a mother's membranes (placental tissues) and her amniotic fluid that happens in about 1 to 2 percent of all pregnancies, but is much more common when mothers give birth prematurely. It can lead to a blood infection in the mother (bacteremia) and serious infection in the newborn baby.

The organisms usually responsible for chorioamnionitis are those that are normally present in the vagina, including *E. coli (Escherichia coli)*. Group B streptococcus may also cause the infection. Chorioamnionitis can develop when the membranes (amniotic sac) are ruptured (broken) for an extended period before labor begins. This allows the vaginal organisms to move upward into the uterus.

The symptoms of chorioamnionitis are fever, an increased heart rate in both mother and baby, a tender or painful uterus, and amniotic fluid that has a foul odor. If you are suspected of having this infection, you may need to have laboratory tests for infection, or a test of your amniotic fluid. Antibiotics are used to treat it and are usually continued after delivery as well. Your baby may be delivered early to prevent complications for you, or if your baby is thought to be in danger.

Another serious maternal infection, *postpartum endometritis*, an inflammation of the lining of the uterus, doesn't usually set in until a few days after delivery. It is caused by one of a series of organisms including forms of Strep infections. It occurs in 1 to 3 percent of all deliveries. Mothers are more at risk of having endometritis if they have had a cesarean section or *premature rupture of the membranes* (PROM). Symptoms are fever, a tender uterus, pain in the abdomen, and foul-smelling *lochia* (the discharge after birth).

HIV/AIDS

Women with HIV infection should have their prenatal care supervised by healthcare providers experienced in caring for HIV infected pregnant women. If you have HIV or AIDS, or test positive for it during your pregnancy, your baby will be vulnerable to catching it from you.

Having a vaginal birth puts your baby at a higher risk for catching the virus from you because of the presence of the virus in the secretions inside your birth canal.[44] Taking HIV/AIDS medication during the second half of pregnancy can help to reduce your baby's risk for catching the virus by less than one in one hundred by cutting in half the load of the virus in your body. Having a cesarean section may also help to reduce your baby's risk of contracting the virus.

Should you give birth vaginally, your baby should not have an electrode from an electronic fetal monitor inserted in his scalp or have fetal blood sampling before birth, which increase his risk of infection.

A four-hour IV infusion of zidovudine (AZT, ZVD) just before delivery can further reduce your baby's risk of catching your infection. Your newborn may also be given the drug for the first six weeks starting eight to twelve hours after delivery.

A PCR (polymerase chain reaction) test will be used after birth to tell whether your baby is going to share in your HIV infection. It will be performed three times: during the first week of life, between two weeks and two months, and after four months. If the results of all three tests are negative, the chances of your baby developing HIV is less than three out of one thousand (0.3 percent).

Life-threatening pregnancy complications

Between 1991 and 1999, 4,200 deaths were found to be pregnancy-related. In 1999, 525 mothers died during or after pregnancy from pregnancy-related complications according to the Centers for Disease Control and Prevention. This becomes a ratio of about 12 pregnancy-related deaths occurring for every 100,000 live births.

An analysis of maternal deaths between 1979 and 1972 found *hemorrhage* to be the leading cause of mother's dying (1.6 per 100,000), followed by *embolism* (1.9 per 100,000) and preeclampsia and *eclampsia* (preeclampsia with seizures).[45] Infection and anesthesia-related complications are also associated with maternal deaths.

A major racial disparity has persisted for more than sixty years, with African-American women having three to four times the risk of pregnancy-related death than Caucasian women do. This striking difference in the pregnancy-related mortality ratio is the largest disparity in the area of maternal and child health. The mortality ratio for U.S. African-American women between 1991 and 1999 was 30 per 100,000 live births, compared with 8.1 for Caucasian women.

Here is an explanation of these three leading causes of maternal death:

Preeclampsia and eclampsia

Sometimes pregnant women develop a special form of high blood pressure caused by pregnancy itself. Approximately 10 percent of pregnancies in the U.S. are complicated by pregnancy-related hypertensive disorders known as pregnancy-induced hypertension. Other names are preeclampsia, eclampsia (which is preeclampsia with seizures), or toxemia.

Pregnancy-induced hypertension is a serious body reaction to pregnancy that usually shows up during or after the twentieth to the twenty-fourth week of pregnancy and can become more severe as weeks pass.

This condition of pregnancy called by a number of names: preeclampsia, eclampsia (preeclampsia with seizures), toxemia, or pregnancy-induced hypertension, and they account for about 18 percent of maternal deaths, or about seven hundred women. (See www.preeclampsia.org for more information.)

The symptoms are swelling in the hands, legs, and feet, headache, vision disturbances, high blood pressure, and protein in the urine. Although there have been numerous studies about this condition, there is no known cure, although some medications may keep the condition from worsening. If you're suspected of having preeclampsia, you'll be given careful monitoring to make sure you and your baby are all right. Birth usually, but not always, cures the condition.

Embolism

Sometimes blood clots can form after birth in the deep veins inside a mother's body. A piece of the clot may break off from a vein in a mother's legs or her pelvic area and travel back to her heart, where it is eventually pumped into the arteries of the lung. This is called *pulmonary embolism*, and it is the leading cause of pregnancy-related death, accounting for one out of five deaths (20 percent).

The risk for having this kind of blood clot during pregnancy and after birth is 5.5 times greater than that for non-pregnant women and nine times greater with a cesarean delivery. The risk of blood clots is increased during pregnancy because the weight of the uterus on veins impairs the speed of blood flow from the legs.

A woman with deep vein thrombosis (DVT, or embolism) may have leg pain and feel heat or have swelling in the area where the clot is forming, but she may have no symptoms at all until the clot reaches her lung. When that happens, she may develop a fast heartbeat, shortness of breath, have sharp chest pain that gets worse when she breathes, or she may cough up blood. If the clots are large and block one or two major arteries in the lungs, a mother's blood pressure will plummet, and she may pass out and possibly die from lung or heart failure. Moving around soon after birth is thought to help prevent clots from forming. If you are suspected of having DVT, you may be given special diagnostic tests or medications to help dissolve the clots.

Amniotic fluid embolism (AFE) is a very rare life-threatening event that happens immediately after birth. Seventy-five percent of the time, it occurs with first-time mothers. AFE causes severe collapse of a mother's cardiopulmonary system, and 87 percent of mothers die when it happens. It is thought to be related to a powerful immune reaction in the mother when the blood vessels surrounding her uterus are exposed to amniotic fluid. AFE is estimated to happen in one in eight thousand to one in eighty thousand pregnancies.

Hemorrhage

Hemorrhage, or rapid, massive bleeding, during or after childbirth is also a leading cause of pregnancy-related death in the U.S. and one of the most common reasons mothers die during childbirth. Mothers who have had more than five babies are the most at risk, as are those who have had trouble with hemorrhage in past pregnancies. Hemorrhage is responsible for 17 percent of maternal deaths, or claiming the lives of approximately 365 mothers every year in the U.S., or approximately 8 mothers out of every 100,000.

Postpartum hemorrhage (PPH), a mother's severe bleeding after a baby arrives is defined as losing more than 500 mL of blood after vaginal delivery, and more than 1,000 mL after a cesarean delivery. But measuring how much blood a mother has lost is not a very accurate science. Sometimes, a blood test is the best way to detect the loss. The problem becomes severe and life threatening when a mother loses too much blood too quickly.

The causes of hemorrhage include a weak uterus that fails to contract and close off blood vessels after the placenta is expelled; when the placenta fails to separate from the wall of the uterus; tears in the cervix or vagina during birth; or when a mother's blood has problems thickening around a wound (coagulopathy). Sometimes, medical interventions can contribute to hemorrhage, including induction of labor, or using high doses of oxytocin for more than twenty-four to thirty-six hours.[46]

Mothers are thought to be more at risk when there is placental abruption (the placenta pulling away from the wall of the uterus), placenta previa (the placenta attaching in front of the opening of the uterus, which impedes birth), polyhydramnios (having too much amniotic fluid), prolonged labor, precipitant labor, difficult forceps delivery, prolonged oxytocin administration, and breech birth.

If you hemorrhage, your healthcare provider will immediately begin to administer fluids through IVs.

Your blood may be sent to the lab for typing and cross matching and to determine your blood-clotting speed (coagulation). You may be given packed red blood cells or whole blood. If your uterus has failed to contract, you may be massaged or given oxytocin or other drugs to help it contract.

If parts of your placenta have been retained, your caregiver may try to remove them by exploring the uterus with a swab or by hand, or surgery may be required. If you've been cut during a c-section, have a wound, or your uterus has turned inside out or ruptured, then you may require emergency surgery. In some cases, your uterus may be packed or a saline-filled balloon inserted to help the uterus seal off. Severe hemorrhage that can't be controlled may require that the uterus be surgically removed (a hysterectomy).

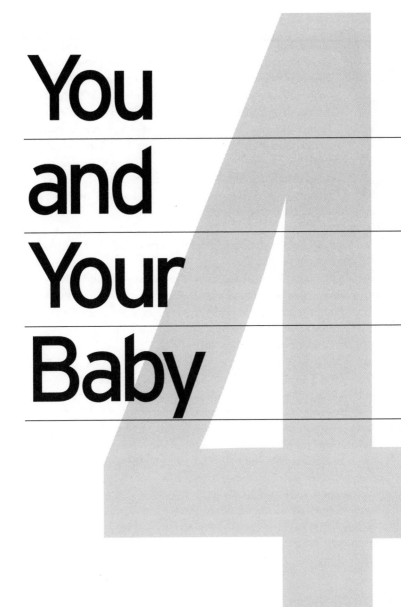

You
and
Your
Baby

You made it! Your labor is over, you've given birth, and now it's time to return home to start recovering and exploring life with your new baby. During the nine months of your pregnancy, your every physical shift was carefully monitored by your healthcare provider who stood by to reassure you that your fears, cravings, aches, pains, and mood swings were all normal.

Now that your baby has arrived, you may find yourself vying for attention with your new child. Most likely you are awed by this tiny, soft, sweet-smelling creature who has entered your life, but you may also find yourself struggling about what to do (or not to do) when it comes to the stresses of baby care and your own body pains.

As you'll soon discover, getting over childbirth and coping with a newborn is quite challenging, but very do-able.

This section of our book covers the span of time between your arrival home with your new baby and the six months that follow. We offer detailed descriptions of how pregnancy and birth recovery feel; suggestions for coping with post-pregnancy aches and pains, and practical tips on how to feed, dress, bathe, and understand your newborn.

This part of the book is divided into two distinct sections.

Section 1: **Your Complete Mother's Manual** is just what it says— a total guide to help you adapt to becoming a new mother and to help you as your body recovers from pregnancy and birth. Section 2: **Your Baby Care Guide** gives you all you need to know to make it through the first six months of caring for your baby.

If you're reading this while you're still pregnant, all the better. It will help you think ahead about the new-mother experience, especially about getting the help and support you're going to need.

Your Complete Mother's Manual

Having successfully gotten your baby out is a great feeling, but it can also be shocking. For most mothers, the postpartum weeks feel more like baby boot camp than those beaming diaper commercials. When the initial feelings of celebration, relief, and joy begin to fade, most mothers crash. The heaviness of the around-the-clock responsibility for their babies begins to exert its weight.

Face it: In Babyland, there is no *normal*. The only language spoken here is crying (sometimes your baby's, and sometimes yours). As you wade through feeding, diapering, burping, rocking, sleeping, feeding, *ad exhaustium*, clocks are useless and only make you aware of how much sleep you're *not* getting. You find yourself falling deeply, exhaustedly to sleep, only to be

roused again an hour or so later. Even when you do sleep, it's not the kind of sleep you're accustomed to. It's as though a fog has slipped over reality—two days seem like two weeks.

Part of the reason for your newborn's continual waking up is that his stomach is so small. He needs nourishment every few hours day and night just to thrive. An overly sluggish baby who doesn't awaken his parents very much and allows them luxurious hours of sleep is far more of a concern to healthcare providers than one who demands his meals day and night.

While some babies "settle" into day/night routines during the first few weeks following birth, it's perfectly normal for settling to not happen until eight to twelve weeks of age. Newborns typically awaken every few hours day and night for a total of about sixteen hours of sleep in a twenty-four-hour period.

Most new parents finally figure out that it is better to "let sleeping dogs lie," that is: to not wake a baby out of concern that he's got a wet diaper, or that he's too cold and should be dressed in something warmer, or because you think he needs to eat. Some babies are sluggish in the first few days, especially if they had a difficult delivery.

As long as your baby gets nourishment eight to twelve times in twenty-four hours, there's no need to worry. Most babies will teach their parents in no uncertain terms with a whimper or a scream if they're hungry, uncomfortable, or just need to be held and comforted.

Remember too, that all babies should be placed on their backs for sleep. Recent research has shown that doing so can lessen the risk of your baby dying from Sudden Infant Death Syndrome (SIDS). You should also keep suffocating sheets, blankets, pillows or stuffed toys away from his face.

> *"Even when I can sleep, I can't sleep. My mind races ahead to all that I didn't get done today, and I lie awake anticipating the next baby call."*

Until your baby sleeps more and becomes more predictable (which usually happens before the first three months are up), you're likely to be bleary-eyed, irritable, and praying for at least four straight hours of sleep just to stay functional. It's no surprise that sleep will now become the most precious commodity in your home, and it will seem more luxurious than lying on the beach in the Bahamas. (More about baby sleep on pages 391–393.)

If you can, sleep when your baby does. If sleeping during the day is difficult for you, turn the bedroom clock to the wall, and unplug the phone. Then, try tricking your body by pulling down the shades and rolling into bed with your nightgown on. The hours of your baby's nighttime sleep will gradually increase and times of being awake will grow. When that happens, most mothers begin to feel that life is getting more "normal."

It's important to not expect too much of yourself for at least the first month of life with baby, or even the first half year, or more. Doing so will only exhaust you, make you crabby, and lower your resistance to illnesses.

If you can't swing a full month for recovery, we suggest spending as long as possible at home nestled in your bed, cuddling with your baby and just snoozing. Turn over the jobs of grocery shopping, meal preparation, washing dishes, laundry, answering the phone, and keeping unwanted guests away to your partner, your relatives, or hired help.

More often than not, it's all the unfinished jobs around the house that make a mother feel overbur-

> *"Who do you turn to at 3:45 a.m. when your newborn is crying, your stitches are throbbing, your nipples are on fire, and your husband has to get up to go to work in a couple of hours? I've never felt so lonely!"*

dened and stressed, not the baby. Stay in your bathrobe. Use paper plates. Microwave frozen dinner entrées. Do just enough laundry and house maintenance to get through. Keep in contact with your employer and try to arrange to stay home from work as long as you can.

But just a reminder: While you're recovering, relax and try to cherish the payoff moments that having a baby in the house brings. There's the almost overwhelming sense of wonder and joy as you peer down upon your sweet-smelling, soft-skinned child with his exquisite fingers and toes, and the tuft of silken hair.

You'll swear your baby smiled at you, even if all the books say it's too early. You'll soon be convinced that your baby is the most beautiful one on earth, and you'll find yourself bursting with pride at having "made him yourself."

POST-BIRTH BODY DISCOMFORTS

During the postpartum period, your body will be undergoing a huge series of changes and making radical hormone adjustments. Most new mothers report feeling exhausted, swollen, sore, and drained for the first few weeks. So don't be surprised if you're not up to planning the big celebration party you so deserve. Even if the birth was uncomplicated, resting

Five Postpartum DON'Ts

Once you and your baby get home, make an appointment with your healthcare provider right away for your first checkup. Usually it happens within the first few weeks after giving birth. You may need to be seen sooner if you develop problems. Until your post-birth appointment, here are the basic five don'ts suggested by most healthcare providers:

1. **Don't try to drive.**

2. **Don't lift anything heavier than your baby.**

3. **Don't try sex before you've healed.**

4. **Don't use douches or tampons.**

5. **Don't do heavy household chores.**

Five Postpartum DO's

1. **Seek support from others.** Having help with the baby can keep post-partum blues at bay—or at least make them less severe. It will provide you with a window of time and energy to sensitively respond to your baby. It will ensure you're eating and getting enough fluids. It will also help you not feel lonely or lost. On the other hand, we would caution you to shield yourself from support that isn't all that "supportive": Postpone demanding houseguests, and put off visitors until you're sure you're up for playing hostess.

2. **Sleep.** Trudging back and forth to the nursery all night long will probably interfere with going back to sleep. Consider a bedside sleeper or bassinet. Have your partner do diaper changing and then bring the baby to you for nursing. Put a changing pad or changing table in your bedroom, and do the diapering there. Install nightlights or very dim bulbs in lamps and down the hall, and leave them on through the night so you won't have to truly "wake up" when baby calls. (More about baby sleep on pages 391–393.)

3. **Eat to energize.** Skipping meals will only drain your energy in the long run. Now's the time to eat like an athlete-in-training. Eat well-balanced meals as often as possible, especially if you're breastfeeding. (It burns calories fast, so you'll feel hungrier than normal.) If you're tempted to snack, make it nutritious foods that really count. This is not the time to count calories, be seduced by the promises of diet pills, or put yourself on a crash diet. Later, there will be time for a solid exercise and nutrition program that will lead to healthy, gradual weight loss.

4. **Drink plenty of water.** Your body will need lots of water and healthy beverages to recover and to keep hydrated. The experts recommend six to eight glasses daily, and if you're nursing, you'll notice your thirst is related to feeding times. (More about hydration on page 381.)

5. **Exercise.** It may seem counterintuitive, but even a simple walk around the block can help you feel less tired. Doing simple stretches, or a brief workout during the day will help you tone up and sleep better at night. But be careful not to overdo it if your recovering body isn't ready yet. Start your *Kegel exercises* (contracting and releasing your vaginal and rectal area) as soon as you can. (See our exercise suggestions starting on page 159, and Kegels discussed on page 35.)

and keeping your baby clean, fed, and comfortable is truly all you should ask of yourself.

Physical recovery from childbirth is gradual. It generally takes about six to eight weeks, or sometimes up to six months if you've had a c-section. And it may take as much as a year to feel as though your "life force" has fully returned. Below are some of the post-pregnancy body changes that could crop up during the first six to eight weeks after giving birth.

- **Hormone changes.** Once your placenta is delivered, your estrogen level plummets and won't return to normal until your first period following birth. Not having estrogen flowing around causes rapid-fire changes in your moods and can put a damper on your sexual interest and drive. It can also make your vaginal lining more delicate and less lubricated. Expect spells of being momentarily weepy or oversensitive, otherwise known as *baby blues*, which sometime play a part in triggering "postpartum depression." (See our discussion on page 371.)

- **Weight changes.** Your body will probably lose about ten pounds during delivery. It will drop another ten or more in the first three weeks after pregnancy. Within two to three weeks, you will likely lose about one-quarter of your pregnancy weight, but after that, your "baby fat" is apt to cling like a half-deflated inner tube around your hips and midsection. Nursing mothers tend to lose up to one and a half pounds a month for the first four to six

months after giving birth, and they continue to lose weight, but more slowly after that. If you are a calorie counter, note that your nursing body will require between 2200–2700 calories a day. If you're active, and eat foods high in nutritional value, your pregnancy weight gain will decrease in a gradual, healthy way. (See exercise on page 157.)

- **Lightheadedness.** Your blood volume that increased twenty percent during pregnancy will return to its normal level within a week after birth. You may temporarily feel lightheaded when you sit up or stand quickly. Drink lots of fluid to help compensate for the rapid decompression going on inside.

- **Sweating.** Sweating after pregnancy is common during the first two to six weeks after birth. It appears to be one strategy your body uses to shed extra fluids. Your kidneys will be working overtime, and that may translate in having to urinate more than usual. Your pores also work overtime to shed the extra water you retained. Breastfeeding also stimulates perspiration. As a result, nursing mothers tend to sweat more than bottle-feeding moms. It's important to keep your fluids coming in to prevent dehydration and to help your kidneys with housecleaning. If you're sweating and have a fever, that's a sign of an infection. Check with your healthcare provider.

- **After pains.** Your uterus begins shrinking right after the placenta is delivered in order to shut off open blood vessels. Within thirty minutes after birth, it reduces to the size of a large grapefruit. It will return to a more normal state within six weeks after birth. In the meantime, especially in the first three to four days after birth, you'll experience what feels like "after contractions," or mild menstrual cramps. Your healthcare provider is the person to suggest the best medication to take for the cramping. Whatever medication is recommended, check to be sure it's safe for nursing mothers if that's what you are, and to follow the instructions about the recommended dose and frequency.

- **Breast discomfort.** Your breasts are likely to become heavier, more tender, and hard during the second to sixth day after birth. This is called engorgement. It's caused by extra blood and lymph fluids and milk building up in your breasts as your milk begins to flow. Engorgement can be particularly uncomfortable if you elect not to nurse, and it can be made worse if your baby's not positioned correctly at your breast. After your baby nurses for a while, your nipples may feel painful and "sunburned" from the stretching and friction of your baby's mouth and tongue action. (We talk about sore nipples on page 410.) You may discover that your unused breast drips milk during a let-down, even if your baby isn't around. These are all normal startup problems that ease once you get into the swing of nursing. (See our discussion of breastfeeding starting on page 408.)

- **Breast changes.** Will your breasts ever be the way they were? For some women, the changes in shape, size, and stretch marks stay around. Others find their breasts became more "normal" after a year or so. As long as you're breastfeeding, your breasts will be full and the same cup size as they were a few days after the baby was born. After you wean, your breasts will gradually lose weight. They'll become flatter, and they may hang lower than they did pre-pregnancy. This "deflation effect" can even make them appear smaller than before. The flop happens to mothers who bottle feed too. Fortunately, the changes may be so subtle that no one notices them but you, especially if you have small breasts. Stretch marks on your breasts will gradually fade to a lighter color, although they may never disappear completely. After you wean, your nipples will return to their normal size and color over time. Your *Montgomery glands*, the white spots on your nipples, will stay enlarged for a while. Eventually they'll shrink, but may remain more visible than before you became pregnant.

- **Sore incision or tear.** If you had a vaginal birth, the area around your vagina and rectum will probably be swollen, distended, and tender for several weeks after birth. If you were given stitches from an episiotomy, have a tear, or had a *cesarean section*, you may have swelling, soreness, scabbing, and possibly bruising where you were cut and sewn. Your sore places could make lifting your baby, changing positions, and going to the bathroom temporarily intense and painful.

- **Achy bones.** If your baby was very large or arrived in an odd position, or your pelvis was very narrow or oddly shaped, your tailbone (coccyx) could have been injured during delivery. There is no way to splint a broken or injured tailbone, so it will simply need time to heal on its own. In the meantime, keep pressure off the bone by lying sideways, or sitting on a hollow pillow. Applying an ice pack on the area during the first twelve to twenty-four hours may help to reduce swelling and pain. If you find the pain unbearable, you may need stronger pain medication, but make sure the drug is baby safe if you're nursing. Some mothers also experience temporary or enduring pelvic pain from a stretched pubic bone. (See *symphysis pubic dysfunction* on page 385.)

- **Vaginal bleeding and discharge.** Lochia is the name for the extremely heavy period-like discharge that starts immediately after birth and stops sometime between four and six weeks. During the first two days after birth, you will be changing one blood-soaked pad after another. Basically, it's the wall of your uterus sloughing off stuff from the placental site so it can grow a new lining. Sometimes the fluid will pool inside and not gush out until you get out of bed and stand up, but don't panic, it's not a sign that you're hemorrhaging. You may experience more flow while you're nursing too, from the hormonal stimulation to your uterus.

Put on a fresh pad before you sit down for a feeding. From the third to the tenth day, the discharge will begin to lessen and turn pink or brown, and finally, it will turn yellow. There may be occasional clots the size of dimes or quarters, but bright red bleeding that requires changing a pad more than once an hour, or clots larger than silver dollars may be a sign of active bleeding. Contact your healthcare provider immediately. Some doctors wipe down the lining of a woman's open uterus during a c-section. If that was done to you, you'll have lighter flow that disappears more quickly than mothers who haven't had it done.

- **Anemia.** Symptoms of anemia may include paleness, tiring easily, breathlessness, rapid heartbeat, and sometimes a headache in the forehead, or between your eyes. Continue to take your prenatal vitamins for the next six months while your body recovers, and talk with your healthcare provider about taking supplemental iron tablets. (Severe headache may also be an aftereffect of an epidural. See page 320.) A severe headache in the first week after birth may be a dangerous symptom of preeclampsia especially when it's accompanied by blurred or double vision. See "preeclampsia," on page 215.)

- **Hemorrhoids.** The pressures of pregnancy and birth can make hemorrhoids (swollen veins around your anus) larger and more uncomfortable, and sometimes they may bleed after a bowel movement. Hard stools are your enemy. (See "Three Ways to Make BM's More Bearable" on page 375.) Practical comforts: a topical cream or suppository supplied by your healthcare provider; sitting in warm water for ten minutes several times a day; and compresses—either using Tucks®, unscented feminine cleansing cloths, or frozen witch hazel–saturated maxi pads. Sleeping on your side may help to relieve hemorrhoid pressure, as can moving around rather than standing or sitting for long periods of time. Eventually most hemorrhoids shrink, and they are likely to completely disappear. (See our discussion of hemorrhoids during pregnancy on page 133.)

- **Hair loss.** Many mothers experience hair loss soon after pregnancy ends. Typically, hair starts falling out about twelve weeks after birth and stops three months later. Hormones during pregnancy keep your scalp from shedding hair as it normally would, which leads to a more luxuriant head of hair. Once your baby is born, hormones shift, and hair loss increases temporarily as hair growth slows down. You may feel as though you've got more hair on your hairbrush than on your head. Consider getting an easy-to-care-for shorter hairstyle, such as a blunt cut that will appear to have more volume. Also take advantage of thickening shampoos, hair gels, and leave-in rinses that will thicken the appearance of your hair.

- **Ovulation and your period.** It makes sense to plan your contraception strategy with your obstetrician as soon as you're ready to resume intercourse. It is possible to ovulate before your period returns, and in very rare cases, mothers have become pregnant before it started again. Breastfeeding your baby may offer some protection from conception during the first six months after birth, but it's not completely failsafe. You're more likely to be protected if you're not supplementing your milk with formula, and if you're nursing your baby on demand at least once every four hours in the daytime and every six hours at night. Whether you breastfeed or bottle feed, your returning period may be different than what you're used to. It may last longer or be shorter than before. Gradually, it will normalize again, but you may discover your menstrual cramps are less painful, or that they've disappeared completely.

THOSE "NEW MOTHER" FEELINGS

You may be surprised at the strength of some of the feelings that creep up after you've gotten back home with your baby. The following are some normal reactions to the post-baby period. Fortunately, all of these feelings are usually temporary.

- **You've "lost" yourself.** Suddenly it feels as though you have no identity of your own.

Comfort Measures for Your Perineum

Go baggy. Avoid tight-fitting jeans or zippered pants. Wear big, comfortable tie-front pants (or even pajama bottoms), or return to maternity jumpers and generously sized muumuus for a while.

Wear fat underwear. Roomy underwear knitted from 100 percent cotton is a must.

Toilet tips. Keep your stitches clean by spraying or pouring warm water over your perineal area following urination. Then gently pat dry from front to back. Use a small footstool to reduce the strain on your stitches, or sit backward on the seat so you're facing the tank top. Some mothers find that urinating in the shower is the most comfortable for them.

Pat, don't rub. Pat, don't wipe, with toilet paper, or better yet, use wipes pre-moistened with witch hazel, or damp, warm washcloths.

Cool down. If you have pain and swelling, apply an ice pack to your perineal area. A bag of loosened frozen peas wrapped in a kitchen towel works, as does applying a maxi-pad that's been doused in witch hazel and frozen.

Pick your seats wisely. If sitting hurts, try an inflatable doughnut-shaped peri pillow available in pharmacies. Some mothers find sitting in a hard chair more comfortable than in a mushy one.

Tuck and hold in. Tense your buttock muscles before you sit down or stand up so that you pull your sore parts in and up. Start your Kegels as soon as possible. (Kegels are discussed on page 35.)

- **Invaded or violated.** Your body doesn't feel like your own anymore. It belonged to your healthcare practitioner and now it belongs to your baby. Couple that with any impersonal treatment you may have received at the hospital, and you may experience weepiness, sadness, or rage. Strong emotions are usually temporary, and your sense of self will return in time.

- **Body image problems.** You thought you'd be slender after the baby was born, but you're not, and you wrestle with feelings of being unattractive, or worry that your breasts or vagina have been ruined forever. Think of all those glamorous movie-star mothers with stretch marks under their gowns! A soft and rounded look can be beautiful. Rest and cope. There will be plenty of time later to get buffed. (See our section on postpartum exercise and nutrition starting on page 381.)

- **Bad advice.** Everyone wants to jump on the bandwagon and give you baby-care advice. You should breastfeed, or you shouldn't breastfeed. You should let your baby cry it out in the crib, or you should never let him cry. All this "noise" can make you feel as though you're being nagged and diminished by friends and relatives. Ignore, or pull out the royal "WE," as in "WE have decided that this is the best way to raise our baby, and WE would appreciate your honoring that."

- **Like a slob.** Your house is a mess; you look like the bride of Frankenstein; your life is going to hell in a handbasket. Relax. You've got years ahead to get yourself and your house in order. Baby time is rare and short, and babies don't stay small long. Enjoy the intimacy and beauty of this moment.

- **Loss of independence.** You feel tied down, as though you'll never again be able to be spontaneous or leave the house on your own to sip coffee and read the paper in the neighborhood café. You will someday. In the meantime, strap your baby to your front, and take a long afternoon walk.

- **Like a failure.** It feels as though your baby's crying is an indictment of your awkward mothering style. Your personal goals have slipped away, and now they loom as impossible. You'll soon get the hang of all this. Funny how old goals recede and don't seem so important anymore.

- **Overwhelmed.** You feel you're in over your head, as though the responsibility of this baby is more than you bargained for. In your fantasies, you dream of going back to your pre-pregnancy days, or you're plagued by scary nightmares of something happening to you or your baby. Acknowledge the powerful change you're undergoing. Be extra kind to yourself: get more rest, eat wonderful foods, take walks, and make appointments for massages and makeovers.

- **Angry and frustrated.** You find yourself mumbling "If this were a paying job, I would have quit a long time ago." You don't want to blame the baby, so you become rejecting and enraged at your partner for the slightest failing. Yes. Babies are demanding, but they're also really worth it. Show your partner how best to help you. Start your own weekly support group with other mothers.

Believe it or not, you will begin to feel normal again, but totally accepting your new role as a mother may take a year or two. By then, your baby will be a little person who can communicate; you'll have your routines down pat; and your personal goals will be back on track. You may even get eight hours of sleep in a row.

Meanwhile, don't back yourself into a corner with your negative thoughts, or try to hold in your feelings. Make an effort to reach out and communicate with friends and family who've already had babies and young children. They'll understand what you're going through and will probably tell you that they felt the same way too.

NEW BABY "BLUES"

Society expects mothers with newborns to express nothing but happy sentiments about parenthood and babies. Yet, 60 to 80 percent of new moms suffer from baby blues, a mild, temporary depression that lasts for hours, a couple of days, or a week, at most.

"Baby blues" are so normal, they're not even classified as a disorder. For most mothers, the blues visit during the first week or two after birth.

While some mothers have only one or two feelings in the list, others experience almost all of them. Then again, a few lucky women don't report feeling unpleasant at all.

Symptoms of the blues include:

- insomnia
- periods of weepiness or sadness
- diminished interest in almost all activities
- difficulty concentrating
- change in appetite

Steps for Dealing with New-mother Feelings

Sometimes trying to cope with a new baby can verge on being overwhelming. Here are our suggestions for keeping yourself in balance.

1. **Recharge your batteries.** Prevent meltdowns before they happen: build at least an hour every day into your routine where you're left alone to do whatever you choose. You may prefer just to sleep, to sit quietly and read a good book, take a long bath, or take a walk around the block.

2. **Reduce other stresses.** Don't consider returning to work until you absolutely must. Stop worrying about your post-baby pounds until a month or two after your baby is weaned. Make use of all the conveniences you can afford: takeout meals, frozen dinner entrées, and extra hired help for the house. Release non-baby worries for a while.

3. **Keep things in perspective.** Remind yourself that you may not be getting much confirmation for the hard work and love you're pouring out right now, but trust in the fact that the work and care you invest now will result in a happier, healthier child later on. You are cementing your relationship with your baby. Hopefully, that will make your child easier to communicate with and more pleasant to be around in the years ahead.

4. **Remember that this is a temporary situation.** Sometimes it may appear that your dreams have been permanently deferred, or that you're stuck forever in a tiresome domestic situation, or that you'll never get the chance to blossom. It is true that you may have to postpone some things for a time to fully respond to your baby, but the experience of motherhood will make you a stronger, smarter, and more "together" person than ever before. Trust us on this: You will still have wonderful life choices in the future. The major difference is that you will have a companion along with you for the ride.

- anxiety

- feeling like you're going crazy

- moodiness and irritability

If your blues don't go away, or you find yourself going into depression, or having more serious emotional problems, see our discussion of postpartum depression, post-traumatic stress disorder, and postpartum psychosis starting on page 386.

Postpartum depression

Ten to twenty percent of moms settle into clinical depression, which has the same symptoms as baby blues, but with bouts that last longer—usually from three to six months after the baby's born, and sometimes as long as a year. Some mothers develop even more serious emotional problems that require psychiatric intervention.

Why are the numbers so high? In part, the depression is thought to be related to the sudden drop in *estrogen* and *progesterone* after birth, and the increase in prolactin, the milk-making hormone that can be sedating. Add to that the possible traumatizing experiences in the hospital that might have made you feel diminished and injured, and the dramatic shift in your reality. It sometimes can feel like taking on a job overnight where you have all of the responsibility and very little control.

Family interaction can affect how you feel too. Women who have negative relationships with their own mothers and those with financial and/or marital problems are at a higher risk of the blues becoming deeper and lasting longer.

Throw in a dose of sleep deprivation, the possible loss of sexual desire, isolation and loneliness, particularly after your partner returns to work, and the lingering physical discomforts following birth, and it's easy to see why mothers sometimes become overwhelmed.

PPD doesn't always happen right after birth. It can occur up to one year after giving birth. Symptoms may be mild or severe. Contact your healthcare provider, and ask for a referral for professional help.

Here are some symptoms:

- overwhelming sadness and uncontrollable crying

- prolonged irritability and moodiness

- nervousness, anxiety, and/or panic attacks

- sluggishness and excessive fatigue

- appetite and sleep disturbances

- confusion and memory loss

- difficulty concentrating and mental confusion

- overly worried, or having no concern for the baby

- crippling feelings of guilt, inadequacy, or worthlessness

- ongoing feelings of hopelessness and helplessness

- fear of harming your baby or yourself

NEW DADS HAVE FEELINGS TOO!

Witnessing someone they love go through the physical pain and bloodiness of childbirth, while at the same time feeling helpless to do anything about it, can feel disempowering and shocking to even the most stable and stalwart of men.

Just as coming home with your new baby can be an emotional and physical upheaval for you, your baby's father is likely to be reeling himself from his own version of post-birth shock and recovery. Both of you need rest and time to process what you've just experienced and to adapt to the new stresses and demands that your baby is putting on the two of you.

To your partner, you probably seem pale, exhausted, teary-eyed, testy, and sometimes incoherent and disoriented. And to you, your once loving and attentive partner may seem withdrawn, aloof, selfish, and not helpful enough.

In the early days of adjusting to a new baby, most fathers have feelings of being left out or abandoned. Pangs of jealousy are normal. The breasts have now been traded to a small and demanding intruder. Although he may not be able to openly express it, he may worry that the baby has permanently usurped his place in your world.

In time, most men adjust to sharing their partners, especially as they begin to fall in love with their babies themselves. New fathers, just as new babies, need affection and reassurance, but you may find yourself resenting having to deliver that when your own energy stores are so depleted. Fortunately, recovery does happen, but it takes time.

At first, many dads have a strong urge to withdraw from the scene for a few hours at a time, just to reassess this powerful life change that's going on. Some dads vacillate between being loving and responsive to their partners and baby and being preoccupied with other thoughts.

Some men are not comfortable in expressing their feelings because it may appear to them as an admission of weakness or failure. The responsibility of being a father can sometimes feel very heavy at first, and some dads secretly panic at the nearly overwhelming sense of responsibility they feel both protecting and providing for their mate and baby.

For some men, the new responsibility of fatherhood translates into a sudden feverish devotion to work, and shouldering more, rather than less, outside responsibilities. That, in turn, may make you feel he's emotionally distant at the very moment when you're feeling the most vulnerable and needy. Here are some practical coping strategies to help you and your baby's dad make it through this powerful transition into parenthood.

- **Encourage your partner to relate to the baby in his own way.** Your baby and his dad have to form their own relationship separate from you, and mothering and fathering styles are usually very different. Your baby is sturdier than you think and perfectly capable of adapting to both. Even though your partner may appear brusque, physical, or loud around the baby, and he may move the baby around in a way that makes you cringe, you'll probably be surprised how readily your baby adapts.

- **Show your partner how to handle the baby.** Some new dads are baby-handling pros based on their family experiences from the past, but many go through an initial awkward phase when it comes to how to manage their own baby. One way to model baby skills without threatening your partner's ego is to simply voice to your baby what you're doing while he's nearby, as in: "Now I'm going to support your little head while I pick you up. Let's keep you covered with a blanket so you won't get cold. I'm going to lower you slowly so you won't think you're falling."

- **Explore new ways to express affection.** It's not unusual for new mothers to lose all sexual interest for a long time following birth. Typically new moms feel "all touched out" by their babies, so what they want more than sex is to be left alone to get a few good hours of sleep. Most couples find it helps to explore other ways of expressing physical affection than sex, such as holding, hugging, giving back scratches, or sharing impromptu events, such as a pizza picnic on the bed.

- **Ask for help in the sleep department.** One of the biggest ways a new dad can help a mom is to share baby care duties so she can rest as she recovers. On the practical level, this translates into offering to fetch the baby

when he cries, diapering and dressing, rocking the baby between feedings, strapping the baby into a soft carrier for walks, and letting the baby sleep on dad's chest when you need time to rest and restore yourself.

- **Divvy up responsibilities.** Most dads are willing to do what they can to help out, but it helps to be clear who's supposed to do what. A list of duties—who's washing the dishes, running loads of laundry, paying the bills, or vacuuming—helps. So does openly expressing gratitude and acknowledging each other's contributions, no matter how small.

- **Recognize that the situation is temporary.** Life changes like a new baby can sometimes bring out the worst in most relationships. It's best to take the longer view of the situation: Babyhood is temporary. And even though the baby may be completely mother-centric at the moment, children alternate attachment to each parent as they grow up, so both of you will have your turns.

- **Make time to mingle with other parents.** Hanging around with other new moms and dads can help parents of babies adjust to their new roles. Experienced fathers and mothers can be a treasure trove of practical coping advice and humor. It helps, too, to see how their helpless babies have grown into more self-reliant toddlers and children. Talking, sharing, and laughing with other couples may be just the release of steam needed to take the pressure off your relationship.

PHYSICAL RECOVERY FROM BIRTH INTERVENTIONS

If you've had tears or an episiotomy, a cut in your perineal area to widen it during birth as the result of a large baby, rapid birth, or to repair a tear, you'll take some time to recover. How much discomfort you'll experience depends on the depth of your cut or wound.

Tears in the perineum are called "third-degree lacerations" when they reach the muscle around your anus, and "fourth degree" when they enter the lining of the rectum. These lacerations can be very painful during recovery, and you may still experience some pain months after giving birth. In addition, about 5 percent of mothers report having *fecal* or *urinary incontinence*, difficulty containing feces, urine, or holding back gas, which can be temporary, or, sometimes more long term.

Stitches to repair tears or episiotomy incisions dissolve on their own in about two weeks, so they won't have to be removed. The scar will start to heal in two to three weeks. In the meantime, you may find going to the bathroom to be an excruciating experience. Some mothers experience itching as their stitches heal, and as the stitches disintegrate, you may find harmless, small particles in your underwear. In the meantime, Dermoplast® spray or Bactine® spray may help to temporarily blunt the pain.

If sitting on the toilet puts "splitting" pressure on your sore spots, try positioning yourself backward on the toilet seat ring so you're facing the tank. A mild pain reliever such as Advil® or Tylenol® may help with pain, but follow your healthcare provider's instructions to the letter for when to take them and how much, since overdosing can be harmful.

Three Ways to Make BMs More Bearable

Here are our tips for making bowel movements less painful when your lower parts are sore and swollen from giving birth, or your hemorrhoids are enlarged and uncomfortable.

Eat fiber-filled foods. Veggies, fruits, and whole grains are nature's way of making stools soft and keeping things moving. Dried plums, prune juice, or bran cereals can help.

Drink more fluids. Sip water throughout the day. It will help with the breastfeeding thirsties that start in the minute you have a letdown. Keep a jug of water or bottled water at arm's length.

Use stool softeners. Hopefully, your healthcare provider will send you home with stool softener in a tablet form. If not, the old standbys—prune juice and milk of magnesia (now in new fruit flavors)—still work. You can turn prune juice into a mock soda by pouring it over ice with seltzer water or any sparkling beverage. Add a touch of lemon or lime, or a sprinkle of almond or cherry flavoring, close your eyes, and pretend.

What's a sitz bath?

Most mothers are sent home with an oval, plastic "sitz bath." We're almost positive that no one actually knows how to use one. All we know is that a sitz bath is designed to rest under, or maybe over, the toilet ring, or maybe on the floor, and is supposed to somehow facilitate soaking your privates in warm water. If, like us, you just don't get it, ask your care provider for advice about taking "sitz baths" in the tub. If you aren't allowed to tub yet, shower instead. Keep yourself clean by using a "peri bottle," which is like a ketchup squeeze-bottle filled with warm water or a cleansing solution, or use a large measuring cup to pour warm water over yourself while toileting. Then pat (don't rub) dry with tissue or a washcloth. Consider buying a stack of cheap, dark-colored washcloths you can throw away for the gentlest patting experience.

HEALING FROM YOUR C-SECTION

Recovery takes longer following a cesarean section than from an uncomplicated vaginal delivery. Recovery will be gradual and generally requires about six months of slow body changes. The first twenty-four to thirty-six hours after your surgery will generally be the most painful and challenging.

There are various ways physicians close the top incision. You may have staples that will be (almost) painlessly removed a few days later, or stitches that will be pulled out after four to five days. More commonly, top stitches are the dissolving kind, and "Steri-Strips™" may be used that can be loosened and peeled off in about ten days with the help of warm water. In total, your incision will take about six weeks to heal.

You will be offered pain medication immediately following your surgery in the form of pills or an injection, or through an IV attached to a pump that you can control by pushing a button (patient-controlled analgesia). You'll also be given pills and instructions to take home. It will help to reduce swelling and may even speed up healing.

Accepting pain medication to use for a while after your c-section is a good idea. It will allow you to rest and build up your strength so you're less tense holding your baby and moving around. Just make sure the painkillers are safe for your baby if you're nursing.

After two to three weeks, most post-cesarean mothers will advance to normal activities with some pain and with reduced energy and stamina. It may take a while for your abdominal muscles to regain their strength and flexibility, so don't expect to spring back right away into normal exercise.

Some healthcare providers recommend not climbing stairs for the first few weeks, more for ensuring you get adequate help and rest rather than from the danger of hurting your stitches. You will also be advised not to drive for two weeks or even longer. Your c-section bruising and stitches could interfere with your reaction time during an emergency situation. Plus, pain medication could affect your alertness.

The stitching of your incision isn't just one layer, but a series of layers underneath your scar. Until the incision area heals, it will be swollen and a bit sticky and may have bruises that change color from blue to brown to yellow over time. Usually, the most painful part of the incision is at the corners.

During healing, you may experience patches of numbness around the scar site, and possibly itching, burning, or odd "pins and needles" sensations. Internal stitches are self-dissolving and will be gone within a couple of weeks. Notify your healthcare practitioner if you develop a fever or your incision site feels hot, is red, remains painful, has pus-like discharge, or swells— all signs of an infection.

Your abdominal muscles were stretched and spread apart to get to your uterus. You will probably feel soreness and pain in your abdominal and pelvic region, similar to the sore feeling of a pulled muscle in your shoulder or calf. That will

"I really worried about how to get the 'Steri-Strips' off my c-section wound. We weren't looking forward to ripping them off. Last night, I got into a warm tub for a soak, and they pulled right off with no problem."

gradually resolve over the period of three to four weeks.

Because your bowel was moved aside to get your baby, and exposed to air and anesthesia, you may experience a slowing down or temporarily stopped bowel function. That can cause painful gas to build up inside, and you may experience sharp belly cramping for the first few days after surgery.

You'll be given instructions about eating and drinking, but it makes sense to limit the volume of liquids and food and to avoid gas-producing foods, such as beans, onions, cabbage, and broccoli. Also avoid carbonated beverages and dairy products that might cause more gas. You may be given medication to help break up the gas or be offered an enema or suppository in the hospital.

Just as with a mother who gives birth vaginally, you will feel cramping from your uterine area as it begins to shrink, and you will have lochia, the afterbirth period. How heavy it is depends upon whether your healthcare provider wiped out your uterus lining before sewing it up, or not. If so, your period will be lighter.

You will also be experiencing the same hormonal changes as mothers who had vaginal deliveries. That means temporary tearfulness, sadness, and mood swings. If your heart was set on having your baby vaginally, you may also experience feelings of remorse or sadness related to undergoing unwanted surgery.

Talk over your feelings with other mothers who've had c-sections in your circle, or visit an online post– c-section bulletin board to find

Symptoms That Shouldn't Be Ignored

If you have any one of these signs, seek the guidance of your healthcare provider:

Excessive bleeding. If you're using more than a pad an hour for bright red blood, or passing clots larger than a ping-pong ball, your uterus could be bleeding. Also report post-birth discharge that lasts longer than six weeks.

Unpleasant-smelling vaginal discharge. Could mean that parts of your placenta didn't come out or that you have an infection.

Fever higher than 100.4°F. A high fever in the weeks that follow childbirth could be a sign of a uterine or strep infection. Or it may signal a breast infection (see next entry). In any case, contact your healthcare provider.

A tender spot, redness, or a sore lump in your breast. If you're breast-feeding, it could be a sign of mastitis, commonly called a "plugged duct," or a breast infection. Often *mastitis* brings a mild fever, and flulike symptoms, such as feeling achy or run down. If you have cracked nipples with pus or blood in your milk, or red streaks that run from the site of the infection back into your breast, you may have a bacterial infection. Your healthcare provider will likely prescribe antibiotics. Your baby will be perfectly safe, and there's no need to stop nursing.

Trouble having a bowel movement. Sometimes, the painkilling drugs used during labor can slow down your colon, but that problem usually resolves itself before you're sent home. Some mothers postpone having a bowel movement simply because they're afraid of the pain. If you go longer than twenty-four hours without a bowel movement, ask your healthcare provider for suggestions on what to do.

Trouble urinating. Your bladder and ureter could have been damaged during delivery. Drink water to make sure you're not dehydrated. If you find you still can't "go," it's serious, and needs attention.

support. You'll discover that most mothers make their peace with the procedure in time. They emphasize that having a healthy baby was the most important outcome.

Expect to not be interested in physical workouts and exercise routines, or even using your new jogging stroller, for six to eight weeks or longer. Most mothers don't find themselves fully recovered and energized until six months have passed.

Remind yourself, too, that each mother's c-section experience is different; so don't feel bad if your friends appear to be recovering more quickly than you. Everyone's body is unique, and you may have had a different birth experience.

For example, if you were wheeled in for a c-section at the last minute, you may be more tired and recover more slowly than a mother whose c-section was performed before labor started or happened early

Pain in the calf of your leg. If you feel tenderness in one of your calf muscles located behind the bone of your lower leg, or if the sore spot is reddened and warm, it could be a sign of a blood clot forming that could be life-threatening if it breaks loose and travels to your lungs or heart. A second cause is *thrombophlebitis*, an inflamed leg vein. Either way, make an urgent call.

Inflamed incisions. If you had stitches in your perineum and the area becomes redder than normal, starts to swell, feels tender to the touch, or there is a foul odor or a discharge from the wound; or if you have a cesarean-section cut that opens, smells bad, is red, or has a discharge, you'll need to be treated right away.

Stomach or uterus pain that doesn't go away. Could be signs of internal bleeding, an infection, or other serious physical problems. Again, make the call.

Swelling. In very rare cases, **preeclampsia** can strike in the first week after birth. Symptoms are excessive swelling, especially in the face and fingers, headache, and blurred vision. If not treated immediately, this malady can lead to seizures and even death. (Note: your headache could also be a reaction to your epidural; see page 320.) See our discussion of eclampsia on page 215.

Breathlessness. Sudden panting not related to exertion could mean you have a clot in your lungs or a heart problem. Or less seriously, it could mean you are having an anxiety attack. Call your healthcare provider.

Severe emotional reactions. It's normal to have feelings of sadness, being afraid, or not being able to cope in the first two weeks after having a baby. If those feelings don't lighten up, and you're sad to the point of not being able to care for your baby, or you find yourself being obsessed with negative thoughts about hurting yourself or your baby, seek professional help right away. (See "New Baby Blues," page 371.)

during labor. You may also have a more demanding baby who's keeping you awake in the night.

YOUR SIX-WEEK CHECKUP

Most care providers schedule a postpartum visit for their patients a few weeks after birth to make sure they're healing properly. Don't hesitate to call or visit your healthcare provider sooner if you have any gnawing questions or things don't seem to be going well for you.

Believe it or not, by this time, you'll probably be well on your way back to your old self—physically, anyway. Your postpartum bleeding will have begun to disappear, and your perineal incisions or any tearing should be healed. Bring your baby along in a carrier if you want to—your care provider and the office staff will be happy to see her!

Your First Exam After Birth

During this exam, your care provider will

• Check your perineal area to make sure any tearing or incisions have healed

• Examine your breasts for any lumps, which may signify a clogged duct

• Check your incision, if you've had a cesarean

• Feel your stomach to make sure that your uterus has returned to its normal size (about the size of a pear)

• Give you the go-ahead to resume exercising (or not). You should ask if you need to restrict or modify your activities for any reason. You may also want to ask your care provider to suggest local postpartum exercise classes.

• Give you the go-ahead to resume sexual activity

• Discuss birth control options with you. We recommend that you not leave your healthcare provider's office without a plan to prevent pregnancy until you feel mentally and physically ready for another child. Remember that many birth control pills aren't recommended for breastfeeding mothers.

Quick Steps for Getting Your Groove Back

Here are some quick fixer-uppers to help you start feeling better about your recovering self:

• **Pamper yourself.** After your month of wearing nothing but a bathrobe, consider a facial, a manicure, or a pedicure. Get a massage. Let someone else care for you—you need to have TLC, too.

• **Buy some new duds.** If you don't have them already, you'll need nursing bras. While you're at it, get roomy drawstring pants and a new pair of comfortable, slip-on walking-around-with-baby shoes. Throw in a colorful soft carrier, like a Baby Bjorn, so your arms are free, and you can exercise and walk with baby. (We discuss baby carriers on page 524.)

• **Fake housecleaning.** If it drives you crazy to have your house in chaos, try just keeping one room clean. That will fake you into believing the whole house is in order. If you have to, hire a teenager, and pay him or her by the hour to do laundry and vacuuming.

• **Rest. Rest. Rest.** Overdoing it during the first weeks after birth can lower your resistance to illness and slow down your recovery.

• **Get out with your baby.** Fresh air, sunshine, other babies and mothers— do anything but stay inside with a pile of dirty dishes in the sink.

Once your exam is over, your yearlong, close relationship with the person who delivered your baby will come to a close. If everything checks out okay, you won't need to see your care provider again until your next annual exam—or ever, if you choose.

NEW MOTHER NUTRITION

After your baby arrives, you'll need excellent nutrition and hydration, just as you did when you were pregnant. This is especially important if you feel tired and drained all the time, or you're recovering from a c-section. The only problem is that you'll probably discover you don't have the energy or the free hands to get up and fix meals for yourself. Carry-out food, meals frozen ahead of time (like stews, lasagna, or quiches), and your partner's (or parents') cooking can be lifesavers.

If you're breastfeeding, simply follow the same nutritional requirements you did during pregnancy (see our suggested foods on page 382), and plan to continue taking your prenatal vitamins for the next six months. Also consider a DHA supplement (discussed on page 152). As during your pregnancy, reduce your intake of heavily sweetened beverages, and sugar-loaded snacks and breads which can cause spikes and drops in your blood sugar. Beware drinks that appear to be "healthy" but list high fructose corn syrup in the top five ingredients.

Breastfeeding or not, eat frequent snacks featuring high-quality protein, such as chicken, turkey, or fish, cottage cheese, beans, or eggs balanced with fiber-rich complex carbohydrates, such as grilled vegetables, brown rice, and whole grain breads, and combine these with small sources for nutritionally useful, monosaturated fats, such as olive oil, nuts, and avocado.

Start eating in the morning as soon as you can after your baby's first feeding, and then continue to nosh your way through the day with small, but potent meals and snacks so that you don't go longer than three hours without food.

If you do take to the kitchen to cook, plan ahead, and prepare a larger-than-usual amount of the dish to create your own frozen entrées from the excess, and store them in meal-size portions for freezing. It helps to use disposable storage containers so you won't add to your pile of dishes waiting to be washed.

Keeping hydrated

There's no evidence that forcing yourself to drink milk or water will increase your milk supply; in fact, drinking too much water (more than twelve glasses a day) can actually make you feel sick and cause "water intoxication," and it can also decrease your milk supply. The routine recommendation is six to eight glasses of water each day, but most of us find that a bit daunting. The better strategy is to sip small portions of water throughout your day, rather than loading up one full glass at a time.

The color of your urine is a simple test of whether you're getting enough fluids or not. It should be pale and barely yellow. Urine that's concentrated and dark, especially

CHECKLIST: Fast Foods for Moms

Effective new-mother eating is mastering the art of eating on the run. Stock up on healthy snacks, and keep them where you can easily grab them in the scant moments you'll have between sleeping, feeding the baby, diapering the baby, bathing the baby, feeding the baby, putting the baby down...well, you get the picture. Here are some quickies to have on hand:

Fruits. Bananas, oranges, berries, grapes, a peeled apple slathered with peanut butter.

Snack-size vegetables. Raw broccoli, cauliflower, carrots, grape-sized tomatoes, roasted green beans, salad in a bag.

Quality carbs. Guacamole dip and whole wheat crackers; a yogurt smoothie made with blended fruit and protein powder; a bowl of fortified cereal with milk topped with frozen strawberries, blueberries, or raspberries; whole wheat crackers topped with cheese; whole wheat toast spread with peanut butter. While you're at it, substitute whole wheat pasta for white; brown rice for white; sweet potatoes for white potatoes.

Easy proteins. Precooked baked chicken fingers; slices of cheese; boiled or scrambled eggs; a sardine sandwich using whole-grain bread; a cup of cottage cheese sprinkled with nuts and fruit; a handful of unsalted almonds or walnuts; fish filets or meatballs painted with olive oil and baked at 400°F for ten to twelve minutes; overnight Crock-Pot specials, such as beef, lamb stew, or chili.

when it is accompanied by hard and dry stools, is a sign that you need to increase your fluid intake and to eat more fiber-rich foods, such as vegetables, fruits, or nuts. But note: It's normal for the first urine of the day to be more concentrated than at any other time. Your prenatal vitamins will probably turn your urine fluorescent yellow.

The easiest way to keep the fluids flowing is to start your morning with ice water in a large jug (the kind sold in convenience stores) with a straw then tote it around, and sip on it wherever you sit to nurse. A second strategy is to invest in a case of bottled water, and station the bottles next to the toilet, on the bedside table, and around the house so there's always water within arm's reach.

GETTING YOUR SHAPE BACK

Your first look at your postpartum body in a full-length mirror can be a scary experience. Put it off for as long as possible if you have body-image issues. You'll be flabby all over, have the waistless figure of a sack of flour, have loose skin and a paunch, wide hips, and possibly stretch marks on your stomach, thighs, and breasts that you didn't notice as much during your pregnancy.

The good news is it's all uphill from here, and you can indeed get your old body back, more or less. You can even become fitter than you were before. The bad news is that it won't happen overnight. It may not happen for a year. The adage about pregnancy weight, "nine months to put it on, nine months to take it off," is more or less true, depending on how much you gained and how fast your metabolism is. In the meantime, it's going to be really hard to squeeze into your favorite pair of jeans without having to lie down and throw your legs up in the air just to get the zipper up.

Even if you've carefully monitored your nutrition during your pregnancy, and your weight gain was a healthy twenty-five–thirty pounds, it will still take some doing to get back into shape.

When it comes to getting enough exercise, build up your energy output gently, and don't make the mistake of trying to do too much too early. Doing so will only discourage you by leaving you exhausted and achy. The easiest way to begin your re-entry into exercise is by doing simple stretches and workouts with various parts of your body, such as leg and arm lifts, shoulder crunches, and neck stretches while you're in the midst of carrying out everyday routines—lifting the baby, vacuuming, watching television, or standing over the sink. Adding weights to your wrists or lifting lightweight barbells can start making a difference in muscle density.

Sitting and moving around on a sturdy, inflated exercise ball (your old "birth ball") can be a wonderful way to loosen your hips and stretch your thighs and legs and strengthen your back. Try varying air pressure to harden or soften the ball until you find the tightness that is the most comfortable.

The back-and-forth motion of walking and rocking, officially known as vestibular stimulation, not only soothes most babies, but is thought to speed up their development. Have fun dancing with your baby to your favorite CD or taking a vigorous afternoon walk with him strapped on your front in a carrier. If it's too hot, too windy, or too cold, do chores and stretches with him attached. Most babies love being fastened to their mothers' bodies, and the carrier will free your hands, balance your baby's weight, and strengthen your legs.

You'll also need a routine of stretching exercises to tone your body to ease out all of the kinks from its adapting to its huge weight burden during pregnancy. Many childbirth education and mothers' groups and gyms offer exercise sessions for mothers with their babies, which is a great opportunity to get out of your den and socialize. It's one way to build a support group and to get great advice from other new moms.

When you're ready to get serious about exerting yourself, then start with three or four exercise sessions per week beginning with brief spurts of ten minutes each and gradually building to thirty-minute stints rigorous enough that you can talk, but not sing.

Joining a postpartum exercise class is a great way to tone up as well as make new friends. You can usually locate a class by making a few telephone calls. Here are some possible sources: your local information and referral source, such as United Way or the public library; your childbirth instructor; a nearby health club, Gymboree®, or the YMCA or YWCA. You may also be able to find yoga classes designed specifically for women with babies.

Make sure your instructor is well trained to work with postpartum women and that the class can accommodate women at different fitness levels. The facility should let you try a class at no charge so you can evaluate whether or not it's for you.

If you don't find a class especially for mothers and babies together, consider joining a gym with excellent child care where the staff will come and find you immediately if the baby starts to cry. You may find that you go to the gym just to take a peaceful shower! You certainly don't need to join a gym to get fit. Invest in a jogging stroller (see page 526) for walks, walk vigorously around the mall, find mother–baby yoga classes in your neighborhood, or put on a postpartum exercise video.

Whatever you do, be especially kind to your feet and joints. You definitely don't need an injury right now. Warm up and stretch for at least five minutes before you start exercising, and cool down for at least five minutes afterward. If you lift weights, never, ever "lock" your arms or knees. Perform all exercises in proper form and alignment, and check your alignment in a mirror, or have someone check your posture for you if you're not sure. Invest in new walking or jogging shoes—your old ones will probably be too small, and the ones you wore during pregnancy may be too big, now that you aren't swollen anymore.

Ab training and your postpartum belly

Some mothers discover they have *diastasis recti,* a separation of the long muscle that runs down the center of the abdomen. While some mothers discover they have it during pregnancy (see our discussion on page 593), others don't find out until after birth. It happens to mothers whether they deliver their babies vaginally or with a cesarean section.

Here is a way to tell if your abdominals have separated: Lie on your back with your knees bent and your feet flat on the floor. Gently lift your head and shoulder blades off the floor as though you were hardening your abs. Place the fingers of one hand on the abdomen underneath your belly button. If your recti muscles have spread apart, you'll be able to feel the soft space in the center with hard muscle running from the top down on both sides. If the gap in the center is more than an inch or so, then your muscle has split, a common occurrence during pregnancy, and you may be able to do special exercises to help it come back together.

There are some simple exercises that can help you coax your split "rectis" back together. Lie flat on your back with your knees up and your feet flat on the floor as though you were planning to do ab crunches. Place your fingertips on the center of your belly just below your belly button. Raise your head, exhale, and gently press your fingers toward each other. While you're down on the floor, do simple leg stretches, one side at a time while exhaling.

RARE POSTPARTUM PROBLEMS

Postpartum thyroiditis

All new mothers feel run-down and tired for a while. Approximately 5 to 10 percent (one out of ten to one out of twenty) women are thought to suffer from postpartum thyroiditis, temporary or permanent problems with thyroid functioning. Having thyroid problems can sometimes be an inherited disorder. The thyroid glands become inflamed, not from infection, but from the body's becoming hypersensitive to its own secretions after birth.

The condition may not appear until three, or so, months after birth, and can begin with temporarily having too much thyroid hormone (hyperthyroidism), followed by thyroid depletion (hypothyroidism).

The hyperthyroid stages includes these symptoms: feeling warm, muscle weakness, feeling shaky and tremulous, unexplained anxiety, rapid heartbeat, having trouble concentrating, or sudden weight loss.

The hypothyroid symptoms that come later include tiredness and sluggishness, constipation, memory loss, intolerance of cold weather, muscle cramping, dry skin, feeling of physical weakness, or weight gain.

Talk with your healthcare provider if you suspect your thyroid is acting up. The condition can be detected by special tests, but the condition may heal itself within the first year. If it is severe enough to interfere with your care of your baby or if your thyroid glands fail to begin to readjust, your provider may recommend taking supplemental thyroid hormones.

Symphysis pubic dysfunction (SPD)

Some new mothers suffer prolonged pain after giving birth caused by a gap in the two pubic bones in the front of the pelvis, which normally stretches apart during birth. Sometimes the pain can start before birth in the third trimester from doing exercises that place a lot of strain on this joint, such as using stair-climbing exercise devices.

If you have SPD, the center of the mons pubis, the bony, hairy mound below the belly button will be painful if pressed. You may experience dull pain while walking, and there may also be related pain in the lower back, nearby joints, the groin, or inner thighs. The condition is known as symphysis pubic dysfunction (SPD), or symphyseal separation.

If you have this condition, the pain will get worse when you walk, bear weight (such as carrying your baby), spread your legs, lift one leg, such as during stair climbing, or when you change position in bed. Turning over in bed will be painful. It will be hard to stand on one leg to put on pants. Rarely, a mother may be in such pain that she requires elbow crutches to get around. You may be given pain medication, but if you're breastfeeding, make sure it is safe for your baby. Physical aids, such as a bath seat, a tall stool for "perching," and a grabber that helps in picking things up from the floor may be useful.

While the joint heals, avoid stair climbing, or move up steps sideways. Also avoid squatting or yoga positions that involve separating or spreading the legs. Some mothers tie a band around their thighs for support while dressing. Warm baths and swimming (but without the frog kick) can be soothing. Putting a foam "egg carton" pad on top of your mattress and using soft pillows to support your top leg when you lie on your side can help to make sleeping more comfortable. Physical therapy and deep tissue massage may be useful.

A support belt may be able to temporarily ease discomfort, while gentle stretching exercises may help to strengthen core muscles and help with alignment. High impact exercises such as aerobics and jogging may only increase pain. A physical therapist specializing in pregnancy and postpartum pain may be able to suggest specific exercises.

Post-traumatic stress disorder

Studies show that after childbirth, about three to six percent of women experience post-traumatic stress disorder (PTSD), a condition first recognized in soldiers returning from Vietnam. While one survey found that 33 percent of women who recently gave birth (one out of three) described giving birth as traumatic, you may not need to have a traumatic birth experience to enter into PTSD. The condition is more common in women whose births were complicated or who perceived that their hospitals or care providers had made mistakes during delivery. It is also more apt to happen with women who carried vulnerabilities prior to giving birth, such as a history of emotional, physical, or

sexual abuse. Here are some of the symptoms you may experience:

- feelings of panic when near the site where the birth occurred
- obsessive thoughts about the birth
- feelings of numbness and detachment
- disturbing memories of the birth experience
- nightmares
- flashbacks
- unexplainable sadness, fearfulness, anxiety, or irritability

Not all healthcare providers are aware of PTSD, but if you experience these symptoms, it is important to get help. Your provider may be able to help you find a counselor, such as a psychologist or psychiatrist who is familiar with the disorder. Your treatment may involve one-on-one talk therapy, group therapy, medication, and in some cases, watching videos of similar birthing experiences, or going back over the details of your own experience to help you in processing your experience. The sooner you can work through these feelings, the more energy and attention you will be able to devote to your baby.

Postpartum psychosis

Postpartum psychosis (PPP) is extremely rare, affecting about one-tenth of one percent of new mothers. If you're sane enough to be reading this and wondering if you have it, you don't. Symptoms could come on quickly in the first two to three weeks after birth, or they may be more gradual. A mother's family usually has to pitch in to find the best help for her.

Here are the symptoms:

- delusions (false beliefs; e.g., you think you're the Virgin Mary)

- hallucinations

- refusal to eat

- extreme confusion

- incoherence

- frantic activity

- paranoia

- irrational statements

A woman who is diagnosed with PPP may be hospitalized until she is in stable condition, and then she may continue in therapy afterward. Doctors may prescribe a mood stabilizer or antipsychotic or antidepressant medications to treat the psychosis.

Your Baby Care Guide

The following is a manual for basic care of your baby. It is designed to be read while you're still pregnant in order to help you plan ahead about how to manage the first months of life with your baby.

The first section describes some common characteristics of newborns and addresses some of the most common immediate concerns of new mothers about their newborns: appearance, first basic physical response, crying, and the best place for the baby to sleep.

"Your Baby from Head to Toe" describes your baby's body from top to bottom, offering information on practical baby care and suggestions about when to contact your baby's healthcare provider.

Because adequate nutrition is essential to your baby's health, a special section, entitled "The Complete Guide to Feeding Your Baby," contains all of the information you need to successfully breastfeed or bottle-feed your baby.

Other topics in this chapter include skin care and rashes, how to bathe your baby, common illnesses, immunizations, air travel with your baby, and a discussion about the experience of losing a baby during or soon after birth.

Although we've attempted to cover the most important points of caring for your baby, it's important to discuss any concerns you may have about your baby's health or well-being with your baby's pediatrician or family physician. (How to choose a pediatrician is discussed on pages 57–59.)

YOUR REAL BABY VS. YOUR "DREAM" BABY

Newborns are rarely winsome and beautiful to look at after they're born. If they are, it's usually because they were a little overdue and their cheeks have had time to become pudgy. Babies born by cesarean section will have rounder heads; babies delivered vaginally may have elongated heads.

Remember that the baby models you see on television and on greeting cards are usually pudgy six-month-olds. Typically, a newborn looks splotchy and puffy, with a face like Winston Churchill's in his later days, which is darling in its own way.

Normal body position for a newborn is to hold his arms folded tightly into his chest and his legs drawn up to his belly. His tiny hands will be clasped in tight fists, although he may relax more when sleeping. When the baby cries, his arms and arms and legs may flail outward and then return to the belly with his fists opening and closing.

It's normal to feel a bit awkward about picking up and carrying your newborn. After time and practice, you'll realize that your baby is less fragile and far more resilient than you might have thought. So you needn't treat your baby as though he were a porcelain doll that you might drop and shatter if you're careless, though it is important to support his head, which for about the first six months is much heavier than his neck can support.

Your baby may feel upended and complain if you move him around too quickly. So before you pick him up, get into a calm state by breathing deeply and relaxing all over. Then use slow, deliberate motions that will physically convey to your baby that "all is well."

YOUR BABY'S BASIC BODY LANGUAGE

Reflexes are the physical responses your baby makes when touched in a certain place or way. No one knows for sure why babies are born with the reflexes they have, but all newborns have certain reactions in common.

Rooting, also known as the search reflex, is worth noting: If anything touches your newborn's cheek, he will automatically turn to that side, open his mouth, and extend his tongue in readiness to nurse. This is important to note if you're trying to breastfeed. You

may try to guide your baby to your nipple by touching his cheek, but he'll turn towards the touch of your hand, not the nipple. This is why for a good latch, you need to guide the back of the baby's head, and touch his face only with your nipple.

Rooting also helps to explain why babies become agitated when you try to fasten a hat on them that has a ribbon that touches a cheek, or why they can become upset when their cheeks brush your clothing or the edge of a blanket.

Your baby also has a *dive reflex* that makes them hold their breath under water. That's why underwater birthing can work: the baby's throat will shut down for about half of a minute until he reaches the surface. They also have a swimming reflex: When placed in water on his tummy, he'll move his arms and legs in a swimming motion. These reflexes last for about six months.

By four weeks of age, your baby will adopt what's called the **tonic neck reflex**. Most babies sleep on their back at this stage and will spend about 85 percent of that time with their head turned to the extreme right and the other 15 percent of that time with their head turned to the left. About half that time, the arm on the side to which the head is turned stretches out in that direction and the other arm bends upward, like Zorro in a fencing pose. This reflex lasts about four months.

Other reflexes worth noting include:

- The **Babinski reflex**: When you touch the sole of his foot, he spreads his toes.

- The Palmer reflex: When you touch the palm of his hand, he'll grasp your finger.

- The stepping reflex: If you hold him upright on a flat surface, he'll make stepping motions.

- The crawling reflex: When placed on the floor on his tummy, his arms and legs will make crawling motions, even though he won't be able to crawl until about seven months.

- The *Moro reflex*: If he has a sense of not being supported, his arms and legs will flail out.

- The righting reflex: If he is held in an upright position and is tilted, his head will move in the opposite direction to the body tilt.

WHY BABIES CRY

Crying is the only reliable signal that your vulnerable baby has to summon you to the rescue—and what a sound it is! For a new mom, it can be really shocking to discover how that sound can drown out everything else in the world. It is comparable in volume and intensity to the noise of a nearby jackhammer, but there's more to it than the noise level—hearing your baby cry can scramble your brain to the point that it's downright impossible to focus on anything else.

Hearing your baby cry can make your heart race, your blood pressure go up, your palms sweat, and your milk start leaking. If you're driving in the car with your baby and your baby starts to wail, pull over. It's simply not safe for a mom to be

driving with a screaming baby in the car. There's simply nothing that compares to how upsetting and distracting your baby's cry can be.

There's no need to worry that you will spoil your baby by attempting to soothe his cries. The concept of baby spoiling is an old doctor's tale based on the writings of Luther Emmett Holt, a rigid and unlovable physician and author of *The Care and Feeding of Children*, published in 1894. Holt cautioned mothers not to cuddle their babies, as it leads to overstimulation and gives them germs. He told mothers not to pick up crying babies, either, claiming that crying was good for a baby's health and was a form of baby exercise.

Modern-day research has shown that the faster parents respond to their baby's cries, the more easily and rapidly the baby can be quieted. A slow response can triple or quadruple the amount of soothing time required.

Babies whose parents respond consistently and rapidly are more likely to expend their vocal energies in learning how to coo and make other pleasing vocal sounds. On the other hand, babies who have to scream for every meal show slower developmental progress in communication and the nuances of language and sound.

That being said, it's also important to note that most, if not all, babies have periods when they cry for no discernible reason. Some baby experts theorize that babies sometimes simply need time to let off steam, just as some adults do.

If your newborn isn't hungry, but starts screaming, it could be gas pain, uncomfortable clothing, an oncoming cold, or you could have set off his Moro reflex.

Here's what happens: You lower your baby backward too quickly; your baby throws his arms backward into the air with his palms wide open, then he clutches forward with flailing arms as if reaching for something. Then comes a deep gasp and screams of terror. Basically, his body is telling him he's being dropped, and he had better grab onto something quickly or fall.

If you're diapering him or putting him in the crib, lower him slowly backward and downward while securely supporting his head and neck, keeping him covered all the while.

If your baby cries excessively for hours on end, day after day, he may be expressing pain, or he may be labeled as having *colic*, a broad term used for the one out of five babies who scream their way through their first months of life with no explainable cause. (See our discussion of colic on page 425–429.)

SLEEP TIGHT, BABY, *PLEASE*?

As you will discover, babies make a lot of weird noises when they sleep, from snorting to whimpering, and they may even appear to smile. Sometimes their bodies jerk. That means the baby is in REM (rapid eye movement) sleep, which babies do more than children or adults.

A typical newborn sleeps for about 16½ hours a day. Unfortunately, those sleeping hours are not all grouped together,

but are broken up into small irregular units of sleep and wakefulness.

Rarely do babies sleep through the night right from birth. In fact, if they do, their healthcare providers will be concerned that the babies are too sluggish—not a good sign—and not receiving adequate, regular nourishment sufficient to thrive. A healthy "sleeping through the night" for a newborn is about five hours. More than six hours may be a cause for concern, and you should notify your pediatrician.

Newborns typically sleep for one- to two-hour spans with more frequent waking at night than in the daytime. Occasionally, sleeping hours will double up, causing parents to race to a baby's crib in fear he has perished when they weren't paying attention. The baby will be fine, the parent relieved, and the old pattern of waking up an hour later will return.

When other parents brag that their newborn babies are "sleeping through the night," they're usually embellishing the "through the night" part, and Junior is going to bed at midnight and waking up at 5 a.m.

Regular sleep patterns develop slowly over time for most babies. They usually become more predictable at about three months of age or later. In the meantime, you may feel like a soldier in basic training, slogging through. Work with your partner and any support that you have to make sure that you get at least seven or eight hours of sleep in a twenty-four-hour period, because sleep deprivation can be dangerous and lead to accidents. Driving while sleep-deprived can be as dangerous as driving drunk.

PUTTING BABY DOWN TO SLEEP

Where your baby sleeps at night is purely a personal choice. Some parents elect to tuck their babies into a crib from the very start, which prevents having to transition them into a crib later on but also means stumbling down the hall to the baby's room a few times every night.

Other parents place small cribettes or bassinets in their own bedrooms so they won't have to move as far to tend to their babies' nursing needs and can monitor breathing and sounds to reassure themselves that the baby is all right. (See our discussion of sleeping equipment starting on page 501 of the *Baby Gear Guide.*)

Another group of parents, the so-called "co-sleepers," sleep with the baby in the family bed.

It's estimated that about 13 percent of babies share their parents' beds every night, and 50 percent of babies co-sleep with their parents for at least part of the night.

Advocates of co-sleeping feel that making a baby sleep alone in a crib prohibits parent–baby bonding, and that co-sleeping helps to regulate the baby's sleep patterns, reduces the risk of SIDS (Sudden Infant Death Syndrome), and makes parents be more responsive to their babies' signals.

If you're breastfeeding, your baby will want to nurse about every three hours. In that case crib sleeping means barely an hour or two of sleep in a row for mom, whereas co-sleeping breast-feeders can learn to nurse without opening an eye.

Crib-sleeping advocates claim that sleeping in the adult bed can be dangerous for the child, with the risk of the baby suffocating when a parent rolls over or becoming trapped in gaps in between the headboard and the bed. Parents have a need for privacy, they also argue, and when the parents are ready to reclaim their bed, the baby's transition to sleeping in a crib will be that much more difficult.

Who's right? Everybody.

Co-sleeping pluses

Each type of sleeping arrangement has its own merits. Here are some factors to help you weigh your choices:

It may be more restful. If you're breastfeeding and co-sleeping, you'll soon master the art of breastfeeding while lying down. Eventually you'll be able to do it while hardly waking up at all. So having your baby right next to you can ultimately be a lot more restful than having to get out of bed, turn on the lights, trudge into the baby's room, and sit up to nurse.

Lower risk of SIDS. According to at least one international survey, babies are much less likely to die of SIDS if they co-sleep. Sleeping in the same room with adults is thought to lower babies' risks of SIDS by 20 percent.

The theory is that being close to a parent may help to entrain the newborn about breathing rhythms. Others believe it's because co-sleeping moms are more likely to breastfeed, and breastfed babies are five times less likely to die of SIDS.

U.S. studies, however, appear to show that co-sleeping slightly increases the risk of babies suffocating or strangling in soft bedding. Parents who smoke or go to bed under the influence of drugs or alcohol make co-sleeping equally or slightly more dangerous than crib sleeping for babies.

Co-sleeping minuses

It may interrupt your own sleep. Babies don't sleep peacefully—sometimes they thrash, snort, squeak, and make other sounds or movements. If you or your partner is scared of rolling over on the baby, you may find it hard to sleep comfortably.

By the way, it's hard to roll over on a baby—they'll usually make plenty of noise in protest, and they're pretty lumpy. Rolling-over-on-the-baby deaths are almost always the result of a parent being under the influence of drugs or alcohol.

Less privacy. It's hard to have time, space, and a feeling of privacy and intimacy with a baby between you, and some parents sleep more lightly because they're listening to their babies' noises and breathing patterns.

Baby will have to sleep alone some day. A lot of parents avoid co-sleeping because they don't want their child to get used to the big bed, then have to readjust to sleeping in a crib.

Some healthcare providers suggest that if you choose to co-sleep with your baby and don't wish to do so forever, you should begin putting the baby in the crib at age eight to twelve months, when babies are learning how to put themselves to sleep and have the stomach capacity to sleep for five hours or longer.

Co-sleeping precautions

If you decide to co-sleep with your baby, check your bed and mattress for possible gaps, such as between the mattress and headboard, where a baby's head or body could become caught. If you want to be extra safe, remove your bed's mattress from its springs and place it directly on the floor. Wedge the mattress up against two corner walls. Never co-sleep on a soft surface, such as a waterbed or a couch. Keep blankets, sheets, bedding, and pets away from your baby's face, and keep your baby on his back for sleep. Keep blankets minimal to avoid overheating the baby.

POSITIONING YOUR BABY IN THE CRIB

The best way to position your baby in his crib is with him on his back near the crib's end board, so his feet almost touch it. Make sure there are no soft toys, pillows, or soft bedding in the crib. Tuck in the blanket or sheet at the bottom of the mattress and then fold it so it only comes under his armpits, no higher.

Or instead of using a blanket, you may choose to simply dress your baby in a warm, footed sleeper, or a drawstring "Maggie Simpson" (a nightgown with an enclosed bottom), and forgo extra coverings completely.

During the first few weeks, most newborns need a small cap and some booties, or some type of foot covering if it's chilly. After that, most babies adjust and are comfortable at the same temperatures you are. (For information on how to choose a safe crib, see our *Baby Gear Guide* starting on page 454.)

Your Baby from Head to Toe

This section is designed to give you a quick and logical reference to your baby's body, starting with the big items: his weight, his temperature, and his skin. It will then move from his head downward to discuss various body parts.

WEIGHT

Your baby's weight will probably seem like a big deal to caregivers and relatives. Healthcare providers are concerned about babies who don't weigh enough or who weigh too much.

The average newborn weighs in somewhere between 5 1/2 pounds and 8 3/4 pounds. If your baby doesn't fit into this standard and is smaller or larger than 90 percent of babies his same gestational age, it could be that you and your baby's father are very small or large people, or it may signal a physical problem. (See "When a Baby Is Too Large or Small" on page 407.)

Most babies lose weight after they're born. The loss is usually about 10 percent of birthweight or less and results from the loss of excess body fluid, plus not getting very much to eat until feeding skills are mastered. Within two weeks or sooner, your baby should build back up to his original birth weight.

After that, he will likely gain at a rate of approximately two-thirds of an ounce per day, and grow about one to one-and-a-half inches in length during his first month.

Growth spurts announce themselves with a baby's increased appetite and the strong demand to nurse more frequently. They usually occur when a newborn is seven to ten days old and later at three to six weeks of age.

TEMPERATURE REGULATION

Babies have only primitive mechanisms for maintaining their body temperatures. After all, they've been living for nine months at about 98°F, and suddenly it's at least 25 degrees colder outside. Plus, most babies are bald, which means they lose a lot of heat out of the top of their heads. That's why nurses put tiny caps on them.

A normal temperature for a baby is between 97°F and 100.4°F (36° to 38° Celsius). A temperature higher than that signals your baby has a fever and may have an infection requiring medical attention. (Fever and taking a baby's temperature are discussed on pages 436–438.)

When they're cold, babies will shudder or tighten their arms and legs into a tight ball. You can help to keep your newborn feel more comfortable by not exposing him to drafts or placing him in the blowing air of air-conditioning vents.

Generally, though, after the first few weeks, most babies are comfortable at the same temperatures as adults.

It's important to not overheat or overdress your baby. Use just a light blanket in the summer if you have air conditioning, or a diaper, T-shirt, or "onesie" (an all-in-one T-shirt and diaper cover combined). In the winter, let your baby wear a footed sleeper or a sleep sac to bed and forego a blanket.

SKIN

A newborn's skin is very thin, almost translucent, and changes color with shifts in temperature. It may appear cherry red, mottled, or sometimes bluish or even bruised from his trip down the birth canal.

Your baby will redden all over if he has been crying, if you're changing his diaper and clothes, if he's urinating or straining at a bowel movement.

You may glimpse blue veins underneath his skin that are transporting blood back to his tiny heart and lungs for oxygen. All babies, even if they have dark skin, appear pinkish and fair-skinned at first until the skin's natural pigment develops.

At birth, your baby's skin will probably be coated with streaks of a creamy white substance called vernix, especially in folds and creases. It served as a protective ointment while your baby floated in his mildly salty amniotic bath during your pregnancy. If left alone, the vernix will naturally be absorbed into your baby's skin or get rubbed off.

Science is only now beginning to appreciate the role of this natural cream in protecting newborns from skin infections. It has antibacterial properties that help to protect from infection. Ask your healthcare practitioner if you can gently massage the vernix into the skin of your newborn, rather than having it roughly toweled off by caregivers immediately following birth.

Babies who arrive earlier than expected are often wrinkled because they haven't had time to develop a fatty layer beneath their skins. Some newborns develop peeling skin after birth, especially on their palms and soles, and some are born covered with a downy layer of hair called lanugo on their shoulders, down their backs, and sometimes on their faces, too. It will soon disappear.

A newborn's skin is very sensitive to dryness and may peel and be vulnerable to rashes, particularly if his skin comes in contact with irritants, such as the chemicals and perfumes in detergents used to launder his clothes and sheets or those found in pre-moistened diaper wipes and baby skin products. (See "Skin Rashes" starting on page 431.)

Babies sunburn very quickly, so keep your baby covered and out of direct sunlight, especially between 10 a.m. and 3 p.m. when the sun's rays are the strongest, and use sunscreen on any exposed skin.

During hot weather, use loose, absorbent all-cotton shirts, or dress your baby only in a diaper during hot weather if you don't have air conditioning. Frequent, lukewarm baths also help your baby cool down on extremely warm days after his umbilical stump and circumcision have healed.

Some babies are born with birthmarks, skin discolorations or semi-permanent bumps that generally go away on their own.

Stork bites, sometimes called salmon patches, or angel kisses, are reddish or pink patches that often can be found above a baby's hairline, at the back of his neck, on the eyelids, or between the baby's eyes. They are caused by collections of tiny capillary blood vessels close to the skin that darken when your baby cries. They generally fade within the first two years.

Mongolian spots are large, blue-gray, bruise-like marks, often on the lower back or buttocks, most often found on babies with dark skin. They generally fade over time, although in some cases, they never disappear entirely.

Café-au-lait spots are permanent birthmarks that are light and coffee-colored and usually occur on a baby's torso, arms, or legs, while ***strawberry marks*** are soft, raised marks that will turn red usually at about a month of age. Sometimes strawberry marks grow larger over time, but they almost always disappear before a child reaches age 10.

HEAD

Some babies are born with a full head of hair; others come into the world completely bald. The hair your baby is born with is likely to rub off in patches a few months after birth, and it could grow back a completely different color. Unless your baby's scalp develops scales or a rash, your baby's hair won't require any special brushing or shampooing. (Baby skin rashes are discussed on page 431, and bathing techniques on pages 429–431.)

If you had a vaginal delivery, your baby may have an elongated head from the pressure in the birth canal. This is called molding. After the first few days, his head will return to a more normal, rounded shape.

You will notice two sunken places on your baby's skull. They're called ***fontanels***, or soft spots, and are where the bones of the skull have not yet fused. You will see a diamond-shaped indentation on the top of the head and a smaller triangle-shaped one toward the back of the skull. The soft spot may have a pulse, but the membrane and skin over the fontanels are pretty tough, so you need not worry about it getting punctured. The triangle-shaped one will fuse together first, at between two to twelve weeks of age, while the larger one on the top of the head will close between nine to eighteen months of age.

Parents are now being cautioned to always place their babies on their backs for sleep, a position that helps to reduce the risk of Sudden Infant Death Syndrome (SIDS). (SIDS is discussed in more detail on page 398.)

This on-the-back positioning can cause the back of the heads of some babies to become flattened in appearance. Sometimes babies also flatten one side of their heads by the habitual position they assume in their car seats.

You can help to even out your baby's head shape by gently alternating your baby's head from left to right to center while he sleeps or change his orientation in the crib. His instinct will be to face out towards the room. A "U"-shaped headrest can also be used to support your baby's head while he is

SAFETY WARNING: Shaken Baby Syndrome

A baby's head is large and heavy in relation to his body. Every year, thousands of babies and young children are seriously injured when they are violently shaken, usually because they are crying. One out of four children shaken that way die from internal neck and brain damage and more than 60 percent will suffer permanent, lifetime injuries. Always support your baby's heavy head and vulnerable spine, and warn all family members and babysitters about the dangers of baby shaking.

riding in his car seat. It should be designed specifically for the model of car seat your baby is using, and it should not interfere with the shoulder harnesses that help to safely restrain him in his seat.

It's also important to give your baby lots of "tummy time" when he's awake to strengthen his neck muscles and take pressure off the back of his head.

EYES

You may notice that your newborn's eyes are very sensitive to glare. Shielding his eyes from the lights in the delivery room may encourage him to open his eyes wider to gaze at you.

During the first weeks after birth, newborns don't generally shed tears when they cry. After three to four weeks, your baby's eyes may start to appear glassy and there may be a tear or two when he cries. In time, he will shed copious tears, mostly when crying.

A newborn's eyes can appear puffy and swollen for a day or so, the result of natural fluid accumulation from having lived in the amniotic sac for so long coupled with the pressures of birth. You may also notice red streaks in your baby's eyes

caused by broken blood vessels from birth pressures. All of these eye problems quickly disappear.

Most, but not all, Caucasian babies are born with dark gray-blue eyes. It may take months for your baby's true eye color to emerge.

Many African-American, Asian, and Hispanic babies are born with dark gray-brown eyes that don't change color significantly, but some start out with hazel eyes that darken as they approach six months of age. After six to nine months, your baby's eye color will settle into its natural state, although sometimes blue eyes may turn green after a few years.

While your baby was able to perceive light and dark inside your body, after birth he will temporarily be color-blind except for red tones. Beyond twelve inches from his face, everything will appear blurry—the exact distance for focusing on your face when he's nursing.

Your baby's ability to understand visual signals and to focus his eyes matures rapidly during the first few months of life.

By the time he is six or seven months old, his vision will have sharpened from 20/500 (legal blindness) to 20/50. Then he will be able to recognize you when you walk into the room, tell the difference

SIDS—The Silent Killer

Sudden Infant Death Syndrome (SIDS) is the sudden, unexplained death of a baby who is less than one year of age. SIDS usually occurs when babies are sleeping. For babies less than a year old, it is a leading cause of death after the first month.

The exact cause of SIDS is still unclear, but there are numerous theories about what happens. One is that babies at risk for SIDS have underdeveloped carbon dioxide sensors in their brain that fail to arouse the baby to change positions while sleeping, so the child suffocates. One study found that SIDS babies had different heart rates than those not at risk. It has also been found that babies at risk of SIDS move the muscles of their upper airways in a different way than normal babies. High levels of certain chemicals have been found in the spinal fluids of some babies who have died from SIDS.

Some babies, especially if they were premature or small for gestational age, may have **sleep apnea** which causes them to stop breathing for a while during sleep and then snort themselves awake again. Even healthy, full-term babies can stop breathing for fifteen to twenty seconds with no harm done.

There is no sure way to protect your baby from SIDS, but studies have shown that positioning a baby to sleep on his back, rather than face down on his stomach have significantly reduced the risk of SIDS.

Babies can suffocate in soft bedding, so it is also recommended that you keep soft quilts, stuffed toys, and pillows out of your baby's bed, and that you never put your baby down on a beanbag chair, sofa, waterbed, or couch for sleep.

between day and night, and be able to discern whether objects are close or far away.

Some newborns have eyes that don't appear to work well together. One eye may wander in a different direction than the other, or both eyes may appear crossed.

True crossed eyes are rare in babies. If your baby's eyes are actually crossed, light will not reflect the same way from both eyes. More often, the appearance of crossed eyes is an illusion caused by having a wide bridge between the eyes and thick folds on the upper eyelids.

Most eye alignment problems resolve themselves in the first twelve weeks of life. After the first twelve weeks, if one eye appears crossed or turns outward while the other doesn't, your baby may have weak eye muscles on one side. If after the first four months you suspect your baby's eyes are crossed or not working together, confer with your baby's healthcare provider.

If a visual problem is suspected, your baby may be referred to a vision specialist (ophthalmologist). In rare instances, a baby may be given small glasses to balance the visual input from both eyes so that the brain learns how to process signals evenly, or, more rarely, surgery may be suggested to correct more serious eye coordination problems. (Eye cleaning techniques are discussed on page 431.)

NECK

Your baby's head will appear to be attached almost directly to his chest at first, and as he matures, his neck will begin to elongate.

Some babies have uneven neck muscles that causes them to hold their heads cocked to one side. This is called *torticollis*, and it may result in an oddly shaped head from uneven pressure in the back. It can be caused by the baby's cramped quarters inside the uterus, or it may result from injury during birth.

The shortened neck muscle that pulls the head to one side may seem swollen in the weeks that follow birth, or it may have a small lump the size of an olive. After two or three months, this condition usually resolves on its own.

Sometimes babies develop torticollis following birth from remaining in the same position while sleeping or riding in the car. You can help your baby's shortened neck muscle to lengthen and become more flexible by gently changing his head position during sleep or in his car seat.

NOSE AND BREATHING

A newborn's nose is flat, which helps him to breathe and nurse at the same time, even when a mother's breasts are pillowy and large. Babies' breathing may be noisy even though it is perfectly normal.

While young children normally breathe twenty to thirty times a minute, newborns breathe twice as fast—forty to sixty times a minute. Your baby's breathing will naturally get faster if he has a fever, which is his body's way of trying to cool down.

There are certain signs of infant breathing problems, but these symptoms are normal for a crying baby: flaring the nostrils with each breath; contracting and releasing of the muscles of the neck with each breath with pulling down (sinking) between his ribs while struggling for breath; and the belly moving up and down in an exaggerated way with each breath. If you sense your baby is having serious breathing problems, or his lips become blue around the edges, contact your healthcare provider or 911 immediately. Do not try to feed him anything until you get help.

FACIAL EXPRESSIONS AND HEAD CONTROL

Newborns don't have control of their facial muscles as older babies do. They can grimace and yawn, and there may be spells of hiccuping. (Remember those bounces from inside when you were pregnant?)

Between birth and four weeks of age, most babies are able to briefly gaze at their parents' faces before blinking or dozing off to sleep. You're most likely to elicit this response from your baby if you position him face to face with yourself with about twelve inches of distance between the two of you.

Sometime during that first month, your baby will also master briefly holding his head up when he's in a facedown position lying on his stomach.

You also may notice that your newborn suddenly pauses at the sound of your voice or music, or he may awkwardly turn his head in the direction of your voice as you speak to him, as if he is trying to locate you.

Baby smiles or cooing when you smile, talk, or play with him don't usually appear until between three weeks and two months.

Between five weeks and three months of age, your baby will be able to hold his head up for a long time when lying on his stomach and he may turn himself over, at first by accident and then on purpose, between two and five months of age.

Your baby will gain head control when supported in an upright position sometime between six weeks and four months of age, but he won't be able to sit up on his own without toppling over for several more months after that.

Your baby may laugh and squeal by six weeks to four-and-a-half months of age. Keeping a journal of your baby's emerging body skills and antics could be something you'll treasure in years to come.

HANDS AND FINGERS

You may be able to get your newborn to grasp your finger or a rattle or other object in his tiny fist, but he probably will be oblivious to what you're doing. A baby's toes can grasp too, especially if you elicit the Babinski reflex by gently caressing his arches.

A newborn's grasping skills are probably left over from more primitive times, enabling a baby to cling tightly to the hair of the caregiver who is toting him. A hungry newborn has the power to propel his body toward your breast, and babies also change positions in their cribs by digging their small heels.

Your baby will be able to bring his hands in front of him between six weeks and three-and-a-half months of age, and to grasp a rattle placed in front of him by about two-and-a-half and four-and-a-half months.

Some babies are born with scratchy fingernails. Until you can cut them, baby gowns with fold-over mittens may help to protect baby's face from getting scratched. Use baby-size fingernail clippers, and clip his nails when he's asleep.

To make fingernail cutting easier, sit in a chair with a good light. Position your baby with his back to your chest so that his fingers will be in the same position as your own.

Some parents, afraid of cutting tiny fingers, elect to file the nails with an emory board.

BREASTS

Newborns of both genders may have puffy-looking breasts and can even secrete fluid from their nipples during the first weeks of life. This so-called *witches' milk* is a reaction to the massive dose of hormones babies get near the time of birth. These hormonal effects will disappear in the first few weeks after birth.

UMBILICAL CORD

All during pregnancy, your baby was nourished inside your uterus by the umbilical cord that fastened him to the placenta. When the baby is born, the cord is cut an inch or two out from the baby's body, and it may be bandaged.

The fleshy stump that remains will begin to dry up and darken in the days after birth. In about two to three weeks, it will fall off on its own. You shouldn't tamper with it or try to do anything to make it come off before it's ready. That could cause unnecessary bleeding and could lead to infection.

The best way to prevent infection is to keep the cord clean and dry. Use a cotton swab dipped in warm water to gently wipe away any moist debris and scabbing material that forms next to the belly. Give the cord lots of fresh air by keeping the diaper peeled away from it to help it dry up and heal.

Some babies are born with "outies"—belly buttons that are destined to stick out rather than turning inward. There's nothing you can do about that, so there's no need to fuss or worry. It's futile to use bandages, wraps, or other gimmicks to make it stay inward. They don't work and may irritate your baby's belly.

HIPS

Newborns don't have hipbones with sockets like those of children and adults. The socket for their hipbone is nearly flat, and the head of the hipbone must stay in the right position for the joint to form around it.

About one out of every 100 babies is born with flat hip sockets that may not form correctly as the child matures. Your baby's healthcare provider will check your baby's hips by holding your baby's knees and pressing down on the hipbones and then rotating the bones in their sockets. It's not painful, but if a "clunk" sound is heard, it means that the baby's bone (femur) is not in the appropriate place because the socket is too flat. This condition is called developmental dysplasia of the hip, or DDH.

If your baby is diagnosed as having DDH, an X-ray or ultrasound exam may be recommended in order to determine a course of treatment. It may be as simple as double-diapering your baby, or a special harness to hold your baby's hip in place. In more severe cases, a cast or surgery may be recommended.

GENITALS

Your newborn baby's genitals may be swollen and red from the rush of maternal hormones that your baby experiences as birth nears. Female newborns may also have a whitish vaginal discharge. All will return to normal size and condition in the first few weeks after birth.

If you chose to leave your son uncircumcised, his penis will require no special care. Don't try to pull back your baby's foreskin to clean underneath it. Doing so could damage this sensitive penis area and lead to infection.

Sometime during the early years of your son's life, the foreskin will start to loosen on its own and will retract naturally. Once that happens, your son will be old enough to be shown how to gently wash himself with plain, warm water without soap. Do remember to clean the crease behind your baby's scrotum.

Just as your son's penis does not require a lot of attention to cleanliness rituals, under normal circumstances your infant daughter's vagina does not require extraordinary care either.

Girls form a white substance in the folds of the vagina, called *smegma*, and it's beneficial and necessary. If fecal matter gets into the vaginal folds, wipe from front to back with a warm, damp washcloth or baby wipe, or if the umbilical cord site has healed, dip her bottom in a warm bath.

One important thing to remember about changing your daughter is to always wipe from front to back. Fecal bacteria *(E. coli)* in the urinary tract can lead to painful urinary tract infections in girls of any age. (See our discussion about diapering on page 425, and circumcision on pages 402–406.)

CIRCUMCISION

Circumcision is the surgical removal of the prepuce, the part of the shaft skin of the penis that folds over the glans when the organ is in a flaccid state.

If you choose to have your son circumcised in the hospital, the surgery is typically performed the day after birth, before you leave the hospital. The surgery can also be performed in a private doctor's office, or if you are Jewish, by a mohel who is medically trained to perform circumcisions as a part of a Jewish ceremony known as a bris.

Postponing the circumcision a few days will give your baby a chance to recover from birth. Doing so also enables you to choose who performs the procedure. In many hospitals, whichever medical professional is free at the moment— the pediatrician or obstetrician on duty, or even a resident, performs the procedure. If you elect to have it done before you go home, we strongly suggest you request to personally meet the person who will perform it and that you also ask to send your partner to be with your baby during the procedure.

For a hospital circumcision, a nurse will come by before the procedure to make sure that you've signed the proper consent forms and to pick up your baby. The procedure should only be performed on healthy babies in stable condition. (The pros and cons of circumcision can be found on pages 404–406.)

Your baby's penis may be numbed, using a cream similar to Novocain which is applied to the penis half an hour to an hour before the procedure. This cream, however, is thought to have limited usefulness when extensive tissue trauma occurs, such as during the breaking away of adhesions inside the foreskin or the tightening of the clamp used to hold the skin in place for cutting. A dorsal penile nerve block (DPNB) uses a needle to inject numbing agents around the base of the baby's penis.

A newer method, called a subcutaneous nerve block, injects the painkiller directly into the penile shaft and has been found to be very effective in blocking pain with fewer side effects than other methods. Ask the person who plans to perform circumcision what numbing agents will be used; if none is planned, refuse the procedure.

Your baby will have his diaper taken off, and he will be strapped onto a board, called a "circumstraint," that spreads his legs and covers his body so that only his penis area is exposed.

Since a newborn's *foreskin* is not fully developed and is tight, the doctor will stretch the skin away from the penis head and pull it forward. A metal clamp will be used to capture the skin to hold it in place so that the foreskin can be slit and trimmed away. There may be bleeding following the surgery, usually no more than a drop or two, and the device purposely remains in place long enough for it to stop. Following the surgery, your baby may be fussy and not interested in eating for a few hours. The end of his penis will be red, and after awhile, a yellowish crust may form around the penis head.

Depending upon the procedure used, your baby's penis may have a dressing and gauze on it that will need to be changed when you change the baby's diaper. You'll be given written instructions about what to do. Normally, a baby's circumcision site will heal within eight to ten days. In the meantime, don't bathe him, other than with a washcloth or sponge. You may be instructed to apply a dab of petroleum jelly to the tip of his penis to keep it from sticking to the diaper.

Call your baby's healthcare provider if you see any of these signs of infection: swelling, redness, and a white, yellowish, or greenish discharge resembling pus with a foul odor.

History of circumcision

The practice of circumcision is commonly associated with Semitic religions (Islam, Judaism, and Coptic Christianity), but it predates all of these and has been serving a religious and cultural purpose in societies all around the world for at least four thousand years. Egyptian farmers would ritually offer their foreskins in burnt sacrifices to the god Bes, in exchange for abundance and offspring. The practice also developed independently in various warmer climates around the globe, from the Aztecs and Mayans of South America to the Adnjamatana of South Australia. None of these groups had metal—the cutting was done by a sharp flint and served as a rite of passage for adolescents. In ancient Bedouin tribes, circumcision was part of the wedding ceremony, performed by the bride on the groom.

Circumcision was unheard of by Christians in Europe or America until after 1841, when Queen Victoria's doctor (who had traveled through Africa and the Middle East) advised her to circumcise baby Prince Albert. Victoria did, was happy with the results, and the British royal family has kept the tradition ever since.

In the 1870s, the practice was introduced around America by a physician, Dr. Lewis Sayre, who claimed he cured a boy of paralysis by cutting his foreskin off. Over the next hundred years, circumcision began to catch on in the United States. Today, 65 to 70 percent of males in the U.S. don't have a prepuce, compared with about 15 percent worldwide.

Why is it done today?

Religious Reasons

Judaism

No boy is considered Jewish without a circumcision ceremony—a bris is on par symbolically with Christian baptism. In Judaism, the prepuce is removed on a boy's eighth day of life in a ceremony called a *brit mila* (*bris*), literally, ritual circumcision, followed by a party where the baby is passed around and welcomed. Jewish ritual circumcision is performed by a *mohel*, a specially trained circumciser who may also be a rabbi and/or doctor, in a family ceremony, usually at the parents' house. If you're planning a *bris*, talk to your rabbi to find a qualified and experienced *mohel*, and ask your pediatrician to prescribe an analgesic cream that can be applied to your son's penis beforehand.

Islam

Circumcision isn't mandated by the Qu'ran or required for membership in Islam, but one interpretation of the scripture asserts that when Muhammad was told to follow Abraham, it was implicit that circumcision was part of the deal, as Abraham is famous for circumcising himself at an old age. Muhammad himself, according to narrators, was circumcised and favored the practice for both men and women for aesthetic reasons, saying "circumcision is a tradition for men and an honorable deed for women." In America, most Muslims have it performed at the hospital without ceremony.

Health and hygiene

One in eight boys is circumcised for religious reasons. The remaining parents cite health and hygiene as a motivator. It's true that an uncircumcised penis does need to be kept clean by being washed with water for a few seconds a couple of times a week, or a man will be more at risk for a urinary tract infection. While this is important in hot climates with no running water, it's not as essential in modern cultures today.

There's no evidence that a circumcised penis is healthier than an uncircumcised one. The surgery itself can cause problems, such as pain, bleeding, and more rarely, swelling, and infection, and in 1999, the American Academy of Pediatrics (AAP) issued a policy against the routine circumcision of babies.

The Academy noted that the chance of an uncircumcised baby getting a urinary tract infection as the result of not having circumcision is less than one percent. Circumcised men are thought to have lower instances of penile cancer, but the disease is so rare (about nine in one million) that the benefit doesn't outweigh the risk of a newly circumcised baby having bleeding and contracting an infection as a result of the procedure (one in two hundred to one in five hundred). Babies may also incur lifelong damage to the penis as a result of the accidental cutting off of more than the tiny foreskin, or from infections. There is also an argument that circumcision may reduce the incidence of cervical cancer in the female partners of circumcised males, but research results aren't in agreement on that finding.

Aesthetics

In America, many women are used to, and prefer, the circumcised look, and we can only assume that they assume their son's future girlfriends will too. Some dads worry that their sons will be teased if their looks don't conform to the majority of boys in the locker room. We know that guys with foreskins don't grow up to be social misfits or unable to get dates.

REASONS NOT TO CIRCUMCISE

Ethics

Many parents feel that having cosmetic surgery performed on a child before he is able to consent violates his human rights and the principles of medical ethics. It's impossible to speculate on what your son, when he gets old enough to understand such things, would want. Unfortunately, deciding to let your son decide when he becomes old enough to consent isn't an easy compromise, because for adults, the surgery is much more debilitating, requiring more than a month of bed rest and painkillers.

Not wanting to cause a baby pain

In years past, babies were not given any painkillers for the surgery, though in 1999, the American Academy of Pediatrics began recommending for the first time

that painkillers be given for the surgery. Research demonstrated that newborns circumcised without analgesia showed significant changes in their heart rate, blood pressure, oxygen saturation, and cortisol levels, indicating severe pain. In addition, the circumcision experience appeared to influence the pain responses of babies to immunizations later on. Today, a topical cream called EMLA® is typically applied thirty minutes before the procedure, though it has shown to not be effective during foreskin separation and incision.

According to the most recent research, the best pain-relief method is the penile ring block, where lidocaine is injected into the spaces next to the suspensory ligaments, near the pubic bone. A dorsal block, where lidocaine is injected into the nerve at the base of the penis, is also more effective than topical cream, though it is thought to not be as effective as a ring block. Circumcised boys are fussier, have disturbed sleep patterns, and often have a hard time eating for a day after the procedure.

Loss of sensation

There's no doubt that circumcised men have less sensitive organs. This is what the Victorians liked about it. Until the 1970s, medical textbooks still advocated circumcision as a way to prevent masturbation. Back then, before AIDS changed the national dialogue, masturbation was considered a seriously nasty and shameful thing to do. Circumcision removes twenty thousand nerve endings and 50 to 80 percent of penile skin and makes a callus form on the glans (head) of the penis, which naturally has the sensitivity of the inner eyelid.

Religion

For Christians, Baptism replaced circumcision as a ritual. Saint Paul said, "In [Christ] you were also circumcised, in the putting off of the sinful nature, not with a circumcision done by the hands of men but with the circumcision done by Christ, having been buried with him in baptism and raised with him through your faith in the power of God, who raised him from the dead." Three popes have opposed it, most recently Pius XII in 1952, who said that it was only permissible for specific medical reasons. Nurses at Catholic hospitals nationwide have refused to assist in the procedure.

The practice is condemned in the Book of Mormon and opposed by the Quakers (Religious Society of Friends).

BOWEL MOVEMENTS

Baby bowel movements can change from one day to the next, and can be very different from one baby to another. Most babies will have their first bowel movement, called meconium, soon after they're born. It will be dark, sticky, and tar-like. In the weeks and months that follow, your baby may have a bowel movement eight times a day, or he may not have a bowel movement for days on end. As long as his stools are soft, rather than hard like pellets, everything is probably okay.

How bowel movements look and smell depends upon whether a baby's breastfed or bottle-fed. A breastfed baby's stools are almost liquid (but not the same as diarrhea). They aren't smelly, resemble small curds, and range from mustard yellow to light brown in color, sometimes with small speckled solid pieces that look like mustard seeds. Breastfed babies will pass stools almost every time they nurse. In the early weeks, that may mean as many as eight to ten stools in one day.

A bottle-fed baby's stools are usually green, but they can be yellow to brown. They are usually firmer than a breastfed baby's, similar to thick pudding, and they may change appearance if your baby changes formula brands. The stools will have a stronger, more unpleasant odor than those of a breastfed baby.

Your bottle-fed baby will pass fewer stools than a breastfed baby, too, and the stools will be larger. Stools may change color temporarily if your baby becomes ill, but contact your baby's healthcare provider if they turn bright red, are filled with mucus, are white, bloody, or have a coffee-grind discoloration. (See the discussion of diarrhea on page 439.)

Around four to six weeks of age, your baby's pooping pattern may slow down, and by the time he reaches a year of age, bowel movements and diaper changes will be much less frequent. By that time, breastfed babies will have about four bowel movements a day, while formula-fed babies will have two a day.

Some babies may go three or four days before having a movement and be perfectly normal. If you're concerned that your baby hasn't had a bowel movement in a long time, or the stools are hard, then contact your baby's healthcare provider.

Once your baby begins eating solid food, at about six months, his stool colors will change in response. Stools may be green, orange, yellow, or brown depending upon the foods your baby has eaten. Some foods that the baby can't digest will be passed intact, which can be odd and sometimes surprising to parents. A breastfed baby's stools will likely get firmer as he moves to solid foods, while a formula-fed baby's stools may do just the opposite and become looser.

WHEN A BABY IS TOO SMALL OR TOO LARGE

Babies who are born smaller than normal are called *small for gestational age (SGA)*. That means the baby is smaller than 95 percent of all babies born that same number of weeks of pregnancy.

The baby may be small because he has small parents. But in some cases this small size can signal that the baby did not get adequate nutrition during pregnancy. If poor nutrition is the cause, the baby will be said to have *intrauterine growth retardation (IUGR)*.

IUGR can be caused by chromosomal abnormalities, poor functioning of the placenta, or the mother's illness or smoking during pregnancy. A tiny baby may have trouble breathing and low oxygen or blood sugar levels, or trouble keeping warm, and he may require support in a neonatal intensive care unit (NICU).

Exceptionally small babies are sometimes more vulnerable to breathing problems and other complications, while a larger-than-normal baby may signal a problem with blood sugar levels and need extra feedings to help control the problem.

A baby is labeled as *large for gestational age (LGA)* when he is larger than 95 percent of babies the same gestational age. Some babies may be too large to safely be birthed by their mothers, and a cesarean section may be required.

Most babies are big because their parents are large, too. Besides inheritance, the most common cause of LGA is a mother with diabetes, which causes her to pass high blood sugar levels onto her baby. This causes the baby's body to produce extra insulin, which results in excessive baby weight and size. After delivery, the baby's blood sugar may rapidly drop, which may make the baby fussy, jittery, and ravenous for feeding. A heel prick may be recommended to test the baby's sugar level, and the baby may be given sugar water, or formula, or fed through an intravenous line.

The Complete Guide to Feeding Your Baby

Breastfeeding your baby is one of the best birthday presents you can give him! That's because human breastmilk is more than food—it's a gift of living tissue to your baby that will build his brain and help to protect him from disease.

The American Academy of Pediatrics recommends babies be breastfed for at least twelve months, and thereafter for as long as mother and child desire. If you aren't able to pull that off, every month that you do breastfeed adds to your baby's health.

Mother's milk is powerful. It can transfer immediate and potentially lifesaving benefits to a baby, and it can even build a lifetime buffer zone to help protect from diseases and viruses long after breastfeeding has ended.

There is strong evidence that breastfed babies have fewer cases of severe diarrhea. They have fewer colds and flu bouts and fewer ear and urinary tract infections.

Human milk helps to protect babies from SIDS, juvenile diabetes, some childhood cancers, obesity, allergies, and chronic digestive diseases. As an extra bonus, children who are breastfed appear to have higher intelligence scores (about three to five IQ points) on the average than bottle-fed children.[1]

Breastfeeding isn't just good for babies; it's also good for moms. Immediately after birth, breastfeeding increases the level of oxytocin in a mother's body, which helps to stop blood loss and increase the tone of the uterus. For many mothers, it helps to speed the loss of weight during pregnancy during the early months, and, when babies are solely breastfed, it can offer temporary protection from getting pregnant again, as long as you solely breastfeed your baby and offer no formula (although you shouldn't rely on this). Some studies appear

Six Practical Reasons to Breastfeed Your Baby

1. It's portable: always there, and ready to go.
2. You don't have to mix it, heat it, refrigerate it, or sterilize it.
3. It's free; you don't have to buy formula, bottles, or nipples.
4. It helps you and your baby to bond.
5. You don't have to get out of bed do it.
6. Breastfed baby poop is less smelly.

> *"My nipples were so sore at first I had tears rolling down my cheeks. Fortunately, the pain went away after about four days, and after that there was no discomfort at all."*

to show that it can also help protect a mother from future breast and ovarian cancer.

COMMON WORRIES ABOUT BREASTFEEDING

1. I'm afraid I'll fail.

Many moms who have never breastfed are afraid that they won't succeed, even if they try. They give up quickly before things have time to get started. It can take a while for you and your baby to get used to what you're doing together. In the meantime, you can trust that the same body that grew your baby also knows how to feed him. Plus, there are a lot of well-trained people who want to help you succeed, including the nurses at the hospital, lactation consultants whom you can hire, and volunteer leaders from La Leche League International who offer mothers advice, sometimes available around the clock, at no charge. (See the *Resource Guide* on page 538).

2. I'm worried that my breasts won't make enough milk for my baby.

Very few mothers have problems producing adequate milk for their babies. Women with large breasts may be able to store more milk, but women with small breasts produce milk equally as well during nursing times.

The best way to make sure you have enough milk is to let your baby nurse whenever he wants to, day or night. Most newborns need to nurse about eight or nine times in a twenty-four-hour period.

Don't worry about baby weight: All lose weight during the first three to four days after birth and start gaining within ten days to two weeks. After the first three to four days of nursing, your baby should be having about five to six wet diapers and three to five soiled diapers a day, a sure sign that the milk is working.

At two weeks of age, about the same time your breasts start to get smaller, you can expect your baby to go through a temporary period where he seems to want to nurse all the time. This is called a growth spurt; it's normal and not a sign that your breasts are failing their jobs. It's just your baby's way of building up your milk supply so he can start growing more.

3. I'm embarrassed to expose my breasts in front of others.

Breastfeeding doesn't have to be embarrassing. It won't take long to figure out how to use a big T-shirt, a large scarf, or special nursing shirts with side vents to cover your front while your baby nurses, so no one is the wiser about what's going on under there.

4. *Help!* My nipples hurt!

If your nipples hurt when you nurse in the early days, you may feel discouraged and find yourself dreading nursing. Nipple pain peaks during the first week of nursing and then goes away about a week later. The pain is the sharpest in the first few sucks, and then the moisture of the milk makes it more bearable. Once your breasts have adjusted, the pain goes away, as long as you have a good feeding position, and it's smooth sailing after that. If nipple soreness doesn't go away, don't give up on breastfeeding just yet. Contact your healthcare provider or a lactation consultant for help.

Cures for Sore Nipples

The friction of your baby's nursing may cause your nipples to feel sunburned. Sometimes nipple soreness may get even more painful than that, and your nipples may develop scabs or bleed slightly. There are several things you can do:

Check your position. Change your nursing position often. Your baby should be well supported at breast height with the baby's whole body against your stomach and chest. His head should be cocked upward, with his nose turned upward so his lower lips and chin are the first parts to contact your breast. Most of the dark ring around your nipple should be stuffed into his mouth with his chin pressed upward against your breast. (See positioning suggestions on page 412.)

Infection protection. Apply a thin layer of antibiotic ointment, such as Polysporin® after each feeding to help reduce infection.

Start the milk early. Once your milk has come in, wash your hands, try to relax, and express some milk so that your milk is already flowing when the baby latches on.

Avoid harsh cleaning. Use only water, not soap, to clean your nipples.

Cure with breastmilk. Apply your own milk to your nipples after nursing, and allow them to air dry. Human milk has antibacterial properties that can help your nipples to heal.

Use a lubricant. Apply USP-modified lanolin, such as Lansinoh to soothe your nipples between feedings.

Wear absorbent materials. Avoid bras or breast pads with synthetic fabrics or plastic liners.

Try tea. Apply warm, wet black tea bags as a compress. They contain tannin, which soothes the skin.

Get help. Persistent or toe-curling pain may mean you've got an infection. If your nipples are cherry red, you may have thrush, a yeast infection that causes sore, cracked nipples. Your healthcare provider will recommend medications, such as an antibiotic or antifungal ointment.

Six Tips for Breastfeeding Success

1. Get help. Study a few good breastfeeding books in advance or attend La Leche League meetings while you're still pregnant to learn how to breastfeed. After birth, request the help of a lactation consultant or an experienced labor and delivery nurse. Call the on-duty La Leche League leader to coach you through your first nursing experiences or if you encounter problems.

2. Start right away after birth. Breastfeed as soon as possible after birth, ideally immediately or within at least the first two hours.

3. Keep your baby with you. Room in with your baby in the hospital. Get others to help you put your baby to your breast if your stitches are sore.

4. Don't give your baby formula. Newborns sometimes have "nipple confusion" that makes it hard for them to adapt to breastfeeding after they've been introduced to an artificial nipple and become used to nursing from a bottle. (See our discussion about formula and breastfeeding on page 416.)

5. Feed your baby whenever he wants. Your baby will let you know when he needs to nurse. Don't try to schedule your baby.

6. Breastfeed a lot and without time limits. Newborns need to nurse eight to twelve times every twenty-four hours.

They may suggest for the first weeks that you try taking low doses of acetaminophen, biting on a teether or pacifier, or distracting yourself with a magazine or network television until the pain eases.

5. I don't want to be trapped. It's true that if you breastfeed, you shouldn't supplement your own milk supply with formula. This means that either you or the milk that you've pumped need to be available for the baby at all times. Pumping will let you get out of the house for more than an hour at a time, but still, the burden of feeding the baby is undeniably solely on you.

GETTING STARTED WITH BREASTFEEDING

Your nipple and areola, the dark circle that goes around your nipple, are the perfect shape for fitting between the gums and into the mouth and palate of your baby when he nurses.

Your breasts have muscles that enable the nipple to stand up and harden when they're stimulated, so your baby can grasp on for nursing. When your milk begins to flow, you will discover that your nipple doesn't have just a single hole in the center but a series of five to ten pores that project the milk outward.

Breastfeeding Technique

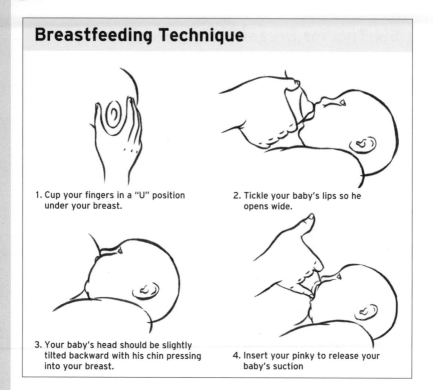

1. Cup your fingers in a "U" position under your breast.

2. Tickle your baby's lips so he opens wide.

3. Your baby's head should be slightly tilted backward with his chin pressing into your breast.

4. Insert your pinky to release your baby's suction

How you position yourself and your baby for nursing can make the difference between success and frustration for both you and your baby.

A newborn is a heavy weight to hold for long periods of nursing. Use every pillow you can find to support your back, your arms, and even under your knees. A "Boppy®"— a firm, doughnut-shaped cushion available in many baby stores—is useful for the early days of nursing.

Pay attention to how your baby is positioned as you get ready to nurse. Your baby's whole body should be aligned facing yours with his face and head aimed straight toward the breast, rather than his body being turned to the side.

If you nurse lying down on your side, your baby should be on his side too, so his body is aligned face-to-

face with yours. Let the baby's head rest on the bed or on your arm. To change sides, pick up your baby, and hold him to your chest, and roll the two of you over together.

There are a few tricks of the trade that mothers pass on to one another. During the early days of nursing, you can help your baby grasp your breast by cupping your fingers in a "U" shape around your breast. Your thumb should be on the outside, your forefinger on the inside. Keep your fingers off your areola, and squeeze your fingers toward each other so your breast gets longer.

Pressing backward toward your chest with your fingers will make your nipple stick out even further.

Once you've mastered the hand tricks, tuck your baby in your arm so his head is above the crease in your elbow. Face his body and head toward you. Using your opposite hand, squeeze your breast into a cone shape, and move your fingers back and forth so your nipple tickles your baby's lips. Wait for your baby to open his mouth wide. Then, bring your baby toward your chin first rather than nose first, so his mouth is at nipple level.

If you're having problems getting your baby interested in nursing, try spreading a little colostrum, the fluid that is secreted by a new mother's breast, on the tip of your nipple. A baby bonds to the smell of his own mother's breast, so don't put cream or other substances on them until breastfeeding is well established.

When you bring your baby in for nursing, his head should be slightly tilted backward with his chin pressed into your breast tissue. The concept is to have your baby take in as much of your areola as he can. There should be more areola in his bottom jaw area than in the top of his mouth. If your baby's chin is tilted too far downward, it will make his tonguing action and swallowing harder.

Allow your baby to complete nursing on one side before moving him to the other. You'll know when he's had enough because his sucking will slow down and he'll relax and start to snooze.

You may be surprised at what a strong vacuum hold your baby has on your breast.

To take your baby off the breast, press down on the areola part that's near your baby's mouth, pull down on your baby's chin, or insert your pinky finger in the corner of the baby's mouth. Don't attempt to pull the baby off your breast without breaking the suction seal.

"I found that a bunch of bed pillows tucked around me worked well for the baby's nursing after my c-section. It was challenging at first, but once I got the hang of it, it was a lot easier and less work than trying to bottle-feed; plus, my baby could go wherever I went with no hassle."

Alternate breasts with each feeding so one breast won't become larger than the other, and don't try to change breasts midstream in the hope that it will keep your nipples from being sore. It won't.

Waiting to change breasts until your baby has totally nursed all he can from the starting side will ensure he's getting the important milk fat, called hindmilk, that comes at the end.

A football hold is a good alternative way of holding your baby if you've had a cesarean and your lower belly hurts. Tuck the baby underneath your arm on one side, so his body goes around the side of your rib cage. Support your baby at breast-height with your hand holding up the base of your baby's head. This position allows you to watch the baby carefully and to control his position better than other positions.

WHEN THE MILK STARTS FLOWING

Breastfeeding your baby soon as possible after birth and frequently when he is awake is especially important for both you and the baby. Nursing will help your uterus to contract back to normal size. It will deliver to your baby important protective factors against infection, and it will keep you from experiencing painful engorgement, which signals your breasts to reduce milk production. So the secret is to let your baby nurse soon, often, and for as long as it takes to empty your breast.

Every baby is unique, and different babies have different nursing patterns. Most newborns latch on and keep sucking for a long time. It's normal for a baby to want to nurse continuously for as long as more than an hour and then to sleep for several more hours before waking up to nurse again. Others will breastfeed for only ten minutes at a time and then sleep for only thirty to forty minutes, then want to nurse again.

Babies are more likely to nurse in the evening and into the wee hours of the morning and less likely to nurse in the middle of the night and early morning. Feedings will be sporadic throughout the day.

It usually takes three to four days after birth for your milk to come in. When it does come in, it may feel like a warm rush of fluid that fills up your breast, and you may have leaking out of the breast that isn't being nursed.

Until your milk arrives, your baby won't be drinking milk but small amounts of colostrum, a nutrient-rich liquid that is yellow or golden in color. It has high concentrations of protein, nutrients, and immune agents to protect your baby from infection.

The most important way to get your milk copiously flowing is to allow your baby to nurse a lot starting right away after birth, preferably within two hours, and then, once your milk comes in, to let your baby stay latched onto your breast long enough so it gets completely emptied.

Your Baby's Basic Feeding Signals

There are several ways to tell your baby's hungry. Your baby will turn his head back and forth (called rooting) as he searches for your nipple. He may try to suck his hand, make sucking movements with his lips, or open his mouth when you touch his lips. If he gets desperate, he'll start crying.

You can tell when your baby's drinking milk because his jaw motions will become rhythmical, and you'll hear him swallowing or clucking.

You can tell when your baby's full because the rate of his sucking will slow down. He may pull away from your breast and release your nipple. Your baby may look around and seem relaxed or contented, but most babies fall asleep at the breast. Most newborns nurse a little, sleep a little, and then nurse a little more.

When your breasts are emptied of milk, your body understands this as a signal to produce more. The proof of this is that mothers who habitually favor one breast over the other when nursing their babies will serve up copious milk on the favored side and scant milk on the ignored side.

If your newborn is sluggish and sleeps a lot, he may need to be awakened to nurse. Dehydration is rarely a problem for newborns because they come into the world filled with fluids. The symptoms of dehydration are listlessness, sluggishness, dry mouth, a weak cry, only one or no wet diaper a day, and fever.

You will reach your maximum milk-making capacity within a month after your baby is born. After that, your baby's need for milk doesn't increase. In fact, it will gradually decrease when you introduce solids around five to six months of age. Your body will change the protein balance in your milk to suit your growing baby's needs.

During your baby's first month, when his stomach and digestive system are still immature, your body will deliver heavier concentrations of whey protein and less of casein-based protein.

As your baby matures, the amount of casein-based protein will increase, while the amount of whey-based protein will decrease. Finally, during the last stages of nursing, the protein ratios are about equal. Infant formula that uses cow's milk, on the other hand, delivers about eighty percent of the casein type of protein, regardless of a baby's stage of development.

> *"I really loved the tender, quiet moments I shared with my baby while nursing. I wouldn't give a million dollars for that tender experience. I think it formed a close bond between my baby and me."*

THINGS THAT AFFECT NURSING

Sometimes your baby's experiences during labor and afterward may affect his ability to nurse. If you've had a c-section or a long and difficult labor, your baby may be sluggish and want to sleep instead of nurse, and his sucking may become weaker too.

If your baby has undergone painful procedures, such as having his heel punctured for a blood test, being given a shot, circumcision, or if he has a sore throat from overly vigorous suctioning at birth, he may refuse to nurse for a while.

Certain pain relievers can affect a baby's nursing behavior. For example, meperidine (Demerol®) used for labor pain has been found to delay and depress a baby's skill at rooting and sucking if it's given to the mother near the time of delivery.

WHY FORMULA AND BREASTFEEDING DON'T MIX

Some mothers who intend to continue breastfeeding may inadvertently wean their baby by feeding him formula in bottles.

One study found that 30 percent of mothers whose babies were given bottles in the hospital later reported severe breastfeeding problems, while less than half of mothers had breastfeeding problems if their babies had *not* been given bottles.[2]

Feeding a baby artificial milk affects his demand for human milk, which in turn initiates the progressive shutting down of a mother's milk-making system. Her breasts become engorged, which causes milk to back up, which signals milk production to slow and then shut down.

Some babies who are less than a month old will completely reject their mothers' breasts after being given bottles. This is because the nipples on bottles can cause *nipple confusion*. The baby adopts an incorrect sucking style and then has trouble changing back to suckling at the breast, which requires an entirely different mouth and jaw action. The same problem can occur with pacifiers. Once a baby has decided to stop nursing, it's hard to coax him back into doing it again, because bottle nipples simply require less work.

Glucose water supplements given in bottles have been found to contribute to babies losing more weight in the early days after birth. Unlike colostrum, water doesn't stimulate the baby's bowels to pass the meconium.

STORING BREASTMILK

After the first four weeks, when your milk supply is well established and your baby has bonded to your breast, you can hand express or pump an extra bottle of milk by using the milk from the opposite breast from the one your baby is nursing on. That will allow your partner to feed your baby while you rest or run an errand. (But remember not to introduce a bottle nipple to your baby in the first month, since it could lead to nipple confusion—having trouble or being unwilling to nurse at the breast.)

Human milk has built-in antibacterial properties that make it keep well. One study even found that after eight days of storage in the refrigerator, some milk samples had fewer bacteria than the day they were expressed.

Breastmilk can be stored in the freezer compartment of your refrigerator for two weeks. If your refrigerator has a separate freezer section, milk can be stored safely for three to four months. It will last for six months or longer if you have a deep freeze that can hold the temperature at a constant of 0°F.

When you're gathering milk to be stored, make sure that your hands are clean, and, if you use a breast pump, that the components and bottles have been washed in hot, soapy water and allowed to air dry.

Milk can be stored in a plastic or glass bottle with the top sealed and screwed on tight, or you can purchase freezer bags designed specifically for milk storage. You can add fresh milk to frozen milk as long as there is less fresh than frozen.

Remember that the milk will expand when it freezes, so allow adequate space. Date the bottles or bags by writing on masking tape with a marker or ballpoint pen. Defrost the milk under warm running water.[3]

SMOKING AND BREASTFEEDING

It's definitely better if you not smoke if you're a breastfeeding mom, because your baby will be exposed to nicotine in your milk.

But if you smoke, don't stop breastfeeding in the belief that formula feeding is safer for your baby. Doing so will deprive your baby of the valuable protective powers of human milk.

Breastfed babies whose mothers smoke are less likely to have acute respiratory illnesses and a lower risk of dying from SIDS than babies whose mothers smoke and feed their babies formula.

If you are unable to give up smoking, but want to breastfeed your baby, here are some hints for how to do that:

- **Smoke for shorter times and less often.** Your baby is very vulnerable to passive, secondhand smoke. Direct exposure to cigarette smoke, whether from you or someone else in your home, increases your baby's chances of getting pneumonia and bronchitis, and dying from SIDS. Step outside to smoke, snuff out the cigarette after an inch or less, and cut down on the number of cigarettes you smoke each day.

- **Smoke after feeding.** It takes approximately an hour and fifteen minutes for nicotine to clear from your body, so try to limit your smoking to immediately following a feeding to allow as much time as you can in between smoking and nursing.

- **Use iodized salt on your food.** Recent research appears to show that smoking reduces the transport of iodine through breastmilk. Iodine is critical for a baby's thyroid hormone formation during pregnancy and the first years of life, and insufficient iodine has been associated with developmental brain damage. Using iodized salt on your food and eating iodine-rich foods like fish may help. (See our practical ideas for giving up your smoking habit on page 21.)

- **Use patches only in the daytime**. If you're trying to stop by using a nicotine skin patch, your baby will get less nicotine than if you smoke. Remove the patch at night when you least need it so your baby will get less nicotine during night feedings. (For more help on stopping smoking, see our suggestions on page 22.)

DRUGS AND BREASTMILK

After birth, let your healthcare provider know that you are breastfeeding. Many drugs have never been licensed for use during lactation. That means manufacturers have not undertaken research to confirm whether or not their drugs are safe for nursing babies. Data may be available on the amount that gets into breastmilk. Simply because trace amounts of a drug show up in a mother's milk does not mean the baby is being harmed.

Most drugs taken by mothers pass to their babies through their milk, but usually it is in very small doses, less than one percent of what the mothers take. Most pain medications are safe to take, and it is usually considered safe to continue breastfeeding when taking most common medications. If there is not enough information on the safety of a specific drug, your caregiver may be able to substitute another drug that will work equally as well.

Your baby's age may be an important factor. A premature baby, for example, may be more vulnerable to even trace amounts of drugs in breastmilk, while an older baby or toddler will have a mature elimination system able to detoxify and get rid of drugs.

Sometimes a mother and her physician may have to weigh a mother's requirement for medication and the slight possibility of side effects for the baby against the excellent immune and health benefits of human milk.

One rule of thumb is that if the drug is available in a formulation for children, then it is likely to be safe for babies.

Your pediatrician is a good place to start when you are exploring whether the drugs you plan to take will be safe for your baby. In addition, there are numerous Web sites that also offer lists of safe and unsafe drugs for babies. La Leche League International can suggest references for more information on breastfeeding and drugs.

WEANING FROM NURSING

As we mentioned earlier, the American Academy of Pediatrics and every major healthcare organization in the world recommends breastfeeding at least for the first year, which can confer huge health benefits on your baby. But the only best answer is how you (and your baby) feel about it.

Experts agree that the best strategy for weaning is gradual and gentle. Stopping too quickly can cause you to experience painful engorgement for a few days, and it may be distressing to your baby. Introducing formula is probably the easiest way to begin weaning. Gradually eliminate one daytime feeding at a time while maintaining the early morning and go-to-sleep feeds in the evening. Finally, you can drop the morning feed and, ultimately, the last feed of the evening.

Rock and hold your baby, and continue the bond of physical closeness even though you're bottlefeeding. Some babies wean themselves around nine months.

BOTTLE-FEEDING BASICS

Most babies can thrive solely on drinking formula for the first half-year or more. Babies' bodies aren't able to absorb straight cow's milk because it doesn't contain the right mix of nutrients and proteins the baby's digestive system needs. For the same reason, skim milk won't work either, and it doesn't contain the fat babies require in order to gain weight and insulate nerve cells in their brains.

Baby formulas continue to improve every year as more is learned about the components of human milk. Modern-day formulas could be called artificial human milk. They're created from homogenized vegetable and animal fats, oils, and skim milk to closely imitate the fatty-acid content of human milk. Liquid formulas may also contain thickening and stabilizing agents for uniform consistency.

Most formulas come in three versions: powdered, ready-to-feed bottles, and concentrated liquid. Powdered is the least expensive, and ready-to-feed bottles are the most expensive. There is really not

How to Turn the Milk Off

If you choose not to nurse your baby after birth, or if you nurse for a while and then decide to stop, expect that you're going to have some pain at first. The best advice is to take it easy and wean slowly. Your breasts will become swollen and hard for two to four days, and you may run a slight fever. The official name for this tightness and congestion is engorgement, and it can be unpleasant, if not painful. Here's how to help ease your discomfort:

• **Bind your breasts for twenty-four to forty-eight hours.** Use an extra-wide elastic (ACE) bandage. Wrap it tightly around your breasts three or four times, and pin it in place. This will compress your breasts and slow down milk-making.

• **Apply ice packs.** Or use a towel-wrapped bag of frozen vegetables for 15 minutes on and 45 minutes off. (If you leave the ice pack on for longer than 15 minutes, it may cause your breasts to swell even more.)

• **Wear a bra.** Wear a supportive bra at all times. A snug sports bra is best, and an underwire is the worst. Avoid extra pressure anywhere on your breast.

• **Don't take a drug to stop the milk.** If you're offered any drug to suppress lactation, refuse it. In 1990, the FDA recommended that lactation-suppression drugs not be prescribed, because they're no more effective than icing and binding and expose women to side effects, including headaches, dizziness, and stroke. Currently, no drug is approved by the FDA to suppress lactation.

• **Keep warmth away from your breasts.** Stand with your back to the shower.

• **Apply cabbage leaves.** An often-used home remedy for breast swelling is to place raw cabbage leaves under the ice pack. Cabbage is thought to have anti-inflammatory properties.

• **Don't express milk.** Though it will relieve the pain temporarily, it'll encourage more milk production.

a difference between the major brands—just make sure that the formula is fortified with iron.

Be careful to follow the formula manufacturer's instructions to the letter when you mix formula. Formula that's too concentrated can put a strain on baby's kidneys. Formula that's too diluted with water can keep your baby from getting critical nutrients.

Only prepare formula in small batches, so that you're sure it's fresh. Keep it refrigerated, or use an ice pack in your diaper bag so it can't spoil. Discard leftover formula rather than serving it a second time. Baby's mouth and saliva can cause the formula to become contaminated with bacteria.

There's no medical reason for heating formula, but babies appear to prefer it at least at body temperature. Most parents opt to immerse baby's bottle in the warm faucet water for a few minutes until it becomes comfortably lukewarm. You can also buy bottle warmers for the same purpose. (Note: Adult fingers and hands aren't sensitive enough to sense heat differences. Always test a sprinkle of the milk on your wrist just to make sure it's not too hot.)

If you use powdered formula and your tap water comes from a well, be sure to have the water tested periodically, especially during hot weather, for the presence of *E. coli* bacteria and other contaminants. You may want to consider investing in a quality water filtration system if you suspect that your water contains nitrates, lead, or other contaminants.

If you want to save money, it helps to let formula companies know that you'd like to be put on their mailing list for samples and money-saving coupons. You can do this by calling their toll-free customer service numbers. Another way to save on formula is to buy it by the carton from baby-discount stores. Just be careful to examine the labels on the cans to be sure that the formula's fresh and the use-by date won't expire before your baby's able to consume all the cans.

In rare instances, a baby may have an allergic reaction to the proteins or sugars in the cow's milk portion of a formula. Rarely, a baby's allergic reaction to formula can be serious—life-threatening vomiting, hives, bloody diapers, poor weight gain, and/or breathing problems.

If a baby is allergic to formula proteins, there are alternative formulas made with soy protein (*not* the soy milk found in health food stores), and more refined, predigested formulas, called protein hydrolysates.

Your baby's healthcare provider may prescribe one of these alternative formulas if your baby shows symptoms of being allergic to regular formulas. Ask about recent research that links soy formulas with an increase in vulnerability to peanut allergies and the way soy could affect your baby's processing of certain minerals.

BOTTLE-FEEDING SUPPLIES

Baby bottles can be found in a variety of shapes and designs. Whatever you opt for, pick one shape and stick to it, because having a drawer of different bottle and nipple sizes to be matched up is enough to drive a parent crazy.

When it comes to cleaning, the simpler the bottle shape, the better. Bottles should be dishwasher safe and come with easy-to-read ounce markings on the side for measuring. The more transparent the bottle, the easier it is to watch what's going on inside. Glass bottles are the easiest to get squeaky clean, but they're also breakable. If you decide to use them, make a mental note not to let your toddler walk around with one.

Angle-necked bottles are the newest baby-bottle inventions. They're designed to keep baby from swallowing too much air, which leads to uncomfortable gas. Angled bottles are more comfortable for parents to hold, especially when a baby's trying to suck out the last dregs of formula. They help by collecting the last of the formula in the nipple so baby isn't sucking half air and half liquid.

> *"I'm really proud of myself for breastfeeding for three months, because honestly I found it very challenging. I felt a lot of pressure from everyone to do it. For myself, I was relieved when she finally went on the bottle."*

Bottles with built-in straws aren't very usable inventions. That's because it's next to impossible to scrub the entire milk residue from the inside of the straw. Also beware bottles shaped like doughnuts, bears, animals, soda bottles, or sports equipment. They're cute, but spoiled milk residues stuck in hard-to-reach nooks could pose a health hazard.

Using a disposable bottle system is another alternative. Usually, you can buy the whole system in a box. It contains bottle-size plastic rings for holding throwaway liners that resemble plastic sandwich bags and special nipples or nipples and plastic rings for securing the liners inside the holders. Once you've used up all the liners in the initial box, you'll have to buy replacements that come in a roll. While the system saves dishwashing hassles, it's a lot more expensive than recycling regular bottles. The bottles aren't all that easy to set up, measure, and fill, and there's always the problem of running out of liners.

All in all, standard, reusable bottles are still the best and most economical solution. You'll also want to buy a baby bottle-brush and a small, plastic cage for holding nipples in the dishwasher, or a drying rack for the bottles if you plan to hand wash them. If your baby's bedroom is upstairs, and your kitchen is downstairs, you may also want to invest in a small refrigerator and a bottle warmer with a thermostat for upstairs.

NIPPLE KNOW-HOW

Babies seem to have their own preferences about the shape and feel of the bottle's nipple. Nipples, like

SAFETY NOTES

Never heat baby's formula in a bottle using a microwave oven.

The formula will heat unevenly and develop hot spots, which can burn baby's mouth. This can also cause disposable bottles to rupture. Instead, use a bottle warmer or immerse the bottle in a bowl of warm water.

Don't prop your baby or the bottle

Some parents believe that the sooner their baby can hold his own bottle and feed himself, the smarter and more independent he is. And every year, another couple somewhere in America invents a contraption for holding a bottle in a baby's mouth so parents don't have to do it. Not only do these less-than-loving contraptions not work, they can also be dangerous if your baby begins to spit up or choke on formula.

bottles, come in a variety of shapes and materials. In addition to the standard nipple, other models are designed for special uses: for premature babies with sucking problems, for pulpy juices, or for feeding toddlers formula thickened with cereal.

So-called orthodontic nipples are elongated, almost hourglass-shaped. Advertisers claim they're better for baby's jaw development, but the center of the nipple is hard to get clean, and if it's made of latex, it may rot over time, causing it to become sticky and interfering with milk flow.

Start first with a standard, newborn-size nipple, and then experiment with other versions if your baby seems confused at feeding time.

Be sure to read the directions for the nipples after you get them home. Some nipples come with special breathing holes on the base to help adjust the amount of milk flow according to how tightly you screw on the plastic bottle ring. All nipples should be boiled about five minutes before using them for the first time to be sure that dust and chemical residues are removed. Note: There is no need to boil or sterilize nipples after the first time.

Most nipples are molded from latex, a form of rubber, or from silicone. Silicone nipples are made from a clear material used widely in the medical world. It's durable and isn't likely to cause allergic reactions. Latex, on the other hand, can cause allergy problems in babies. Latex nipples also tend to rot over time from exposure to saliva and the acids in milk. On the other hand, silicone nipples can rupture and tear if your toddler chews on them, and they're slippery, which may cause difficulty for young babies. Whatever kind you choose, inspect nipples closely every few days for tears or abnormalities, and replace old nipples with new ones every three months or so.

BURPING

While breastfed babies don't need burping very often, bottle-fed babies can get air in their bellies and stop drinking temporarily. The rule of thumb is to burp your newborn about every one to one and one-half ounces of formula.

Remove the bottle from your baby's mouth and sit him upright while patting him gently on the back. Usually that will bring up a big burp along with some milk, and baby will be happy to settle back to drinking.

Another way to bring up air is to place baby up on your shoulder. (Be sure to cover your shoulder with a diaper or towel first.) After a few pats, air usually comes up.

THE DIFFERENCE BETWEEN SPITTING UP AND VOMITING

All babies spit up. Your newborn's stomach is the size of a walnut at birth and it grows to the size of a golf ball by the first three to four weeks of age.

Babies have very immature muscles inside their throat, which makes it difficult to hold milk inside. Most babies spit up during feeding or after they're finished. Spitting up is made worse by a baby's being upset and crying hard before getting fed; eating too fast; or from swallowing air while feeding.

Milk sometimes comes up with an air bubble when a baby burps, and sometimes milk may come out his nose too. Most spitting up usually resolves itself by the fourth to sixth month.

If your baby arches his back and starts to cry before he spits up, if he seems to be in pain when it happens or when you lay him down after a feeding, he may have GERD (which stands for gastroesophageal reflux disease). The milk the baby swallows gets mixed with stomach acids, causing a burning sensation in the baby's throat when the milk comes back up.

If your baby has GERD, you can help him to be more comfortable by keeping him upright for ten to fifteen minutes after eating. Sometimes an infant-only car seat can provide the best angle for the baby.

Just be sure to stay with your baby to make sure the seat isn't tipped over by a pet or sibling, which can be dangerous. Feeding your baby smaller amounts but more often may help to reduce his discomfort, too.

Most problems with spitting up will resolve themselves as your baby matures, but in the meantime, you will need to make sure that your baby doesn't become dehydrated from the loss of fluids. Dry lips are a common sign of dehydration. If it worsens, the inside of the baby's mouth will also become dry, his urine will become stronger and darker, and he will become sluggish with sunken eyes.

Your baby's healthcare provider may suggest a way to thicken your baby's formula to make it stay down better and may explore whether your baby is having an allergic reaction to his formula. If so, a pre-digested version that will be easier for his body to absorb may be suggested.

There are also a variety of medications that can be used to make your baby more comfortable by treating the acid in his stomach; speeding up the emptying of his stomach; and easing throat discomfort.

Projectile vomiting is when large amounts of milk shoot out of your baby's mouth and travel two or three feet or even more for two or more feedings, and your baby seems ill. Contact your baby's healthcare provider right away if your baby is vomiting repeatedly and/or the vomit is red, dark brown, black, or green from bile.

BABY BOTTLE MOUTH

Never put your baby to bed with a bottle. Babies can get an unusual form of tooth decay from being put to bed with a bottle. The acid and sugars in formula and juices pool in the sleeping baby's mouth and begin to erode tooth surfaces. The problem is usually difficult to detect, because it starts with chalky spots on the inside of baby's front teeth where you're not likely to look. The teeth eventually begin to break down and crumble.

Some parents don't consider it a problem since preschoolers will lose their baby teeth anyway. But dentists warn that a baby's jaw development and the angle at which permanent teeth emerge can be affected by the premature loss of baby teeth.

If your baby can't stand to go to bed without a bottle, try a small bottle of water.

PACIFIERS

Babies have an instinct to suck, even when they've had enough to drink. Pacifiers have both good and bad points. On the plus side, babies have a need to suck, and at least one recent study appears to show a connection between the regular use of a pacifier and the reduced chance of a baby dying from SIDS. And if you're breastfeeding, it's just not advisable or possible to be a human pacifier day and night.

On the down side, prolonged pacifier use in childhood has been associated with jaw deformities and may contribute to speech impediments. One important warning: Never tie a pacifier around your baby's neck using a ribbon or string. Your baby could strangle if the string gets caught in the crib or playpen and tightens around his vulnerable neck. Also inspect pacifiers frequently to be sure the shield hasn't cracked and the nipple hasn't started to pull loose.

Just as with bottle nipples, pacifiers come in a variety of materials and shapes. You may want to buy several types to try with your baby. Again, boil them for five minutes before letting your baby suck on one.

DIAPER DUTY

In the first year alone, you'll be doing diaper changes about two thousand times. Newborns hate to have their diapers changed. It upsets them. So watch out, there are apt to be howls of protest and chin-quivering cries.

UNDERSTANDING COLIC

Rarely, there are babies who cry around the clock, which can be exhausting and even devastating for their parents who spend their days and nights searching wildly for some special technique that can help their tense, miserable babies relax and go to sleep.

Some babies cry so much that they earn the label of suffering from colic, an old British word for bad indigestion. The term is now used to describe inconsolable baby crying for long periods of time for which there is no apparent cause. Approximately one out of five babies earns the label of being colicky, or excessively fussy, as a result of their daily crying jags.

You may be surprised to learn that colic doesn't actually exist as a specific medical condition with a defined set of symptoms or indicators. Instead, it is a broadbrush term, just as headache is, used to cover a panoply of baby ailments. Typically, baby-crying episodes start

Diaper Changing 101

If you've never changed a diaper in your life, here's what to do. (We'll assume that you're among the 95 percent of parents who use disposables.)

1. Prepare by getting out a clean diaper and a wipe or two. Usually the design on the diaper will indicate where the front is.

2. Lay the baby down on his back on a changing pad or towel, being sure to support the head and neck at all times.

3. Remove the old diaper. If it has Velcro tabs, you can roll it up, and use the tabs to make it a tidy package.

4. Use a damp washcloth or a pre-moistened baby wipe to clean off the baby, being sure to wipe from front to back, and keep all fecal material out of the urinary tract area.

5. Apply diaper rash ointment or kaolin clay powder if your baby's bottom looks red.

6. Lift up the baby by the ankles, and slide the new diaper under his rump.

7. Peel off the tabs that cover the tape, pull the diaper firmly around your baby so it will stay on, and press the tape into the soft, patterned area of the diaper. *Voilà.* You'll become so expert at it that you can do it in the dark with your eyes closed.

within the first two to three weeks and peak at around six weeks after birth. Most, but not all cases of so-called colic resolve themselves on their own before the baby reaches his fourth month.

The symptoms of colic—the distressed screaming, the wide-open mouth with lips that almost turn blue, the frowning brows, the flailing arms and legs, and the rock-tight belly—are identical to any expression of extreme baby pain although the baby may or may not be in pain. And many parents discover that what was labeled as colic was really an ear infection, an allergy to dairy products or baby vitamins, an immature and dysfunctional digestive system, or other actual physical problems, such as a hernia or an undetected physical condition. Sometimes sudden-onset crying can be caused by an oncoming illness, or something as simple as a string or hair wrapped around a baby's finger, toe, or penis.

If the crying doesn't go away, and you're worried, it makes sense to have your baby thoroughly examined by his healthcare provider to try to uncover what's causing all the pain. Before you go, document a sample of your baby's crying

> *"If you wonder whether your baby has colic or not, he doesn't. Colic is real. Colic is pain. And it's living hell for his parents!"*

episodes by keeping a journal about when it happens and how long it lasts. You might want to consider videotaping an episode so your healthcare provider can actually see and hear your baby's behavior, since babies have an uncanny way of being calm and sleepy when their appointments roll around. A blood sample may be needed as well as a urine sample. Bring along your baby's most recent poopy diaper too.

If your baby seems to have sieges of dire distress, that you feel are not taken sufficiently seriously by your healthcare provider, you may want to seek help from a baby specialist, such as a neonatal gastroenterologist.

It helps to keep reminding yourself that as overwhelming as your baby's crying may feel at the moment, the situation is temporary. Research has shown that colicky babies are far more likely to turn out to be sweet and amenable toddlers, while passive, so-called good babies are much more likely to transform into demanding hellions after a year or so.

When it comes to their everyday discontents, most babies appear to be disappointed that they've been booted from their warm, cozy womb world and are no longer at "home." The sounds and motions that duplicate life in the womb are the very ones that are most likely to calm a newborn who is upset. For example, vigorous rocking while your baby is resting on your shoulder works great, probably because it mimics the familiar motion your baby felt every time you took walks during your pregnancy.

Droning sounds, similar to the sounds of your heartbeat and the flow of blood through your arteries,

Baby Symptoms You Shouldn't Ignore

- **Excessive crying.** It's normal for a newborn to cry when he is hungry, needs to be burped, is cold, or needs a clean diaper, and for a period of time in the early evening. But if your baby's cry sounds different than normal or seems to go on for an unusually long time, then it could be a signal that your baby is in pain.

- **Fever.** Make an emergency call to your pediatrician if your baby is less than eight weeks old and develops a fever of more than 100.4°F (rectally), or if he's eight weeks or older with a fever above 104°F.

- **Jaundice.** More than half of full-term babies and about 80 percent of premature babies who are otherwise healthy develop a yellowish discoloration of their skin and the whites of their eyes soon after birth called jaundice or neonatal *jaundice*. Jaundice is not a disease, but a symptom that usually signals that a baby's liver simply isn't mature enough to process a substance called *bilirubin*, which is created as the body recycles old or damaged red blood cells. It isn't painful or dangerous and usually disappears in one to two weeks. Exposure to sunlight or artificial light can help jaundice, and your healthcare practitioner will probably want to monitor your baby and may recommend exposing your baby to special treatment lights.

- **Constipation and dehydration.** If your baby is formula-fed, he may develop constipation. Stools may be hard and resemble small pellets. If your baby is breastfed, it's impossible for him to be constipated—lack of stools could mean that he isn't getting enough milk, so be sure to tell your pediatrician if your newborn doesn't poop for two to three days. Dark urine or dryer-than-usual diapers may also be signs that your baby isn't eating enough, or is becoming dehydrated.

- **Sluggishness.** It's normal for a newborn to spend a lot of time sleeping, but if your baby is rarely alert and doesn't wake up for feedings, or seems too listless to want to eat, contact your healthcare provider right away.

- **Infected umbilical cord.** If the stump from your baby's umbilical (belly button) cord gets pussy or red, swollen skin at the base or if your baby cries as though in pain when you touch the cord or skin, the site may be infected and you should contact your healthcare provider.

- **Infected circumcision site.** Call your doctor if your son's penis isn't healing, or the tip of your baby's penis is red, swollen, oozy, or foul smelling.

can sometimes lull a fitful baby into relaxation and sleep. Other things to try when you're at your wit's end:

- Running the vacuum cleaner or dishwasher.
- Parking the bassinet next to a whirring window-unit air conditioner or fan.
- Putting the baby in a carrier on top of a running washing machine or dryer (don't leave baby alone).
- Taking the baby for a drive in the car while playing percussive bass-heavy music, like hip-hop or military marches.
- Taking baby to a new climate, like an ice rink or arboretum.

- The one-arm hold. Drape your baby on your arm, facedown, with his head resting in your palm, and sway.

Shushing your baby loudly in his ear while moving him rhythmically and swaddling him is also a maneuver worth trying. To swaddle your baby, wrap him firmly in a blanket. You might think that babies would naturally want to be nude and free, but not so—it seems that most feel comforted by being wrapped up tight, with hands and arms immobile in a little bundle, imitating the feeling your baby had inside your body. Some parents find that just holding down one arm of an upset baby can

Three Baby Soothing Strategies

Experienced parents suggest that no matter what technique you use, continue to do it long enough to bore the baby, instead of hopping around from one thing to another before baby can acclimate to what's happening. However, if your baby's hungry or truly in pain, nothing will help for very long.

- **Vigorous rocking.** The rocking chair is a great invention. Put your baby to your shoulder and really rock vigorously, almost abruptly. Or if no chair is available, you can rock back and forth, or raise your baby up high and then swoop him down. It works, but it's tiring. Introduce baby to your exercise ball. Cover it with a towel, and rock him gently back and forth in a face-downward position to help him quiet down during a crying jag. Just make sure the baby's nose is never covered by the ball's surface.

- **Colic carry.** Rest your baby on your arm with his body facing downward. His cheek should be at the crease of your elbow with your hand holding onto one of his legs. Take the fingertips of your free hand, and gently and rhythmically massage his belly. While you're doing that, gently rock back and forth from one foot to the other.

- **Chest rest.** This is a good one for your partner to try. Lie on your back on the sofa, in a recliner, or in the bed, and place your bare or diapered baby facedown on your chest. Rest your hands on baby's back. Cover your baby's back and your arm with a sheet or blanket. Your baby will smell your scent, hear your heartbeat, feel the up-and-down rhythm of your breathing, and he may just calm down.

help to stop the flailing and encourage the baby to stop fussing.

Walking into a new environment, like taking baby outside so that he feels a change in air and light, or momentarily placing a cold washcloth on his face, can also be startling enough to break through a crying cycle.

WHERE TO GO IF YOU'RE OVERWHELMED BY BABY CRYING

Intense, unrelenting baby crying can sometimes provoke parents into committing baby abuse, particularly with babies whose cries appear to fall outside of the normal range of human tolerance. There's a particular danger of such abuse occurring when parents are isolated and not getting sufficient help and human support. If you find this to be your case, it's critical that you marshal all available resources to get help that will allow you to get some time off from around-the-clock baby care in order to maintain your own psychological balance.

If you have the urge to hurt your baby, seek counseling or some other forms of professional help. Try calling a local or national counseling hotline for support, visit a pastor, priest, or rabbi, your childbirth educator, your pediatrician, or La Leche League leader, or call a friend or someone you love.

Your library or your local United Way can also help you find the telephone numbers of agencies, or you can search in the Yellow Pages™ of the telephone directory under "Social Service and Welfare Organizations."

Meanwhile, if you find yourself isolated with your baby and about to explode with nowhere to turn, put the baby somewhere safe like the carseat or crib, ask a neighbor to baby-sit for a while, and be sure to arrange your schedule with adequate breaks so you won't ever be pushed that far again.

BABY BATHING BASICS

New babies really don't need baths—they don't sweat, they don't crawl around, and they just don't get very dirty. Furthermore, temperature changes, such as those caused by the cooling of water as it evaporates off their wet skin, usually will arouse screams of protest.

It will be easier on both of you if you hold off an immersion in a bath for as long as possible, and definitely until after the circumcision and umbilical cord sites have healed. Even then, your newborn won't need a daily bath—once every two or three days, or even longer, is sufficient. Too much rigorous cleaning will deplete your baby's natural skin oils and cause dryness.

There are ways to keep your baby clean during the pre-bath days. Brush his hair from back to front with a soft brush to stimulate the scalp and help prevent cradle cap, and clean up after bowel movements using a damp, lukewarm washcloth, a pre-moistened baby wipe, or a spray bottle filled with warm water. Remember: Rubbing a newborn's tender skin with a regular washcloth is harsh—wipe gently with a soft, knit baby washcloth instead.

Anyone who claims that giving a new baby a bath is "fun for you and baby" either never had a baby or forgot how new babies tend to hate being undressed and messed with. The best timing for your baby's bath is when he is alert but not hungry. Go slowly. Babies react to being lowered quickly and to sudden changes in temperature—especially when you undress them, and they feel bare and cold. The trick for those early days is to keep your baby wrapped loosely in a warm towel or blanket while you gently wipe down his body and folds with a warm, soft washcloth.

There are a variety of products to help you with bathing. A hooded towel and several baby washcloths will come in handy. You can also purchase a baby bathtub or a bathing insert that looks like a small hammock seat lined in terry cloth or other absorbent materials to prop in a sink or the big bathtub. Large, thick baby-shaped bathing sponges are inexpensive and help to cushion baby's back and bottom in a tub or sink. (We discuss how to choose a baby bathtub in the *Baby Gear Guide*, on page 454.)

Many parents opt to use the kitchen sink, with extra cushioning for baby's first bath. If you don't have a propper or a big sponge, simply fold a thick bath towel and line the bottom of the sink with it. Then add a few inches of warm water. Keep a measuring cup full of warm water within reach for pouring over your baby's body to rinse off soap.

Another practical bathing option to consider is taking your baby in the tub with you. Sit yourself down in waist deep, mildly warm water in the bathtub and let your partner hand the baby over to you. (Don't try to do this on your own—you could slip and hurt both of you.)

In the seated position, bring your knees up to support the baby, so his buttocks are resting against your belly with his head aimed toward your knees. Then soap, and rinse. Have your partner take the baby and wrap him in a big, warm towel while you finish bathing and getting out of the tub. The advantage to this whole-body approach to baby bathing is that most babies are soothed by skin-to-skin contact, and you can nurse him if he gets upset.

BABY'S FIRST BATH

When your baby's healed and ready for the first real bath, make sure the room's toasty warm. Your hands aren't good thermostats when it comes to judging the hotness of your baby's bathwater. Use the underside of your wrist instead. And before you take hold of your baby, wash your hands to remove any germs.

Gather together everything you'll need so it's within arm's reach. On the list are a clean gown or T-shirt; a fresh diaper; a gentle, non-perfumed soap such as Aveeno® or unscented Dove®; a soft baby hairbrush; a plastic or glass measuring cup to hold warm rinse water; a baby washcloth; and a big, soft towel.

Babies are as slippery as eels when they're wet. Hold your baby so his head is supported on the wrist of one hand with the fingers of that same hand holding baby's arm. Remember, never take your hands off your baby or leave him unattended—even if the telephone rings or someone comes to the door.

Babies can drown in less than an inch of water in only a minute or two.

It really doesn't matter where on your baby's body you begin the job, just be gentle about it, or simply use your fingertips and palms to do the job. While most advice books suggest you wash the baby from the top downward, we suggest doing his body first. That's because his head is more vulnerable to heat loss from evaporating water.

Most babies and young children hate having their faces washed. Be careful not to cover your baby's nose or mouth with a washcloth, and clean just one side of the face at a time. Better yet, just use your own gentle hands. Remember to keep soap away from his eyes; it can burn and make him start crying.

Once you've cleaned and rinsed all parts except your baby's scalp, you may want to pick baby up and wrap him in a towel with just his head uncovered. Then put him in a football hold, and gently lather his scalp using a few drops of tearless, baby shampoo. Hold his head in a downward direction and use the measuring cup filled with warm water to rinse so the water flows to the back of his head and away from his forehead and eyes.

After you're done, use an edge of the towel to gently pat his head dry. Then it's time to put on a fresh diaper and clean clothes. Note: If your baby screams and protests being bathed the traditional way, try keeping him wrapped in a warm, soft blanket or towel and damp-mopping his body, one part at a time with a warm washcloth. You can also do this cleaning while holding your baby in your lap. Later, after a few baths this way, you can try lowering your baby— blanket or towel and all—down into the warm water of the tub before gently starting the unwrapping and washing process.

EYE CLEANING TIPS

You may notice a white, yellow, or greenish discharge that collects in the sides of your baby's eyes on the side nearest the nose. This usually means that the baby's tear ducts are still too small to handle the pool of tears.

You can gently clean away the mucus by wiping from the corner of eye, starting near the nose, toward the outer edge of the eye. Use a damp cotton ball dipped in warm water, but inspect the wet end of the ball first to make sure there are no loose cotton fibers that could be irritating.

If the discharge doesn't go away after a few days of gentle cleaning, or your baby's eyes look bloodshot, you may want to contact your healthcare provider.

SKIN RASHES

Most babies develop odd rashes from time to time, and there are hundreds of different varieties. Everyday rashes are caused by a baby's sweat and oil glands not functioning normally for the first few weeks after birth. You may see little whiteheads (known as *milia*) on his face, or tiny pimples on his face between the third and sixth weeks. The bumps will disappear on their own and require no special care. Don't pick at them, as doing so will cause infection. Also keep baby's nails short to prevent scratching, which may also lead to infection.

Sometimes rashes are caused by the baby coming into contact with harsh chemical and perfumes in their clothing or in sheets. We suggest laundering all of the fabrics that come in contact with your baby in an unscented detergent and not using a fabric softener or perfumed softening sheets in the dryer.

Heat rash, sometimes called prickly heat (its medical name is ***miliaria rubia***) is an itchy, red rash with small bumps or fluid-filled blisters that is caused by plugged sweat glands. It usually shows up in hot, humid weather, but sometimes babies get it in the winter, particularly if they are overdressed. You'll usually find it in the creases or skin folds around a baby's neck, on his back, in his armpits, or in the diaper area.

You can help to prevent heat rash by keeping your baby in the shade or indoors during the hottest part of the day, giving frequent lukewarm baths, using clothing made of absorbent cotton, and avoiding greasy ointments or skin lotions that hold your baby's sweat in. If your baby seems ill and cranky or has a fever, or if the rash spreads to other parts of the body, contact your baby's healthcare provider.

Cradle cap (medical name seborrheic dermatitis) is a harmless, scaly, crusty area, usually on a baby's scalp but sometimes at the hairline or on the nose, behind the ears, or in the eyebrows. It is not an allergy, and it isn't caused by a lack of bathing. The patches of cradle cap can be yellow, pink, or brownish in color and usually show up in the first few weeks of life and disappear after a few months. The condition

is very common and affects one out of two newborns.

It's not clear what causes cradle cap, but it's probably related to your baby's oil glands, which aren't yet fully developed. The condition will usually disappear without needing treatment. Gently massage olive oil or mineral oil into the crusts to soften the scales, then wipe with a washcloth to take off the crusts. Swaddle your baby with just his head out, and then gently rinse his scalp with lukewarm water using the kitchen sink and a watering can or a measuring cup. Shampoo with a gentle baby shampoo, then rinse thoroughly. Contact your baby's healthcare provider if the rash spreads to other parts of your baby's body, if it bleeds, or if it appears red, swollen, or infected.

Eczema is a broad term for dry, itchy, inflamed skin. The first signs usually develop in the first three months of life. The baby with eczema will have red, scaly skin, and there may be red patches on his cheeks, followed by an inflammation of his scalp, arms, and legs. The patches will be itchy, which may make your baby restless and cranky. Babies and children with dry, very sensitive skin are more vulnerable to it, but allergies, such as to formula ingredients, pollens, or house dust can cause an outbreak or make it worse. Heat, excess humidity, chafing, and soaps, or the strong chemicals and perfumes in detergents and fabric softeners can also aggravate it.

The causes of eczema are not completely understood but are probably genetic. Notify your baby's healthcare provider, who may prescribe medications to help with the itching and a moisturizer to make your baby more comfortable. Also, protect your baby from those who have active cold sores caused by herpes, which might cause serious complications if your baby becomes infected.

PARENT–BABY COMMUNICATION

Your newborn is acutely aware of your voice and is prepared to respond to it. Even when he is only a few days old, he will turn his whole body around to orient to the sound of your voice calling his name from across the room.

Your baby will move in synchrony with your voice's inflections. Only a few weeks after birth, he will move his lips and tongue in response to your talking. In moments of alertness, he may imitate you when you make a facial grimace, stick out your tongue or shape your lips into an "O." He is capable of responding to your speaking to him by changing his breathing and making cooing noises.

It's important to always talk to your baby when you are interacting with him. Greet him in the morning, and continue a running conversation throughout your day together. Name body parts. Warn him when you're planning to pick him up, and explain when you're going somewhere or what you're thinking. This will help to enable him to master the rhythms of human language.

As you move close in toward your baby's face, slow down your speech, make your voice higher, and exaggerate your facial expressions to get your baby's attention.

He will respond by arresting the movement of his legs and arms, and,

if he's not hungry or sleepy, he will likely orient his body toward you, and eventually, he will coo back to you or give you a grin.

Since your baby can't walk away or tell you, "I'm sorry, Mom, but I'm tired and need a little peace and quiet," it can he hard to tell if your baby is being over-stimulated. Your baby will signal that he's ready to stop playing by glazing over, hiccuping, yawning, getting a distraught look on his face, or by turning his head to the side. Gaze aversion, as this baby maneuver is called, is his way of trying to make you disappear when you threaten to become overwhelming. Experts suggest that parents imitate the reaction by turning their heads to the side too. Often, the baby will re-engage and face forward after a brief pause. Then, you can try a few more gentle interactions.

SILLY BABY GAMES

The limited attention spans of young babies means that they will only be able to attend to you for moments at a time. As your baby matures, the amount of time he can spend paying attention to you will expand. But there are some tricks that even babies less than a week old can do that might be fun to try once your baby's fed and diapered but is still awake and staring:

- **Rattle watching.** Babies are attracted to movement if it's close enough (about twelve inches from the face) for them to focus. Slowly pass a bright rattle, ball, or other toy back and forth in front of his face and watch how his eyes try to track it. Your baby's eye movements may be jerky, and he may seem cross-eyed, but still you can see that he is trying to watch.

- **"Monkey see, monkey do."** Babies sometimes will imitate the facial gestures of adults. Again, move into an eye-to-eye position, about twelve inches from baby's face, and stick out your tongue, or open your mouth widely. Do this slowly and deliberately, and see if your baby returns a similar facial gesture.

- **Marching.** Babies only hours old will make marching steps if they are supported in an upright position. Hold your baby with your hands around the chest, under the arms. Hold the baby over a tabletop so that the soles of his feet are pressed gently onto the surface. Then tilt your baby a little to one side and then the other so that one foot and then the other touch the table. Your baby will lift alternate legs.

- **Palm trick.** Pressing your thumbs gently into your baby's palms will likely cause him to open his mouth.

YOU AND YOUR BABY'S HEALTHCARE

It's important to choose your baby's pediatrician before giving birth. This lets your baby get personalized care from the very beginning; plus, most health insurance policies will pay for your baby's first exam in the hospital. (For help in choosing a healthcare provider for your baby, see pages 57–60.)

The first checkup can be as soon as within forty-eight hours of discharge from the hospital if the mother is breastfeeding, had an early discharge from the hospital, or if there are other complications that need to be monitored. The American Academy of Pediatrics recommends well-baby checkups at the following ages: two weeks old and at months one, two, four, six, nine, twelve, fifteen, eighteen, and twenty-four of age. It's important to keep an ongoing record of your baby's appointments, illnesses, and immunizations and to carry them with you, along with a warm blanket for the examining table when you head off for your baby's appointments.

If this is your first visit with your baby, you may need to fill out forms and present your insurance card. Your healthcare provider may provide a waiting room for well children that is separate from the one for sick kids.

Once you've been escorted back to an exam room, your baby will be measured and weighed and your baby will then have a complete physical exam.

You will be asked a series of questions about your baby's feeding, wetting, and sleeping patterns, and you may be asked about how you and your family are coping with your new arrival.

Your baby may remain calm during the process, or he could protest loudly at the change in temperature or the pain from an immunization.

Most babies cry when they are given a shot, which may be surprisingly upsetting to you now that you've begun to bond with your child.

If you're nursing, ask your provider if you can nurse your baby through the experience, or immediately afterward to help distract him from any discomfort. If you're bottle-feeding, carry along a comforting pacifier or bottle of formula.

Rather than trying to race home if your baby's upset, ask your healthcare provider if there is an available room where you can sit quietly and feed your baby until the two of you are calm again before trying to put him in his car seat to drive home.

State-mandated newborn screening tests

The uniform screening of newborn babies mandated by states began in 1962, with blood tests to identify babies with *phenylketonuria (PKU)*. Since then the program has expanded to test for a variety of potentially serious diseases. These tests vary from state to state. Now, over four million newborns a year are tested which helps to identify about three thousand babies with serious diseases that can usually be treated early, even before symptoms develop.

If your state requires testing, your baby will have blood drawn before going home from the hospital, usually using a heel stick, and the blood specimen will be placed on a special filter paper that is sent to a centralized lab for testing.

A repeat or second newborn screen may be required, often after your baby's first checkup, especially if the first test was done in the baby's first twenty-four hours of life. Some states, such as Texas, mandate by law that two screens be done.

Sometimes normal babies may have erroneous results that appear to show an illness when there is none. A positive test should always

be redone to make sure your baby has the illness. Which tests your baby will be given depends upon the state where you life.

Phenylketonuria (PKU) and congenital adrenal hyperplasia (CAH) are screened for in all states, and other states require tests for other diseases as well. Six states, for example, test for cystic fibrosis, and New York tests for HIV.

If you would like to know more about the tests, don't be shy about asking your baby's pediatrician for more information.

Immunizations

Your pediatrician will recommend the proper immunization schedule for your baby. Prior to starting your baby's routine immunizations, you may want to ask the doctor for information about the potential mild and rarer serious side effects of vaccines, the best timing for them, and the prevalence and dangers of the diseases from which the immunizations provide protection.

Some, but not all, immunizations cause mild, temporary aftereffects, such as fever and irritability for a few hours afterward. In rare instances, immunizations can have more serious consequences. Ask your provider what to expect and if there are any medications to help your baby's symptoms. Also ask how to tell if symptoms are serious enough to warrant a call to the office.

Most likely your baby will be given three separate *hepatitis B* immunization shots, including one in the hospital, especially if tests show you to be hepatitis B positive.

Your provider will also recommend the DTaP (diptheria, tetanus, and pertussis—whooping cough),

MMR (measles, mumps, and rubella—another form of measles), varicella (chickenpox), HIB (haemophilus influenza B), and PCV-7 (pneumococcus). The small-pox vaccine has been discontinued.

Baby illness

It's likely that your baby will get sick at some point, though if you're breastfeeding, your baby will be just as immune to germs as you are. Still, help prevent illness by making sure that all visitors who hold the baby wash their hands, and politely ask anyone with a cold to delay their visit until they're well again.

Most common illnesses are caused by invisible bacteria and viruses transmitted from one person to another. Coughing, kissing, or hand contact can transmit illness. In rare cases, signs of sickness, such as a fever, sluggishness, rashes, or a runny nose can be the start of some-thing serious, but, in most instances, it just means your baby's caught a more common bug, like a cold.

Any time you suspect your baby is coming down with an illness, it's important to contact your baby's pediatrician immediately. That's because your baby's body is begin-ning to develop antibodies to illness, so sickness can be much more serious than it would be later on when your baby's internal defenses have become stronger. Sometimes, serious problems may at first look like an oncoming cold but then quickly worsen.

A baby's symptoms may take hours or days to develop after germs have been passed on. Symptoms of oncoming illness can include demanding to nurse more often or less often than usual, or the opposite, refusing to eat; a fever of greater than 100.4°; crankiness or excessive sluggishness; and vomiting or diarrhea.

HOW TO TAKE YOUR BABY'S TEMPERATURE

A fever is a sign that your baby may have an infection. A fever in a baby under two months of age may be especially significant and should be reported to your baby's healthcare provider right away. The easiest way to tell if your baby's running a fever is to kiss his forehead. If it feels hotter than normal, you're probably right.

A normal temperature for a baby is between 97°F and 100.4°F (36° to 38° Celsius). A rectal temper-ature higher than 100.4°F in a baby under two months of age, should be reported to your baby's healthcare provider.

The American Academy of Pediatrics (AAP) recommends that pediatricians and parents no longer purchase and use glass thermome-ters that contain mercury. Mercury is poisonous, the glass can shatter, and the thermometers are hard to read. Instead, purchase an easy-to-read digital thermometer from a pharmacy or on the Web. Most cost less than $10. Ear thermometers cost more and may not be as accurate.

Don't try to get your baby's temperature by mouth; it probably won't work and you might injure his delicate tissues. Your best two choices are by placing the sensitive part of the thermometer in your baby's rectum, or putting it directly beneath his armpit and gently

Basic Baby Medical Supplies

You'll find these items, all of which are available in a pharmacy, helpful when your baby gets sick:

- **A medicine spoon or dropper.** It should have easy-to-read markings on the side to help measuring doses.

- **Saline nose drops or sprays.** These drops in baby strength will help to break up stuffy noses for babies.

- **A bulb syringe (nose bulb).** It will have a bicycle-horn looking bulb on one end and a rounded suction tip on the other. It's for suctioning out baby's nose mucus.

- **Thermometer.** Ask your baby's healthcare provider what type of thermometer to use and the recommended way of taking the baby's temperature.

- **Baby-strength acetaminophen.** Tylenol® (or other brand) for treating your baby's fever in concentrated drops if your baby is over eight weeks old. Consult with your physician before administering acetaminophen; too much acetaminophen can hurt your baby's liver.

- **A memory-jogging card.** While you're at it, create a card for recording the date, the time, and how much of the medication you've given your baby to share over the telephone with your doctor.

- **Petroleum jelly.** Use it for lubricating the thermometer if your doctor wants a rectal reading.

- **Diaper rash cream or kaolin clay powder.** For when baby's bottom gets red and looks raw.

holding his arm down. The armpit method, called axillary temperature, is about 2° cooler than a rectal temperature.

A rectal temperature is usually more accurate and not as uncomfortable as it may sound, for the baby, anyway. If your pediatrician asks you to take your baby's temperature rectally, you can take it while diaper changing by holding your baby's ankles, spreading his buttocks, and grasping the thermometer between your middle and index finger with your other hand. Gently insert it in about one inch. Don't use a digital thermometer if it has a sharp, pointed probe that could injure your baby's rectal area.

A second way is to place your baby facedown on your lap with his legs dangling from your thigh. Support the thermometer with your cupped hand so that it sticks out from the base of your fingers. Either way, the thermometer should be lubricated with petroleum jelly. Newer thermometers with flexible tips are safest. The thermometer will beep when it's ready. (Have some tissue on hand: Your baby may poop when the thermometer's on the way out.)

Write down your reading and the date and time you took it. When you call your pediatrician, make sure he or she knows the method you used to get your baby's temperature reading.

TREATING A FEVER

During an illness, babies and toddlers can suddenly spike a high fever that would seem very dangerous for adults, and some babies may even go into a convulsion when a fever rapidly rises over 101°F.

While conventional wisdom used to be that fevers should be brought down right away, more recent research suggests that fevers serve a purpose. Contact your baby's caregiver immediately if your baby gets a (rectal) temperature higher than 100.4°F.

If your baby does have a fever or a seizure, it's important to contact your doctor immediately to get instructions about what to do next. In the meantime, try to cool your baby by undressing him to his diaper and gently wiping him off with lukewarm water.

If your baby has a convulsion, it will look like odd, spastic movements in his body for a very brief time, and then he may fall into a deep sleep. Your job is to simply protect the baby from hitting his head or limbs on anything. Don't try to put anything in his mouth. It could cause injury.

Your doctor may recommend a fever-reducing medication, such as acetaminophen (e.g., Tylenol®) for babies. It will be a concentrated

liquid that comes with its own dropper. It's critical to give the *exact* dosage as recommended! Administering too much medication is a common mistake that parents make because the gradations are so tiny when you're using a small dropper. Measure the liquid in a bright light, so you can see what you're doing.

Ibuprofrin (Motrin®) is not approved for babies under six months of age. Aspirin is usually not recommended for babies and young children with flu-like symptoms of illness because it has been linked to a rare, but serious disease called Reye's syndrome. The illness most often affects children between the ages of three to twelve. It begins with cold-like symptoms and then progresses to frequent vomiting and changes in consciousness—going from extreme sluggishness to agitation or delirium, and more rarely followed by coma and death.

COLDS AND RSV INFECTIONS

Colds are especially hard on young babies. They can only breathe through their noses when they nurse and not through their mouths like children and adults can do. The colds begin with irritability and eating changes, clear fluid running from the nose, sneezing, and possibly a low fever.

Our grandmothers used to say: "You can treat a cold, and it will be over in a week, or you can do nothing, and it will end in seven days." There's some truth to that. But sometimes colds can develop into something more serious.

RSV stands for *respiratory syncytial virus* (pronounced sin-SISH-al), one of the most common sources for serious pneumonia and other infections of baby's nose, throat, and lungs. Every year, 90,000 babies are hospitalized with RSV-related illnesses.

It's believed that nearly half of all babies catch some type of RSV every year, usually in winter. Its symptoms are like a cold: stuffy, runny nose; a low-temperature fever; and a cough. Sometimes bacteria come along to cause an inner-ear infection at the same time.

Preemies and babies with serious diseases, such as HIV, congenital heart disease, or lung conditions are more vulnerable to the serious side of RSV. It may begin as a simple cold and then become more serious.

Symptoms include a fever higher than 100.4°F for a baby under three months of age, or higher than 102°F for older babies and toddlers. Other serious symptoms include fast breathing or difficulty getting breaths, a whistling noise in the chest when breathing out (wheezing), a deep or frequent cough, disinterest in nursing, and listlessness or unusual irritability. Contact your baby's pediatrician for instructions about what to do.

INNER-EAR INFECTIONS

Next to colds, inner-ear infections (*otitis media*) are the reason most parents take their babies to the pediatrician. As many as three out of four babies have some form of ear infections by age three. Typically, the infection will set in a few days after a cold has started. You can't see that the baby has the infection; it's on the other side of the eardrum.

If your baby has an ear infection, he's likely to be cranky (you'll think it's colic), and he may bat at his ear, or a baby may temporarily lose some hearing and scream in extreme pain.

Your doctor will want to examine your baby's ears and may suggest a painkiller such as acetaminophen or ibuprofen along with a course of antibiotics if a bacterial infection is suspected.

In the meantime, you might try keeping your baby in a semi-upright position, such as in a car seat that's carefully supported on the sides so it can't tip over. And you can outside a mildly warm, moist towel to your baby's cheek near the ears. Usually, these infections get better after several days of treatment.

DIARRHEA

Diarrhea is dangerous for babies during the first four months of life. It can be brought on by an illness, a change in formula or vitamins, and taking antibiotics. Although a baby's normal stools may resemble diarrheal disease, it is rare in babies fed only breastmilk. A baby's having more stools that are liquid and sometimes foul-smelling signals true diarrhea. You may see solids sitting on top of the diaper core with a ring of staining where the semi-liquid part of the diarrhea has soaked in.

The risk of diarrhea is that it will quickly deplete your baby's fluid stores, and that can quickly lead to dehydration—a serious threat to young infants. A dehydrated baby may be more sluggish than usual and harder to rouse, may have a dry mouth, and may go for hours without wetting a diaper.

If your baby is getting dehydrated or you see blood in the stool, you should contact your healthcare provider immediately.

THRUSH

If your baby's tongue and cheeks stay coated in white patches that won't wipe away, he may have thrush, a fungus-caused problem. This yeast infection grows in moist places, and it may also appear as red, irritated patches in the folds of your baby's skin, such as on the neck or in the armpits and thighs. Sometimes a cherry red diaper rash that doesn't clear up easily can also be caused by yeast. A mother's red, itchy, cracked nipples, sometimes with white patches, may also be yeast-related. Both the mother and baby may need to be treated to prevent re-infecting one another. Your healthcare provider will suggest medication to treat it.

MENINGITIS

Meningitis is a rare and deadly infection of the tissues that cover the brain. Babies under two months old are especially vulnerable. The signs are subtle and not very different from those of a bad cold. A blood test to check for a bacterial infection may be called for, and possibly a spinal tap to see if the spinal fluid is infected. If meningitis is treated aggressively and quickly with antibiotics, the crippling and long-lasting effects of the disease can be avoided.

The symptoms of meningitis mimic those of other serious baby illnesses: fever, decreased appetite, listlessness, or increased crying and irritability. Babies over two months of age may have the same symptoms plus vomiting. Crankiness will be extreme, and your baby will be hard to comfort, followed by such sluggishness that you have trouble rousing him. Older children with the disease will complain of headache, pain in the back, or a stiff neck, and they may feel pain when looking at a bright light.

EMERGENCY BABY LIFE SUPPORT (BLS)

Basic baby life support is designed to keep your baby alive and breathing until help comes. It is very rare for a baby to need emergency resuscitation, but it's a very good idea to take a course in life support or CPR through your local American Red Cross chapter or the American Heart Association.

In the meantime, here are some basic instructions to rehearse:

1. Make sure to check if baby is breathing or moving. Mucus, blood, vomit, a solid piece of food or candy, or the tongue can easily obstruct the small airways of a baby, and your baby may become unconscious.

2. Shout for help.

3. Have a second person call 911.

4. If there's been an accident, try to see how seriously your baby is injured and whether he is unconscious, in which case he will not respond to gentle motions or to tapping his feet.

How to Do Baby CPR

Place your baby on his back, and try to open the airway by tilting his head back and lifting his chin. Place your mouth over your baby's mouth and nose and give two slow, gentle breaths. If breathing doesn't start, try two more slow breaths, one breath every two to three seconds with one to one and one-half seconds per breath (about twenty breaths per minute). Pause in between to take air. If your baby is still not breathing, and there are no signs of movement, place two fingers between your baby's ribs on the lowest place on your baby's chest (the sternum). Press down in cycles of five compressions followed by one slow breath in the baby's mouth and nose with your mouth. Continue five compressions and one slow breath until your baby revives or help arrives.

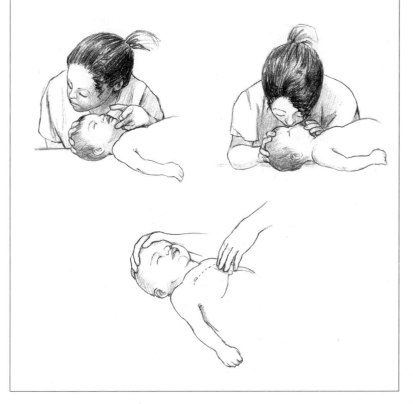

5. Take special care if you suspect that your baby has a head or neck injury so that you don't move his body, which could make the spinal cord vulnerable.

6. Look, listen, and feel your baby's chest to see if he is breathing. If there is no one to help you, and your baby is obviously not breathing, or is turning blue, perform CPR for one minute before calling for help. Remember, a baby's lungs are tiny, and so are his air passages.

YOUR GUIDE TO CHOOSING GOOD CHILDCARE

Finding a responsible caregiver for your baby is an important job. Babysitters, babysitting co-ops, day care centers, home day care settings, nannies, and au pairs—there are a huge variety of ways to find help in caring for your child. The important thing is that your child receives loving, responsive care that is stimulating and offers opportunities for learning and growth. Below are your options for finding childcare.

Hire a babysitter

Babysitters are for occasional childcare needs. You can use members of your family, hire an adult neighbor or teen, or you can go through a formal agency that provides professional babysitters for a fee.

What's needed is a responsible person who is mature enough to think clearly in emergency situations, who can follow your directions to the letter, and who will show up as promised. When it comes to caring for a baby, kindness and gentleness are to be preferred over a rigid, disciplinary approach.

Your local chapter of the American Red Cross may offer "Babysitters Training," a special course for kids eleven to fifteen that teaches basic first aid, feeding, and diapering, and other useful skills. You can find your local chapter, where you can call for information on qualified babysitters, online at www.redcross.org. Guidance counselors in junior highs and high schools can sometimes offer help in finding just the right young person for your needs.

It's important to have the sitter visit you at home with your baby before leaving your baby at home alone with her. That's when you can teach the sitter your basic routines and rules. Diapering, feeding, and sleeping routines should be demonstrated, even though a sitter may claim to be familiar with all of these skills. Formula preparation for your baby may require careful directions plus written instructions.

You'll want to come to an advance agreement about payment, transportation, and hours needed for the job. Some teens, for example, may not be able to stay out past eleven on school nights.

Before you go out, be sure to post important telephone numbers: how to reach you in an emergency, a nearby relative or neighbor who can be called upon if there's a problem, the number to call for emergencies (911), and the number of your baby's doctor.

Use babysitting co-ops

If you're only seeking occasional baby-sitting, you may want to join with other parents in forming a babysitting cooperative. Usually, a co-op consists of four to five families who agree to exchange babysitting duties with each other in exchange for points instead of money. Co-ops that have been around a long time can grow to be much larger—fifty or more families. Running a successful co-op requires good organizing skills. The larger the group, the more organizing that will be required. During the initial planning stage, you'll want to decide together to limit the number of families that can participate, and, perhaps, a list of the values or qualities of the families you want to have as members; otherwise, you may find members you don't wish to use.

You'll need a chairperson to oversee the running of the co-op and a secretary whose job is to keep records of people's points. You can either give your officers extra credit for their duties, or you can rotate responsibilities, but organizational and follow-through abilities are important qualities for your leaders.

The chairperson's job is to oversee the running of the co-op, to plan regular co-op meetings so everything runs smoothly, to help in setting up basic rules (such as delivery and pickup of children, not sitting sick children, and a point scale), and to intervene in conflicts between members (e.g., when a member fails to carry out his babysitting duties).

The secretary's job is to locate an available sitter when a request comes in and to negotiate with the requesting family the number of points involved in the job. In addition, the secretary keeps a ledger on each family, listing the names and ages of their children, their address and directions to their home, telephone number, e-mail address, etc.

Below the basic information should be a column giving the date

of service, points of credit or debit, and the remaining balance of points. The secretary periodically informs members of their accumulated credits, and updates and distributes membership lists.

Hire in-home care for your baby
If they can afford it, most parents would rather have their babies kept in their own homes, rather than having them watched in some other setting. The advantages of keeping baby at home are the additional security for your child of being in a familiar setting and the lessening of exposure to childhood illnesses, including colds and chronic ear infections.

To achieve in-home care, you may want to consider having (or hiring) a relative, such as your baby's grandmother, to care for your child or using a worker who provides childcare, or childcare plus housekeeping for a living.

A more costly option is to hire a nanny or au pair person using a professional agency that subcontracts with a person, paying them to work for you. Most agencies handle recruitment, hiring, and the financial aspects of salaries and health insurance. These agencies often charge top dollar for their services, and those whom they hire may only be available for limited spans of time, but some families with the resources find that nannies are a wonderful solution for in-home childcare.

If you aren't able to manage the costs of having your child cared for in your own home, you may want to consider finding a mother or older person who would be willing to care for your baby in their home. The best solution is usually an at-home mom who wants to supplement her income by caring for one or two

Qualities of a Good Caregiver

There are very special characteristics that make for a good caregiver. He or she should genuinely love children. The ideal person is self-confident, affectionate, and positive in the way that he or she interacts with children.

Not all caregivers are suited for caring for babies. While a firm disciplinarian might be suitable for an active, unruly preschooler, babies thrive in a flexible, responsive environment where a baby's needs are more important than set rules.

Consistency is important. In interviewing potential homecare providers, try to determine the stability of the person and the situation. High turnover in sitters can cause a child distress and affect his security. At the same time, don't be afraid to change caregivers at any point if you find yourself feeling uncomfortable.

other children besides her own. The closer to your home, the better. Look for a neat, orderly house, safe baby equipment, plenty of baby toys, and a person who seems to genuinely enjoy talking and playing with babies and tots. Too many kids in one house can mean that your baby has to cry for attention, and he may be vulnerable.

Find a commercial childcare center

Not all childcare centers will accept infants. For that reason, centers that care for babies are in high demand, often have long waiting lists, and charge premium prices.

Providing quality care for babies requires an intense relationship between babies and caregivers, and the best centers have a low ratio between staff members and babies (three to one or better). Also remember that staff members can call in sick—so a large baby-to-staff-member ratio means your baby may end up with less attention on some days, simply because there aren't enough people on hand to care for everyone.

The number-one quality to look for in a center that cares for babies is an atmosphere of warmth and affection. Good caregivers genuinely love babies and relate to them as people, not simply charges to be routinely fed and then put to sleep. Observe how the staff relates to individual babies, especially babies who are unhappy.

Staff training is important too. Teachers and aides should have degrees in early childhood education or other infancy areas, or at a minimum, one year of specialized training in caring for babies. Ask about ongoing staff training as well.

Visiting a center more than once is an important way of determining how well babies are cared for. The center should have open doors when it comes to parents' visits, and you should be welcomed to visit the center and your baby whenever you wish.

The facility should be brightly lit, immaculately clean, and offer safe equipment and a variety of playthings for babies.

Sanitation and infection control are critical issues. So it's important to take a look at how babies are being diapered, since feces and saliva are two ways that serious infections can be passed from one baby to another. Observe staff hand washing and food handling, and ask about the sanitizing of toys. A good center will routinely sanitize baby playthings that have been mouthed and touched by a baby.

What are the center's sick baby policies? Will you need to keep your baby at home, or is there a sick bay where sick babies can be cared for without spreading germs to other babies? Remember, if the center lets sick babies come, then your baby will be exposed to illnesses too.

Look for daily educational and exploration activities that are suitable and safe for infants. Your baby should have a chance to play with a variety of materials with baby-conscious outdoor opportunities as well. Toddlers and babies should play in separate spaces. (See the *Resource Guide* on page 538, for Web sites with lots of information on childcare issues.)

Some state-of-the art centers allow special cameras so you can check in on your baby at any time during the day using your computer and a Web-cam. Some businesses also offer minicams for hidden, at-home use, so you will know what's happening to your child. Those are very costly options, but if you can afford it, and the monitoring gives you more peace of mind, you may decide doing so is worth the price.

TRAVEL WITH YOUR BABY

A special event is coming up for your family, or the holidays, or your mother's birthday, or a sister's wedding, and you're duty bound to board an airplane or drive a car to get there. Here are our suggestions to help you and your baby survive the travel stress.

It's amazing how much stuff you'll end up packing to cover your baby's travel needs! And most of your baby gear should be carry-on luggage and not checked ahead of time.

If you're planning to fly with your baby, book your flights for the least-crowded times of day. You may want to fly a day or two early if you're coming up on a holiday when there will be heavy crowds in the airport. Try to get the bulkhead seats if you can—it will give you more legroom, and your tot will have squirm room.

Plan to arrive at the airport $2\frac{1}{2}$ hours early, instead of just one. That gives you plenty of time for diapering and feeding your baby and keeps you from experiencing last-minute panic when cabs don't show up, parking is a hassle, or long lines slow down your check-in process.

Most airlines will allow you to carry your baby's car seat onto the airline if it's been approved by the Federal Aviation Administration (FAA). If it has been, there will be a sticker on the seat that says it. (Note: Most booster seats are not FAA approved.) The only problem with fastening your baby down during the flight is that the airlines will probably expect you to purchase an extra ticket for your baby. Talk with the airline representative in advance.

Although in-flight injuries to babies and toddlers are rare, they do happen. Usually, they're injured when a plane hits turbulence and the baby flies out of his parent's arms, striking seat backs or luggage compartments.

The easiest way to install your baby's car seat in the airplane seat is to push the rear seat back as far as you can first. That gives you more leeway for fiddling with the belts.

Most babies cry during takeoff and landing. There's a simple explanation: Babies have huge middle ear canals on the inside of their eardrums that allow air to expand as pressure builds, causing pain. Letting your baby nurse or drink formula may help, but don't overfeed your baby! That can cause vomiting. Be prepared for that, or for getting your lap soaked, by bringing along a lightweight change of clothes for both your baby and you.

When the fasten-seatbelts sign gets turned off, consider taking your baby for a brief walk or two in the aisle if the refreshment cart isn't too near. You may need to change your baby's diapers on the closed lid of the toilet seat. Bring your own changing pad for sanitation. A flight attendant may let you use her fold-down seat at the rear of the plane for the job.

When you arrive at your destination, the car rental company will insist that your baby ride in a car seat. Most will promise you a rental seat when you call to make your reservation, but if you're traveling during peak vacation and holiday periods, you may find yourself at the airport with no seat for baby, and, thus, no car. Play it safe by bringing your own. (Some of the big baby equipment stores sell zippered car seat carry cases.)

What to Pack

- **Your doctor's telephone number.** Make sure you have it at all times in case baby gets sick, and you need medical advice. (And don't forget your medical insurance card.)

- **Car seat.** You can use it on the airplane if it is approved by the FAA. Rental car companies require that you use a car seat, but sometimes, especially during holidays, they run short. Just bring your own.

- **Sun shield.** Use a suctioned shade for the window nearest baby to prevent glare and sunburn.

- **Heat protection.** Take a thick blanket or beach towel to cover your baby's seat when your car's parked. Babies are far more vulnerable to heatstroke than children or adults, and they can die from it. Don't ever leave your baby inside the car without the air conditioning and an adult during the summer. Interior temperatures soar to 120°F and higher!

- **Diapers.** Newborns wet the most of babies at any age. They use up a minimum of ten diapers in twenty-four hours. Plan ahead just in case you end up stranded with car trouble, or sitting in an airport because a flight's been canceled.

- **Formula.** If you're not breast-feeding, the same goes for pre-measured, powdered formula and bottles.

- **Clothing.** You'll need a collection of baby T-shirts or gowns to make sure you're covered for all the wetting and spit-ups that babies routinely do.

- **Pacifier.** If your baby uses a pacifier, then pack three or four new ones that you've boiled out of the package for at least five minutes to remove chemical residues. A pacifier can help to balance air pressure changes in plane cabins.

- **Cloth diapers.** A handful of cloth diapers make great milksops on airplanes and for burping baby.

- **Sealable plastic bags.** Carry along three or four zippered plastic bags in the two-gallon size if you can find them for storing wet diapers and soiled clothing until you can get to a washing machine. Also carry smaller, sandwich-size bags for odds and ends.

- **Wipes or washcloths.** Put several folded, damp washcloths (or disposable baby wipes) for damp mopping jobs in one of the sealable plastic bags.

- **Clothes for the weather.** If it's winter, you'll need to pack a soft, warm blanket for carrying baby outside, and a knitted hat and booties for extra warmth. If you're going into warm weather, baby will need a brimmed hat.

- **Skin protection.** A tube of zinc oxide or a jar of petroleum jelly may come in handy as bottom protection if a rash shows up.

- **Medications.** Baby-strength Tylenol and a thermometer will be useful if baby spikes a fever. But don't use any medication without your healthcare provider's approval.

- **Stroller or front carrier.** A lightweight, easy-to-fold stroller with a good canopy, or a clip-on, gooseneck umbrella will come in handy for sightseeing and strolls, however, these types of strollers are not recommended for newborns younger than four months old (see page 526, *Baby Gear Guide*). But if you're flying, be careful about checking your naked stroller as a piece of luggage! The frame may get bent unless you secure it into a protective box like those used for golf bags.

- **Sleeping options.** If you're driving and have to bring your own baby bed, then consider purchasing an easy-to-fold travel play yard. It should have a firm mattress pad that's fastened down well. Don't waste your money on models with bassinets or diaper-changing add-ons—those features aren't worth it, and they may be unsafe if there's a chance baby could roll overboard or get caught between the tubular components. (See "Play Yards," on page 520.) Your other option is to rent a crib at your destination from a local rental service store. Inspect the crib when it arrives to make sure it's in good working order with no loose hardware or missing bars—both can cause deadly strangulation accidents. Plan to bring your own mattress protector, blankets, and fitted sheets.

Don't be surprised if you find yourself more tired when you get back home than before you left! Many parents say they return home feeling like they need a vacation *after* their vacation. One solution is to purposely plan an in-home family retreat for a few days after you get back home—carry-in dinners in the bedroom in front of the TV, leisurely walks in the park or nearby woods, hiring a neighborhood teenager to wash the dirty clothes. Downtime is critical before day-to-day work pressures inundate you again.

WHEN A BABY DIES

According to national statistics, there were 6.9 deaths per 1,000 live births in the U.S. in the year 2000. The leading causes for babies dying were: congenital anomalies (5,743 babies), being pre-term or low birthweight (4,397 babies), sudden infant death syndrome (SIDS) (2,523), problems related to complications of pregnancy (1,404), and respiratory distress syndrome (999).

It's normal to worry what it might be like if something were to happen to your baby. For most parents that fear does not materialize, but for parents of premature babies, or those born with serious birth defects, losing a baby sometimes becomes a heart-rending reality. Losing a child at any age can be hard, and it is profound when it happens with a newly born baby.

When a baby dies inside its mother, or an unexpected death occurs at birth—just when you are eagerly looking forward to the arrival of your new baby—you may find yourself plunged into a timeless place of intimate sorrow.

Your body will still be undergoing the powerful process of recovery from birth: stitches, bleeding, and swollen, engorged breasts, but you may also be burdened with a lonely, deep feeling of emptiness and sadness that's partly the huge disappointment of not having the joy you expected, but also it's hormonal from the readiness of your body to receive and nurture your baby.

Dr. John Bowlby, a British researcher, first identified the phases of grief that seem to apply to the death of a baby: numbness, yearning and searching, despair, and disorganization, followed eventually by hope and rebuilding.

Many parents who lose their babies experience both physical and emotional symptoms. Physical symptoms can include exhaustion, nausea and physical pains, headaches, an overwhelming feeling of emptiness or heaviness, not being able to sleep, or, the opposite, wanting to sleep all the time.

You may cry a lot, or, then again, you may find yourself in a trancelike state and not cry much at all. Some mothers feel an intensely poignant yearning to hold their babies in their arms. You may experience anger toward your healthcare providers if you feel they are somehow at fault for your baby's death. And, you may feel an almost overwhelming sense of guilt that your baby's death could have been averted had you just done things differently.

With all this going on, it's not unusual to wonder if you are going insane.

After a baby dies, his or her body may be pale or discolored, cold or stiff. In the past, when a newborn died, hospital caregivers often moved quickly to dispose of the baby before the parents had the chance to see or hold him or her, on the thought they were sparing the parents of grief.

It's natural to want to avoid facing the death of your baby and the feelings seeing the baby may engender, but holding and touching your baby can be an important part of telling your baby goodbye. It can help you to acknowledge the loss of this precious being who has been such an important part of your thoughts and experiences over the past nine months.

Even if your baby is stillborn, or only lives for a little while, you should give him or her a name. That will allow you to talk more easily with others about your experience, and it will confer human status to your baby as a person who truly existed for you, who has died, and who now must be mourned.

You may be asked whether you want an autopsy for your baby that may help to determine the cause of death. Autopsies are usually done at the hospital, and it will require the person performing the autopsy to look at your baby's internal organs. If having this done to your baby is emotionally distressing to you, you can decline having it done.

If you have questions about whether your baby's death could have been averted, or if you have a compelling need to know what went wrong, which might affect your having more children, then the results of the autopsy, which usually come back as a report weeks later, may give you some answers.

Dealing with Others' Reactions

Your parents, friends, and co-workers may find your baby's death hard to acknowledge, and may not accept how real your baby was to you, or the extent of the depths of feelings and grief you are experiencing.

Medical professionals may also have a hard time being open to you and your pain. Sometimes it's because they take the loss of the baby as a professional and personal failure, but don't want to show you their interior feelings about it. As a

consequence, they treat you curtly, or as though they have no feelings about what happened as their own, very human way of buffering themselves from the pain of your situation.

If the baby was born with a serious, long-term medical condition, friends may attempt to reassure you by telling you your baby would be better off than if he or she lived, but that does nothing to assuage your sorrow and loss.

"My baby was born dead. At first I was afraid to hold him, but I'm glad I did. A gentle nurse took a family picture of us together that I cherish now. I never felt such grief and loneliness as I did that night. My arms ached to hold my baby, but all we could do was cry."

Sometimes thoughtless people will try to convince you that you "can always have another baby," without understanding that it is this specific baby you loved and looked forward to taking home and caring for. At the same time, it can be heartbreaking to watch other mothers caring for their babies when you no longer have yours, and sometimes mothers who have suffered the loss of a baby are moved to a different wing to try to buffer them from the stark reality of that loss in the face of others' celebrations.

Rituals to Help You Mourn

Having a memorial service and a burial may help to provide you a way of connecting with others who love and support you so you won't feel quite as lonely during your grieving process.

Think about where you want to have your baby buried. If you move away later, it may be hard to leave the baby behind. There are a wide range of costs and options for cemeteries. You may choose one because you find it beautiful or soothing or because other family members are buried there.

Make sure you chose a plot that allows you to have a marker for your baby's name. A funeral home will help you in making arrangements, and some funeral directors even provide services free of charge or at a reduced rate.

Rather than having your baby's body picked up at the hospital, you may choose to carry the baby yourself, but you may need a special permit or death certificate. You may want to enclose small stuffed toys, or dress the baby in clothes that you bought in anticipation of bringing your baby home.

You will always remember your baby's birth day and death day, and you will probably calculate how old your baby might be if he or she had lived every year until you die.

Getting counseling, and finding a support group for grieving parents can help you to cope with your loss and to move toward recovery.

There are numerous parent-support organizations online. Your healthcare provider or hospital may also be able to provide the names of support groups.

A FINAL WORD

For most mothers, there's a gap between the birth of their baby and the time when the deeper, more meaningful rewards of parenthood start to set in.

Unless you've had a baby before, it's hard to imagine what life might be like with a baby. Even if you are an experienced parent who has been through pregnancy, birth, and baby care before, no two babies are ever alike. That means having to adapt to a whole new set of baby rules each time.

We promise that at some point, your body won't hurt any more, you'll get eight hours of sleep—give or take a few—and your baby will gradually transform from being a need machine into a human being. Not merely any human being, but the most interesting, entertaining person you can ever hope to know.

It will take about two years before your child can begin to communicate with you in words you can understand and about that amount of time to get out of changing poopy diapers. And those two years can seem like a long time.

Rest assured, though, that in time, and after you've recovered from pregnancy and the demands of a newborn, you'll start to discover the joy, rewards, and fulfillment of parenting. You can expect worthwhile, intensely valuable moments will come, one small moment at a time.

Someday, having a child in your life will feel as natural to you as having fingers. Life before baby will be as hard to recall as trying to picture your parents' lives before you were born. You won't wish your old life back for anything in the world, at least most of the time.

Bonding is a lifelong experience, not made in a single day, month, or year. It doesn't matter if you feel how you're "supposed" to feel, or if you do what you're "supposed" to do in the way experts say you should. What truly matters is that you and your baby not only survive, but thrive.

The joys will outweigh the pain, and all of the attention and affection you've poured into your baby will reap positive results. Even though pregnancy has caused your body to undergo subtle (and not so subtle) changes, your mind and heart will be stronger for the experience.

You may hear people say that "there's no such thing as a perfect mother." We may have even said it at some point in this book. But it's not true. You are your baby's perfect mother. Whatever your choices are, you are your baby's only, best mother, and no one can do your job better.

Your love for your baby may take the form of tenderness or affection so huge that you fear it may overwhelm you, or sometimes your love may feel more like duty.

It doesn't matter if you're single or married, sad or serene. Your love for your child will not be any less if you go back to work the day after delivery or stay at home until he or she leaves for college.

What does matter is that you do your best to do what's right for your child. Your love is perfect and whole because you are your baby's only mother, the best and only mother your baby will ever have.

Baby
Gear
Guide

5

urprise! Equipping, feeding, and outfitting your tiny offspring is likely to cost between $3,000–$5,000 during your pregnancy and the first year of your baby's life. Our guide is designed to help you figure out what to buy and what to avoid so you can save yourself hundreds or even thousands on your baby's gear. We'll help you determine in advance what is absolutely necessary to own immediately, which items you can wait to purchase until later, and what you may not need to buy at all. We'll also give you the best, state-of-the-art, category-by-category information on how to pick and choose products, and our handy illustrations will show you the major components of the most important product categories, so you'll know what you're looking at in the store.

Keep in mind, though, your newborn couldn't care less how much you spend. Your adorable little creature's primary motivation will be to get held, keep warm, get fed, be rocked, and have wet diapers changed. Then, repeat.

Starting Your Layette

"Layette" is the traditional word for all the baby stuff parents "lay up" before their baby arrives. Baby magazines and stores love distributing long, detailed layette lists for the sole purpose of driving guilt-ridden parents into the stores.

The lure of the baby product world is so strong that it's hard to resist piling up your shopping basket with everything that catches your eye, especially when you're in the throes of feeling "hormonal." Expect to feel a bit overwhelmed by the thousands of baby items lined up on store shelves. The best way to start is by hauling in only the barest of baby necessities that you choose because they're been proven to be useful, safe, and durable.

"The stores will still be open after your baby arrives" is excellent, grandmotherly advice. By postponing the purchase of items your baby won't use right away, you'll increase your savings.

OUR TWO-MINUTE, MONEY-SAVING ROUNDUP

Here's our quick list on how to save more than two thousand dollars in baby costs. It takes less time to read than it takes to browse a baby store.

- **Ask other parents.** Your friends who have kids will be great advisors. Before you buy, ask them what they liked and didn't like about their stroller,

high chair, crib, etc. Check out baby books with what-to-buy sections from the library. Make copies, and go home to study them. Copy, and print out parents' product reviews from www.epinions, www.baby-bargains.com, and other Internet sites featuring parents' product reviews. Good keywords for finding the review sites using www.froogle.com or another search engine: "comments" or "advice" and "baby products." Some big parenting sites offer product reviews from parents too. (See resource guide on page 538.)

- **Window shop first.** Don't buy a stroller, car seat, or other big-ticket item until you've taken a studious look at what's in the stores. Pull down the products from the shelves, and give them test drives. If it folds, fold it. If there are removable items, remove them. This way, you can troubleshoot for potential problems. Write down model names, numbers, and prices so you can comparison-shop later.

- **Don't buy anything until after the baby showers are over.** People love buying for babies. Spread the joy (and expense) by giving your relatives, friends, and grandparents a chance to outfit you with what you need. And, of course, save gift slips and tags, so you can return or consign what you don't need. (See "Getting the Word Out" on pages 459–461.)

- **Find your neighborhood kids' consignment shop.** Consignment shops sell used clothes and goods on behalf of clients, and then split the profits with them. Not only can you find great clothing and gear deals, but you can also recycle your own kids' unwanted or unused stuff later.

- **Beware of salespeople.** Don't trust salespeople to be straight with you. When you're ready to start buying, remember that even mild, grandmotherly shop clerks are experts at subtly (or not so subtly) guiding you toward buying more than you need. Don't let them "upsell" you into things like expensive mattresses, matching bedding sets, pricey car seats, and video baby monitors.

- **Shop the big guys.** Kmart, Wal-Mart, Target, and Costco sometimes offer good deals on no-frills baby products. Watch for sales and specials at the big megastores for babies too, such as Babies-R-Us and Baby Depot (sometimes found inside Burlington Coat Factory stores), but make sure you're given more than thirty days to return products.

- **Know what you're looking for.** Have your shopping list down in writing before you enter one of those giant baby emporiums, or you'll just feel dizzy and over-whelmed. The little doodads that you throw in at the last minute can really add up.

- **Buy a new, not used, crib and car seat.** New safety features hit the market all the time, as do product recalls for design flaws. A used car seat could have been in an accident and have invisible cracks in the frame that could compromise its ability to protect your baby. The glue that holds used cribs together deteriorates when it's been stored in a super-hot attic or a damp basement. Important pieces of hardware often get lost, or bent, and screw holes wear out. So to avoid potential injury the car seat and crib are best bought new.

- **Buy a "convertible" car seat.** It will be good for infants and kids from six to thirty pounds. These seats can ride facing backward or forward and will remain useful for two to three years. Babies should ride in the rear seat of cars, facing the back seat until they weigh twenty pounds or more. Try to install any seat you buy in the store's parking lot, so you can exchange it right away if you don't like it—you'll be using this piece of equipment for a while. Be sure to read your car owner's manual and the car seat directions. Also consider taking your car and seat to your local fire or police station to have them install it for you.

- **Nix bulky stroller/car seat combos.** Don't buy a stroller/car seat combo: They're bulky and awkward, and the small car seat is only good for a short time. Get a hands-free soft carrier such as the Baby Bjorn for shopping, and get a long-lasting car seat for riding. As for the stroller, get something that's lightweight with a reclining back that can handle a little gravel, rather than a giant baby bed on wheels.

- **Breastfeed your baby for as long as you can.** You can save your family about $1,000 a year in the cost of formula and bottles. Breastfeeding is also more convenient—you'll have less stuff to cram into your diaper bag, and you can go anywhere on a whim with your baby and have nice warm milk ready and waiting.

- **Buy or rent a breast pump.** You can purchase a good breast pump for less than $250, and this is still a great bargain compared with the costs of formula feeding. Pumping and storing milk will allow your partner and family to share the joy of feeding your baby. Pumps can also relieve painful pressure if your breasts become too full when your baby isn't hungry, and they can help you keep up your milk supply if you're separated from your baby.

- **Get a comfy carrier.** All your baby really longs for is to be kept close to you—to be nursed, rocked, carried around, and talked to. So, forget about baby toys, and instead buy a soft baby carrier you wear on your front—either a hammock-like sling or a little fabric baby seat with straps. Baby will get to ride with you and feel the soothing motions of your walking, and you'll get the use of your arms back.

Our Baby Shopping Primer

Most novice parents make the mistake of assuming that by paying a huge price for designer baby gear, they're getting better quality and safety. That's simply not the case. Middle-of-the-line products often hold up equally well, and sometimes they perform even better than pricey top-of-the-line models.

If you buy the highest-priced stroller, for example, you're most likely paying for a larger frame, thicker padding, and more accessories—all of which make the stroller heavier, bulkier, and less portable.

Sometimes manufacturers rent well-known logos and brand names from other companies just to make their products sell better. If you buy car seats or strollers labeled "Eddie Bauer," "Jeep," "Carter's," or "Oshkosh," it doesn't mean the products are any less vulnerable to serious flaws and safety recalls. You can save money and get equally durable products sticking to plainer, more generic models from the same manufacturers.

EXPECT "EXPECTANT PARENT" MAIL

Now that you're expecting, you're probably going to be targeted for baby product marketing. Most reputable marketers currently make an effort to protect consumers' privacy by giving them choices about the use of their personal information. This could be a checkmark if you wish more information, or agreeing to the privacy policy of an Internet site with the option of not signing up if you disagree. Even with caution, your name will probably migrate to lists for getting baby-related junk mail.

Even if you are planning to exclusively breastfeed your baby, you may find a carton of formula propped at your front door. Manufacturers know if they can get you on board and build what they consider brand loyalty, then you'll buy not just one product from them, but a whole series of products, including thousands of diapers in the course of your baby's long wetting career.

Manufacturers of formula, disposable diapers and baby wipes can offer free samples and money-saving coupons, and sometimes they have useful giveaways, such as free diaper bags. Deep-pocketed companies also underwrite numerous mailouts, free parenting magazines, and Internet sites offering what appears to be factual information. Whether you're surfing on the Web or delving into parenting pamphlets or magazines, keep your eyes open for biases that favor sponsors more than readers.

GETTING THE WORD OUT

It makes sense to postpone your shopping until you've had a baby shower (or two). Not only are baby showers fun, but they can help you stockpile what you need for Junior.

You have a couple of choices about getting the word out about what you need so you won't be inundated with cute, but not-so-usable stuff. First, don't be shy about hinting, and in fact, people will probably ask what you need.

If you need something, say so! If you're close friends with the hostess of your shower, give her a list, and tell her to relay suggestions. Some gift givers might be willing to pool their gift money to come up with a big-ticket item, such as a car seat. Or you can take the safe route, and simply ask for clothes and packages of disposable diapers in size 1. Hopefully, everyone remembers to put a gift receipt in the bottom of the box so you can discreetly return unwanted items.

"We decided to wait until the baby was born to see what we needed. It worked out well: We ended up buying very few of the things we thought we just had to have. Now we know we couldn't tell what was important ahead of time."

Another way to make your baby needs known is by using a baby registry at a major store, such as Babies-R-Us, JC Penney, or Target. Similar to bridal registries, expectant parents can create their wish lists by filling out forms and walking around the store with sales associates.

In some large chains, you will be given a computerized wand so you can wander through the store zapping the product code for anything that strikes your fancy. Your gift selections will then be downloaded into a gigantic database that can be accessed online nationwide or in store kiosks by anyone who walks in and wants to buy you a gift.

One advantage of a registry is that it will usually signal items that have already been purchased, which helps to avoid your receiving duplicate gifts.

List of unusual (but useful) shower gifts

• **Scarf for Mom.** Consider a generous, large wrap-around scarf for discreet breastfeeding or covering up Mom and baby during naps. You could even pair it with color-coordinated baby cap and booties.

• **Blankets and hand towels.** Collect burp cloths and absorbent, small baby blankets for catching spit-ups and keeping laps dry. Also consider making a double-sided flannel blanket (40″ × 40″), or two, that you cut and edge with stitching.

• **Baby care kit.** Put together your collection in a bathtub or a square wicker storage basket with a lid: baby shampoo, baby soap, a nasal aspirator, a digital thermometer, baby fingernail clippers, baby-dose Tylenol®, Vaseline®, A&D® diaper rash cream, two baby washcloths, and a hooded towel.

• **Dinner "in."** Set a date for a few weeks after the baby's born for an at-home catered dinner for the couple. You can cook yourself or hire someone else to do it. (Just be sure everything's cleaned up afterward.) Also consider gift certificates to local delivery and carryout restaurants.

• **Seasonal baby outfits.** For winter: a zip-front, cozy baby bunting with slots for car seat straps in a small size. For summer: a set of small baby hats and a tiny pair of sunglasses.

• **Stroller accessories.** For summer: a small, gooseneck umbrella to fasten onto the stroller to protect baby from glare. For winter, a Velcro™ fastened fuzzy "boot" that covers baby's legs and feet.

• **Baby bouncer.** A springy baby seat that also has a battery-operated vibration feature.

• **Comfort aids.** A crescent-shaped nursing pillow ("Boppy ®") and a small footstool in a carry case for toting to the hospital.

• **Privacy.** You'll have to have a deep pocket for this, but find out, and write a check for, the difference between a shared room and a private room in the hospital for two nights if the couple's health insurance doesn't cover it.

• **A clothesline of baby duds.** Gather a collection of colorful baby shirts and onesies. Use bright plastic clothespins to fasten them to a cord for pulling out of the box one after another.

• **Five big, extra-firm pillows.** It will make her final days of pregnancy a lot more comfortable and breastfeeding easier. Cover them in a cheery mix of colors and patterns, and stuff them into a bag tied together with a big ribbon.

• **Magazine subscriptions for Mom.** Some options: *Mothering, American Baby, Baby Talk, Parents, Parenting*, and *Child*. Wrap samples in a roll with gift-wrap and a bow. (See subscription information in the *Resource Guide* on page 538.)

• **Cleanup help.** A few weeks of maid service.

• **A baby swing.** Babies love to snooze in them. A small travel model will work great. (See our discussion on page 473.)

• **Nappies.** A package (or two) of newborn-size diapers.

• **Pet help.** A gift certificate for pet-sitting services for the week after birth.

BABY SHOWER GAMES

Having a baby shower thrown for you is one of the most fun things about being pregnant. Traditionally, they're women-only events, but men are showing up more often these days.

Spare a square.

With rolls of toilet paper, have guests guess how many "squares" you are around your pregnant belly. The guess that comes closest wins a prize.

Critter relay.

Have a diaper relay with stuffed animals or dolls. Contestants must undress the doll, hand it over to a team member for changing, and to another team member who puts its clothes back on.

Name that poopy.

Microwave different types of bite-sized chocolate bars of different flavors, and put them at the bottom of a diaper. Guests reach in and try to guess the candy bars by feel. Winner gets the "doody" prize. (Okay, so it will get lots of laughs.)

Baby-themed yummies.

Serve drinks in baby bottles or disposable sippy cups and snacks on teething biscuits or Zwieback. Gifts for all. Wrap little gifts—soaps, candles, picture frames, etc., and place them in a basket. Announce to your guests that a timer will go off every few minutes while you're opening your baby gifts. Whoever's gift you are opening when the timer goes off gets a favor from the basket.

Start a betting pool.

Have guests wager on the baby's birth weight and length or arrival date and time with a promise to pay off after delivery.

The $10,000 Diaper Pyramid.

Write the names of baby items on a card, and tape them on the backs of guests as they arrive. Give everyone five minutes to offer hints to one another about what's on their backs. Give gifts to the first four guests who guess the name of the item.

Baby bingo.

Use the computer to create your own bingo sheets with names of baby items. Or, if the baby's sex is known, but the name hasn't been decided, use boy or girl names to fill the card. You can use small tabs of paper to cover the card, or let guests use highlighters. Draw the items or names from a basket or bowl. The first person to get a row wins the game. (And you can keep going until the second and third person win prizes too.)

Essential Products for Before Baby Arrives

PRODUCT	OUR RECOMMENDATION
CAR SEAT	A "convertible" seat that faces rearward during the first year and forward until forty pounds, or a less adaptable rear-facing, infant-only seat.
CRIB	Mid-priced, JPMA-certified model with a quality wood finish to match your home décor.
CRIB MATTRESS	A mid- to upper-priced foam or innerspring.
SHEETS	Three or four fitted bottom sheets.
BLANKETS	Three or four small cotton blankets, plus one thicker polyester weave blanket (for winter).
DIAPERS & CLOTHING	(See list on pages 480–482.)
DIAPER WIPES	One carton.
BOTTLES & NIPPLES	Four, four-ounce size for storing breastmilk or formula.

IMPORTANT FEATURES

PAGE FOR MORE INFO.

Simple five-point harness system—
one strap for each shoulder, one for
each side of the waist, and one
between the legs.

491-498

Smooth, splinter-free wood with well-
attached bars, and one easy-to-lower
dropside.

501-503

FIRM. Thick upholstery (ticking) and
double-stitched edging.

504-506

Elastic on all sides to hold to the
mattress without coming loose.

NO PUFFY QUILTS. All-cotton is
absorbent and washable. Get one
dense polyester blanket if it's winter.

482-483

(See list on page 480-482.)

478-484
509-513

Any brand. A wipe warmer is optional
but makes for more baby comfort.

Clear plastic or glass. Easy-to-read
measurement lines and a set of
silicone nipples.

486-487

Optional Products for Before Baby Arrives

PRODUCT	OUR RECOMMENDATION
FRONT CARRIER	One
ROCKER & FOOTSTOOL	One each
SUPPORT PILLOW	One
AUTOMATIC BABY SWING	One
NURSERY MONITOR	One
BREAST PUMP	One electric
STROLLER	One midweight
HIGH CHAIR	One adjustable-height
CRIB MOBILE	One
BABY TOYS	One or two rattles or teethers
STATIONARY EXERCISER	One
SAFETY GATE	As many as needed when baby begins to crawl: one for top and one for bottom of each staircase

BEST FEATURES	PAGE FOR MORE INFO.
Washable, simple to put on, sturdy buckles, snaps and straps.	524
Comfortable with moisture-resistant upholstery.	521-522
A firm doughnut shape for supporting baby during feeding.	522
Windup or battery operated for soothing a cranky baby.	473-476
To listen for baby sounds. 900 MHz with rechargeable batteries.	518-519
An efficient electric model for storing extra breast milk.	487-490
Sturdy, easy to fold, reclining seat, ample storage bin.	526-530
JPMA-certified. One-hand tray release, sturdy belt, easy-to-clean upholstery.	516-518
Windup or battery operated. Whirling objects should face baby.	531
Bright colors, sized for tiny fists.	531-533
Optional, but fun, for a six- to twelve-month-old baby.	533-535
Easy to open and shut. Mounted to the wall with hardware.	522-524

Who's that baby?

Have everyone bring their own baby pictures. Place all of them on a bulletin board, numbering them, but not identifying them. Ask guests if they can guess who the other guests are from their baby pictures. The person who can guess the most wins a prize.

"Before I had a baby, I always went for cuteness when it came to baby shower gifts, but after I had a baby, I decided to give my friends only practical gifts: a teething ring, some tiny, side-tying T-shirts, a dozen cloth diapers, and a bath toy for the baby."

WHERE TO SHOP FOR THE BEST BARGAINS

Discount chains.

Huge discount chains like Wal-Mart, K-Mart, Sam's Club, and Costco are great places for saving money on everything. Although their baby-product lines are frequently limited to rather basic, no-frills models, their prices are often better than you can find anywhere else; plus, you can buy disposable diapers in bulk at great savings.

Baby superstores.

Gigantic baby superstores are next in line for savings. The list includes Toys-R-Us, Babies-R-Us, Baby Superstore, Buy Buy Baby, and Baby Depot sections found inside Burlington Coat Factory stores. Most carry a huge inventory of products, with advertised models at a substantial savings.

Retail chains.

Mainline retail chains such as JC Penney and Sears carry limited stocks of mainstream baby products, such as cribs, strollers, and clothing items. Prices are generally reasonable. Occasionally, you may be able to grab a great bargain during special discount days, such as baby week, or with end-of-season, or change-of-model markdowns. (New baby product models usually debut in late fall and the first of the year.)

Internet stores and manufacturers' sites.

Baby product e-tailers on the Internet sometimes offer huge discounts, but e-tail outlets come and go quickly, so make sure you're dealing with a reputable, enduring firm. Don't agree to back order if the product is not presently in stock, or you may get stuck with long delays. (See *Resource Guide*, pages 542–544 for Web addresses.) Some manufacturers offer periodic warehouse sales through their Web sites. (Also see *Resource Guide* for manufacturers' Web addresses, page 567.) In both cases, don't forget to factor in shipping and handling costs when comparing prices.

Specialty baby stores.

Independent baby stores usually carry upscale products and accessories not available at huge discounters. You're likely to find excellent customer service there with managers willing to respond to every nagging product question. Pricetags are usually higher, but so are service levels.

Baby product catalogs.

Direct mail catalogs carrying baby goods make for interesting browsing, but by the time you add shipping and handling costs, you probably haven't saved very much at all.

Yard sales and consignment shops.

Clothing and toys are great finds at yard sales, but cribs and car seats aren't. Ever-changing federal regula- tions make each new generation of car seats and cribs safer than those manufactured even a year earlier.

FATAL PRODUCT FLAWS

Just because a product appears to be designed for use by babies, there is no guarantee it's going to be safe. Every year baby products injure tens of thousands of babies seriously enough to require hospital emergency room treatment. The three biggest causes of baby-product related injuries are poor design, misuse, and product deterioration after use.

The competition among baby product manufacturers is fierce. When an innovative product design makes a big profit in the marketplace, other manufacturers quickly follow with nearly identical clones. The only problem is that fatal flaws get copied and reproduced.

Over the decades, products that might have once appeared to be wonderful contraptions for babies have only later been discovered to have serious, baby-threatening flaws.

Sometimes parents misuse baby products by relying on them to serve as babysitters. Many babies have died when they were left alone in a device and got into trouble with no one to there to help them. They've fallen over in suctioned bathtub seats and drowned; gotten strangled in the frame strollers when they were supposed to be napping; or strangled when their necks got captured on the partially collapsed side of a playpen while their parents were somewhere else in the house.

Parents often fail to follow manufacturers' age and weight guidelines, unintentionally putting their babies at risk. A too-big baby could overload a car seat and could be killed; a toy meant for an older child could have small parts that a baby could chew off and choke on; a curious toddler could open the battery compartment of a kid's toy, and choke.

All baby products eventually break down from the wear and tear that parents and babies give them. Wheels fall off strollers, safety latches get bent, and stop holding, seatbelts fray, buckles break—and sometimes these product failures can be a life-threatening hazard for a baby. The worst offenders are old, malfunctioning cribs with missing bars or broken hardware that are responsible for the deaths of nearly a hundred babies every year in the U.S.

WHAT "CERTIFIED" MEANS

All baby products have to meet minimal product safety standards set by the federal agencies listed in the box to the right. But, some baby products display a certified seal on their frames. That means they have met voluntary safety guidelines overseen by manufacturers themselves, the JPMA (the Juvenile Products Manufacturers Association).

When a product carries a certified sticker, the product complies with certain safety guidelines, and the manufacturers' product line has passed rigorous tests for durability and safe design.

Currently, the JPMA certification program includes bassinets and cradles, bath seats, carriages and strollers, full-size cribs, gates and enclosures, handheld infant carriers, high chairs, infant bouncers, infant swings, non-full size cribs and play yards, portable hook-on chairs, stationary activity centers, and toddler beds and walkers.

But note: Not all baby products and baby product categories are certified. And manufacturers can choose not to participate in the voluntary sticker program, or its products can fail, so they will not wear the sticker. Often, imported products, even though they may be perfectly safe, will not be certified. It's too bad baby products aren't required to be certified!

Protecting your baby from baby product dangers

1. Shop carefully. Make sure the product is right for your baby. Check out the manufacturers' recommended age and weight recommendations, and read all the warnings before you buy.

2. Follow the directions. The manufacturer's directions contain information that is critical for your baby's safety and detail who to contact when there's a problem. Put all your baby product receipts and literature in a single file so you can find them when you need them.

3. Mail the registration card. Even though it may make you a target for junk mail, it's also the primary way that manufacturers locate customers who have bought bad products to inform them there's been a recall.

Recall Reconnaissance

Federal agencies have the power to recall baby products that pose dangers, and literally millions of baby products have been banned, pulled off shelves, or undergone corrective actions to retrofit the unsafe parts of a product.

In spite of federal actions, product-related accidents and injuries continue to happen, killing hundreds of babies every year, and sending more than ten thousand babies to emergency rooms for treatment.

New products introduce new baby dangers into the marketplace; old and worn-out products fail and greedy importers ignore federal regulations by selling shoddy goods that fail federal standards.

Keep on top of recalls, and report baby product problems by frequently accessing these federal sites:

U. S. Consumer Product Safety Commission (CPSC)
Washington, D.C. 20207–0001
Toll-free consumer hotline: 800-638-2772
Web site: www.cpsc.gov
Regulates the safety of most baby products, clothing, bedding, and toys. (Car seat recalls generally come from the National Highway Traffic Safety Commission—below.)

National Highway Traffic Safety Commission (NHTSA—"nit'-sah")
400 Seventh Street, SW
Washington, D.C. 20590
Toll-free auto safety hotline: 888-327-4236
Web site: www.nhtsa.dot.gov
Regulates and recalls children's car seats and rates their installation instructions.

Food and Drug Administration (FDA)
5600 Fishers Lane
Rockville, MD 20857
Toll-free general information number: 888-INFO-FDA (463-6332)
Web site: www.fda.gov
Regulates baby food, medicines, and cosmetics, such as bathing products and diaper rash creams.

Potential Dangers

PRODUCT	FATAL FLAW	WHAT HAPPENS
CRIBS	Hardware could bend and break. Bars work loose. Decorative posts capture baby's clothing.	Babies' vulnerable necks get caught in gaps between the mattress support and the crib, or between the bars when their bodies slide out. Clothing forms a noose and strangles.
CAR SEATS	Parents fail to follow directions. They place seats in the front seat of the car in front of killer air bags; seats are installed incorrectly; children aren't safely secured in the seat; or the child is put in the wrong seat for his weight.	Front seat airbags deploy during a crash, killing the small occupant in front. The seat isn't fastened down, or the baby isn't correctly strapped into the seat, or the baby is too large for the seat, leading to serious injuries during a crash.
PORTABLE PLAY YARDS	Sidebars may not click into place when they're set up, forming a loose V shape.	Toddlers attempt to climb out, and strangle when they get their necks captured in the V.
STROLLERS	Large legholes or gaps in the frame might allow the baby to slide out. Sharp hardware could capture small hands and fingers, especially when the frame accidentally collapses.	Napping babies are left unattended. Strangulation occurs when the baby's body slides through legholes or out gaps, leaving the head behind. Frames fail to lock in the open position, capturing children's fingers and hands in sharp hinges.
BEDDING	Puffy, soft surfaces on quilts, loose sheets, and stuffed crib toys could suffocate or strangle a baby.	Babies suffocate in soft surfaces when placed face downward, or when their necks get wrapped up in loose sheets.

PRODUCT	FATAL FLAW	WHAT HAPPENS
BABY TOYS	Small parts, such as eyes, buttons, or wheels could work loose. Sharp points and edges might injure. Loose fur or hair can get chewed off. Balloons could pop, and catch in the throat.	Small parts and loose fur are swallowed and get stuck in babies' throats, cutting off the air supply. Sharp points injure during falls. Fur and hair gets caught in the throat. Pieces of latex from popped balloons are inhaled and shut off the baby's air supply.
SUCTIONED BATH SEATS	Suction cups on the base of self-standing tub seats don't always hold.	Parents leave the baby unattended. The seat falls over, pressing the baby's face into the water, and the baby drowns within several minutes.
WHEELED WALKERS	These small seats on wheels sometimes move faster than parents anticipate.	Walkers tumble down open staircases, causing severe head trauma. They propel babies into hot stoves, fireplaces, and outdoor swimming pools where they drown.
DIAPER PAILS AND LARGE WATER-FILLED BUCKETS	Toddlers might drop a toy into the water and then reach down to try to retrieve it.	The baby's heavy head causes him to fall in headfirst and drown.
SAFETY GATES	Accordion-style gates have X-shaped joints that could work like scissors when they close. Some models have holes in center mesh panels that a toddler could use for climbing. Stoppers on the side of the gate sometimes fail.	Babies get their hands or fingers crushed when the gate opens. Toddlers use holes in the gate panel to climb over and fall down stairs on the other side. Stoppers on pressure-mounted gates don't hold, causing the gate to fall down stairs with the baby.

4. Keep up with recalls.
Periodically check the Web sites
of the Consumer Product Safety
Commission and other federal
agencies that regulate baby products
to see if you own recalled products.
(See page 469.)

5. Use straps. The seat straps
in strollers, car seats, high chairs,
booster seats, swings, and changing
tables are there for an important
reason: They protect babies from
falling out or getting strangled.
Use them every time you put your
baby inside.

6. Stay nearby. Stay in the same
room if your baby is in a holding
device, such as a stroller, high chair,
play yard, car seat, or stroller. Feed
your baby in your arms instead of
using a bottle-propper, and always
hold your baby during bathing
instead of using a suctioned bath
seat that could topple over and
drown your baby in only a matter
of minutes.

7. Keep baby away from dangers.
Keep your baby out of range when
you're installing, opening, closing,
assembling, or doing other things
with baby products. You're distracted, and sharp corners, hinges,
and edges could cause injuries.

Baby Gear
A to Z

Here's our prep course on choosing great baby gear along with our recommendations. We'll be covering not only the basic equipment you'll need before your baby arrives, but also the big-ticket items you're likely to acquire later, such as strollers and high chairs. Everything's in alphabetical order to make it easy to find what you need.

AUTOMATIC BABY SWINGS

If your baby appears to be quickly soothed by rocking and rhythmical motion, then an indoor, automatic swing may be just the answer for wooing him into a peaceful, hypnotic state so the rest of the family can eat dinner in peace. These devices come with baby-size seats mounted on a frame that tick-tocks the seat back and forth after you wind it up, or with a switch that turns on a small, battery-operated motor.

Keep in mind, though, most swings take up a lot of floor space and are the most useful up to about six months of age. After that, there's a danger that your tot may reach out and grab the bars and cause himself

to get hurt. A folding travel swing may be a good buy if space is a problem. Or, you may want to consider a rocking baby seat as an alternative. (They're described on page 478.)

There are basically five styles of automated swings: windup A-frames; battery-operated A-frames; open-front models; multi-use models; and small, travel swings.

Windup A-frames are equipped with an internal spring that tightens with a hand crank. The spring loosens gradually with each successive swinging motion. They are the least expensive swings you can buy. While some models offer only fifteen minutes of rocking time per windup, others will run up to thirty minutes with cranking—a better choice.

Battery-operated swings have small motors inside to push the swing arm, and usually require approximately six C-cell batteries that can run the swing for about two hundred hours before the juice runs out. Most versions offer on/off switches and allow a choice of several swing speeds. Some come with built-in computer chip music, which is more likely to drive you nuts than soothe your baby.

The Skinny on Swings

Here's what to look for when you go swing shopping.

Seat belts and between-the-legs post. A sturdy, easy-to-operate seat belt and a permanent post that goes between baby's legs will help to prevent your baby from falling forward into the front bar or slipping out between the seat's legs.

Front play tray. A front play tray can help to hold your baby safely inside, but models with front bars that open and swing out may make it easier to put your baby in the seat. Toys mounted in the tray are nice, but certainly not worth paying extra for.

Age and weight limitations. Be careful to note the age and weight ranges for use of the swing, and do not allow toddlers to swing who exceed the recommended weight limit.

Windup running time. If the swing is a windup model, get the one with the most minutes of swing time.

Battery life. If battery-operated, check how many batteries it requires, what type are needed, and how long the swing is expected to run before the batteries have to be replaced.

The frame. Measure the amount of floor space the swing requires. If you live in a cramped apartment, choose a miniaturized version, or a rocking baby seat, instead. Newer models have open tops that make installing a baby easier, but the extra price may not be worth the convenience. Check to see if the frame folds for storage.

Seat reclining options. Try out the seat's reclining feature, and check how many positions it offers. A deep recline will be the most comfortable for small babies and for napping.

Seat covering. Choose a seat cover pattern you like, and make sure it's removable and machine washable.

Extra features. Manufacturers add sound, vibrations, lights, deep headrests, suspended moving toys, and even seat height adjustments to induce parents to spend more. Remember: Your baby's swing will likely only be used for a couple of months, so save your money, and buy a basic, no-frills model.

While traditional swings have an A-shaped frame to support the swing assembly, some newer designs are configured with an open top, allowing easier access to the seat portion when you're putting baby inside or removing him. Folding travel swings are small, tabletop versions of swings that fold readily for travel. They use batteries and may offer sound and music options. Multi-use swings are equipped with both a seat and an interchangeable bassinet (baby bed), either of which lock onto the swing's arms.

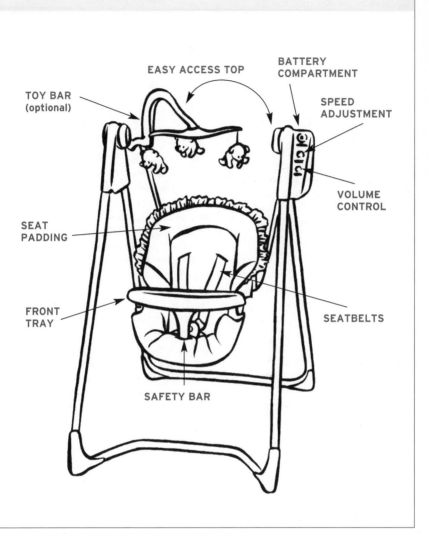

EASY ACCESS TOP

BATTERY
COMPARTMENT

TOY BAR
(optional)

SPEED
ADJUSTMENT

VOLUME
CONTROL

SEAT
PADDING

FRONT
TRAY

SEATBELTS

SAFETY BAR

Windup

(+) The least expensive option.
Babies like the tick-tock sound
they make. Models fold easily
and are usually very simple, but
adequate for the job.

(−) They hog a lot of floor space.
Winding the swing may be noisy
enough to wake up the baby.
Sometimes the spring assem-
blies break from overwinding.

Battery-operated

(+) They're quieter than the windup models, but they cost more; plus, you'll have to pay for the batteries. Seats may be more comfortable and offer recline features that the windups don't.

(−) They take up a lot of floor space. Sometimes their small, whirring motors slow down or break. Their batteries and motors make them heavier and more cumbersome to move or store. The computer chip music that adds to the price of the swing can be annoying.

Open-topped, battery-operated

(+) They're easier to use, and some offer side-to-side rocking in addition to front-to-back motion. Most offer reclining seats.

(−) They generally cost more than A-frame models and take up a similar amount of floor space. They don't fold for storage as compactly as A-frames.

Folding travel

(+) They don't take up much space, yet offer rhythmical movement that babies love. They're easy to move from place to place.

(−) Don't offer the full range of motion of larger versions.

Multi-use with bassinet

(+) Gives a young baby an alternative place to snooze without having to sit upright.

(−) These systems are huge, and the bassinet section isn't always comfortable for small babies. When rocking, it will knock the baby from one side to the other. There have been recalls when the bassinets have broken loose from the swing's arm.

BABY BOUNCERS

Baby bouncers are miniature baby seats on a frame that perch a baby where she can watch the action going on around her. Usually the seat portion is made like a fabric sling. They may make baby more comfortable after a big nursing by putting her in a semi-upright position, and bouncers give baby a place to watch family members work and play.

Most models jiggle each time a baby moves. Some come with a small, battery-operated motor for soothing vibrations (like a massaging bed). Others have rockers on the bottom, or offer lights and/or music shows to entertain the baby.

Safety is an important issue. Don't ever leave baby alone in the seat, even for a few minutes, and be sure to follow the manufacturer's suggested weight guidelines for use. The safety belt is critical too. It will keep the baby from flipping out of the seat.

A non-skid surface on the seat's base will prevent it from "walking" off table or counter edges. But for maximum safety, seats should be kept on low surfaces to prevent falls. Frames are flimsy and can buckle, so never try to carry your baby from one place to another while she's in the seat.

The Skinny on Baby Bouncers

Stable frame. Try placing your hand in the center of the seat to test how easily it tips sideways, forward, or backward. Look for a sturdy frame that's larger than the seat, which indicates better stability.

Good seat belt. The bouncer should have a good seat belt to hold baby safely inside.

Recline options. Extra reclining positions will give you some options in finding the most comfortable position for baby.

Non-slip base. Skid-resistant pads on the bottom of the seat are essential and help to keep the baby from walking the seat off a table or countertop when he jiggles.

Seat comfort. Colorful, deeply padded seat covers are a plus, but read the label to make sure they are removable and washable.

Toys. Baby will have fun batting at playful toys suspended from a front toy bar. Just make sure the bar and the toys are well secured and can't work loose.

Entertaining extras. Vibration, music, and rocking are extras that may help to soothe a fussy baby. Buy an extra pack of batteries.

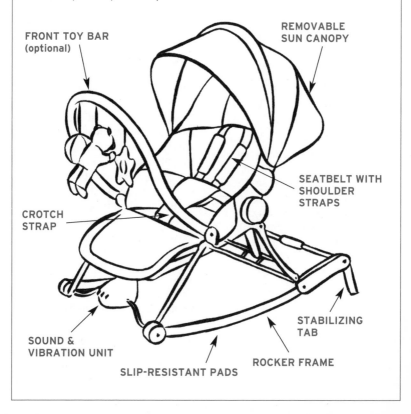

FRONT TOY BAR (optional)

REMOVABLE SUN CANOPY

SEATBELT WITH SHOULDER STRAPS

CROTCH STRAP

SOUND & VIBRATION UNIT

STABILIZING TAB

ROCKER FRAME

SLIP-RESISTANT PADS

Don't confuse a baby seat with a car seat. The former is lightweight, reclines, and is for use in the house; the latter is a heavy shell with padding to be used only when a baby is strapped into the car, a specially equipped stroller, or in a grocery cart. Don't substitute a car seat for an in-the-house baby seat. It is extremely heavy and can be toppled over by pets or siblings, possibly injuring the baby inside. (For more on car seats, see page 491–497.)

Bouncer

+ A baby seat is a handy place to hold your baby while you work in the kitchen or do housekeeping chores. Those that jiggle offer vibrations, or rocking can substitute for a baby swing and take up a lot less space. Suspended toys or interesting sounds can be momentarily entertaining, but the noise can irritate others.

− They're only useful for a small time before the baby can sit up on his own. Baby seats sometimes fall from countertops and tables, resulting in serious head injuries. Don't try to carry your baby in the seat; frames can sometimes bend, toppling the baby out.

BABY CLOTHES

Babies have very tender skin, and most little ones hate getting dressed and undressed. Their biggest complaint is when parents pull things over their heads. It makes them think they're suffocating, and they will fuss every time. Other than that, your baby will be oblivious to what you make her wear. Using your baby for a fashion statement in cuteness is your own doing.

When it comes to buying baby clothes, you basically get what you pay for. Inexpensive baby clothes tend to be thin, almost transparent, and their finishing may be so poor that there are loose strings and scratchy seams, and they will fade and come apart after a couple of washings.

On the other extreme, designer brands in upscale department stores and from the Internet will be dense and buttery soft. The only problem is that your baby is going to grow like wildfire, practically doubling weight in the first four months. Investments in tiny luxury just won't pay off, especially if the duds have to be dry-cleaned (though you may be able to minimize your loss by reselling at a consignment shop).

Rather than dressing your baby to the hilt, think simple comfort instead. The best baby duds are super-absorbent and soft. Avoid shirts or clothes with scratchy seams, especially around the arm and leg holes. Also avoid appliqués that are rough on the inside and can cause skin irritation. Watch out for garments with sharp metal-backed snaps. They can scratch, and if they aren't enameled, the raw metal surface may cause a skin rash. Avoid unshielded metal zippers that could scratch or capture a baby's fragile skin. Plastic zippers are better. Constantly monitor all garments for loose threads that could wrap around a baby's fingers or toes and cut off circulation.

There is no uniform industry standard for sizing baby clothes, and there are wide differences among brands. Most prepackaged baby garments have a weight chart on the back to help you choose the right size for your baby, but it's always better to err on the large side. Don't hesitate to open packages to look at the size or to compare the quality of garments from different manufacturers.

Although it's nice to have several shirts in a baby's actual, newborn size, you'll quickly learn to buy shirts, onesies (shirts that snap at the crotch), and nightgowns in six- and twelve-month sizes so they'll last longer. Sleeves can always be rolled up.

Most babies hate having shirts or other pieces of clothing pulled over their heads. Shirts should either open from the front or have generous, wide necks, or neck flaps to make pulling them on and off a quick and easy task.

Everyday baby shirts usually come in either all-cotton, or cotton-polyester blends. Cotton-polyester blends are less likely to wrinkle, and they're often cheaper, but pure cotton knits are more absorbent and less likely to stain.

Cotton garments tend to shrink and become denser and more absorbent with laundering. Most manufacturers have compensated

> *"Unless you just love dressing and undressing, dressing and undressing (repeat ad nauseum), keep your baby's in-the-house clothes simple. A diaper and shirt will do."*

for that by making the cut of their garments larger. If you go the all-cotton route, buy items that are at least one or even two sizes larger than your baby's current weight just to get more wear out of them.

Babies soil clothes several times a day. So how many shirts, onesies, or gowns you buy depends mostly on how easy and convenient it is for you to do laundry. If you live in an apartment with all the washers and dryers in the basement, then stock up on lots of baby shirts so you can wait longer than a day before being forced to take that long trek down to the laundry room.

Baby nightgowns can be handy in the early days, especially those gowns with small flaps to cover the baby's fists. This feature will keep the baby from scratching his face with his fingernails until you gain confidence in fingernail filing or cutting. (Look for fingernail clipping hints on page 400.) Softly elasticized bottoms on gowns will help to keep them down over the baby's legs

Minimum Clothing to Have on Hand

TYPE OF GARMENT	DESCRIPTION	NUMBER	COMMENT
Baby T-shirts	All-cotton baby T-shirts that snap on the side, or slip over the head with wide necks.	6	Your baby will outgrow them quickly. Buy two in the newborn size just to have something that fits perfectly, but buy the rest in the six-month size, or larger. Get short sleeves for warm weather and long sleeves for winter, or a combination of the two, and use the short-sleeve versions for undershirts. Check for soft inside seams, and inspect for loose strings after every laundering.
Onesies	All-cotton knit shirts with wide neck openings that snap at the crotch. Choose three- or six-month sizes.	4	Choose long sleeves for winter, short sleeves for summer.
Nightgowns	Full length, all-cotton, or cotton-poly blends with an open or gently elasticized bottom.	4	These keep babies' legs covered in the night. Fold-over cuffs for the hands can keep baby's fingernails from scratching his cheeks.
Footed sleepers	Stretchy, baby-style pajama suits with long sleeves and covered feet.	3	Buy the six-month size, and roll up the sleeves. Avoid metal snaps if the skin side is not enameled. Inspect the inner seams after every washing to make sure there aren't any loose strings that could wrap around tiny toes.

Useful duds and baby stuff that will come in handy during the first six months of baby's life.

TYPE OF GARMENT	DESCRIPTION	NUMBER	COMMENT
Sleep sac (baby bunting)	A baby sleeping bag made from fleece or quilting for cold weather.	1	Use it instead of a blanket and a cover sheet in the crib in cold weather. Look for the six-month size with a shielded zipper down the front, or flat snaps that give access to the diaper area. Avoid versions with scratchy appliqués on the front.
Socks	Cotton knit with soft cuffs.	4	They stay on better than booties and help to keep a baby's feet warm. Tie the socks together in a knot, or stuff them in a zippered lingerie bag for washing so they won't get lost in the machine.
Baby sweaters	Choose tightly knit cardigans that zip or snap up the front. Use for winter warmth or in buildings with air conditioning.	2	Get the six-month size, and roll up the sleeves. Should be washable and without extra lace, appliqués that could scratch, or that use a loose knit that could capture tiny fingers.
Hat	A small, knitted toboggan if it's winter. For summer, a brimmed hat with a neckband to hold it on and a flap to cover the back of the neck for protection.	2	Most babies hate wearing hats, but they can help to keep a baby from losing heat in the cold, and shield the baby from sunburn in warm weather. Expect to lose one overboard.
Bibs	Small, washable bibs with easy-open neck closures.	4	Babies constantly drool and spit up, so use them to protect clothing.

Clothing to Have on Hand

TYPE OF GARMENT	DESCRIPTION	NUMBER	COMMENT
Receiving blankets	Choose the twenty-eight-inch or thirty-six-inch size in a soft, absorbent cotton flannel or a waffle weave.	5–6	These handy, washable blankets are great for protecting your shoulder, or for swaddling up a fussy baby.
Waterproof pads	Small fabric-backed with waterproof (rubber) pads.	4–5	Use them under the baby in the crib to protect the sheet from wetness, and on your lap or shoulder for spit-up protection.
Reusable diapers	Thick, soft, prefolded terry or flannel with outer covers that use Velcro™ side closures.	12 diapers, 4–5 outer covers	Handy when you run out of disposables in the night. Also handy for cleaning spit up.
Cheap washcloths	Buy several large packs.	1 to 2 dozen	Use them to wipe baby's messes. If they get stained and won't wash clean, just toss them.
Baby snowsuit (for cold climates)	The suit should have insulation, a hood, legs, and a zipper to the ankles for diapering.	1 (winter)	If your baby is born in late summer or early fall, go for the twelve-month size to take your baby through the entire winter. For a midwinter baby, buy the six-month size. For a late-winter baby, a sac (see above) may work, but only if there are slots inside the garment to adapt to the shoulder and crotch straps of the car seat.

while he sleeps.

Since babies outgrow clothes so quickly, consider loading up on baby shirts and garments at thrift stores and tag sales. Or beg on your hands and knees for the cartons of used baby duds stored in friends' attics when they're through with baby making. Almost all baby hand-me-downs are likely to have formula stains down the front that can usually be removed by a soaking in bleach, using oxy-based cleaners, or spotting with stain removers.

Hidden fire and heat hazards

When it comes to sleepwear, the U.S. Consumer Product Safety Commission (CPSC) has issued several warnings: One is against using loose-fitting, all-cotton garments as pajamas because they ignite rapidly if exposed to a flame.

As a result of burns to toddlers, the commission has required that children's loose clothing labeled as sleepwear be flame resistant. Form-fitting clothing is considered safe. Unlike toddlers, newborns are not likely to wander near flames, but if you or someone in your household smokes, you use a wood stove or kerosene heaters, or have open-flamed stovetop units, flame retardancy in your baby's clothing could be an issue to consider.

Smoke detectors are critical lifesavers. Make sure all of them are operational before you bring your baby home. Install a carbon monoxide detector as well. Ask your local fire department about putting a special sign on your baby's window indicating a child is there, and make sure your house number is brightly displayed at the bottom of your driveway.

Babies can be seriously burned by hot water coming from the faucet. Lower your water heater's thermostat to no hotter than 104°F, and if your sinks and bathtubs have a hot and cold knob, make it a practice to always turn the hot water off first.

The sac option instead of blankets

The CPSC also warns against using loose top sheets and blankets to cover your baby at night. That's because babies can strangle when they've become entangled in them. One suggestion is to place baby with his feet nearly touching the end of the crib, and then to carefully fold sheet and blanket so that they are only to the level of your baby's armpits.

A clothing option for safe sleeping is to use no top coverings at all, but to place your baby, face up, in a sac, a one-piece bag that encloses baby's legs. Sacs can be found in large retail baby product stores. A small, strapless knit cap can help your baby to conserve body heat if you turn down the thermostat at night, or if it's drafty in his bedroom.

After the first few weeks, your baby will adapt to home temperatures that are comfortable for you. Babies' feet are always colder than the rest of their bodies, but some parents have found that keeping small socks on a baby's feet helps him to feel safer and more comfortable.

It's important to not overdress your baby if he is ill and has a fever. The concept of sweating out an illness is dangerous and can even be fatal for a sick baby. A baby's internal thermostat is primitive, and a baby doesn't sweat like children and adults in order to cool down. Some babies have died from heatstroke when they had fevers and were purposely overheated by their clothing.

BATHING AIDS

All new parents are a little scared of giving that first bath to their babies. As long as the baby's umbilical cord is healing, you shouldn't try to bathe the baby, and you probably won't need to, anyway. Eventually, the time for bathing will come around, and you're going to have to face the suds challenge.

It's really demanding to try to prepare everything in advance and then have to deal with a slippery and not-very-happy newborn at the same time. (For instructions on how to carry off that first big bath, see our instructions on page 430.) The easiest thing is probably to just take the baby into the bathtub with you on your lap, and have your partner help you pass the baby in and out of the tub so you can get in and out safely yourself.

As for baby bathtubs, they're virtually all the same. They're huge, bulky, and hell to manage when they're filled with water that sloshes over the side with the least misstep. Although you may feel more secure using a baby-size bathtub at first, you'll probably soon convert to washing the baby in the kitchen sink lined with a folded bath towel, or taking the baby into the tub

with you where you can hold him securely in your lap.

Bath supports are baby-size wire frames shaped like lounge chairs that are lined with a terry or absorbent fabric sling. Once your baby's been bathed, set it out to dry.

Foam bath supports for babies can be useful. They're inexpensive, thick slabs of foam shaped to fit into a baby bathtub that help to hold the baby in place. Once a toddler becomes curious and starts pulling foam pieces off, they should be thrown away. Mildew causes a problem, so wring the foam out and put it in a warm, sunny place to dry.

Extra bathing supplies

Does your baby need special baby soaps for his tender skin? Probably, or at least something very gentle without the harsh chemicals contained in most soap bars. Aveeno® and Dove® brands are often recommended for baby skin, as are castile soaps labeled specifically for babies.

Other than special soap and shampoo, your baby doesn't need a lot of cosmetics—powders, oils, lotions, and ointments that are supposed to be for baby's cleanliness and skin care. They're a waste of money, and some products, particularly those containing perfumes or strong chemicals, may irritate a baby's tender skin. Use a tearless baby shampoo for your baby's scalp instead of soap that leaves a residue. (See "Baby Bathing Basics" on page 429.)

Baby powders containing talcum

The Skinny on Baby Bathtubs

Sturdy sides. The tub should be made from thick, rigid material with smooth rims so it won't scratch or spill water when you lift it.

Small is better. Miniature, body-shaped tubs are easier to manage with newborns than large, one-size-fits-all models. Get one that will fit into your kitchen sink, or simply line the sink with a folded, wet bath towel. (Toddlers usually prefer using the regular bathtub.)

Safety features. A gentle seat angle with crotch support and slip-resistant surfacing will help hold the baby in place.

Tight plug. A leak-resistant plug on the base makes emptying easier.

Folding feature. Tubs that fold in half for storage take up less room when not in use. Just make sure there are no seams that could pinch a baby or gaps that could leak.

Nix bath seats. Baby bath seats with suction cups on the base have been implicated in more than thirty baby deaths. The suction cups don't hold, and babies drown. **Don't buy or use one.**

have been connected in some cases with a rare form of baby pneumonia. If the baby spills the powder onto his face, and inhales the dust, fine particles irritate the lungs and make the baby seriously ill.

If you do use powder, try a talc-free version, such as one made from kaolin clay powder, and gently dust it onto your palms first before applying it to your baby's diaper area.

Keep your baby dry with your family's regular terry towels laundered in a non-irritating, fragrance-free liquid detergent. Knit baby towels aren't very absorbent.

BIRTH ANNOUNCEMENTS

There are literally hundreds of choices for announcements to let the world know that your baby has finally arrived. Most card stores have clever preprinted cards with a place for you to fill in the blanks about your baby's name, date of birth, and weight. Enclose a snapshot if you wish. Office supply stores offer formal announcement cards, similar to wedding announcements, but be prepared to wait a week, or so, for delivery.

Anne Geddes' Web site (www.annegeddes.com) offers adorable announcement cards and snoozing cherubs with simple borders that you can download and print on your own computer, and you can also find numerous sites on the Internet that sell customized announcements. (You can find additional baby announcement Web sites in our *Resource Guide* on page 545.)

BOTTLES AND NIPPLES

Standard baby bottles usually come in four-ounce and eight-ounce sizes. They can be made of glass or molded, transparent plastic. Most newborns get along well with the four-ounce size for the first few months. Clear bottles with easy-to-read measurements are the easiest to use. Whimsical bottle shapes, such as those shaped like bears, doughnuts, or baseballs make it hard to wash out all the milk residue.

Most bottles come with an adjustable, screw-on collar to hold the nipple in place. How tightly the collar is screwed on affects how much air the nipple lets in. A loosened collar will speed up milk flow, a tightened collar will make baby have to work harder to get the milk out.

Sterilizing bottles and nipples is no longer considered necessary. Just use warm, soapy water, a bottle brush, and a small nipple brush to help get out the slimy film that forms on the inside of bottles and nipples. Then, drain them, or place them in the dishwasher. Small, plastic cages are available for holding nipples and other small baby feeding items together for the dishwasher.

Disposable bottle systems include a circular sheath, vinyl inserts shaped like condoms, a nipple, and a retainer ring. The advantage of vinyl throwaway inserts is that you don't have to wash bottles, but their disadvantage is that they are more expensive. You can run out of liners in the middle of the night; they may carry a fine vinyl residue that might not be healthy for a baby.

Don't plan to warm your baby's formula in a microwave. Microwaving can cause boiling hot spots that will scald your baby's mouth, and disposable bottle liners have been known to rupture, spewing hot milk on babies. (We discuss choosing baby formula on pages 418–420.)

Nipple styles

Nipples come in rubber and silicone. Silicone is the best material of the two, because it's more sanitary and less likely to rot or absorb milk residue. But sometimes silicone nipples can develop tears. It is recommended that new bottle nipples be boiled for two to five minutes to remove any chemicals involved in their manufacture. Replace nipples every few months just to be safe.

Nipples come in different sizes: small for preemies, and standard for most babies. Some nipples are designed with big holes or cross cuts in the outlet expressly made for feeding baby thickened cereals. Nipples also differ in how firm or how soft they are. If a nipple's too soft, it will collapse when baby tries to suck on it; if it's too firm, it could make your baby have to work too hard for a drink. Some nipples come in an hourglass configuration (orthodontic shape) that allegedly evokes a more natural sucking motion from a baby's tongue. These nipples are difficult to clean, which can lead to rotting in the rubber versions.

The type of nipple you use is mostly a matter of preference. Try out different styles until you find one that seems to be the most comfortable for your baby.

BREAST PUMPS AND BREASTFEEDING AIDS

A breast pump is a hand-operated or motor-driven device that creates suction. You could compare a breast pump to a vacuum cleaner but with a gentle, rhythmical action that collects mothers' milk into a baby bottle. Most pumps contain a small motor that creates the suction, a breast shield, and a tube or channel to flow the milk into a collection bottle.

If you're planning to stay around home, you'll soon discover your baby is the only breast pump you'll need. So, the concept is to master breastfeeding techniques first; then worry about pumping later.

No pump will work well unless a mother has a *let-down*, that rush of milk that comes a few minutes after nipple stimulation. In time, an experienced mother can learn to create a let-down by gently massaging the breasts while simply imagining the act of nursing. (Breastfeeding is discussed in detail on pages 408–418.)

With practice, most mothers can become proficient at expressing (squeezing out) their milk by hand without a pump. The technique is called manual expression, and can be learned from various breastfeeding books and online at breastfeeding sites such as www.breastfeeding.com.

If you know in advance you'll be returning to work, or you expect daily separations from your baby, or if your baby arrives early and could benefit from the disease-fighting powers of human milk, an effective breast pump may help to keep your milk supply going and allow you to collect it and store it in the freezer until it can be fed to your baby.

The most effective pumps are those that are able to mimic the gentle, repeated tugging of a baby during nursing. The most sophisticated pumps have knobs that allow you to adjust both the strength of the suction and timing of the length of time between each suction.

Comfort and efficiency are the two most important qualities to look for in a breast pump. Whichever style you choose, it should be simple to use, easy to clean, and not too much trouble to handle. The best source of information about breast pumps and how they're used is a lactation consultant—a specially trained breastfeeding expert. (See *Resource Guide*, pages 547–548.)

There are five basic kinds of breast pumps on the market, some more efficient than others: inexpensive bulbed models; hand-operated versions; small battery-operated versions, midsize pumps; and, large, hospital-grade models. Midsize models are the most popular with most breastfeeders.

Bulbed pumps

These are no longer recommended, because their strong suction can cause bruising and damage to breast tissue. These are the old-fashioned models found in pharmacies that

The Skinny on Breast Pumps

Efficiency. The best pumps are those that are the most effective at getting the job done. A well-designed manual pump can do the job, but is tiresome. Look for suction control and cycling speed control in electric models.

Quietness. If you plan to pump at work, and there's no private place to do it, the more silent, the better.

Cleaning ease. You'll be cleaning the pump daily, so look for easy-to-wash components.

Electric adapters. Don't just rely on batteries. Get a pump that offers an adapter for electrical outlets, and consider purchasing an optional adapter for the cigarette lighter outlet in your car.

Shield comfort. If you have large breasts, the standard shields that fit on the breast may not fit comfortably. Try special adapter inserts.

Portability. Unless you're only pumping at home, the pump should come with an easy-to-tote carry case and be lightweight enough so you can carry it to work each day.

Trusted manufacturer. Some companies offer poor-quality pumps just to fill out their baby feeding lines. Buy from a trusted breast pump manufacturer, instead.

resemble a bicycle horn with a rubber ball on one end to produce the vacuum. The rubber ball is fastened to a glass or plastic milk catcher.

➕ They're compact and easy to carry in a purse, and they're easy to clean.

➖ They don't work very well and can damage breasts.

Hand-operated pumps

These rely on your hand action using either a fitted cylinder or a squeeze-grip handle to produce a syringe-like tugging action. Most are designed to screw onto a baby

bottle for milk collection and storage. Some offer adjustable suction controls and soft shield adapters to fit most breast sizes.

➕ They're lightweight, silent, and easy to tuck into a purse or briefcase. Those with pistol-grip action and adjustable suction strength work well to collect milk once there's a milk let-down.

➖ They require a lot of effort from you, and your hands and arms can get fatigued. They're simply not as efficient as mid- and large-size electric pumps.

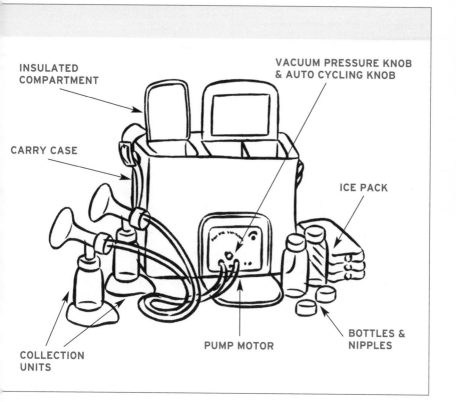

INSULATED
COMPARTMENT

VACUUM PRESSURE KNOB
& AUTO CYCLING KNOB

CARRY CASE

ICE PACK

COLLECTION
UNITS

PUMP MOTOR

BOTTLES &
NIPPLES

Small, battery-operated pumps

These small pumps are usually sold as kits in baby stores and drugstores. They come with a pistol-grip handle, a place for batteries, shields for the breast, a collection bottle, collection tubes, and a carrying case. Some may offer adapters for electrical outlets or for the cigarette lighter outlet in your car.

(+) They're small, fairly quiet, easy to carry around, and less expensive than larger, more professional versions.

(–) They don't work as well as larger pumps, and their small motors have a history of breaking down. They usually have only one milk receptacle instead of two, which makes pumping slower than being able to pump both breasts at once.

Midsize electric pumps

These are the work horses of the breast pump world. Some are designed for pumping a single side, while others are able to pump both breasts simultaneously, which saves time. They are normally sold as a kit that includes a small motor encased in a zippered, insulated carry case. Also included are washable tubes that lead from the motor to the breast shields, and collection bottles. Units offer adjustable speed and vacuum levels and can run either on batteries or an electrical adapter. Some cases also have a special freezer-pack section for holding bottles of breast milk until they can be refrigerated or frozen. Breast shields (horns) may have adapters for larger breast sizes. An optional cigarette lighter plug is usually available for pumping in the car and on trips.

(+) Although not very lightweight, nor very quiet, these units offer excellent efficiency when it comes to collecting milk, and they stimulate the breasts adequately to keep up a mother's milk supply. They're expensive, one hundred to two hundred dollars, but if you're planning to express milk at work every day, the investment will be worth it over the long haul.

(−) They eat up batteries in a hurry, so you will probably need an electrical outlet nearby. They're noisy, so people drifting in and out of the ladies' room or health suite at work will know something's going on. Occasionally, mothers have problems with the fit of the breast shields, and cleaning the tubes and components can be time-consuming.

Large, hospital-grade electric pumps

These are huge, heavy units, about the size of a car battery, that are used in hospitals and cost five hundred dollars or more. They can also be rented week by week very economically from most lactation consultants for personal use at home. They do the most efficient job of all breast pumps and are especially useful if you've got a preemie that is dependent on your milk for survival.

(+) They're highly effective and rapid in gathering milk, and they're useful for emergency situations, such as for providing milk for a hospitalized baby when nursing is interrupted temporarily. (Your breasts need continual suckling to keep producing milk.)

(−) They're heavy and not very portable, and prohibitively expensive for purchase, but short-term rentals are available. They require an electrical outlet, and make a noticeable churning sound that may feel indiscreet in non-private settings.

PREEMIES AND CAR BEDS

The American Academy of Pediatrics recommends that all infants born earlier than thirty-seven weeks gestational age be observed in their car seats before leaving the hospital to make sure they don't have potential breathing problems in the semi-reclining position of car seats. If your baby does have the problem, you may need to bolster underneath the seat base to make your baby's position more reclined, or to purchase a baby car bed (see below).

CAR SEATS FOR BABIES

Your baby's safety zone

All babies weighing less than twenty pounds and younger than one year of age should ride facing rearward in the back seat of your car.

Why? Because babies have very weak spines and necks and overly large heads in proportion to their bodies, which make them vulnerable to whiplash.

During a crash, a baby's head and body will be thrown forward in seconds and then slammed backward. By placing your baby's car seat facing rearward, you are offering firm, solid support to the head and spine to help prevent head, neck, and spine injuries.

Plus, being a backseat passenger provides your baby with a buffer zone of airspace between his seat and the shattering glass and crushing metal of the front seat's windshield and dashboard. More important, front seat air bags, usually located in or just below the glove compartment, deploy with such force they are capable of killing a baby or toddler in a seat, even during a minor fender bender in a parking lot.

Federal laws and LATCH

All fifty states and the District of Columbia have laws that require young children to be restrained in a proper safety seat for their size. Even with these laws, most parents (as many as eighty percent) don't install their children's car seats correctly. Part of the problem is getting the seat strapped into the car and in properly fitting the car seat's belts on the child.

In 2001, federal laws were put into effect by the National Highway Traffic Safety Administration to help remedy the issue of correctly installing a car seat. The restraint systems that the law requires are referred to as LATCH, an acronym that stands for Lower Anchor and Tethers for Children.

Since the fall of 2002, car manufacturers have had to install special U-shaped bars, called anchors, in the crease of the rear seats of every passenger vehicle in two positions—one for each window seat. Children's car seat manufacturers are also required to provide devices, such as hooks, on the backs of car seats so they can fasten onto these pre-installed anchors.

If you own an older model car, it won't have LATCH, but all children's car seats can also be safely fastened into the car by threading the shoulder and lap belts through special slots in the car seat. Follow the directions supplied by the owner's manual for your car on how to use its particular belting system, and be sure to follow the directions that come with the car seat, usually found in a leaflet fastened on the back of the car seat.

Unfortunately, there are no laws that address the second serious problem: parents not installing their children correctly in the seat.

A key to car seat terms

Buckle A metal fastener used to latch all of the straps together in the center of the baby's body, just above the thighs.

Three-point harness Found on some models of infant-only car seats. There are three straps: the two that restrain each shoulder and buckle together with a between-the-legs strap.

Five-point harness Found on some models of infant-only car seats and all convertible seats. There are five straps: one strap for each shoulder, one for each side of the waist, and one for between the legs.

Harness clip (or harness tie) A plastic fastener resembling a large hair clip, positioned at the level of a baby's armpits to keep the two shoulder straps together so baby won't be ejected between the straps during a crash.

Harness slots Slits cut in the rear of the car seat's back and upholstery for adjusting the height of shoulder harnesses to fit babies as they grow. Straps should be threaded into the frame at, or below, a baby's shoulder level.

Metal locking clip A flat, H-shaped metal piece that can be found tucked in back of a baby's car seat. It is used to cinch retracting, one-piece lap-and-shoulder belts in some newer car models. Using the clip may be the only way to firmly hold a car seat in place.

Tether A black, nylon strap that attaches in the rear of convertible seats when they're used in the forward-facing, upright position. It mounts using a hook to bolted hardware into the shelf above the rear seat of the car, or to the hardware on the floorboard of a van or station wagon. The strap stabilizes the seat in the upright position if there's a crash.

What kind of car seat to buy

There are basically three types of car seats suitable for newborns through the first six months of life: rear-facing, infant-only seats; convertible seats; and baby beds for special circumstances.

Infant-only seat

Rear-facing, infant-only seats are shaped like small tubs with a slanted, padded seat inside, and a folding, U-shaped carry handle. They're made to protect babies who weigh five to twenty pounds, or sometimes up to twenty-two pounds, depending upon the brand.

Some models use a three-point harness system, while others have five-point harnesses. A harness clip latches the shoulder straps together at armpit level. Most harnesses can adjust to several heights using slots in the seat back. Many of these seats come with a separate base that fastens down in the car either with LATCH hooks or by using the car's shoulder and lap belts so the seat can simply be lifted out leaving the base behind. Federal regulations require that infant seats be equally as safe with or without their bases.

The Skinny on Infant-only Car Seats

Here's what to look for when you shop for a rear-facing, infant-only car seat:

Five-point harnesses. Models with a five-point harness system (a strap for shoulders, waist, and between the legs) offer more security than models with three-point systems (only shoulders and crotch).

Higher weight range. Seats that safely carry larger babies are a better value. Look for a model that can restrain a twenty-two pound, or even heavier, baby. That way, if your baby is larger than average, you won't have to change seat models before his first birthday.

Carry handle. A curved carry handle with dense foam cushioning will make toting the car seat on your arm more comfortable.

Canopy. A generous, adjustable sunshade will help to keep your baby protected from glare and bright sunlight.

Base. Most seats come with a separate base to lock the seat in place using your car's LATCH anchors (see below), or by threading adult seat belts through the base. Get a base that has an adjustable presser foot so the seat angle can be adjusted according to the slope of your back seat.

Directions. Follow the directions that come with the seat and the installation directions found inside your auto owner's manual.

Avoid used seats. Don't buy a used infant seat unless you're sure it hasn't been on a recall list, and that it's never been in a crash.

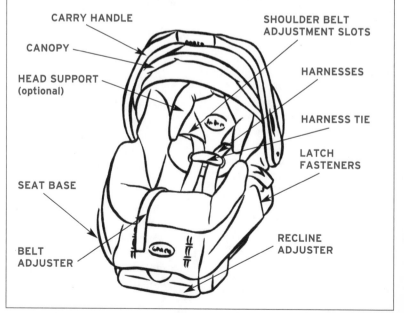

CARRY HANDLE

SHOULDER BELT ADJUSTMENT SLOTS

CANOPY

HARNESSES

HEAD SUPPORT (optional)

HARNESS TIE

LATCH FASTENERS

SEAT BASE

RECLINE ADJUSTER

BELT ADJUSTER

(+) They're the most lightweight, most portable, and least expensive car seat option for babies under a year of age. Models with five-point harnesses are thought to be safer than those with only three straps. The seat is angled well for the needs of babies born after thirty-seven weeks' pregnancy and it is relatively easy to put the baby inside. The base of the seat has latches on the bottom that lock it into grocery carts or specially equipped stroller frames. You may be able to purchase an additional base for a second car. Some handles are more comfortable than others: The best ones have thick padding or a rotating handle grip to allow the seat to swivel into a comfortable position for carrying.

(−) This style of seat has been in a number of recalls, particularly when the baby seat portion hasn't attached securely onto the seat's base because of hardware failure. Heavy and awkward when there's a baby inside, they're comfortable only for carrying short distances. Sometimes the sharp pitch of a car's back seat can make the car seat's angle too sharp, causing the baby to flop forward; although most seat bases have a presser foot underneath to adapt for that. A rolled-up towel under the foot of the seat will work too. Most seats offer a small guide that shows if the angle is correct. You may have to invest in another, better-fitting seat if your baby becomes too tall or too heavy before he reaches one year of age.

Convertible seats

Larger than infant-only seats, these restraints have an upright back and resemble an upholstered chair without legs. These seats are designed to recline and face rearward for babies weighing twenty-two pounds; then, they convert to face forward in an upright position for restraining toddlers until they weigh forty pounds or are approximately four years of age. Most models use a five-point harness system and offer a series of slots for adjusting shoulder belt heights as baby grows. (Not an easy process.) A harness clip holds the shoulder straps together at baby's armpit level. All seats in this category come equipped with a top tether strap that is only to be used in the upright, forward-facing position to fasten the seat to the car's frame as directed.

(+) You are basically getting two seats for the price of one. Since most of these models can accommodate babies weighing more than twenty pounds, a larger-than-average baby can still face rearward through age one. The frames are all one piece, minimizing the dangers of infant-only seats snapping off their stands during a crash.

(−) The seats are not very portable, and they take up a lot of space when they're slanted in the rear-facing position. That could present a problem if you don't have a lot of space in the rear

The Skinny on Convertible Car Seats

Compatibility. Check out the dimensions of your car's back seat. If you're driving a compact or a sub-compact, you may not be able to fit some of the larger models into your back seat in the semi-reclined position.

Crotch strap. If you're using a convertible with your newborn, make sure the seat's between-the-legs strap is positioned closely enough to the back seat so it will provide direct contact with your baby. (Some manufacturers offer two positions for the strap.)

Shoulder slots. Look for four, or more, shoulder harness slots in the back that allow you to adjust the height of the straps as your child grows. (The straps should be positioned at, or below, your baby's shoulders.)

Recline feature. Examine how the seat reclines. It should offer several recline positions depending upon the needs of your baby and the slant of your vehicle's back seat.

LATCH fasteners. The hardware and straps to fasten your seat to the LATCH anchors that come with your car should be easy to fasten and unfasten.

Tether strap. The tether strap coming from the upper back of the seat is designed only for use when the seat is in the upright, forward-facing position for toddlers weighing more than twenty pounds.

Directions. Follow both the directions that come with the seat, and those that are printed inside your auto owner's manual.

Avoid used seats. Don't buy a used convertible seat unless you're sure it hasn't been on a recall list and that it's never been in a crash.

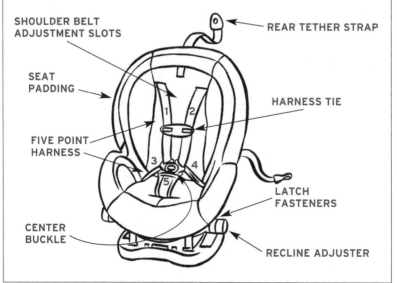

SHOULDER BELT ADJUSTMENT SLOTS
REAR TETHER STRAP
SEAT PADDING
HARNESS TIE
FIVE POINT HARNESS
LATCH FASTENERS
CENTER BUCKLE
RECLINE ADJUSTER

compartment of your car. The distance between the crotch strap and the back of the seat may mean a tiny baby will not get good strap contact. Models with a front shield, rather than a five-point harness system, are thought to be less safe than those relying on the direct body contact of five-point harnesses.

Stroller/car seat combos

Some manufacturers combine their strollers and infant-only car seats together and sell them as a single package. They have matching colors and upholstery. Sometimes buying the stroller/car seat combination costs less than purchasing each item separately. Typically, the carton holding the travel system will contain the stroller, the car seat, the car seat's base, and an adapter bar or railing that fastens into the stroller frame so the car seat can be clicked onto the stroller.

Usually, the car seat is positioned so it faces toward the rear of the stroller where the parent is pushing. Some dual strollers can hold two infant car seats for twins. If you want wheels for your baby's car seat, but don't want to invest in a stroller to support it, consider buying an inexpensive, rolling stroller frame made specifically for infant seats, such as Baby Trend's "Snap-N-Go Lite" series (www.babytrend.com).

(+) A convenient marriage between two pieces of baby equipment that allows you to use a simple snap-out-of-the-car-and-into-the-stroller maneuver. Your baby in his car seat gets to face you in the stroller. You'll probably save money on this two-for-one deal.

(−) Rear facing, infant-only seats have some limitations. You'll use the rear-facing seat for only one year, but the stroller for three to four years, and purchasing the system commits you to the stroller that comes in the package. Most strollers now come with universal adapters that fit all name-brand infant car seats, and the stroller model you're forced to buy with the seat may not be the most compact, lightweight, maneuverable option you could find. Consider purchasing your baby's car seat and stroller separately on their own merits—for example, the car seat because it has a five-point harness system and holds heavier babies, and the stroller because it is lightweight and the best size and wheels for your lifestyle. (Long walks: big wheels; city maneuvering, shopping, and travel: small wheels.)

The test for good car seat installation

Whether you buy a rear-facing, infant-only seat, or a convertible infant-toddler seat, the safety of the seat will depend upon its being tightly fastened down in the rear-facing position in your vehicle's back seat using either the LATCH anchors in the car, or the car's seat belts if there are no anchors.

The ultimate test of a good installation is that the seat won't budge.

If you fail to fasten the seat in correctly, it will wobble to the left, right, or rear when you press down on it. Try grasping the seat near the armrests on either side, and see if you can pull the seat away from the car's seat or make it move from side to side. It should not slide more than about an inch.

Then, without your baby inside, firmly push the top edge of the seat above where your baby's head would be in the direction of the floor of the car. Although the vehicle seat cushion may give, the safety seat should stay firmly in place, and the back of the car seat should stay at approximately the same angle (reclined about halfway back). (It's okay if you can push the top of the seat toward the rear of the car.)

The seat should be so firmly implanted in the auto's seat that it won't budge. You should get someone else to help you so the seat is implanted as tightly as possible. Press the seat deeply into the car's upholstery with your knee while your assistant helps to tighten the straps that hold the seat in place.

If you have an older model car with a retracting, one-piece shoulder and lap belt, you will need to use the H-shaped metal locking clip that comes attached to the back of the car seat. It acts as a cinch to hold both parts of the belt together.

First, knee the seat so it imbeds deeply into the upholstery. Have your helper stretch the seat belt out as far as it will extend. Then, use the metal piece that fastens into the car's seat buckle to thread the seat belt loop through the holes in the back of the car seat for that purpose. Fasten the seat belt buckle; then pull tightly on the shoulder portion of the belt until there's no give. Use the locking clip to fasten the lap section to the shoulder section just above the buckle.

When it comes to installing your baby into the seat, your baby's weight should fall into the stated weight range for the seat; shoulder straps should be taut and allow no more than two fingers of space between the straps and your baby's body; these straps should be at, or a little below, your baby's shoulders; the crotch strap should have contact with your baby's body; the harness tie (see above) should be at armpit level; and the seat should be angled so that your baby lies back, rather than hunches forward (refer to the angle indicator on the side of the seat).

Products to make traveling easier

Travel mirror

If you're worried about not being able to see your baby in the back seat, you may be able to find a mirror that suctions onto your rear window so you can glance at your baby through your rearview mirror. Just make sure it doesn't interfere with your ability to safely negotiate lane changes, and don't get distracted while driving in traffic.

Travel toys

Soft toys and teethers are safe for baby's play during travel, and some can be purchased on a flexible, padded bar. Avoid hard toys that could do their own harm during a crash.

Extra supplies

Keep extra diapers, a box of wipes, several changes of baby clothing, paper towels, a changing pad, an extra blanket, and a bath towel in a bag in the back seat in case your baby vomits or makes a mess. Also use the bath towel to protect the seat from getting too hot or too cold when you're out shopping. If you're not nursing, you should store several bottles of unopened, prebottled liquid baby formula.

Soothing sounds.

Save a CD of children's songs or lullabies from around the world to soothe the savage beast during meltdowns.

DIAPER CHANGING OPTIONS

Changing tables are special stands made just for diaper changing. There are five basic kinds of changing tables: a dedicated changing table with a pad and storage compartments underneath; a folding, wooden top that comes fastened onto a wooden chest of drawers; thick, vinyl-covered foam changing pads that screw onto chests; changing table adapters for cribs and play yards; and thin, lightweight changing pads that come in diaper bags or can be purchased separately.

Dedicated changing tables are somewhat expensive, rectangular-shaped tables that position a baby on top of a cushioned pad. They come with a waist belt to hold baby on the table, and guard rails on two or all sides to help protect babies from falls. They are usually constructed of wood or rattan and have storage shelves or drawers underneath. Some manufacturers have created fold-out diapering tops that come attached to wooden nursery chests and have changing pads and waist belts. The units can be removed by taking out the screws once the baby no longer needs changing.

Vinyl-covered, thick foam hanging pads are available from baby specialty stores. These thick pads are made to screw onto the tops of preexisting chests. They are indented in the center, and usually come with a small, vinyl safety belt.

Some baby specialty stores sell rimmed, plastic changing table shelves that are designed to fit over

The Skinny on Changing Tables

Here's what to look for when you shop for a changing table:

Comfortable height. Get one that is high enough so you don't have to bend over to change your baby, yet not so high that you can't control your baby at all times.

Good waist belt. Look for a sturdy belt with an easy-to-use buckle that snaps together.

Guard railings on all sides. The taller the railings, the better protection for your baby should you neglect to belt him.

Shake test. Give the table a good rattling to test how sturdy the joints are.

Storage. Until your toddler reaches the exploring stage, open storage shelves can come in handy.

Extra safety precautions. Always belt the baby down, and never leave the baby alone on the table, such as to fetch diapers or to answer the telephone.

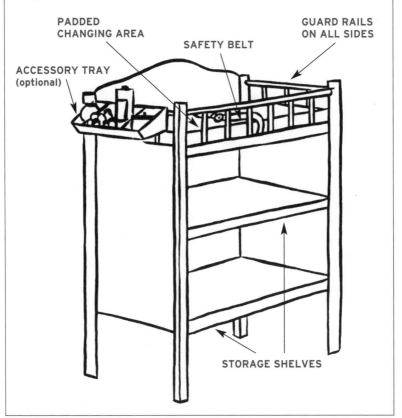

PADDED
CHANGING AREA

GUARD RAILS
ON ALL SIDES

SAFETY BELT

ACCESSORY TRAY
(optional)

STORAGE SHELVES

the bars of a standard-size crib. They come with a pad in the center and a safety belt for baby's waist. Some portable play yards also come with a removable changing table unit that has a pad and a small safety belt.

The most inexpensive option of all is a simple, folding (or rolled up) changing pad, like those that come in diaper bags that can be used on the floor or on a bed, or stuffed in a backpack or purse. They don't offer safety straps, so you'll have to use them on a surface where your baby can't roll off.

What changing option to buy

Here is a comparison of your options for places to change your baby's diapers.

Changing table

(+) They raise the baby to a comfortable height for changing. You can place them wherever it's convenient, or have one for each floor in your home. They come with a waist belt to hold baby in place. Railings on the sides will help to prevent a baby's rolling over and falling out.

(−) Babies are injured when they squirm and roll overboard, falling headfirst to the floor below. Using a retraining belt is important, but it can get in the way of diapering. Open shelves underneath may be an invitation to toddlers to pull things out onto the floor.

Nursery chest toppers

(+) The chest can coordinate with your other baby furniture, and it will adapt for use during childhood.

(−) There have been stability problems with the foldout changer frames that can cause the chest to topple forward. Most chest models don't have a protective railing in the front to prevent a baby from falling.

Changing pad

(+) They present an inexpensive option for adapting any chest for a diaper changing station. They're lightweight, and easy to fold for carrying in a diaper bag, backpack, or briefcase.

(−) They're only safe if they are screwed down on the chest. Seat belts are often flimsy and difficult to thread. Even though they often have an indented channel in the center to hold the baby, none offer the safety of side rails of a standard diaper-changing table that helps to prevent accidents.

Play yard diapering adapters

(+) Diaper changing platforms fit on top of the railings of standard-sized cribs. Some play yards come with a small diaper-changing accessory that fits over the top bars of the yard. Both are less expensive than buying a separate changing table, and both offer cushioned pads and seat belt options.

● The crib shelf may be too high to be comfortable, and an unrestrained baby can easily roll out, which could lead to injury. The attachment will have to be removed each time you put the baby to bed. Portable play yard changers are very small and low, so they will only be useful for a short while, and could lead to a backache. Rollouts are a dangerous possibility for an unrestrained baby.

CRIBS AND OTHER SLEEPING OPTIONS

During the first two years of life, your baby will be spending more time sleeping than being awake. And most babies spend the majority of their sleeping careers in full-size cribs. In the early days after you bring your baby home, though, you'll probably want to keep your baby near you so you can monitor him and make sure he's all right. The problem is that a full-size crib is huge, too large to roll though a doorway, and difficult to assemble and disassemble. So you'll probably want to leave it in your baby's room.

Full-size cribs

It goes without explaining that full-size cribs are the rectangular baby beds with bars on the side that can be found in virtually every baby store. You can buy a crib, or you can buy a whole bedroom suite for baby that includes an armoire and a chest with a diaper-changing platform on top. Note that crib mattresses (discussed on page 504) are sold as a separate item.

The quality and prices of cribs range from less than one hundred dollars for a painted, flimsy wooden model with uneven, and sometimes rough, finishing, up to one thousand dollars or more for an heirloom-quality crib that is actually a fine piece of furniture—huge, finely finished, and fit for a prince (or princess).

But remember: Cribs are the biggest baby killers in the baby product world. Malfunctioning older cribs that parents continue to use even though bars are missing or mattress supports have broken, cause most baby deaths.

All cribs are subject to federal regulations regarding interior dimensions, bar spacing, and safety of components: (1) The interior dimensions of the crib must be uniform so that there are no gaps between the mattress and sides that could capture a baby's head. (2) Bars must be spaced no more than two and three-eighths inches apart so babies can't slide out between them, body first, and get strangled. (3) The regulations also address basic crib safety, such as how high the bars must be even in the lowest position.

Cribs also have a voluntary certification standard overseen by the American Society of Testing and Materials (ASTM) and the Juvenile Products Manufacturers Association (JPMA). To be certified, crib brands must undergo extra testing for sturdiness. Certified cribs will usually have a sticker somewhere on the frame with the words JMPA and CERTIFIED on it. Being certified isn't an absolute guarantee of safety. For example, some certified cribs have undergone federal recalls because

The Skinny on Cribs

Certified. A JPMA-certified sticker means the crib brand passes a voluntary safety test overseen by manufacturers.

Easy-to-use side lowering. Try lowering the side yourself. A simple lift and knee-press action works easier and is quieter than models that require the use of a foot pedal or a spring-action knob.

Frame integrity. Make sure the frame doesn't rattle when shaken. The bars (slats) should be well fastened and should not twist or move.

Finish. All surfaces must be smooth and splinter-free.

Single dropside. A crib with only one side that can be lowered (dropside) will be quieter and more stable than models that have two sides that lower.

Well-glued slats. Slats, or bars, should be firmly attached at top and bottom. Glue residue spilled out onto the wood is a sign of poor craftsmanship.

Teething rails. Most models have a small plastic railing to line the tops of the railings on the sides. Make sure it doesn't have sharp edges and can't be pulled loose.

Mattress supports. The metal support that goes under the mattress should be sturdy with no sharp points that could puncture the underside of the mattress. Make sure it fastens to the crib with strong, thick hardware.

Locking wheels. If the crib has wheels, they should be lockable to prevent a baby's motion from moving the crib.

Underside storage drawer. Storage drawers that slide or roll out from under the crib can be useful, but check their quality before paying extra for them.

of loose bars. A big price tag isn't necessarily a sign of how safe or durable a crib is. Extremely expensive cribs may have a solid feel of quality to them, but could be recalled because of a serious flaw.

Cribs come in a variety of colors and finishes. There are pastel painted versions in light greens or creamy whites as well as models with furniture stains, such as cherry and pale blond, and natural-looking finishes. Lighter wood finishes are less likely to show scratches than darker cherry and mahogany stains,

and often the darker stains are used to cover up visible flaws in less expensive wood cuts.

The best strategy for buying a crib is to shop middle-priced models, choose a smooth finish that goes with your home décor, and examine the quality of crib components, such as well-glued slats, sturdy hardware, and how easily the sides work before you buy. (See the skinny on buying cribs above.)

If the service is available, consider paying the store to deliver and set up the crib. It's a two-person

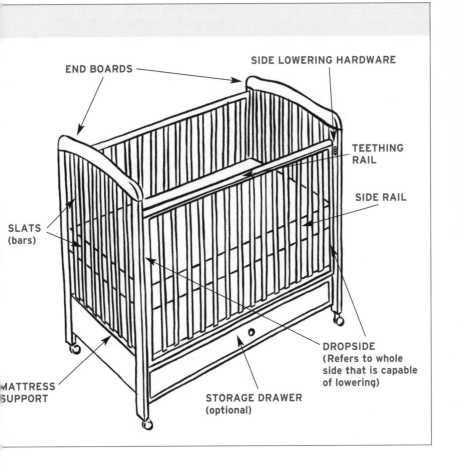

END BOARDS

SIDE LOWERING HARDWARE

TEETHING RAIL

SIDE RAIL

SLATS (bars)

MATTRESS SUPPORT

STORAGE DRAWER (optional)

DROPSIDE (Refers to whole side that is capable of lowering)

job that can last an hour. Make sure you set it up in the room where it is to stay, since cribs are too large to be moved out of rooms without being disassembled.

(+) The biggest advantage of buying a crib, rather than using other baby beds is that they are governed by stringent federal regulations. That means that they are constantly watched for flaws and recalled when they fail to pass the tests and requirements. In addition, they

are also covered by JPMA certification standards, which means that those manufacturers who choose to can have their cribs tested and certified for additional safety compliance.

(–) Full-size cribs are so large they can't fit through doorways. Newborns and young babies don't need all that room. Poorly functioning older cribs and new models with poor craftsmanship can be hazardous.

Crib mattresses

Once you've chosen your baby's crib, you may be surprised to discover that even though mattresses are displayed inside cribs in stores, cribs don't come with them. And salespeople are trained to immediately walk you to their mattress displays while you're in the flush of your crib decision to encourage you to buy the most expensive version in the store.

Your baby will be sleeping on a crib mattress for approximately two years—and maybe a couple of years longer if you buy a pint-sized toddler bed the same dimensions as a crib. Firmness is more critical than internal structure or padding.

Granted, getting a quality mattress is important, but there's no need to pay extra bucks because a sales pitch tries to convince you that your baby needs extra back support. He doesn't. Babies' bodies are quite flexible. It's the grownups who carry them around who need the help.

Federal regulations enforced by the U.S. Consumer Product Safety Commission (CPSC, see page 469) mandate that all crib mattresses be the same length and width so that they will fit flush against the sides of cribs. In turn, full-size cribs must also have identical interior dimensions. But some mattresses may be deeper than others.

There are basically two generic types of mattresses for babies: innerspring and foam. The coverings on crib mattresses, called ticking, come in a variety of colors and materials, such as quilted, moisture-resistant fabric, laminated vinyl, or a combination of fabric and vinyl. Ticking should be thick and resist moisture and stains. The best coverings are triple-laminated, meaning they offer three thick layers of material heat-welted together.

How the mattress ticking is sewn can be important. The binding around the edges of the mattress should be durable and double-stitched to prevent ripping and tearing. And it will help to keep seams from splitting when a toddler jumps around on the mattress. Higher-quality mattresses have fabric bindings all around the seams, rather than vinyl, and the seams are tightly double-stitched so they won't come loose.

Air vents—small, metal-lined holes along the side of the mattress or pocket-style openings at both ends—allow the insides of the mattress to breathe. Inexpensive mattresses may have small metal vents fastened onto thin vinyl on the sides that could be easily plucked off and swallowed by curious tots.

Sometimes manufacturers will claim that a mattress has antibacterial qualities. That means that an antibacterial chemical has been added to the vinyl used in the laminate to help destroy bacteria on the surface of the mattress. Unfortunately, baby's continual wetting is more than any surface material can handle.

Some mattresses claim they are non-allergenic or hypoallergenic. That simply means they're made of foam instead of cotton and other fibers that attract dust mites and can cause allergic reactions.

Manufacturers will also use the selling ploy of a lifetime warranty to get parents to pay more for their baby's mattress. But you'd better comb through the fine print, since the actual warranty may come with lots of loopholes in favor of the manufacturer, such as special conditions and a payback scale that depends upon the age of the mattress.

We suggest using a quality, washable pad to protect the mattress, turning the mattress over frequently, and following the manufacturer's directions for cleaning (usually wiping the surface down with a mild soap solution and then cleaning off the soap residue using a cloth dampened with clear water).

Innerspring mattresses

Innerspring crib mattresses resemble miniature adult mattresses. Underneath the ticking are thick layers of padding, a series of metal coils, and thick metal support wires to hold up the edges of the mattress. As for adults, better innerspring mattresses for babies generally have more coils than less-expensive versions, and the coils are made from higher-quality metal, such as steel.

As the name implies, innerspring mattresses have springs inside, and the quality and price of the mattress often depends upon the number of coils, such as "180 tough steel springs and steel-reinforced edges."

(+) The main advantage of an innerspring mattress is that it offers variable support to different parts of your baby's body as he grows and gains weight.

(−) Their biggest drawback is that they're substantially heavier and less flexible than mattresses made from foam. That makes sheet changing, which you'll be doing once, possibly twice a day, more of a hassle than with a foam mattress. Plus, most tots like to use innerspring mattresses like trampolines, which could lead to falls and injuries.

Foam mattresses

Foam mattresses come in a variety of prices and grades. The higher the quality of foam, the heavier it weighs and the denser it is. Denser versions are less squishy when you squeeze them. Poor-quality mattresses will be lightweight, have a

---

Safety Warning: Old Baby Beds Can Kill!

❗ Nearly one hundred babies a year die in old cribs, heirloom cradles, and bassinets. Rickety beds with weakened screw holes and broken hardware fall apart, entrapping heads and causing strangulation. Loosened or widely spaced bars allow a baby's body to squeeze through, leaving the head behind to strangle. Babies can be poisoned by lead-containing varnish or paint when they gnaw on wooden sides. Poorly fitting or mushy mattresses can lead to suffocation. Protruding carved areas on end boards can strangle a baby if clothing gets captured or small heads become trapped.

single layer of vinyl for a covering, and vinyl bindings.

There are two quick tests for the denseness of a foam mattress. One is to take it down from the shelf (or out of the display crib), and to lean on the mattress with the top edge braced under your arms. A less-dense mattress will bow into a curve under your weight.

The second test is to press your palms together with the mattress in between. A dense mattress will stay put without compressing inward, a less dense mattress will change shape under the pressure of your hands.

Usually, foam mattresses are constructed from a single foam slab, but sometimes higher-quality versions will offer more than one density—a firm surface where baby sleeps, and a tough, non-springy edge to reinforce the outer rim of the mattress.

➕ Quality foam mattresses can be really firm, almost like a brick—an advantage when it comes to preventing a suffocation pocket. They're lightweight too and have clear-cut corners that help keep fitted sheets on.

➖ Inexpensive foam mattresses can compress and sag in the area where your baby lies. Some have only a single layer of vinyl that's poorly bound on the sides, which can lead to tears and stretching. (Stick with a name-brand manufacturer with thick, reinforced upholstery.)

Alternative sleeping options for babies

There are a number of smaller-than-crib options for keeping your baby in your bedroom during the first months after birth.

Bassinets

Bassinets are compact baby beds on wheels. Most frames are made either out of tubular plastic, or from woven rattan with wooden legs. Most have wheels or casters that make them easy to roll.

Their charm is in their appealing ruffles in baby-style fabrics such as lacy white or pastel prints. Canopies are a cute extra, but models without such a topper are simpler to use and may cost less.

➕ While a standard-size crib can't fit through a doorway, bassinets come with wheels and can easily be rolled from one room to another. So, bassinets are one option for keeping your baby close during that first crucial month when you are more likely to worry about your newborn's well being.

➖ Soft mattresses can smother and components including legs and hardware may malfunction, causing the bassinet to collapse.

As with full-size cribs, a baby should always be placed on his back for face-up sleep. And soft quilts, pillows, or stuffed toys should be kept out of the bassinet to protect against baby suffocation or the potential for sudden infant death syndrome (SIDS).

The Skinny on Bassinets

Good mattress. A well-fitted, quality mattress is a must. It should be extra firm and extend completely to the edges and corners of the bassinet's interior.

Rigid sides. Solid sides in the baby's sleep area are safer than soft fabric sides that could allow a small neck or head to get trapped in pockets caused by loose fabric sides.

Washable fabrics. Fabrics and liners should be completely washable. (Read the instructions.)

Leg locks. Folding legs should lock firmly in the open position to prevent accidental collapse.

Locking casters. Wheels are handy. Lockable, multi-direction casters are the best buy. They'll keep siblings from pushing the bassinet around.

Rocking feature. Some bassinets have a rocking option, which could be comforting for a fitful baby. Look for locks to keep the bassinet motionless for sleep; otherwise, your baby may end up pressed into one side when his weight shifts.

Size limits. Follow the manufacturer's weight and age instructions for the best time to graduate your baby to a full-size crib (usually when he is able to roll over or pull up).

Face up for sleep. For safety's sake, always place baby on his back for sleep, and keep out suffocating soft pillows, quilts, or stuffed toys. (See sudden infant death warnings on page 398.)

Bedside sleepers

These are low, small, three-sided cribs with mattress pads designed so that newborns can sleep directly beside their parents. They're made to attach to the side of an adult bed using long straps that go across the adult's bedsprings to strap the sleeper firmly against the side of the bed. The concept of this design is to give parents easy access to their babies without the risk of SIDS, or the suffocation dangers of babies sleeping in their parents' beds.

(+) The beds are handy and allow the baby to be quickly moved back and forth for nursing and feeding with parents not having to get up.

(−) The beds take up a lot of space on the side of an adult bed, and make it difficult for the adult to get in and out of bed herself. Babies tend to fall asleep at the breast, and arousing them by removing them from the warmth of the parent's body to put them onto the cold sleeper surface is likely to awaken them in the same way that lifting them and placing them in a crib or bassinet will.

Cradles

Cradles are the traditional bed for newborns. They come in two basic styles: those with rockers on the base, and those that rock by being suspended on a footed frame by a hook or rocking mechanism at the top.

Unfortunately, small babies have little body control, and they may be rolled back and forth with the rocking motion, or become trapped.

Heirloom cradles with widely spaced bars (more than two and three-eighths inches apart), and those with soft, poorly fitting mattresses can be life threatening. Young babies can slide through the bars leaving their heads behind, causing strangulation, and they can also get wedged between the cradle side and the mattress, causing suffocation.

(+) They have a romantic, all-baby feel to them. They offer rocking that should be soothing to a baby.

(−) Unfortunately, most cradles simply roll a baby's body back and forth from one side to the other, and babies can get trapped against the side that's lowest.

Portable Cribs

An alternative product option is a small-scale crib with wheels. These are actually a safer choice since many models from major manufacturers have passed special safety and durability tests to earn a JPMA (Juvenile Products Manufacturers) certification sticker.

(+) These are simply miniature cribs, small enough to roll through doorways. Most have adjusting legs so that they can later be used as a playpen. They tend to be safer than other bedding alternatives because of the strict regulations they have to follow. Legs may lower to allow the portable crib to sit on the floor like a playpen for use later.

(−) Most do not have lowering sides, so you will have to bend down to put baby in or lift him out. They use nonstandard-size sheets. They may offer only one mattress height. Some models have soft, instead of rock-hard, mattresses. Babies should only sleep on extra-firm versions.

DIAPER BAGS

Going out in the world with your baby will require toting a humongous load of baby gear too. The list of what to pack includes spare diapers, a change or two of clothes, baby bottles, toddler snacks, diaper wipes, and a distracting toy or two.

Diaper bags come in a huge variety of sizes and designs. Outer finishes range from colorful, baby-

The Skinny on Diaper Bags

Sturdy upholstery. A heavy-duty outer covering will resist moisture, dirt, and wear. Dense, moisture-resistant nylon weaves and thick canvas last better than thin cotton quilting or lightweight fabrics.

Handle comfort. Carry handles need to be short enough so the bag won't drag if you're carrying it with one hand. Check underarm carrying comfort too.

Less is better. Light and simple are best. Too many pockets and sections weigh the bag down and make it harder to find lost items.

See-through pouches. The best inside pouches and dividers are clear vinyl or mesh so you can spot what you're seeking.

Zippered closure. Zippering the bag closed will help prevent spills and keep small hands out of mischief.

Reinforcements. The best bags have reinforced stitching or heavy-duty braids where handles and straps join the body of the bag.

Great alternatives. Backpack bags with padded straps and a center carry handle are an advantage: they allow multiple carrying options, including hands-free porting for babes-in-arms. If nothing else works for you, try morphing your favorite large purse or a backpack into a diaper bag by inserting inexpensive waterproof pouches and a lightweight changing pad.

friendly quilted fabrics to serious, down-to-business black and navy bags at home in the office. Most bags offer a wide range of pockets and extras, including removable diaper changing pads, moisture-proof storage pouches, insulated bottle holders, and even loops to hold car keys or snap-on toys.

DIAPERS

Your baby will use up nearly sixty diapers a week in the early months. That rate will gradually slow down until your mature toddler verging on self-toileting will use only a few per day. During your baby's entire diapering career, you'll be changing diapers between five and eight thousand times. Can you imagine? It makes sense to decide on the type of diapering system you're going to use before your baby arrives. Things to weigh: how much a particular diapering option will cost over the process of two years, and how demanding the system will be on your time and energy.

Here are your basic options: reusable fabric diapers, disposables, and in some larger cities—diaper services to launder fabric diapers for you and deliver them to your door.

Each system has its advantages and disadvantages. You don't have to be dedicated to just one solution: You can use a combination of systems, e.g., a diaper service for starters, reusable cloth diapers for most of the time, and disposables for going out. Whichever system(s) you choose, you'll need ample diapering supplies on hand before you bring your little wetter home.

When it comes to diaper pails: You'll need a soaking pail with a locking lid for fabric diapers (or you can simply throw them directly into the washing machine until you have enough to run). If you're using disposables, you can buy a milk jug–shaped pail that takes rolled-up diapers and wraps them in a vinyl sleeve to help keep odor down, or you can simply use a lidded can and throw-away plastic liners.

Fabric reusables

Laundering your own diapers is the most economical option, and you'll probably save over $1,000 during your baby's entire diapering career. But when you compare diapering costs, also try to factor in the wear and tear on your washing machine from laundering fabric diapers every few days, plus your utility and detergent costs, and the value of your time and labor that can translate into hundreds of dollars a year.

Some parents feel that fabric diapers, like woven cotton underwear, are more natural and comfortable. Another group prefers reusables out of concern for the environment, such as the depletion of forests and the impact of disposables on community waste management systems. Whatever system you settle upon, your decision should be based on your judgment about what's best for both you and your baby.

Gear yourself up for a regular, day-to-day laundering schedule to keep on top of the dirty diaper pile that baby will generate. For the most efficient diaper cleaning, it's best to use unscented liquid detergents that won't leave a residue behind. Don't use a fabric softener; its perfumes can be irritating to baby's nose and skin, and it also tends to clog the vent screen of dryers, which slows down the drying process. A sturdy washer and a dryer are essential.

Since cotton is more absorbent than other materials, it's the material of choice for reusable diapers. In decades past, parents could choose from only one or two fabric weaves: mostly birdseye, which resembles old-fashioned white dishtowels, or loosely woven, more porous gauze.

Standard, old-fashioned diapers are usually packaged by the dozen and come in one of three basic models: unfolded, folded, and shaped. Unfolded diapers are simply a single, large square of fabric. The packaging usually gives instructions on how to fold them to fit your baby so that absorbency is concentrated in the middle of the diaper where it's most needed. (Usually they're folded in a triangle: one point for each side of the baby and a point to fit between the legs. The three points are brought together at baby's middle and pinned.)

Prefolded diapers are rectangle-shaped and have extra fabric folds sewn into the center for absorbency. Fitted diapers can be shaped like an hourglass or the profile of an airplane. They're hourglass shaped to leave less bulkiness and chafing between the legs, but you have to stock them according to your baby's size. Avoid plastic pants with sewn-in diaper interiors. They don't launder well, take forever in the dryer, and harbor bacteria that can lead to diaper rash.

Diapering systems that are far more sophisticated than prepackaged cotton diapers are the best (and most expensive) reusable option. Often imported, these systems consist of lightweight, breathable, but moisture-resistant outer coverings that use Velcro™-type closures, and a thick inner core that is smaller, but thicker than a regular diaper and comes closest to mimicking the absorbency of disposables.

These systems are expensive and usually found only in specialized catalogs or on the Web. Usually, you can save money by buying your diapers in bulk, but you may want to survey consumer review sites, such as www.epinions.com to find other parents' suggestions for what to buy. You can also purchase samples of different products to find the system that will work the best for you.

When you search diaper e-tailers on the Internet, try combining the words "diapers" and "cotton" using your favorite search engine; then shop around. It makes sense to order single samples of two or three diapering systems to check out their quality and absorbency before you invest heavily in a single brand. The company will advise you how many diapers you will need to get started, and most company Web sites offer good diaper laundering advice too.

(+) After your initial investment in a fabric diaper system, you can expect to save hundreds of dollars in the years that follow. Some parents consider fabric diapers kinder to baby skin, and

also to the environment; plus, you'll never run out as long as your washing machine and dryer keep chugging along. Fabric versions have other practical uses, too: stuffing in your bra to catch letdowns, soaking up spit-ups on your shoulder, and they'll still be around to use again with your next baby.

(–) They're more labor-intensive to launder and require a hefty up-front investment for getting started. Except for the very expensive versions, most diaper fabrics don't absorb wetness as readily as disposables, nor do they have an outside dampness barrier to protect your clothing and furniture. So, you'll need to buy a supply of waterproof outer pants too—preferably made of breathable materials that won't turn your baby's bottom into a hothouse for bacteria. If not well laundered, they are associated with more diaper rash.

Diaper services
Diaper services flourished in decades past, but they've almost all gone out of business due to the competition from disposables. You may still have the option of using a diaper service if you live in a major U.S. city.

Here's how a diaper service works: You choose the style of diapers you want to use. These diapers, and only these, are allotted to your baby—so the fear of contamination from another baby isn't founded.

Once or twice a week, a truck pulls up and takes away the soiled diapers you've stored in a mesh bag inside a pail furnished by the service. In their place, you're left neatly wrapped stacks of clean, white diapers laundered at extremely hot temperatures that can't be matched by home machines. Most services let you sign up for as long or short a time as you wish.

➕ If there is a diaper service in your community, you can pay a monthly fee to be supplied with weekly stacks of soft, ready-to-use fabric diapers. That frees you from laundering chores, and it may help prevent diaper rash, too. Plus, diaper services are cheaper than disposables.

➖ The service costs more than doing your own laundering. The likelihood of finding a service in your area may be slim. You may not be able to use the sophisticated diaper systems with heavyweight flannel or terry inserts that are the most absorbent. Occasionally, you may run out of diapers before your next pickup.

Disposables

Disposables are convenient and usually effective in wicking moisture away from your baby's skin, a help in preventing skin irritation. Expect to buy about five thousand of them in all for an investment of between $1,200 and $1,500. A good disposable should be snug and not too tight. It should be non-irritating with no redness, rashes, or chafing. And, it should prevent leaks from legholes or around the waistband.

Disposables continue to improve every year, mostly because of the steep competition between Kimberly-Clark (Huggies) and Procter & Gamble (Pampers)— the two giants that manufacture disposables. Over time, these diapers have become more absorbent, fit babies better, and are easier to fasten than ever before. And prices are always changing.

Most parents settle down to a preferred disposable brand after trying a few different versions. They may like a particular type of diaper because it seems to fit better, because it appears to be more absorbent, because they like the way it fastens on the sides, or simply because it's cheaper.

Disposables come in five or six sizes. Some start at a preemie size and go up, others offer the newborn size as the first size. As your baby grows, the diapers get larger too, and that means getting fewer diapers in each package you buy, even though the package prices remain roughly the same.

There are a couple of ways to save some money on disposables. You can purposely get on the company's mailing list to get coupons in the mail. You can sometimes do that by calling their toll-free telephone numbers, signing up on one of their sponsored Web sites, by using a baby registry (discussed on page 459), or subscribing to free baby magazine subscriptions. You can also save a lot by buying your baby's diapers by the case from large discount chains, such as Sam's Club, and watching for special sales.

Generic diaper brands offered by discount stores can sometimes be a real bargain, especially in bulk quantities. But, the quality of these brands sometimes can be inconsistent. It makes sense to purchase several different brands and take them home to actually test them on your baby. You're looking for fit, comfort, leak resistance, plus economy. While one brand may work well on small babies, another may do just fine for toddlers, so remain open to different options.

(+) They're the most convenient of all options and tend to fit babies better than one-size-fits-all diapers. Their absorbency truly does keep dampness away from a baby's bottom, and that may mean fewer diaper rash breakouts. Newer diapers are especially designed to prevent leaks around the legs and waist.

(−) They're your most expensive option, costing more than twice as much as reusables. If you're sensitive to perfume, you'll probably also be sensitive to the strong, undeniable chemical smell of some disposable brands. Some parents nix disposables out of concern for the depletion of forests and environmental issues. Piles of disposables can stink while they wait for garbage day, and, yes, parents do run out of them in the middle of the night.

DIGITAL CAMERAS AND CAMCORDERS

You're going to want to record this time in your child's life for posterity. Digital cameras and camcorders (digital video cameras) are great for creating your own birth announcements and keeping all your relatives and friends posted on your baby's latest antics by e-mail or on your own Web site.

There are hundreds of choices for digital cameras and camcorders out there. The main problem is getting this fancy equipment to correspond with the limitations of your computer software and memory.

Digital cameras

Instead of using film, digital cameras use computer chips to record images. Just as with a computer, your digital camera will let you save, delete, and view images immediately after you take them.

Digital cameras are usually sold according to their resolution: how clear the picture will appear for different-size prints.

A camera offering one resolution megapixel is great for e-mailing small pictures to friends and relatives or posting them on your own Web site. Two megapixel resolution will create up to an 8″ × 10″ print with pretty good clarity, at least adequate for most photo needs. Three and four megapixels are professional-grade resolutions for people who want pristine quality for large prints. As the pixels go up, so does the price, and the amount of memory required inside your camera and on your computer to support them.

Zoom lenses enable a camera to go from extreme close-ups to faraway shots while maintaining clarity. While some cameras say they have digital zoom features, they're really just manipulating the same image by zeroing in on one small section of your print, which leads to grainy results.

We suggest purchasing a camera with an actual optical zoom lens, rather than just a zoom feature. You need a lens that can actually move to focus up close or at a distance without sacrificing image quality. That way, you'll get sharper results on your baby's up-close features, your pet's disdain of your new baby, or the tiny baby duds you plan to sell later on e-Bay.

Digitals offer both a viewfinder like old-fashioned cameras and also a screen that enables you to see exactly what the picture will look like or to examine a series of pictures you've already taken. Look for a large, easy-to-view display (LCD) that shows a clear image before you press the shutter button.

The software supplied with your camera can make a huge difference between easy shoots and feeds into your computer and frustrating problems. You need software that will readily manage your images so you can edit them, change their size, or even offer you a panoramic feature so you can produce longer-than-normal scenes. Unfortunately, the only way to test out the software is to buy the camera. Check on the store's return policy before you pull out your charge card.

The camera's memory demands or software could be incompatible with your computer. Some cameras won't work with Macs, for example. You'll probably need a USB port (a small, narrow plug hole) to unload images into your machine, and a huge amount of free memory space may be required as well as having Windows XP or later for manipulating your images.

If you don't want to run out of picture-taking capacity, plan to buy an extra memory card or two for your camera. These small inserts can make the difference between your camera stopping short at only ten images or being able to digest and hold thirty images or more at a time. You'll probably need between 128 and 266 MB of memory, total, and you may decide to buy more than one card to enable you to capture more images before downloading them. (Turning down the megapixels on your camera enables you to take more pictures.)

Digital cameras are battery hogs. Avoid cameras that will only run on battery rechargers unique to the brand. Instead, buy a camera that adapts to regular AA or AAA batteries. Then, purchase NiMH rechargeable batteries and their recharging unit, if you can find one. These batteries last twice as long as standard batteries and can be recharged nearly one thousand times.

Most color printers will put out usable quality prints. You will need to purchase high-quality photo paper to get the best results.

➕ Digitals allow you to take instant pictures and see exactly what the image will look like before printing it, and you can erase unwanted images with the push of a button. Once you've downloaded the image into your computer, you can easily post it in e-mails to friends and relatives using the "get photo" capabilities of most Internet servers. Most digital software will allow you to doctor your prints. You can remove red eye, take out noisy background images, superimpose multiple images, add frames, captions, or go wherever your artistic leanings lead you.

Digitals are more expensive than most regular cameras, and their results aren't usually as rich and sharp as standard cameras. While you used to run out of film with your regular camera, you will now find yourself running out of battery power and memory. That can be frustrating if you're at a holiday dinner party, or out on the road with baby when your batteries run out of juice or your camera's memory overloads. The only cures are to always carry extra batteries and plan some time for downloading your images onto your laptop.

Camcorders

Just as with digital cameras, camcorders offer you instant images and replay. You can capture moving, video-like footage, complete with sound, or you can freeze an image as though it were a picture for printing later.

The best units are lightweight and compact and can be held and operated with one hand. Consider an affordable model that offers a clear picture without overdoing it in the bells and whistles department. Huge pixel counts and complex editing features add to a camcorder's price tag; plus, they eat up huge chunks of computer memory.

Most off-the-shelf models offer only limited battery life before needing to be charged again. So consider investing in an extra battery pack so you don't run dry during a critical scene.

A full auto switch will enable the camcorder to automatically adjust the color balance, shutter speed, focus, and the camera's iris (called the F-stop or aperture).

Sound quality varies among models. Test mike clarity using both voice and music to see how well it focuses on front sound and eliminates unwanted side noise. A separate, plug-in mike may improve audio performance.

Technical help and responsive customer service are going to be important when you get captured in download or software problems. Read the literature that accompanies the machine. There should be a 24/7 toll-free help line and Web site with around-the-clock technical backup. And don't forget to return the registration card to the manufacturer so you're in line for recall or upgrade notices.

As you pay more for cameras, you also get additional options that may not be worth the extra bucks. Some of these include a remote control when you want to be in the picture or when you use the camera as a playback device; editing features, such as a built-in title generator; a time and date stamp, and a time code; an infrared sensitive device to improve night recording; and an audio/video input jack for transferring images from a VCR or other camera into your camcorder.

Start simple, and work your way up to more sophisticated versions later when you've mastered the basics.

(+) Most are more lightweight and compact than standard video cameras. You can see and hear exactly what you're capturing, and you can go back to enhance or edit later.

(−) Requires huge memory both to run and to be stored in your computer. Images may be grainier and less sharp than with a video camera. Sound may be poorer than with video cameras.

HIGH CHAIRS AND BOOSTER SEATS

High chairs have come a long way from the old wooden models of bygone eras. Now they offer reclining features and almost infinite height adjustments. (But they cost more too.)

Since your baby won't have the strength to sit up on his own until he reaches five to six months of age, you may want a chair that has a recline option so you can use the seat as a baby holder in the kitchen, or you can simply postpone buying a high chair until it's time for baby to start experimenting with eating— at about six months.

There are cheap, bare-bones models with flimsy trays, but they usually can't be trusted to hold up to everyday wear and tear. At the other end of the spectrum are trendy imported chairs priced well over two hundred dollars. Since your baby will be using a high chair three times a day for several years, it might be worth the extra investment to get a quality piece of equipment that can hold up to the day-by-day wear and tear that toddlers dish out.

Scale is important. Some manufacturers have gone overboard with their high chair designs and have made trays and seats so huge that they completely overshadow the small baby seated inside, not to mention eating up a lot of kitchen floor space.

The chair doesn't need a huge tray, just one that has a lip on all sides to catch liquid spills. The tray should also slide effortlessly on and off with one hand and the barest push of a button or squeeze of a latch.

Most chairs now offer adjustable heights so seats can be raised for spoon feeding, lowered to slide up to the dining room table, or even lowered flush with the floor to make a toddler chair. Quality models have seats that effortlessly adjust to numerous positions. Poorly designed models make adjustments difficult and awkward.

The Skinny on High Chairs

JPMA approved. Look for a "JPMA (Juvenile Products Manufacturers Association) certified" sticker on the frame. That means the model lives up to tough safety standards.

Seat belt. The sturdy seat belt should fasten around the waist and between the legs and feature a toddler-proof buckle.

Easy-to-use tray. The tray should be removable with one hand and have a deep, spill-catching rim. It should lock in different positions with an audible click.

Crotch post. A between-the-legs post will help to protect your baby from sliding under the tray (submarining) and getting his head captured, which can be deadly.

Seat adjustments. Multiple seat heights will let the chair fit under a table rim or lower down to the floor for use by a toddler. Reclining positions allow the chair to be used as a baby seat before baby can sit up by himself.

Stability. A wide footprint means the chair will be less likely to tip over when a toddler pulls on the chair or tries to get in on his own. Wheel locks help too.

Washable upholstery. Select a chair with upholstery that's easy to remove and throw in the washing machine.

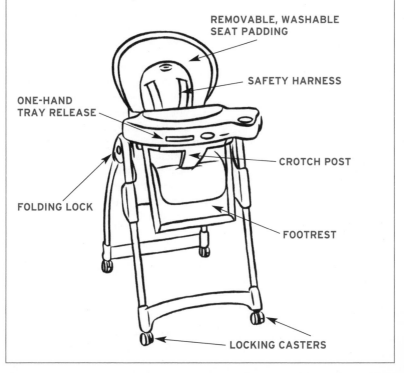

REMOVABLE, WASHABLE SEAT PADDING

SAFETY HARNESS

ONE-HAND TRAY RELEASE

CROTCH POST

FOLDING LOCK

FOOTREST

LOCKING CASTERS

High chairs

⊕ High chairs raise your baby up to your level for feeding, and they give him a bird's-eye view of the kitchen while you're fixing his meal. Some models have adjustable heights so you can lower the chair and remove the tray for pulling baby up to the table during family meals. Trays with deep rims can help to catch spills. One-handed tray removal can come in handy.

⊖ High chairs can take up a lot of kitchen space. High chairs aren't reliable babysitters, so always stay close. Babies stand up and fall out, or try to slip out under the seat when they're not safely belted in.

MONITORS

There are different options for listening in on your baby during pregnancy and also after he arrives. While you're pregnant, you may enjoy tuning into your baby's sounds using a battery-operated amplifier that you place on your belly. If you place it correctly, you may be able to pick up the rapid beating of your baby's heart (120–160 beats a minute) and the whooshing sound of blood moving through your baby's umbilical cord. Some companies now rent sophisticated, handheld Doppler devices for more precise amplification. A "Pregaphone" is a simple handheld device you place on your belly to amplify your voice while you talk to your baby in the womb. Okay, so it's silly, but hey, who knows?

Nursery, or baby, monitors are two-piece electronic devices that allow you to keep tabs on your baby while he's sleeping, and you're in another room. They're like walkie-talkies but most without the talkie part. There are two parts to the monitor. The part that goes in the baby's room is called the transmitter, and it sends out the noise signals. The part that parents carry around with them, usually battery-operated and with a small antenna, is called the receiver. It acts like a radio to amplify your baby's noises through a small speaker.

You may need to try out more than one monitor model to find one with the sensitivity and power that suits your particular environment. Your monitor may lose power if you stray too far. Sometimes barriers, such as brick walls, can block monitor signals. Or batteries can weaken, causing transmissions to dim. Fortunately, most models have a low-battery indicator light.

Parents living in apartments sometimes report that their monitor picks up the sound of another baby, not their own. And some monitors can interfere with cell phone reception, or they transmit annoying sounds from police cars or other passing vehicles.

Most monitors have volume controls so you can listen to baby's every rustle, or you can choose to be signaled only for outright fussiness. Some have light bars that let you see as well as hear your baby's noises, while others borrow from cell phone technology and vibrate to baby's sounds.

Static and interference from cell phones and even crying from a baby in another apartment with a monitor on a similar channel can be annoying.

The Skinny on Monitors

Clear reception. Buy a monitor with a different channel mix, such as channels A plus D, instead of only A and B, and one that uses 900 MHz which is less crowded than the traditional 400 MHz channels and can pick up signals better.

Rechargeable. Monitors gobble up batteries. Rechargeable receivers can save up to fifty dollars a year in battery costs. Also, make sure both the transmitter (baby's unit) and the receiver (yours) have plug-in electric outlet adapters, and a low-battery indicator.

Portability. An easy-to-use belt clip and flexible antenna improve portability. But note: A too-small receiver gets lost quickly. (Search under the couch pillows.)

Sound lights. Indicators that light up to signal the intensity of baby's sound are useful for judging when it's time to head for the nursery, even when you're vacuuming.

Walkie-talkie feature. Monitors that allow you speak soothing sounds from another room or carry on a conversation with your partner are useful.

Useful extras. A light display that lets you see baby's sounds as well as hear them; a warning light or alarm that signals when you're out of range; a night-light feature for baby's room

While most monitors use the crowded 400MHz channels, monitors using 900MHz usually have less interference and promise almost double the sound range. Some monitor brands appear to have better clarity than others. Check parents' ratings of monitors on Web sites that offer product feedback from parents.

You may be able to buy a monitor set that includes an extra receiver so both you and your partner can listen, or you can keep one permanently stationed in the kitchen or your bedroom.

And, at the high end of the monitor price range are monitors that project images on the ceiling, play traditional lullabies or night sounds, or offer not just two channels, but twenty-seven or more from which to choose.

(+) A monitor can give you more peace of mind that your baby isn't crying when you're out of earshot.

(−) Nothing can replace staying close and checking your baby every so often. A monitor can't tell you if your baby has stopped breathing. A monitor may make you more jumpy about normal baby sounds and momentary fussiness that get amplified by the receiver. Static and interference are often problems. Unless your monitor is rechargeable, it can eat up a lot of batteries.

Anatomy of a Portable Play Yard

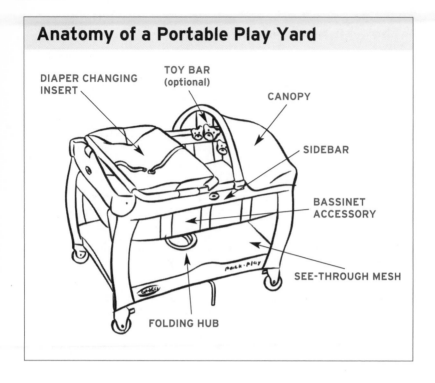

DIAPER CHANGING INSERT

TOY BAR (optional)

CANOPY

SIDEBAR

BASSINET ACCESSORY

SEE-THROUGH MESH

FOLDING HUB

PLAY YARDS

Portable play yards are rectangular like a crib, but instead of being constructed from wood, their frames are made out of tubular metal and covered in moisture-resistant fabric with see-through mesh sides. Instead of having legs, they sit close to the ground on casters, or they may have two legs on one end and two wheels on the other. They're lightweight and fold compactly for storage. Parents use them for travel, or to restrain a baby indoors or outdoors in the shade.

Unlike cribs, play yards are narrow enough to roll through doorways. The hinged sidebars and folding floorboards are padded for baby's safety and comfort.

For safety's sake, it's important to study the manufacturer's directions about how to fold and open the yard before your baby uses it for the first time. Most models squeeze shut like the ribs of a travel umbrella when you release the sidebars using a button and twist and pull up on handle of the flat hub located in the center of the yard under the floor's padding.

Opening the play yard is a challenge—the hinged sidebars must stand nearly upright before the yard will open completely so its sidebars can be firmly locked into place.

While some play yards feature open mesh on all four sides, others have fabric panels on both ends with a storage pocket sewn on the outside. The fabric on the sides and floorboard can be damp mopped with a mild soap and water solution.

Some models offer an optional bassinet feature that fastens to the frame's sidebars, and most companies also offer models with a small, diaper-changing station that fits over one end of the yard's frame.

Safety issues

Over a million portable play yards manufactured in the past decade have undergone federal recalls or corrective actions when the sidebars of some models failed to completely lock in the open position. A "V" shape was formed when the sides were left limp instead of being locked firmly into place, causing babies to strangle when their necks got caught.

The recalls have provided repair kits or other remedies for older models—but for maximum safety, we recommend purchasing a new model if you're not sure about the safety status of an older version.

Don't use a portable play yard as a substitute for a crib. Its loose mesh sides and puffy quilting can be dangerous for unsupervised sleeping. Babies can get entangled in loose sheets and bedding too, so don't add a sheet or pillowcase as a cover for the floor or bassinet section. Remember, all babies should be placed face up and not belly down to lessen the danger of suffocation. (See Sudden Infant Death Syndrome discussion on page 398.)

Older-model play yards may come with a ribbed dome that fits into small holders on the top corners of the yard. The dome comes with warning signs not to use it in direct sunlight because of the danger of serious heat buildup inside.

Most manufacturers have discontinued making the domes because of the danger of babies getting heatstroke.

⊕ Portable play yards are lightweight, have wheels, and fold compactly for storing or carrying in the trunk of the car. Their dimensions allow them to be rolled from room to room. The mesh sides let babies peer out. The bassinet feature allows small babies to snooze, but only with close supervision. Some models come with a carry case that makes porting easy.

⊖ Opening and folding play yards is a hassle, and if the sidebars don't click into place, as with some older models, a toddler's life could be endangered. Mattress pads tend to be soft and cushy, and their moisture-resistance makes them less porous and breathable, which could affect a baby's air supply in the facedown position. Pad covers aren't removable for laundering, and placing sheets or other bedding on top of them can entangle the baby.

ROCKERS AND GLIDERS

Babies and parents both gravitate toward gentle rocking motions for soothing, nursing, and resting together. Surprisingly, if you've got a fussy baby on your hands, the rougher the rocking motion, the better.

You can use a rocker or glider as the center of your "baby nest," which is most convenient when it's near your baby's crib. You'll use the chair hundreds of times for those l-o-n-g, middle-of-the-night feeding sessions while you both snooze.

Put a table beside the chair for your CD player, a book to read, tissues, some fabric diapers for milksops, and a big, trucker-size container of water with a straw for fueling up. Consider stocking your chair with a couple of large, soft pillows and a small blanket to cover both you and baby.

If you're not using a recliner, you may want to purchase a separate footstool so you can prop your knees up to help hold the baby. A semi-circular nursing pillow (Boppy®) can serve to give your arms a rest if you're nursing.

You have three choices for your official baby chair: an old-fashioned rocker made of wood or wicker, a rocker recliner, or a glider. Wooden rockers are usually (but not always) the least expensive option. Sometimes you can find old, but sturdy versions in antique stores. Make sure their scale fits your dimensions: the armrests should be the right height for your elbows, and your feet should rest comfortably on the floor without pitching you forward. You should be able to add your own cushions for seat and back comfort.

Rocker-recliners come in a variety of sizes and upholstery finishes. Needless to say, babies make messes, so it makes sense to choose a moisture-resistant upholstery finish, such as pleather that you can wipe clean with a damp cloth. Make sure the chair fits to your body. Check out the armrests and the ease of reclining. Don't spend a lot of money on a recliner equipped with massage and vibra-tion features; you probably won't use them enough to justify the expense.

Gliders are usually made from wood or metal frames. They offer deeply padded cushioning and a smooth, back-and-forth swaying motion that comes from the chair being suspended underneath the seat portion. Most come with matching ottomans that also rock. Hopefully, cushion covers can be unzipped and can survive numerous machine washings.

Which style of rocker you choose depends upon its fit to your body, how comfortable it is, and your budget. All versions have one flaw: The rockers or the hardware underneath the chair for the reclining or gliding features can be positively hazardous to small exploring fingers or feet. Be careful when using these chairs around toddlers and children, and don't let children play on them.

SAFETY GATES

Safety gates enclose doors and openings to restrain your tot so he won't wander where you don't want him to go—down staircases, where pets sleep, or into your kitchen when you're cooking or loading the dishwasher or the oven door is hot.

Gates are usually made of wood, metal, or plastic, or combinations of these materials. There are three types of safety gates: those that attach to the side of the wall using screws (hardware-mounted gates); those that cling to the wall using rubber gaskets (pressure-mounted gates); and those that are circular fences that can be used to corral kids inside them.

The Skinny on Gates

Use hardware mounting. Gates that screw into the wall are the safest by far. Gates that use thick rubber stoppers to hold the gate in place can be pushed over by a determined toddler, possibly causing falls.

Metal is sturdier. It also makes gates more expensive and heavier. But if you've got a dangerous stairwell to protect, they're the best solution.

Measure first. Look on the packaging for the gate. It will specify the gate's maximum width.

Choose the tallest version. The taller the gate, the more protection you'll get from a climbing toddler or a nosy pet.

Easy-to-open hardware. Try out the hardware that opens the gate. It should be easy to operate and not break fingernails in the process.

No floor interference. Avoid gates that place a bar across the floor. They could cause you to trip.

No toe holds. Avoid gates with sharp holes in the center panel that a tot could hurt his fingers on or try to use for climbing.

Some models close and open like an accordion, while others open and shut like a gate. The centers of gates can be molded plastic mesh, nylon fabric, or clear poly.

Some models also allow the gate's opening direction to go only one way so they won't swing out over stairs. Although a safety gate can't completely stop your determined toddler from vaulting down the steps or getting into other mischief when he sets his mind to it, it can give you a few extra minutes to figure out what's going on.

Hardware-mounted gates are considered the safest—in fact, they're the only type of gate you should use at the top of staircases or to shut off dangerous areas. Pressure-mounted gates can be used in less risky settings since they can sometimes work loose from the wall—especially if your toddler rolls into one in a walker, or if children are roughhousing.

Old-fashioned accordion gates with wooden slats shaped like Xs at the top are positively dangerous and shouldn't be used. They could capture a child's neck or crush small fingers. Most new-version gates are designed to minimize harm, and to help prevent toddlers from crawling over them.

Here are qualities of a good gate: the latches are easy for you to use but hard for your tot to operate; there are no finger-pinching places; and the placement of slats or pattern of plastic mesh won't allow your tot to get a foothold for climbing.

Specialty gates are available to help you shield wide and unusual openings in your home, such as dining room entries or open stairs with iron railings on the side. Taller-than-normal gates are also available for containing super-active kids and large pets. For safety's sake, remember that safety gates aren't foolproof. You'll still want to keep constant watch over your active toddler.

⊕ Safety gates can help to keep your toddler off the stairs and help to keep him out of the kitchen or other places that may be unsafe.

⊖ Sometimes gates give parents a false sense of security about their babies. Parents routinely forget to lock gates; use gates that don't hold well; or trip and fall down the stairs themselves when they try to step over the gate instead of going to the trouble to open it and walk through. Gates with X joints can strangle and kill, and those with sharp parts, such as molded mesh holes, can actually injure babies' hands and feet.

SOFT CARRIERS AND SLINGS

Mothers and fathers have fastened babies onto their bodies throughout human history. Doing so frees parents' arms to do other things and gives babies the rhythmical rocking movements that soothe them by reminding them of life in the womb.

There are basically three types of baby carriers that parents wear on their bodies: soft carriers made of fabric, slings that go over one shoulder and are also constructed of fabric, and hard-framed carriers for older tots that support a baby who rides on a parent's back. Since backpacks are an option to be post-

poned until your baby gets older, we will only cover soft carriers and slings.

Soft carriers usually consist of an inner seat pocket for the baby and an outer fabric covering that also offers a fold-down firm headrest for newborns, padded shoulder straps for the parent, and waist straps to help support the baby's weight.

Slings resemble small hammocks with pleats that are designed to hold a young baby in a reclining or semi-reclining position. Some parents prefer slings because they feel it gives baby rounded back support instead of making the baby sit bolt upright as soft carriers do.

Soft carrier

⊕ They're made of comfortable fabric, which is easy to wear. They put your baby's head at your chin, and you can provide natural warmth and comfort with your hand on baby's back.

⊖ Some models are a complex mesh of straps that makes putting on the baby a challenge. They can be hot in the summer. Poor hardware or too-large leg-holes have led to baby injuries in the past.

Sling

⊕ They allow babies to lie in a more natural, semi-reclined position. The sling can be quickly adjusted to provide coverage for discreet nursing.

⊖ They're difficult to adjust, and you may need coaching from another user on finding the right position and length for

The Skinny on Soft Carriers

Washable. One spit-up can ruin a whole day! Fabric should be sturdy, soft, and able to withstand lots of machine washing.

Simple to use. Avoid models with a jumble of straps to figure out.

Padded shoulder straps. Parents' shoulder straps should be adjustable, densely padded, and spaced so they don't rub the neck or slip off the shoulders.

Head support. A cushioned head support will be needed for the first few months. Fold it down, or snap it off after that.

Adjusting seat. Baby's seat should adjust to different heights using sturdy snaps that won't rub baby's belly. (Extra safety loops or a backup pouch will help to prevent accidental falls.)

Front or rear facing. Some models allow facing outward as well as toward the chest, or riding on the back too—handy options for porting toddlers.

Nursing position. Read the directions on how to nurse your baby while he sits in the carrier.

Great options. Other extras: snap-on, flannel burper bibs; elasticized pockets for carrying small items; adjustments for discreet nursing; reflector strips for evening strolls; breathable mesh or special porous fabric for air circulation.

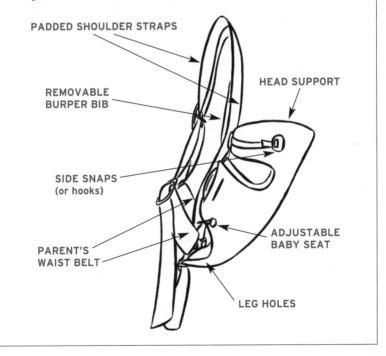

PADDED SHOULDER STRAPS

HEAD SUPPORT

REMOVABLE
BURPER BIB

SIDE SNAPS
(or hooks)

ADJUSTABLE
BABY SEAT

PARENT'S
WAIST BELT

LEG HOLES

your and baby's comfort. There are no straps to hold the baby in, which could be a problem if you lean over to pick something up. Rather than being evenly distributed, all of baby's weight is carried on one shoulder and across your back, which may cause body alignment problems.

STROLLERS

It takes careful searching to locate the best possible stroller for you and your baby-to-be, and other than a crib, it is probably the most expensive piece of baby equipment you'll buy. It is also the most complex baby product, and it can be the biggest investment other than a crib and mattress.

Strollers come in a huge variety of sizes and weights. Most manufacturers offer a basic model, followed by step-up options that drive the price up, making it hard to decide what you really need versus useless extras. You'll have to pay more for those loaded with fancy extras than those offering only basic comfort.

Stroller choices

Here's our breakdown of the different types of stroller models out there. (Mind boggling, isn't it?)

Lightweight and inexpensive. Commonly called umbrella strollers, these are usually flimsy, with single wheels on each axle, hammock-like seats with no padding, an almost-useless canopy, and no reclining options. They're usually priced under $40. Some parents buy one or two in their babies' riding careers just to take on trips or to run fast errands.

Mid-priced and mid-weight workhorses. These are the mainstream vehicles for pushing baby around. They come with dual wheels on the front and comfort features such as reclining seats, thick upholstery, wrap-around canopies, and deep storage compartments. Some offer removable front trays. They're priced in the $40–$150 range.

Lightweight and costly imports. These are the "sports cars" of the stroller world. They're stuffed with gizmos, feature trendy fabrics, luxury padding, and loads of extras, such as padded headrests, cup holders, and sleek folding mechanisms. They're priced between $150 and $400.

Heavy travel systems. These are bulky models with large wheels, mostly designed to support their own snap-out car seats, $80 and up.

Carriage-stroller combinations. Huge, fully reclining carriage/stroller combinations—basically baby beds on wheels, $100 and up.

Jogging and sports strollers. These are even larger, three-wheeled strollers with air-inflated, bicycle-style tires for use by sports and fitness enthusiasts, $100 and up, depending on wheel size.

Price doesn't make perfect

Most parents make the mistake of believing that when a stroller costs a lot, it will automatically deliver more quality, durability, and safety than less expensive models.

That strategy might work with cars, but it doesn't work for baby wheels. Parents sometimes use strollers as status symbols. Instead of bragging about their Mercedes, BMW, or fancy SUV, they brag about their baby's Maclaren, Peg Perego, or Aprica—all imports with price tags starting around $200 and rising to $400 or more.

Never mind the show-offs! The $400 Maclaren is a bummer to open and fold. The Peg Perego is jiggly to a fault. And although Apricas are admittedly plush, you can get the same amenities, feature-by-feature, but perhaps with a little more poundage, from a less expensive Combi, or commonplace Graco, or Evenflo models.

In truth, all strollers are vulnerable to wheel and frame alignment problems and serious safety issues.

Stroller dangers include metal joints and hardware that can crush small hands and fingers during folding as well as legholes and gaps that can cause strangulation if a baby is left alone to nap but isn't belted. Sometimes, stroller latches aren't strong enough to prevent the frame from accidentally folding while in use, tossing the baby out, or capturing and injuring his hands on the sides of the frame during the collapse.

Important considerations

The weight and size of your stroller are important to consider. You'll come to hate the huge, bulky model that eats up your trunk space, leaving no room left for suitcases or groceries.

You'll also despise a giant model that weighs so much you feel like you're breaking your back every time you have to fold it and lift it in and out of the back of your car—an act you'll repeat about one thousand times before your baby can walk.

Super-lightweight models are great for negotiating tight store aisles, but their tiny wheels don't work well for leisurely walking on uneven sidewalks. Your baby will get jolted with every seam in the pavement and practically vault out the front when you try to roll down over curbs.

Some parents ultimately settle for two strollers: a compact, easy-to-maneuver version for shopping, and a larger, sturdier model for taking baby on afternoon walks.

Postpone buying a jogging stroller until your baby is mature enough to have good head and body support (about six months of age). By that time, you'll know whether you have the time and energy to resume your pre-pregnancy exercise program.

Purchase a mid-weight (ten to seventeen pounds) stroller from a mainstream manufacturer. Look for an aluminum frame and a model that isn't burdened with a lot of accessories. The idea is to purchase a competitively priced, sturdy stroller with a variety of options.

Later, consider adding a less-expensive, lightweight umbrella-style stroller (read: throw away) with good brakes and at least one reclining position for running quick errands and negotiating airports. (Be sure to pack the stroller in a box for flying, since the frame is likely to get bent if you check it like baggage.) (For a list of baby product manufacturers, see *Resource Guide* on pages 567–570.)

The Skinny on Strollers

Plan to take a variety of stroller models on a test drive before you settle on the one you want to buy.

Folding. Test how readily the stroller folds up and reopens for locking into the upright position. Expect to feel awkward. In fact, you may need a sales clerk to help you locate elusive release latches. Lightweight strollers are the easiest to open and fold single-handedly and are great for racing to airport gates. They're too lightweight, though, for negotiating sidewalks and steep curbs on long, leisurely walks.

Steering. Try pushing the stroller with one hand. The model should roll straight ahead without veering to one side. Most mid-priced models have swivel wheels with dual tires on the front that lock into a straight-ahead position by a foot pedal on the wheel assembly. A toddler's weight affects stroller steering. A stroller may push straight when you're testing it in the store without your baby, but veer when your baby grows into a weighty toddler. Bring along a friend with a toddler/passenger to help narrow down your choices.

Seat recline. Check out how easy it is to recline the back of the seat and the number of positions offered. The more reclining options, the better, but sides of the stroller should be well-padded to protect the baby's head and arms from slipping through when the seat is in its fullest recline position. Only large, combination carriage/stroller models recline fully into a protected bed. A semi-recline will do.

Seat belt. The seat belt should have straps that come together to click into a center buckle at the baby's waist. Your baby will also require a strap between the legs to prevent slide-outs. The safest models also offer shoulder straps to hold a restless toddler in place. Superior five-point harness systems offer an adjustable strap for each side of a baby's waist, a between-the-legs strap, and adjustable shoulder straps.

Canopy or sunshade. A deep, folding sunshade will help to protect your baby from wind, rain, and glare. Some models offer a small, vinyl window in the back of the canopy that keeps the baby in sight.

Storage bin. A roomy storage bin underneath the stroller seat comes in handy for toting your purse, a diaper bag, or other items. If the bin sags too far down when it's filled with packages, it may scrape the ground when you try to go over curbs.

Weight considerations. An aluminum frame, although a little more expensive than steel, will be sturdier and lighter.

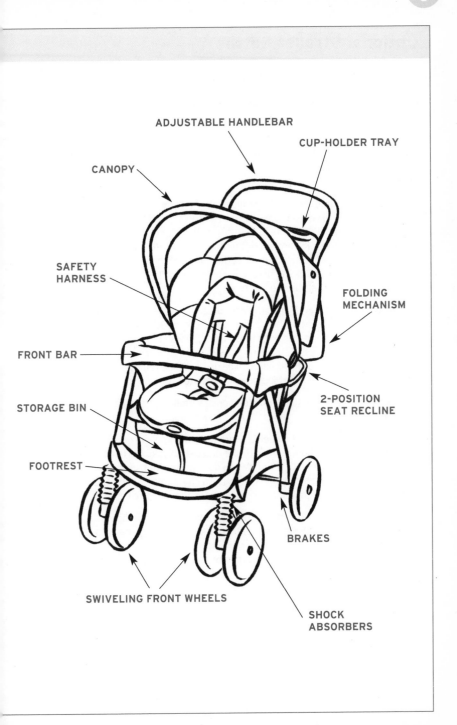

ADJUSTABLE HANDLEBAR

CUP-HOLDER TRAY

CANOPY

SAFETY
HARNESS

FOLDING
MECHANISM

FRONT BAR

2-POSITION
SEAT RECLINE

STORAGE BIN

FOOTREST

BRAKES

SWIVELING FRONT WHEELS

SHOCK
ABSORBERS

Optional Stroller Extras

Here's our list of handy, but costly stroller add-ons:

- **Full recline.** A seat that fully reclines is available only on huge carriage/stroller combinations. Your baby can sleep just fine in a semi-reclined position.

- **Car seat support.** Should you buy a heavier-than-normal stroller just so you can tote baby around in an infant car seat? Only if the supporting stroller is lightweight.

- **Reversible handlebars.** Some strollers offer a frame that allows the handlebar to reverse from back to front of the seat so baby can face toward you or outward. Others have seats that lift off the frame to reverse, and companies are experimenting with stroller seats that can be shifted to allow facing either direction. Most of these features add extra pounds, and, after the first few months, most babies prefer facing the world, rather than their parents.

- **Front play tray or bar.** Many strollers come with trays or padded bars fastened onto the front of the stroller. Some come with attached toys. Although babies like to grip onto these front pieces, mostly they get in the way when it comes to strapping baby in and taking him out. If you buy a stroller with a tray or front bar, make sure it can be removed so your independent toddler can get in and out by himself.

- **Cup holders.** Some strollers come equipped with parent and baby cup holders. This may not be a necessity for your baby.

- **Giant wheels.** Huge sport wheels are great for going over rough terrain, but they add extra weight to the stroller and eat up valuable trunk space when the stroller is folded. If you plan to do a lot of country walking, buy a model with medium-size wheels. If you're a city dweller, go for the most compact and lightweight model you can find in the mid-price range.

- **Snap-on boot.** The most expensive strollers offer a snap-on boot for covering baby's legs during cold weather. The hitch is that you're likely to pay fifty dollars or more for the luxury of it. Consider using a blanket, or buying a baby sac that your baby can use for sleeping in the crib too.

TOYS AND PLAY EQUIPMENT

Do babies really need toys? Parents, grandparents, and other gift givers seem to think so. They spend millions of dollars every year to provide their babies with the latest fads in Toyland. In truth, parents are baby's most cherished toys.

Babies like to slowly track colorful rattles and toys. They like to grasp onto rattles and teethers. They're drawn to sharp contrasts, bright patterns, and bold colors. The best toys are those that respond to some action taken by a baby.

Mobiles

A mobile suspends and rotates toys to music over a baby's head as she lies in the crib. It fastens onto the crib's side bar with a clamp and has a long arm that reaches out into the center of the crib where small stuffed toys or painted images slowly rotate above the baby's head. The best mobiles use very bright, intriguing toys that are faced downward toward the baby.

A mobile should only be used during the first five months of a baby's life or until a baby begins to roll over or tries to sit up. Then, it should be removed from the crib and put away, since a mobile's toys and strings aren't considered safe playthings after that.

Simple mobiles use wind-up music boxes with a small rotator bar to provide both the sounds and the motions. The most sophisticated versions are battery operated, present a huge array of motions and graphics, play classical music, lullabies, or children singing, and may

even offer a remote-control option so you can start it going without baby even knowing you're there.

(+) Mobiles play pleasant music and offer clever, rotating toys for babies who are too young to sit up.

(−) Most babies don't spend much time on their backs staring up at mobiles. When they're awake, they want to be held, diapered, and fed. Mobiles are dangerous for babies who can sit up and pull them over, so they're only useful for a few months, and they may get in the way of lifting your baby out of the crib.

Rattles and teethers

These are the basic items that most babies will play with once they get a little eye-hand coordination, but they really aren't all that interesting to babies until about five months of age, although a newborn will track a brightly colored rattle with his eyes if you move it slowly enough.

Shop for mainstream brands from known and trusted toy manufacturers, and avoid inexpensive imports found in drugstores or airports that are flimsy and could easily break. The best rattles make a lot of noise for not a lot of work and are the right scale for a baby's small fists.

SAFETY TIP

If an item can pass through the center of a toilet paper roll, it's too small and your baby might choke on it.

Never allow your baby to use the tiny diaper-pin or barbell rattles that are used for gift-wrapping shower presents. They could get caught in your baby's throat and cause suffocation. Also avoid versions that are large, heavy, and have a big ball on the end. Your baby could strike himself in the head when he tries to play with it.

Teethers resemble small necklaces or cushioned bracelets that a tot holds in his hand to gnaw on when he gets to the drooling stage. Again, buy from a reputable toy manufacturer, and be careful that there are no small parts that could come loose and be swallowed by the baby.

(+) Babies are intrigued by the sound and motion of rattles. Once they gain some hand skill, they can hold onto it themselves.

(–) Babies like to throw rattles on the floor from high chairs and changing tables. Sometimes their bulbs come loose, or they break, exposing sharp shards of plastic and small objects that can be swallowed.

Soft toys

Your baby is likely to gather a huge menagerie of stuffed toys from well-meaning gift givers. Be cautious about inexpensive stuffed toys like the type you win at the fair or from a vending machine. They may have loose eyes or hair that could choke a baby.

Large stuffed animals should be kept out of a baby's crib because they pose a suffocation hazard, and toddlers will use them as props for climbing out. Probably the best solution is to use your baby's animal menagerie as part of your nursery décor. Sit them on a colorful shelf fastened far away from baby's reach, or suspend them in a mesh hammock, also well out of reach.

Another genre of soft toys is excellent for baby play. They're the worms, flower faces, and baby-size fabric balls that offer a variety of textures, colors, and crinkling sounds to intrigue small explorers. The best versions offer bright colors, whimsical patterns, and a variety of unexpected sounds or textures.

SAFETY WARNING: Toy boxes!

Don't be tempted to use a wooden box with a hinged lid for storing your baby's toys. There have been numerous baby deaths attributed to toy box lids. The baby lifts the lid, peers down into the box, and the lid slams shut on his neck, entrapping him, and leading to suffocation. The best way to store toys is to display them on a low shelf that's been bolted to the wall with an L-shaped bracket so it can't be pulled over by the baby. Rather than put everything out, store toys on closet shelves in boxes so they're out of sight, and then rotate your display from time to time to keep your baby intrigued.

➕ They're cute and appealing just like babies are.

➖ They're not safe in baby cribs because they can lead to suffocation. Sometimes babies can pull off their ribbons, eyes, or fur, and ingest them.

Electronic toys

Increasingly, baby toys are being outfitted with small batteries, sound chips, and flashing lights. Although they are initially fascinating to a baby, most tots enjoy toys that respond to their squeezing or gnawing, rather than those that simply put on a show. (And don't forget the joy of wooden spoons, plastic cups and containers, and pots and pans as freebies that are perhaps more fun because they are things you use, too.)

➕ They offer momentarily exciting stimulation, sometimes fascinating and unexpected to babies.

➖ Some babies are annoyed or frightened by unexpected sounds and lights. These toys eat up batteries too.

Play gyms

These are small play areas designed especially for babies lying on their backs. Arches hold suspended toys, mirrors, and other playthings that babies can bat with their hands and feet. Most gyms fold down compactly into a carrier when you're on the go. Specialized foot toys encourage leg movements, such as presser bars that make noise when a baby's foot taps on them and booties with

noisemakers imbedded inside that sound with every kick.

➕ Babies seem to enjoy the sense of mastery they get from making sounds and motions happen, and it's silly and fun to watch them.

➖ They're sometimes quite pricey, and babies are only interested in them for a short time before they begin to roll over, sit up, and crawl.

WALKERS AND EXERCISERS

Walkers and exercisers are designed to entertain babies who can sit up on their own (around six months of age), but who can't walk yet (one to one and one-half years of age). Both walkers and exercisers are made from molded plastic frames and feature a seat suspended in the center. Some walkers have adjustable, X-shaped metal joints on the side. The difference between walkers and exercisers is that walkers have wheels on the bottom that let a baby propel himself around by pushing on the floor with his toes.

Exercisers have a solid base for a baby's feet and are designed to stay in one place, but offer a baby a jiggling or rocking motion when he moves with his legs and body. Most walkers and exercisers have toys installed on the tray that can help to keep baby entertained. And some models have battery-operated noisemakers and electronic sound and light enhancements.

The Skinny on Exercisers

Adjustable seat height. Offers at least three seat heights so the walker can grow with your baby.

Comfy seat padding. Thick padding, good head support, and smooth seams around the legholes will keep baby comfortable.

Smooth seat rotation. The seat should rotate effortlessly using hidden ball bearings.

Toy joys. The toys should be short enough so they won't block your baby's view, be the right scale for small toddler hands, and offer numerous actions and sounds to keep a baby interested.

Springy motions. Look for spring action that will reward your baby's movements.

Lockable rocking. There should be small flip-down latches that let you lock the rocking so you can feed baby and stop him from propelling the exerciser across slick floors.

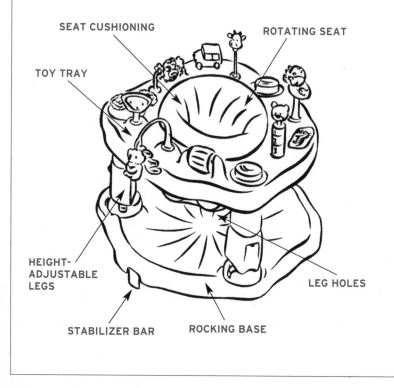

SEAT CUSHIONING

ROTATING SEAT

TOY TRAY

HEIGHT-ADJUSTABLE LEGS

LEG HOLES

STABILIZER BAR

ROCKING BASE

A safety certification program from the Juvenile Products Manufacturers Association (JPMA) and the American Society of Testing and Materials (ASTM) now provides an extra margin of walker safety for those units with the certified sticker. Walkers that get certified must either have a wide-enough base that they won't fit through doorways, or have a stopper foot or other device underneath the walker frame to help halt the walker before it topples down stairs.

So, it's important to buy a new JPMA-certified walker rather than relying on an older, less safe walker for keeping your baby safe—especially if you've got stairs in your house. But, keep in mind that walkers with stoppers and skid-resistant bands on the bottom that are supposed to prevent them from rolling down stairs can go down anyway if your child rolls sideways or backward into the stairwell. Install hardware-mounted gates at the tops of all stairway openings, including the basement, and keep them locked. Or better yet, don't buy a walker at all.

Stationary exercisers, sometimes called Exersaucers after Evenflo's original models, are a much safer alternative than a walker. They stay in one place, but offer jiggling and rocking actions. They've got lots of play toys all around their trays that a baby can manipulate as he rotates his seat around using his hands and feet.

Exercisers

(+) Babies like sitting in them temporarily. The toys are in easy reach of small arms and hands. They get your crawler out from under foot while you're vacuuming, running the dishwasher, or doing other household chores.

(−) Babies at this age shouldn't sit upright for longer than thirty minutes at a time, so use it sparingly, but not as a "baby-sitter." Even though exercisers don't have wheels, some babies can rock them so vigorously that they move across the floor, which could lead the baby into a hot stove, a staircase, or other trouble spots. Use the locking option on the base to hold it still.

Walkers

(+) Before they have mastered crawling, babies seem to delight in mimicking walking. Toys on the tray can be enjoyable.

(−) More babies are injured in baby walker–related accidents than any other nursery product. Walkers have been implicated in thousands of serious baby accidents, usually when they've fallen headfirst down staircases resulting in severe head damage. They also vault babies into swimming pools, and crash them into hot stoves. They don't help babies walk sooner; in fact, they cause babies to adapt abnormal pushing actions with their feet.

Resource
Guide

6

Resource Guide

In recent years, the Internet has developed into a vast and flexible tool for accessing information on pregnancy, birth, and babies. It stores and serves up billions of bytes for almost immediate access, and there are virtually hundreds of sites catering specifically to parents. Some are commercial and sponsored by parenting magazines or by companies trying to promote their products, and others are underwritten by impartial not-for-profit and professional organizations.

Wherever you travel on the Internet, you'll find gigantic collections of pregnancy and parenting information features arranged by topics. Plus, you can choose from a menu of hundreds of bulletin boards and chat groups where parents pregnant within the same month come together to share their concerns, ask questions, or simply make connections with one another.

Some parenting sites have become commercial to the point of frustration. You may have to swim through one irritating pop-up ad after another just to access the information you're seeking. Once you've gotten inside the site, we suggest exercising caution about what information you volunteer just to get ongoing newsletters or

updates dispatched to your inbox. Consider establishing a "junk" mailbox address using a free provider to separate your personal mail from unsolicited e-mail that eats up valuable minutes just to delete.

Many pregnancy and parenting sites sell parents' names, addresses, and private information to mailing list brokers and big manufacturers who are eager to know your due date, your address (to pile junk mail in your mailbox), and even your phone number in order to give you middle-of-dinner calls. Occasionally, though, you may get something more useful, such as a free baby magazine subscription, coupons, or product samples by mail. (We talk more about that in the *Baby Gear Guide* section starting on page 458.)

Most public libraries not only offer e-mail and Internet access on-site, plus they also offer home computer access to major information databases by using passwords that you are given when you sign up for the service at the library. If you're lucky, you may be able to download full magazine and newspaper articles on pregnancy and birth topics from sites that normally charge a subscription rate, such as Infotrac. Major parenting magazines such as *Parents, Parenting, Child, Mothering,* and *American Baby* also have treasure troves of past articles posted on their proprietary sites, which are searchable by keywords.

Major not-for-profit organizations, such as the March of Dimes, the American Academy of Pediatrics, La Leche League, and the Maternity Center Association are valuable sites to bookmark. They all carry well-researched articles of interest to parents on their Web sites. *The New York Times* and other major newspapers also offer news posting services that allow you to have topics of interest e-mailed periodically to you.

How to search for medical information

Finding valid medical research about pregnancy, birth, and babies online can be a task. And it's often difficult to decipher the validity and language of research studies, or to tell which studies are weak, or even misleading. Most full-blown medical studies are obtuse and difficult to understand, especially when it comes to understanding the meaning of their statistics and trying to tell whether their findings were strong enough to be significant when it comes to making an important medical decision. Obviously, the quality of evidence isn't as good if only twenty subjects were used versus a meta-analysis that reports on findings based on studies covering the outcomes for thousands of mothers.

It's easy to become overwhelmed with too much information, particularly when your seemingly infallible sources don't agree with one another. When it comes to making informed decisions about whether to undergo medical tests, what drugs to use or avoid, or how to deal with risk factors, the perspective of a well-trained and seasoned healthcare provider is simply the best place to go for help. In addition, some providers give patients their e-mail addresses so they can post queries that get answered in a day, or so.

PubMed is the most popular Web site for searching abstracts of medical literature. Its main address is www.ncbi.nlm.nih.gov/PubMed. (Note: Abstracts aren't the actual research studies, just brief descriptions and general findings from them.) Using PubMed is free, well, actually, it's paid for by your tax dollars. You can search for specific terms, such as "twins," "labor," "pregnancy," or "breastfeeding," or you can conduct a more formal search based on key terms used by the site, which is called a MeSH (Medical Subject Heading) search.

When you uncover an abstract of an article that appears to address your concerns, you'll find a "Related Articles" option to the right of the article title in PubMed that will uncover even more studies. But note: "Related Articles" will only search starting from the year of publication of your original article, and so it may not bring up the most recent articles first. A number of medical and nursing journals offer on-line access and are linked to the PubMed Web site, but some may require that you register to use them, or pay a huge subscription fee. Biomednet (www.biomednet.com) is similar to Pub Med with numerous links to articles.

One way to obtain research articles without having to pay an arm and a leg for them is to ask your public library. Write down pertinent article information, including the names of the authors, the title of the article, the journal with its volume number, date, and page numbers, and then request that the reference librarian assist you in obtaining a copy through your state's inter-library loan program. You will probably be charged a basic per-page fee, and the biggest drawback is that getting the article may take days, rather than minutes or hours.

Hospitals, medical societies, and medical schools often have libraries open to the public that carry obstetric, pediatric, and nursing journals that can be photocopied for between ten and twenty-five cents per page or copied on a diskette or CD for free. (Bring your own blanks.)

Some medical publishers offer access to their books and journals online. Springer (http://link.springer. de/ol/medol), Blackwell Science/ Munksgaard (www.blackwell-synergy.com), and Elsevier (www.sciencedirect.com) offer fairly open access to their publications and provide a search engine to help readers conduct searches.

Don't forget the books!

We're not just saying that because we wrote this one. A well-researched book on pregnancy, and childbirth, such as ours and others, can serve as a valuable tool for synthesizing information and bringing everything into perspective.

Helpful Web Sites for Parents

Again, just a reminder that Web sites come and go. These listings and reviews were up-to-date at the time this manuscript was completed (2004), but changes are to be expected. If you run into dead addresses, conduct a search using keywords and your favorite search engine such as www.google.com to see if the address has changed. If we've missed any of your favorite sites, or you're with an organization that would like to have your address listed here, please write us in care of our publisher, and we will try to include your address in our next edition.

ALTERNATIVE PAIN RELIEF OPTIONS FOR BIRTH

NAME	DESCRIPTION	WEB ADDRESS
Acupuncture.com	A searchable source for articles on Chinese herbs and the use of acupuncture for relief of discomforts during pregnancy and labor.	www.acupuncture.com

BABY LOSS: MISCARRIAGE & SUDDEN INFANT DEATH SYNDROME (SIDS)

NAME	DESCRIPTION	WEB ADDRESS
The Foundation for the Study of Infant Deaths (FSID)	A UK SIDS (cot death) prevention organization that publishes a range of leaflets and other information.	www.sids.org.uk/fsid
Help after Neonatal Death (H.A.N.D.)	Online support services and downloadable brochure.	www.handonline.org
Hygeia Foundation	On online journal for pregnancy and neonatal loss support and information.	www.hygeia.org
Sudden Infant Death Syndrome Alliance	Research and action for SIDS.	www.sidsalliance.org

BABY PRODUCTS & PRODUCT SAFETY

NAME	DESCRIPTION	WEB ADDRESS
Babies-R-Us	Wide selection of baby products. Occasional specials or free shipping offers.	www.babiesrus.com
Baby Center	Baby clothes, gear, and toys, plus lots of pregnancy and parenting information.	www.store.babycenter.com

BABY PRODUCTS & PRODUCT SAFETY (continued)

NAME	DESCRIPTION	WEB ADDRESS
Baby Mine	Organic cotton baby clothes.	www.babyminestore.com
BabyNet	Sells baby products, but also offers chat-lines and helpful articles on pregnancy, babies, and parenting.	www.babynet.com
The Baby Outlet	A baby gear department store online.	www.thebabyoutlet.com
Baby Style	Large selection of maternity and baby clothes, and a huge selection of upscale, pricey baby products.	www.babystyle.com
Baby Universe	An online department store for a wide variety of baby products.	www.babyuniverse.com
Birthways	A source for belly mask kits to make a lasting mold of your pregnant shape.	www.birthways.net
Breastfeeding.com	Commercial site that sells breast pumps, bras, nursing clothing, video clips about nursing, and answers to common breastfeeding questions.	www.breastfeeding.com
Buy Buy Baby	An online baby product source.	www.buybuyBABY.com
Carseat Data	Supplies detailed information on car seats for infants and toddlers, including important car seat links and a compatibility database to help you in deciding what seat to buy.	www.carseatdata.org
Consumer Federation of America	A nonprofit consumer's organization concerned with product safety.	www.consumerfed.org
Consumer Reports	Site for consumers union. Provides free articles on baby products and subscription-only access to baby product ratings.	www.consumerreports.org
The Danny Foundation	A nonprofit organization concerned with crib and baby product safety. Issues warnings about dangerous products.	www.dannyfoundation.org (800-83-DANNY)

BABY PRODUCTS & PRODUCT SAFETY (continued)

NAME	DESCRIPTION	WEB ADDRESS
Dr. Toy	The site for Stevanne Auerbach, Ph.D., a child development expert who oversees an annual, national rating for the best toys for babies and children.	www.drtoy.com
Eddie Bauer	Sells strollers, car seats, and diaper bags.	www.eddiebauer.com
ePinions	Go there first before you buy to get parents' candid reviews of baby products.	www.epinions.com
Gap	Well-known mall shop offers maternity and baby clothing online.	www.gap.com
Internet Baby	Offers expert advice on baby product selection and a range of products.	www.internetbaby.com
JCPenney	Baby clothes and furniture. Occasional sales.	www.jcpenney.com
The Kids Window	Chic European baby clothes to drool over.	www.thekidswindow.com
KMom	Maternity selections for plus-size pregnant mothers.	www.plus-size-pregnancy .org
Land's End	Excellent diaper bags plus quality baby clothes and carriers.	www.landsend.com
Miracle Munchkins	Clever photo and non-photo birth announcements, shower favors and invitations, and baby mementos, such as handprint kits.	www.miraclemunchkins.com
Nordstrom	Mall store online carries clothes and diaper bags including upscale baby duds from Ralph Lauren and Little Me.	www.store.nordstrom.com
Old Navy	Jeans and tees for expectant moms and babies.	www.oldnavy.com
One Step Ahead	A catalog of carefully chosen baby products with an emphasis on uniqueness and quality.	www.onestepahead.com

BABY PRODUCTS & PRODUCT SAFETY (continued)

NAME	DESCRIPTION	WEB ADDRESS
Organic Bebe	Organic cotton baby clothing.	www.organicbebe.com
Osh Kosh B'Gosh	Sturdy overalls and T-shirts for babies and kids. Great bargains.	www.oshkoshbgosh.com
Rattle & Roll	A boutique of upscale baby products.	www.rattleroll.com
Robeez	Adorable baby shoes for less than twenty-five dollars.	www.robeez.com
SafetyBeltSafe USA	The best source on the Internet for studying car seat safety. Take a look at their technical section.	www.carseat.org
Sears	The old faithful offers clothing and baby products from a limited line of brands.	www.sears.com
Seat Check	A free children's car seat inspection locator service.	www.seatcheck.org
Smarter Kids	A great source for shopping baby toys by age.	www.smarterkids.com
Toy Industry Association of America (TIA)	The professional organization of toy manufacturers. Offers toy safety tips.	www.toy-tia.org
Wal-Mart	Great prices on cribs, strollers, baby clothes, and other gear here.	www.walmart.com

BABY SHOWERS

NAME	DESCRIPTION	WEB ADDRESS
Baby Shower.com	Fun to read other parents' ideas. Announcements, books, clever gifts.	www.baby-shower.com
Baby Zone	A general baby information site that also has a special section on planning baby showers.	www.babyzone.com

BIRTH ANNOUNCEMENTS

NAME	DESCRIPTION	WEB ADDRESS
Anne Geddes	The source for those adorable, pudgy sleeping cherubs.	www.annegeddes.com
Baby Birth Announcements	Clever concepts for anouncing baby, including baby driver's license.	www.babybirth announcements.com
Classic Card Company	Traditional announcement cards.	www.classiccard.com
Stork Avenue	Lots of clever card choices, including "Sports Illustrated" covers for boys.	www.storkavenue.com

BIRTH DEFECTS & DISABILITIES

NAME	DESCRIPTION	WEB ADDRESS
March of Dimes Birth Defects Foundation	A nonprofit organization offering information on birth defects, suggestions for having a healthy pregnancy, newborn feeding tips, and vaccinations. Accepts questions by e-mail.	www.modimes.org
Through the Looking Glass	A non-profit organization offering clinical and supportive services, training, and research for families with disabled children.	www.lookingglass.org
Working Parents (UK)	A British group that produces the newsletter "Waving Not Drowning" for working parents with disabled children.	www.flametree.co.uk

BIRTH INFORMATION

NAME	DESCRIPTION	WEB ADDRESS
ABCs of Pregnancy	An online textbook about pregnancy, childbirth, and early parenting.	www.abcbirth.com
Active Birth	The British site for Janet Balaskas, proponent of active movement of mothers during birth.	www.activebirth centre.com

BIRTH INFORMATION (continued)

NAME	DESCRIPTION	WEB ADDRESS
Birth Balance	Waterbirth, dreamy music, doulas, and balancing chakras during pregnancy presented by Judith Halek.	www.birthbalance.com
Birthing from Within	The site for the birthing approach created by Pam England. Offers teacher courses with an emphasis on awareness during birth. Posts past newsletters and articles on labor pain.	www.birthingfromwithin.com
Born Free!	Site for Laura Shanley, an advocate for the unassisted childbirth movement. Site includes articles on natural birth and birth stories.	www.unassistedchildbirth .com
Brigham & Women's Hospital	The nation's oldest women's hospital in Boston has helpful information on labor, analgesia, and c-sections.	www.brighamandwomens. org/painfreebirthing
Center for Prenatal Music	Offers a bibliography and recommended CDs and tapes for the birthing experience.	www.prenatalmusic.com
Childbirth Solutions	Expert advice and excellent articles on childbirth alternatives including waterbirth, hypnosis, and birthing environment.	www.childbirthsolutions.com
Gentle Birth	Lots of great articles on birthing, comfort measures, fathers' roles. Offers a helpful online brochure, "Planning Your Childbirth," describing commonly used analgesics and anesthetics.	www.gentlebirth.org
Global Maternal/ Child Health Association	Site for Waterbirth International. Information on giving birth in water, including products and referrals.	www.waterbirth.org
Home First	The Web site of a large home birthing practice in Chicago that also offers several home birthing stories from parents and excellent, reviewed links to other sites of interest to families electing home birth.	www.homefirst.com/ main.htm

BIRTH INFORMATION (continued)

NAME	DESCRIPTION	WEB ADDRESS
Mayo Clinic	This famous hospital's Web site offers excellent public information on pregnancy, childbirth, and baby care.	www.mayohealth.org
Motherstuff	"Interventions in Birth" is an especially helpful page of links to follow to study labor.	www.motherstuff.com/html/midwife-inter
Natural Childbirth Organization	A central Florida site for childbirth classes that has a library of more than three hundred articles on childbirth and pregnancy topics.	www.naturalchildbirth.org
National Childbirth Trust	A British site offering a wealth of information about birthing and baby care.	www.nctms.co.uk
Transition to Parenthood	An excellent resource created by a social worker to help parents manage pregnancy, labor, childbirth, and newborn care. The sections on labor are particularly useful.	www.transitiontoparenthood.com/ttp

BREASTFEEDING

NAME	DESCRIPTION	WEB ADDRESS
La Leche League International	The premier, international organization providing education, information, support, and encouragement to women who want to breastfeed. Holds monthly living-room meetings in many communities. Provides a hotline to answer questions and a Web site with publications and has FAQs online.	www.lalecheleague.org
Nursing Mother	Lots of articles on how to breastfeed; plus, nursing clothing and bras and other breastfeeding products.	www.nursingmother.com
Nursing Mothers Counsel	Online pamphlets and articles on breastfeeding, including advice on handling problems. Good links to other sites.	www.nursingmothers.org

BREASTFEEDING (continued)

NAME	DESCRIPTION	WEB ADDRESS
ParentSoup's Breastfeeding Site	More breastfeeding information from one of the largest parent-information sites online.	www.parentsoup.com/ experts/leche

CESAREAN SECTION

NAME	DESCRIPTION	WEB ADDRESS
Baby World (UK)	Site offers answers to frequently asked questions about c-sections including risks, recovery, and anesthesia options.	www.babyworld.co.uk/
Childbirth.org	Good birth information site with a section offering straightforward and objective information on cesarean sections.	www.childbirth.org/ section/CSFAQ.html
International Cesarean Awareness Network, Inc.	A lay women's site containing position papers on c-section risks and VBAC (Vaginal Birth after Cesarean).	www.ican-online.org
Maternity Center Association	Offers a systematic review of more than 300 research studies in an on-line booklet: "What Every Pregnant Woman Needs to Know about Cesarean Section," comparing risks and benefits of vaginal vs. cesarean births and how to avoid unnecessary interventions.	www.maternitywise.org/ cesareanbooklet

CHILD CARE

NAME	DESCRIPTION	WEB ADDRESS
Child Care Aware	Information on finding child care with instant referral to local child care resources using zip codes.	www.childcareaware.org
National Network for Childcare	Sponsored by the U.S. Dept. of Agriculture's Cooperative Extension system, this site offers informative articles about babies including discussions of child care issues and options.	www.nncc.org

CHILD CARE (continued)

NAME	DESCRIPTION	WEB ADDRESS
National Resource Center for Health and Safety in Child Care	Licensing requirements for child care centers, state by state.	http://nrc.uchsc.edu/states.html/

CHILDREN'S HEALTH & SAFETY

NAME	DESCRIPTION	WEB ADDRESS
American Academy of Pediatrics	Valuable information on immunizations, important health issues, and an annual "Family Safety Guide to Car Seats."	www.aap.org
KidsHealth	Created by the medical experts at the Alfred I. duPont Hospital for Children and the Nemours Foundation, the site offers in-depth information on pregnancy and newborns.	www.kidsHealth.org
Mother Risk	Sponsored by the Canadian Health Network, offers information on how to protect yourself and your baby from health risks, including research updates and discussions of occupational hazards, smoking, and substance abuse.	www.motherisk.org/
National Safe Kids Campaign	A national nonprofit organization for preventing unintentional childhood injuries with more than three hundred state and local coalitions, many of which offer safety seat inspections.	www.safekids.org (800-441-1888)
Organization of Teratology Information Services (OTIS)	Teratology is the study of the effects of drugs, medications, chemicals, and other exposures on babies during pregnancy. Fact sheets on a number of different hazards and links to medical providers who provide free counseling for prospective parents and medical providers.	www.otispregnancy.org

CIRCUMCISION INFORMATION & RISKS

NAME	DESCRIPTION	WEB ADDRESS
Circumcision (an online peer-reviewed medical journal)	Research articles on the procedures and effects of circumcision.	http://faculty.washington.edu/gcd/CIRCUMCISION
Circumcision Information and Resource Pages	An online information and resource library.	www.cirp.org
National Organization of Circumcision Information and Referral Centers	Informative articles on circumcision issues.	www.nocirc.org
Nurses for the Rights of the Child	An organization of nurses that posts statements and opinions about why circumcision should be avoided.	http://nurses.cirp.org

DISABLED PARENTS

NAME	DESCRIPTION	WEB ADDRESS
Disabled Parents Network (UK)	British network for disabled parents, offering support in pregnancy, childbirth, and parenting.	www.disabledparentsnetwork.org.uk
Parents with Disabilities Online	Web site offers information, support, and further sources of help.	www.disabledparents.net

FATHERHOOD

NAME	DESCRIPTION	WEB ADDRESS
The Fatherhood Initiative	A federally sponsored program to support and strengthen the role of fathers.	www.fatherhood.hhs.gov
The National Center for Fathering	Numerous articles on the art of fathering babies and children.	www.fathers.com
Slowlane.com	An online resource for stay-at-home dads with lots of helpful postings and links.	www.slowlane.com

FETAL ALCOHOL SYNDROME (FAS)

NAME	DESCRIPTION	WEB ADDRESS
Arium Foundation	Numerous articles and links on FAS.	www.arium.org

HOME BIRTH

NAME	DESCRIPTION	WEB ADDRESS
Birth Love	Approximately 1,800 Web pages on birthing topics, including home birth. Access requires a membership fee.	www.birthlove.com
Home Birth (UK)	A British site providing information about home birth for parents and health professionals.	www.horns.freeserve.co.uk/homebirth1.htm

MATERNITY WEAR & NURSING BRAS

NAME	DESCRIPTION	WEB ADDRESS
Anna Cris Maternity	Wide selection of maternity wear and lingerie.	www.annacris.com
A Pea in the Pod	Fashionable maternity professional and play clothes.	www.apeainthepod.com
Belly Dance Maternity	Trendy tops, bottoms, and dresses for the expectant.	www.bellydancematernity.com
Bravado	Source for comfortable maternity and nursing bras.	www.bravado.com
Fit Maternity and Beyond	Bathing suits and exercise clothing for moms, with great links to pregnancy exercise sites.	www.fitmaternity.com
Japanese Weekend	Trendy looks for the baby endowed.	www.japaneseweekend.com
Maternity Mall	A huge source for maternity wear, including maternity bras, and large-size maternity clothes.	www.maternitymall.com
Milk n' Wild Honey	Clothes for nursing mothers.	www.milknhoney.com
Motherhood Maternity Plus	Maternity duds for the well-endowed mom-to-be.	www.motherhoodplus.com
Nichole Michelle	Upscale seasonal wear.	www.nicholematernity.com
Once Again Maternity	Gently used maternity wear at reasonable prices.	www.onceagainmaternity.com

PARENTING INFORMATION

NAME	DESCRIPTION	WEB ADDRESS
ABCs of Parenting	A comprehensive source: directory of pregnancy, parenting, and child care articles and Web sites. Categories include child care, education, health, fatherhood, finance, nutrition, organizations, safety issues, product recalls, infertility, and online shopping. Accesses chat rooms, discussion boards, support groups, and family home pages.	www.abcparenting.com
Ask NOAH (New York Online Access to Health)	Ask NOAH About: Pregnancy is a well-maintained collection of links related to pregnancy.	www.noah-health.org/ english/pregnancy/ pregnancy.html
Baby Center	Information resource on preconception, pregnancy, baby, and toddlers.	www.BabyCenter.com
Baby Place	A starting point for information on pregnancy, birth, and babies.	www.baby-place.com
Baby Zone	Comprehensive resource with information on each new stage of a parent's life— from trying to conceive to the toddler years.	www.BabyZone.com
The Compleat Mother	Information on breast-feeding, childbirth, parenting.	www.compleatmother.com
CRY-SIS	A UK Web site providing support for parents of babies who cry excessively.	www.our-space.co.uk/ serene.htm
Expectant Mothers Guide	Offers pregnancy, childbirth, and child care information and city-specific shopping and services information for a series of cities and regions.	www.expectantmothers guide.com
iParenting	Product recalls, parenting news, chatboards, experts, and "iParenting University" with subscription courses in pregnancy, breastfeeding, and baby care. Sponsored by *Pregnancy* and *Baby Years* magazines. Also available in Spanish.	www.iParenting.com

PARENTING INFORMATION (continued)

NAME	DESCRIPTION	WEB ADDRESS
Parents Place	This branch of iVillage includes a fully-loaded pregnancy section that features articles, charts, message boards, and a newsletter option.	www.parentsplace.com
Robyn's Nest	A due date calculator, chat rooms, a week-by-week guide, and numerous topics about pregnancy.	www.robynsnest.com
Urban Baby	Offers local Web sites for major cities that include bulletin boards, calendars of events, local resources, and shopping information.	www.urbanbaby.com

PHYSICIAN REFERRAL SERVICES

NAME	DESCRIPTION	WEB ADDRESS
Health Grades	A commercial site offering detailed reports on obstetricians and other specialists as well as hospitals, including hospital c-section rates.	www.HealthGrades.com

POSTPARTUM DEPRESSION

NAME	DESCRIPTION	WEB ADDRESS
Depression after Delivery	Symptoms, treatment options, a bookstore, and help line.	www.depressionafter delivery.com
The Postpartum Stress Center	Site for a treatment center that also offers a checklist, resources, and helpful information.	www.postpartumstress.com
PPD Support Group	Forums, resources, research, chat rooms, and listings of local groups nationwide.	www.ppdsupportpage.com

PREGNANCY INFORMATION

NAME	DESCRIPTION	WEB ADDRESS
BabyCal	This California site offers information on prenatal care, practicing healthy behaviors during pregnancy, and interesting bulletin boards. Some materials in Spanish.	www.dhs.cahwnet.gov/babycal
BirthNet	An Australian site for information on childbirth with discussion forums and useful answers to common pregnancy questions.	www.birth.com.au
Birth Psychology	The home site for the Association for Pre- & Perinatal Psychology and Health with lots of information on prebirth and afterbirth baby psychology. Parent stories of how they have connected with their unborn and newborn babies. Long list of recommended reading material.	www.birthpsychology.com
Childbirth.org	A comprehensive site about pregnancy, labor, delivery, c-sections, fetal monitoring, episiotomy, VBAC, newborns, and postpartum care. Includes an "Ask The Pros" section for e-mailing a doula, childbirth educator, midwife, lactation consultant, or nurse with questions.	www.childbirth.org
ePregnancy	Pregnancy articles, interactive tools, message boards for pregnant mothers.	www.epregnancy.com
Labor of Love	Pregnancy and parenting.	www.thelaboroflove.com
The Midwives' Information and Resource Service (MIDIRS)	British site with excellent information on evidence-based practice for childbirth.	www.midirs.org
Pregnancy Health Center	Sponsored by the University of Pennsylvania Health System, the site provides a "Pregnancy Guide" with a series of helpful articles on pregnancy and childbirth.	www.pennhealth.com/health/health_info/pregnancy/stayhealthy/

PREGNANCY INFORMATION (continued)

NAME	DESCRIPTION	WEB ADDRESS
Storknet	A thorough site on all aspects of pregnancy with calculators, baby names, and expert advice.	www.storknet.com
Visible Embryo	Sponsored by the National Institutes of Child Health and Human Development, it offers images and descriptions of the stages of growth of the fetus. Annotated list of links to other embryology sites and glossary.	www.visembryo.com/baby

PREMATURE BABIES

NAME	DESCRIPTION	WEB ADDRESS
Association for Retinopathy of Prematurity and Related Diseases (ROPARD)	An organization that offers information for parents of premature babies who have retinopathy (retrolental fibroplasia). Includes a bulletin board and useful links.	www.ropard.org
For Parents of Preemies	Detailed information on the preemie experience.	www.pediatrics.wisc.edu/patientcare/preemies/resources
Parents of Premature Babies-L (Preemie-L)	A nonprofit organization for parents of premature babies that offers online information, support, and discussion groups, and publishes a newsletter.	www.preemie-l.org
Sidelines	Multiple resources for high-risk pregnancies.	www.sidelines.org

SMOKING CESSATION

NAME	DESCRIPTION	WEB ADDRESS
American Cancer Society	Offers information on smoking cessation strategies and telephone referrals to "Quitlines," telephone helplines in thirty states for helping smokers stop.	www.cancer.org 800-ACS-2345)
American Lung Association	"Freedom from Smoking ®️ Online" is a free online course consisting of seven modules to help quitters.	www.lungusa.org/ffs/overview.html

TEEN PREGNANCY

NAME	DESCRIPTION	WEB ADDRESS
Alan Guttmacher Institute	This site has an emphasis on teenage sex and pregnancy with statistics, policy papers, law, and public policy on pregnancy and birth, and sexually transmitted diseases.	www.guttmacher.org
National Organization on Adolescent Pregnancy, Parenting, and Prevention (NOAP)	Information on a variety of health and social issues related to pregnant teenagers, teen fathers, and teen sexual behavior. Directories of organizations, lists of print materials, and links to online resources.	www.noappp.org
TeenWire	A source for discussions and Q&As about teen pregnancy, birth control, and sexually transmitted diseases. Sponsored by Planned Parenthood Federation of America.	www.teenwire.com

TWINS & MULTIPLES

NAME	DESCRIPTION	WEB ADDRESS
National Organization of Mothers of Twins	A library of articles, a shopping mall, and lots more for mothers of multiples.	www.nomotc.org
Twins & Multiple Births Association– TAMBAA	British organization offering information and mutual support networks for families of twins, triplets, and more.	www.tamba.org.uk

Nonprofit Birthing and Parenting Organizations

AMERICAN ACADEMY OF HUSBAND-COACHED CHILDBIRTH/THE BRADLEY METHOD

DESCRIPTION	ADDRESS	CONTACT INFORMATION
Based on the philosophy of Dr. Robert A. Bradley, this approach focuses on unmedicated, husband-assisted birth.	Box 5224 Sherman Oaks, CA 91413-5224	www.bradleybirth.com (800) 4-A-BIRTH (818) 788-6662

BACK TO SLEEP CAMPAIGN

DESCRIPTION	ADDRESS	CONTACT INFORMATION
A coalition of groups to disseminate information about placing babies on their back for sleeping to lower the risk of Sudden Infant Death Syndrome (SIDS).	Back to Sleep/NICHD 31 Center Drive Room 2A32 Bethesda, MD 20892-2425	www.nichd.nih.gov/sids/ (800) 505-CRIB (2742)

INTERNATIONAL CHILDBIRTH EDUCATION ASSOCIATION (ICEA)

DESCRIPTION	ADDRESS	CONTACT INFORMATION
The largest childbirth education organization in the U.S. with more than twelve thousand members. Its Web site offers birthing information and a locator for its certified doulas, fitness, and postnatal educators.	P.O. Box 20048 Minneapolis, MN 55420	www.icea.org 952-854-8772 (not toll-free)

LAMAZE ® INTERNATIONAL

DESCRIPTION	ADDRESS	CONTACT INFORMATION
Certifies childbirth educators, locator service for childbirth educators. Articles and bookstore online.	Suite 800 Washington, DC 20036-3309	www.lamaze.org (800) 368-4404

Federal Agencies

EQUAL EMPLOYMENT OPPORTUNITY COMMISSION

DESCRIPTION	ADDRESS	CONTACT INFORMATION
Offers information on the Pregnancy Discrimination Act that is designed to protect pregnant women from discrimination in the workplace. Available in Spanish.	The Equal Employment Opportunity Commission, Office of Federal Operations, P.O. Box 19848 Washington, DC 20036	www.eeoc.gov TEL: 800-669-EEOC

THE FOOD AND DRUG ADMINISTRATION (FDA)

DESCRIPTION	ADDRESS	CONTACT INFO
The branch of the U.S. Department of Agriculture that regulates baby food and baby skin care products. Site offers brochures on baby feeding and health.	5600 Fishers Lane Rockville, MD 20857-0001	www.fda.org TEL: 888-INFO-FDA (463-6332)

FOOD & NUTRITION SERVICE, U.S. DEPARTMENT OF AGRICULTURE

DESCRIPTION	ADDRESS	CONTACT INFO
Administers Women Infants and Children (WIC) programs that reaches 45 percent of all babies nationwide agencies, clinic sites and health departments. Priority is given to low-income pregnant or breastfeeding women and infants at nutritional risk because of dietary problems.	Supplemental Food Programs Division Food and Nutrition Service/ USDA 3101 Park Center Dr., Room 520 Alexandria, VA 22302	www.fns.usda.gov/wic TEL: 800-472-2286 Or, see local listing under "Department of Human Services" or other state services listing in your telephone directory.

HEALTHFINDER

DESCRIPTION	ADDRESS	CONTACT INFO
A federal Web site offering links to organizations, libraries, dictionaries, journals, and government agencies that offer health information, including pregnancy and baby care.	healthfinder®, National Health Information Center, P.O. Box 1133 Washington, DC 20013-1133	www.healthfinder.gov Help desk: 202-401-HELP (4357)

NATIONAL CENTER ON BIRTH DEFECTS AND DEVELOPMENTAL DISABILITIES

DESCRIPTION

Offers tips for a healthy pregnancy, features on developmental disabilities, jaundice, fetal alcohol syndrome, and other pregnancy-related topics.

ADDRESS

NCBDDD
4770 Buford
Highway NE
MS F-45
Atlanta, GA 30341

CONTACT INFO

www.cdc.gov/ncbddd
TEL: 770-488-7160

NATIONAL HIGHWAY TRAFFIC SAFETY ADMINISTRATION (NHTSA)

DESCRIPTION

Oversees the safety of car seats for babies and children. Lists recalls of car seats and offers buying guides, installation tips, and other pertinent car seat safety info. Some offerings in Spanish.

ADDRESS

NHTSA
400 Seventh
Street, S.W.
Washington, DC
20590

CONTACT INFO

www.nhtsa.dot.gov
TEL: 800-424-93939

NATIONAL INSTITUTE FOR OCCUPATIONAL SAFETY AND HEALTH (NIOSH)

DESCRIPTION

Publishes information on workplace hazards that affect female reproductive health. Use the search engine and keyword "pregnancy."

ADDRESS

NIOSH, Hubert H.
Humphrey Bldg.
200 Independence
Ave., SW, Room 715H
Washington, DC
20201

CONTACT INFO

www.cdc.gov/niosh
TEL: 800-356-4674

NATIONAL INSTITUTE OF CHILD HEALTH AND HUMAN DEVELOPMENT (NICHD)

DESCRIPTION

Offers numerous articles on pregnancy and health, including preterm labor, and medical conditions that affect babies before they are born.

ADDRESS

NICHD Information
& Resource Center
P.O. Box 3006
Rockville, MD 20847

CONTACT INFO

www.nichd.nih.gov
Information specialist:
800-370-2943

NATIONAL LIBRARY OF MEDICINE

DESCRIPTION	ADDRESS	CONTACT INFO
Sponsors Medline and Medlineplus, sources for listings, and abstracts of medical research articles worldwide, searchable by topic.	U.S. National Library of Medicine, 8600 Rockville Pike Bethesda, MD 20894	www.ncbi.nlm.nih.gov/pubmed www.nlm.nih.gov/medlineplus TEL: 800-336-4797

NATIONAL WOMEN'S HEALTH INFORMATION CENTER

DESCRIPTION	ADDRESS	CONTACT INFO
A project of the U.S. Department of Health and Human Services' Office on Women's Health. Offers information on pregnancy, breastfeeding, quitting smoking, and other health-related topics.	Office on Women's Health Department of Health and Human Services 200 Independence Ave. Washington, DC 20201	www.4woman.org/ TEL: 202-690-7650

OCCUPATIONAL SAFETY AND HEALTH ADMINISTRATION

DESCRIPTION	ADDRESS	CONTACT INFO
Health and safety primarily as it relates to federal regulations protecting workers from exposure to hazardous and toxic substances.	Occupational Safety & Health Administration 200 Constitution Avenue, NW Washington, DC 20210	www.osha.gov TEL: 202-576-6339

U.S. CONSUMER PRODUCT SAFETY COMMISSION (CPSC)

DESCRIPTION	ADDRESS	CONTACT INFO
The federal agency in charge of monitoring and regulating products, including those for babies and young children. It issues product recalls, and it accepts parents' reports of unsafe products.	U.S. Consumer Product Safety Commission Washington, DC 20207	www.cpsc.gov TEL: 800-638-2772

U.S. DEPARTMENT OF LABOR

DESCRIPTION	ADDRESS	CONTACT INFO
Offers information on work-related questions (during pregnancy)	U.S. Department of Labor Frances Perkins Building 200 Constitution Avenue, NW Washington, DC 20210	www.dol.gov TEL: 800-959-3652

WOMEN'S BUREAU OF THE DEPARTMENT OF LABOR

DESCRIPTION	ADDRESS	CONTACT INFO
Site offers searches of multiple sites for information on the Family Medical Leave Act and other pregnancy and work-related issues.	U.S. Department of Labor Frances Perkins Building 200 Constitution Avenue, NW Washington, DC 20210	www.dol.gov/dol.wb TEL: 800-827-5335

Web Sites of Popular Parenting Magazines

Most of these sites offer searchable archives of past articles on topics of interest to parents.

NAME	WEB ADDRESS
AMERICAN BABY	www.americanbaby.com
BABY TALK	www.babytalk.com
BIRTH GAZETTE	www.birthgazette.com
CHILD	www.child.com
COMPLEAT MOTHER	www.compleatmother.com
EPREGNANCY	www.epregnancy.com
FIT PREGNANCY	www.fitpregnancy.com
MOTHERING MAGAZINE	www.mothering.com
PARENTS	www.parents.com
VEGETARIAN BABY & CHILD	www.vegetarianbaby.com

Professional & Nonprofit Birth-related Organizations

This is a listing of a few of the many organizations for professionals involved in childbirth that offer birth and pregnancy information for parents on their sites.

AMERICAN ASSOCIATION OF NURSE ANESTHETISTS

PURPOSE

Professional organization of trained nurse anesthetists with a public section offering "Anesthesia Options for Labor and Delivery: What Every Expectant Mother Should Know," and a link to a sister site on patient safety and anesthesia.

ADDRESS

www.aana.com
www.anesthesiapatientsafety.com

AMERICAN BOARD OF OBSTETRICS AND GYNECOLOGY

PURPOSE

An independent, nonprofit organization that certifies U.S. obstetricians and gynecologists. Charges twenty-five dollars to release records on board-certified members.

ADDRESS

www.abog.org

AMERICAN COLLEGE OF NURSE-MIDWIVES

PURPOSE

A professional accrediting organization for midwives. Its Web site contains helpful information on pregnancy and birthing and a searchable directory of midwives nationwide.

ADDRESS

www.acnm.org

AMERICAN COLLEGE OF OBSTETRICIANS AND GYNECOLOGISTS (ACOG)

PURPOSE

The nation's largest professional group for obstetricians and gynecologists. Its Web site offers titles of patient education pamphlets and a physician's directory.

ADDRESS

www.acog.com
www.medem.com

AMERICAN MEDICAL ASSOCIATION

PURPOSE

America's largest professional organization for physicians. Its Web site offers doctor searches and public information on pregnancy, child care, and children's health.

ADDRESS

www.ama-assn.org

AMERICAN SOCIETY FOR REPRODUCTIVE MEDICINE

PURPOSE

A professional organization devoted to advancing knowledge and expertise in infertility, reproductive medicine, and biology. Its Web site offers information on infertility and stem cell research.

ADDRESS

www.asrm.org

AMERICAN SOCIETY OF ANESTHESIOLOGISTS

PURPOSE

Offers patient education information on anesthesia in childbirth.

ADDRESS

www.asahq.org/Public

ASSOCIATION FOR IMPROVEMENT IN THE MATERNITY SERVICES (AIMS)

PURPOSE

A British organization working to improve maternity services in the UK, but also with excellent information for parents on preparing for birth.

ADDRESS

www.aims.org.uk

ASSOCIATION OF LABOR AND CHILDBIRTH EDUCATORS (ALACE)

PURPOSE

A professional organization for doulas and labor assistants that offers referrals to professionals on their Web site.

ADDRESS

www.alace.org

ASSOCIATION OF WOMEN'S HEALTH, OBSTETRIC, AND PARENTING ASSOCIATION (CPPA)

PURPOSE

The professional organization of labor and delivery nurses with position statements on birthing practices.

ADDRESS

www.awhonn.org

THE CENTERING PREGNANCY AND PARENTING ASSOCIATION (CPPA)

PURPOSE

An organization that supports mother's prenatal care groups with journaling, group discussions, and educational and self-care activities, in conjunction with prenatal medical care.

ADDRESS

www.centeringpregnancy.org

DOULAS OF NORTH AMERICA (DONA)

PURPOSE

A national organization of doulas; it offers a print library and help in finding a doula.

ADDRESS

www.dona.org

INTERNATIONAL CESAREAN AWARENESS NETWORK

PURPOSE

An organization working to lower the high rate of cesareans and to assist women wanting to have vaginal birth after a cesarean (VBAC).

ADDRESS

www.ican-online.org

INTERNATIONAL LACTATION CONSULTANT ASSOCIATION (ILCA)

PURPOSE

The professional organization of lactation consultants that offers referrals to consultants and information on evidence-based breastfeeding practices.

ADDRESS

www.ilca.org

MATERNITY CENTER ASSOCIATION (MCA)

PURPOSE

MCA is dedicated to improving maternity care. Its "Maternity Wise" program helps pregnant women make informed decisions based on the best available scientific research. Its Website offers information and resources on evidence-based maternity care and women's childbearing rights.

ADDRESS

www.maternitywise.org

MIDWIVES OF NORTH AMERICA (MANA)

PURPOSE

Midwives, student/apprentice midwives, and persons supportive of midwifery. Works to promote basic competency in midwives; develops and encourages guidelines for their education. Offers legal, legislative, and political information and resource referrals.

ADDRESS

www.mana.org

NATIONAL ASSOCIATION OF CHILDBEARING CENTERS (NACC)

PURPOSE

An organization to support and spread information about birth centers. Sets national standards for operation of centers, promotes state licensure and regulation. Has a database of birth centers nationwide for parents.

ADDRESS

www.birthcenters.org

NATIONAL CHILDBIRTH TRUST

PURPOSE

A nonprofit organization sponsoring parent support groups in the UK. Its Web site is a great resource for information on pregnancy, childbirth, breastfeeding, and child care.

ADDRESS

www.nctpregnancyandbabycare.com

NORTH AMERICAN REGISTRY OF MIDWIVES

PURPOSE

The North American Registry of
Midwives (NARM) is an international
certification agency whose mission
is to establish and administer
certification for the credential
Certified Professional Midwife (CPM).

ADDRESS

www.narm.org

SOCIETY FOR OBSTETRIC ANESTHESIA AND
PERINATOLOGY (SOAP)

PURPOSE

A professional site that offers useful
information on anesthesia and
analgesia during labor.

ADDRESS

www.soap.org/patient_education

WORLD HEALTH ORGANIZATION (WHO)

PURPOSE

A division of the United Nations,
WHO works to improve the health
and survival of mothers and babies
worldwide.

ADDRESS

www.who.int

ZERO TO THREE

PURPOSE

A nonprofit organization to promote
the healthy development of babies
and toddlers by supporting and
strengthening families, communities,
and those who work on their behalf.

ADDRESS

www.zerotothree.org

Major Baby Product Manufacturers

NAME	TYPES OF PRODUCTS	CONTACT INFO
ANSA CO., INC.	Baby bottles and feeding supplies	www.theansacompany.com TEL: 800-527-1096
APRICA U.S.A., INC.	Strollers, high chairs, and baby carriers	www.apricausa.com TEL: 310-639-6387
BABY BJORN/ REGAL LAGER, INC.	Soft carriers, potties, and diaper bags	www.babybjorn.com TEL: 800-593-5522
BABY JOGGER COMPANY	Large-wheeled jogging strollers	www.babyjogger.com TEL: 509-457-0925
BABY TREND	Strollers and play yards	www.babytrend.com TEL: 800-328-7363
BEECH-NUT NUTRITION CORP.	Baby food	www.beech-nut.com TEL: 800-BEECHNUT
BRITAX CHILD SAFETY, INC.	Imported car seats and strollers	www.childseat.com TEL: 888-4BRITAX
CARNATION "GOOD START" (SEE NESTLÉ)	Baby formula	–
CHICCO U.S.A., INC.	Strollers, high chairs, soft carriers, play pens, and toys	www.chiccousa.com TEL: 877-4CHICCO
COMBI INTERNATIONAL CORP.	Strollers and diaper bags	www.combi-intl.com TEL: 800-992-6624
CROWN CRAFTS CO.	Baby bedding and soft carriers	www.crowncraftsinfant products.com TEL: 714-895-9200
DELTA ENTERPRISES	Cribs, baby furniture, strollers	www.deltaenterprise.com TEL: 728-385-1000
DISCOVERY TOYS	Developmental baby toys	www.discoverytoysinc.com TEL: 800-462-4777
DOREL JUVENILE GROUP: COSCO & SAFETY 1ST	Large variety of baby products from car seats to strollers, high chairs, and play yards. Manufacturer of "Eddie Bauer" brand baby products	www.djgusa.com TEL: 800-457-5276
EDDIE BAUER (SEE DOREL)	Strollers, car seats, and play yards	–

NAME	TYPES OF PRODUCTS	CONTACT INFO
EVENFLO CO. INC.	Wide variety of baby products including strollers, high chairs, baby carriers, and the famous "Exersaucer"	www.evenflo.com TEL: 800-837-9201
THE FIRST YEARS, INC.	Safety products, baby toys, bathing accessories, safety gates	www.thefirstyears.com TEL: 800-225-0382
FISHER-PRICE, INC.	Baby toys, baby seats, high chairs, and strollers	www.fisher-price.com TEL: 800-828-4000
GERBER PRODUCTS COMPANY	Baby clothing and feeding supplies	www.gerber.com TEL: 800-4-GERBER
GRACO CHILDREN'S PRODUCTS	Wide variety of baby products, including moderately priced strollers, car seats, and play yards	www.gracobaby.com TEL: 800-345-4109
HANDI-CRAFT CO. (DR. BROWN'S)	Baby bottle with a straw inside	www.handi-craft.com TEL: 800-778-9001
HEINZ, H.J.	Baby food	www.hjheinz.com www.heinzbaby.com TEL: 800-872-2229
HOLLISTER, INC. (AMEDA)	Hospital-grade, electric breast pumps	www.hollister.com TEL: 877-99-AMEDA
HUGGIES (SEE KIMBERLY-CLARK CORP.)	Disposable diapers and training pants	–
INFANTINO	Baby toys and soft carriers	(none) TEL: 800-365-8182
INGLESINA USA, INC.	Imported strollers	www.inglesina.com TEL: 877-486-5112
INSTEP LLC	Strollers and bicycle trailers	www.instep.net TEL: 800-242-6110
INTERNATIONAL PLAYTHINGS, INC.	Developmental toys	www.intplay.com TEL: 800-631-1272
JEEP (SEE KOLCRAFT)	Sports strollers and play yards	–
JOHNSON & JOHNSON	Baby bathing supplies, including creams, soaps, and shampoos	ww.jnj.com TEL: 800-526-3967

NAME	TYPES OF PRODUCTS	CONTACT INFO
J. MASON PRODUCTS	Wide range of baby products including inexpensive and moderately priced strollers, high chairs, and play yards	www.jmason.com TEL: 800-242-1922
KELTY K.I.D.S.	Backpacks for wearing baby	www.kelty.com TEL: 800-535-3589
KIDCO, INC.	Jogging strollers and bicycle trailers	www.kidcoinc.com TEL: 800-553-5529
KIDS II, INC.	Baby seats and toy	www.kidsii.com TEL: 770-751-0442
KIMBERLY-CLARK CORP. (HUGGIES)	Disposable diapers and pull-on pants	www.huggies.com TEL: 800-544-1847
KOLCRAFT	Wide variety of baby products including strollers, high chairs, and play yards. Maker of "Jeep" baby products	www.kolcraft.com TEL: 800-453-7673
KOOL-STOP INTERNATIONAL, INC.	Jogging strollers	www.koolstop.com TEL: 800-586-3332
LEARNING CURVE INTERNATIONAL	Toys for babies and children	www.learningcurve.com TEL: 800-704-8697
LEGO BABY/ LEGO SYSTEMS, INC.	Toys for toddlers and children	www.lego.com TEL: 800-453-4652
LITTLE TIKES	Children's climbing and ride-on toys	www.littletikes.com TEL: 888-832-3203
MACLAREN USA, INC.	Very expensive British strollers and carriages	www.maclarenstrollers.com TEL: 800-211-2741
MAYA GROUP/ TINY LOVE	Innovative baby toys	www.tinylove.com TEL: 800-843-6292
MEAD JOHNSON NUTRITIONALS	Baby formula	www.enfamil.com TEL: 800-222-9123
NESTLÉ (CARNATION "GOOD START")	Baby formula	www.nestleusa.com www.verybestbaby.com TEL: 800-547-9400
NORTH AMERICAN BEAR CO., INC.	Baby soft toys and mobiles	www.nabear.com TEL: 800-662-3427

NAME	TYPES OF PRODUCTS	CONTACT INFO
PEG PEREGO U.S.A., INC.	Pricey Italian strollers and high chairs	www.perego.com TEL: 800-671-1701
PRINCE LIONHEART	Soft carriers, feeding devices, and safety products	www.princelionheart.com TEL: 800-544-1132
PROCTER & GAMBLE (PAMPERS)	Disposable diapers	www.pampers.com TEL: 800-285-6064
R.E.I.	Sporty backpacks for carrying tots	www.rei.com TEL: 800-426-4840
ROSS PRODUCTS DIVISION OF ABBOTT LABORATORIES	Baby formula	www.ross.com www.welcomeaddition.com TEL: 800-986-8510
SASSY, INC.	Innovative baby toys, safety devices, and monitors	www.sassybaby.com TEL: 616-243-0767
TOUGH TRAVELER porting baby	Framed carriers for TEL: 800-GO-TOUGH	www.toughtraveler.com

Your Recommended Resources

Use this space to list books, articles, or Web sites you've found helpful,
as well as resources that have been recommended by family, friends,
or medical professionals.

NAME	DESCRIPTION	WEB ADDRESS (if applicable)

Pregnancy
Dictionary

his section supplies you with the best and most complete translation of hundreds of terms available to help you with your pregnancy and after your baby is born. Whenever a topic is discussed in more detail somewhere else in the book, you will find page numbers to guide you there.

Whenever it makes sense, we've used the word "baby," instead of the more formal, medical terms "embryo" or "fetus."

When a word appears in parenthesis immediately after a capitalized HEADING, it is the alternative name for the same word. When you find a word in both bold and italics in the text, it means that the definition can be found elsewhere in the dictionary.

One note of caution: Don't let the strange terms and descriptions of rare abnormalities frighten you. We could have omitted them, but we wanted our guide to be as complete as possible. That was in case you need a down-to-earth companion for translating what a clinician is trying to communicate to you, or you're trying to decipher a difficult-to-understand research article, or make sense out of your, or your baby's, medical records.

A

ABORTIFACIENT

A drug or device that ends a pregnancy within the first several weeks after conception.

ABORTION

Giving birth to an embryo or fetus in the first twenty weeks of pregnancy. Abortion may be spontaneous, called a miscarriage, or induced, when a pregnancy is terminated on purpose. After twenty weeks of pregnancy, it is called a live birth or a stillbirth. Spontaneous abortion in the first half of pregnancy is synonymous with miscarriage.

ABORTION, THERAPEUTIC (See THERAPEUTIC ABORTION)

ABRUPTION (PLACENTAL ABRUPTION, ABRUPTIO PLACENTAE)

Any sudden breaking away. During pregnancy, the term is usually used to refer to the premature separation of the placenta from the uterus prior to the delivery of the baby. When this happens, a woman's body may deliver the baby early. Bleeding is the number one symptom, and there can also be severe, premature contractions.

ACNM (The American College of Nurse-Midwives)

The American professional organization of midwives (midwifery) that maintains the certification process for midwives. (See the *Resource Guide*, on page 562.)

ACOG (The American College of Obstetricians and Gynecologists)

The professional organization of obstetricians and gynecologists who specialize in the care of women's reproductive needs. (See *Resource Guide*, on page 562.)

ACTIVE LABOR (See DILATION AND EFFACEMENT)

The phase of labor when the cervix (mouth of the uterus) is in the process of expanding and thinning—usually between four and ten centimeters (sometimes expressed as fingers). Contractions are usually two to five minutes apart. Typically, the cervix dilates about one centimeter (one finger), or more, per hour.

ACTIVE MANAGEMENT OF LABOR

An approach to managing the labors of a first-time pregnant mother that calls for continuous nursing support; continuous monitoring (electronic fetal monitoring); routinely breaking the mother's waters upon admission to the hospital (amniotomy) when the mouth of the uterus (cervix) is at least three centimeters dilated; and artificially speeding up labor using drugs to make contractions stronger when labor fails to progress within set time limits.

ACUPUNCTURE

The ancient Chinese medical practice of inserting and pulsating thin needles in selected locations on the body that is thought to help balance the body's energy flows and soothe pain. It can be used to help a mother through labor.

AFEBRILE

Not having a fever. A sign that you, or your baby, are not suspected of having an infection.

AFTERBIRTH

The placenta and membranes expelled by the uterus after the baby is born. The "birth" of the placenta is called the third stage of labor. (The first stage is when contractions position the baby to move down into the birth canal for delivery; the second stage is the pushing stage after complete dilation of the cervix that results in the baby being born; the fourth stage is the recovery after giving birth.)

AFTERPAINS (See INVOLUTION)

Cramping caused by the contraction of the uterus while it is returning to normal size.

AIDS (Acquired Immunodeficiency Syndrome) (See HIV)

A virus transmitted from one person to another through the exchange of bodily fluids—primarily through blood, blood products, semen, and vaginal fluid. In women, AIDS is often caught through intravenous drug use or sexual exposure through an infected partner. There is no evidence that pregnancy accelerates AIDS, but women in advanced stages of AIDS may be more likely to give birth prematurely or to have a low-birthweight baby or a baby that dies before or after birth. Most babies born to mothers with AIDS do not become infected, but some do. Mothers who take medicines to fight the disease rarely transmit it to their babies.

ALBUMINURIA

Excess protein detected from testing urine (urinalysis). Sometimes, but not always, it can be one of the symptoms of preeclampsia. It also shows up temporarily as a side effect of vigorous exercise.

ALPHA-FETOPROTEIN TEST (AFP) (a-Fetoprotein test, triple test, triple screen, MSAFP-plus, AFP-plus)

A blood test administered between the fifteenth and twentieth week of pregnancy to screen mothers for increased risk of having a baby with Down syndrome, neural tube defects (NTD), and abdominal wall defects. The test registers levels of Alpha Feto Protein (AFP), human chorionic gonadotropin (hCG), and estriol (uE3). Some tests also register the presence of inhibin, a chemical produced by the ovaries and placenta. A low AFP reading is associated with Down syndrome. The test is used to decide whether a mother should undergo a more invasive test, such as amniocentesis. Most women who test positive for these disorders give birth to a baby without the disorder.

ALVEOLI

Grape-like clusters of glandular tissue in a woman's breast where milk is made. The cells of the alveoli secrete the milk that is then expelled into the tiny tubes (ductules) that deliver the milk to the nipple for the baby.

AMA

Stands for the American Medical Association, the largest professional organization for physicians in the United States. (Also sometimes used by providers for Advanced Maternal Age, as a mother's age at thirty-five or older at the expected time of delivery.)

AMBULATION (See THROMBOPHLEBITIS)

Getting up and walking after surgery or giving birth. Nurses are likely to urge mothers to get out of bed and walk as soon as possible in order to help prevent blood clots from forming.

AMENORRHEA

Absence of menstruation.

AMNIOCENTESIS

The testing of the fluid inside the amniotic sac that surrounds the baby. A long, thin needle is used to obtain the fluid, and the results help to detect fetal abnormalities by examining the baby's skin cells sloughed off by the baby that float in the "waters." (See discussion on page 193.)

AMNIOINFUSION

Injection of solutions into the amniotic fluid in an attempt to cushion the umbilical cord and prevent it from being squeezed during labor.

AMNION (amniotic sac, bag of waters) (See AMNIOTIC FLUID)

One of the membranes that make up the sac, which contains the amniotic fluid in which the baby floats during pregnancy.

AMNIONITIS (CHORIOAMNIONITIS)

An infection of the amniotic sac and amniotic fluid that sometimes happens, usually after the membranes (bag of waters) break.

AMNIOTIC FLUID

A clear, slightly salty fluid with flecks of white skin cells floating in it that fills the sac that surrounds a baby during pregnancy. It protects the baby from being injured from outside, and maintains an even temperature. Approximately one-third of the fluid is replaced every hour. At term, it is primarily composed of the baby's urine and fluid made in the baby's lungs.

AMNIOTIC FLUID EMBOLISM

An extremely rare event, when amniotic fluid escapes into the wall of the uterus or where the placenta is implanted and into the mother's bloodstream usually during labor, causing the mother to go into shock.

AMNIOTIC SAC (See AMNION)

AMNIOTOMY

The intentional rupture of the amniotic sac using an instrument that resembles a long crochet hook. Doing so may speed up labor but may increase the chance of amnionitis. Having an amniotomy commits a mother to giving birth. (See discussion on page 342.)

ANALGESIA

A medical intervention that reduces the sensation of pain.

ANALGESIC

A drug that helps to relieve or reduce the sensation of pain.

ANEMBRIOTIC GESTATION (blighted ovum) (See MISCARRIAGE)

An implanted egg that dies during the early months of pregnancy, which leads to miscarriage weeks later.

ANEMIA

Any condition of the blood in which the number or shape of red blood cells is altered. It is discovered by a blood test. When the red blood cell content is low, it is more difficult for the body to supply sufficient oxygen to the tissues of the body. Anemia is a common condition during pregnancy. (See discussion on page 367.)

ANENCEPHALY

Defective development of a baby's brain combined with the absence of the bones normally surrounding the brain.

ANESTHESIA

A general term for all techniques used to alleviate pain. During childbirth, you may undergo general anesthesia (being put completely to sleep, such as during an emergency c-section), local anesthesia (you remain conscious, but a small area of your body becomes numb), or analgesia (reduction of your pain that allows you to remain conscious and relaxed with discomfort minimized).

ANESTHETIC
An agent or drug that is able to produce partial or complete loss of feeling (anesthesia).

ANESTHETIC BLOCK
Numbing of a part of the body. In obstetrics, this usually refers to an epidural or spinal anesthetic that is used for cesarean deliveries.

ANOMALY
An abnormality, a deviation from the normal.

ANOXIA
A lack of oxygen.

ANTENATAL (prenatal)
Before birth.

ANTENATAL GLUCOCORTICOID THERAPY
Drugs administered to a mother in danger of giving birth prematurely to prepare her baby's immature lungs for breathing.

ANTEPARTAL
Happening before delivery.

ANTERIOR POSITION (anterior presentation) (See POSTERIOR POSITION)
During the descent through the birth canal, the baby's face is turned toward the spine of the mother. This is the most common position for emerging babies.

ANTIBIOTIC
A medication that kills or stops the growth of bacteria.

ANTICIPATORY GRIEF (See GRIEF, STAGES OF)
When a person experiences numbness, shock, and fear, which causes them to emotionally pull away from the dying person. Parents may distance themselves from their premature or sick newborn

out of fear of impending loss and death. They may, for example, postpone naming their baby while they wait to see if it survives.

ANTICIPATORY GUIDANCE
Guidance given in advance of a difficult event. During pregnancy, it is counseling offered to expectant parents in advance to help them in coping with the needs of their newborn, or for how to cope with a baby diagnosed with a physical disorder.

ANTIPHOSPHOLIPID SYNDROME (APS)
Up to five percent of all pregnancy failures are thought to result from this little-known immune disorder that is associated with the formation of blood clots in the body. The body attacks certain fatty molecules (phospholipids) that make up part of a cell membrane, and the result is inflammation and blood clots. Pregnant women with APS are more likely to develop blood clots and preeclampsia and to have repeated miscarriages. When APS causes blood clots in the placenta, it can result in fetal growth problems, fetal distress, preterm birth, or pregnancy loss. There is no known cure, but low doses of aspirin and daily injections of a blood-thinning drug, heparin, may be recommended.

APA
Refers to antiphospholipid antibodies, the antibodies that cause antiphospholipid syndrome (APS).

APGAR SCORE (APGAR rating)
Ratings taken of a baby's condition at one and five minutes following birth that assigns zero, one, or two points for each of the following factors: tone, pulse, grimace, color, and respiration. The maximum total score is ten points, but most babies get around an eight or nine. An extremely low score indicates a baby

that needs immediate medical attention. (See discussion on page 324.)

APNEA (See POSITIONAL APNEA)

A temporary pause or complete cessation of breathing that frequently occurs in premature and low-birthweight babies.

APNEA MONITOR

A motion detector that sets off an alarm when a baby ceases to breathe for a period of time. Portable monitors are available for home use but are suggested only for premature and low-birthweight babies with an apnea problem.

APPROPRIATE FOR GESTATIONAL AGE (AGA)

When a baby's weight falls within normal range based on the actual age of the baby, rather than the date the baby was born.

AREOLA (plural: AREOLAE)

The dark ring of skin that surrounds the nipple of a breast. To milk the breast correctly, a nursing baby needs to latch onto much of the areola as well as the nipple. (See "Breastfeeding," on pages 409–418.)

ARRHYTHMIA

Irregular, abnormal, or missed heartbeat.

ARTERY

Blood vessel that carries blood away from the heart.

ARTIFICIAL RUPTURE OF THE MEMBRANES (AROM) (See RUPTURE OF MEMBRANES AND AMNIOTOMY)

ASPHYXIA, PERINATAL

The lack of oxygen in a fetus or baby that can lead to the excess buildup of carbon dioxide waste, which can lead to death if not corrected.

ASPIRATION

Using suction to draw air or a substance in, out, up, or through the breathing passages. During the birth process, a baby may aspirate meconium, which can block and irritate the airways, potentially causing damage to the baby's lungs. As soon as their faces emerge during birth, the mouth and nose are usually aspirated using a bulb-like suction device to help prevent aspiration of meconium-stained fluids. Aspiration also refers to the extremely rare event of a woman aspirating the acidic contents of the stomach while under general anesthesia, which can potentially harm the lungs. Healthcare providers may administer an antacid to a woman prior to a cesarean delivery to neutralize the acids.

ATONY, UTERINE (ATONIC UTERUS)

When a uterus relaxes and fails to contract during birth, or when it fails to tighten after birth, which potentially leads to excessive bleeding.

ATROPHY

When a part of the body (an arm or leg, cells, organs, or tissues) shrinks and withers from lack of nourishment or use.

ATTACHMENT (bonding, love)

The strong bonds of affection that form between a parent and a baby. Sometimes feelings of attachment are felt immediately, other times, the feeling takes time to develop.

AUGMENTATION OF LABOR

An intervention to make labor contractions stronger after they have already started.

AUSCULTATION

Listening to the sounds made by various organs of the body, including the heart, to determine their condition.

AUTOLOGOUS TRANSFUSION

A transfusion of a person's own blood previously donated by her in anticipation of surgery.

B

BABINSKI REFLEX

An automatic response in newborns that causes a baby to curl his big toe and spread out his other toes when his foot is stroked from the heel upward and across the ball of the foot.

BABY BLUES (postpartum blues) (See POSTPARTUM DEPRESSION)

A feeling of sadness and letdown that affects forty to seventy percent of all new mothers. It usually starts a few days after birth, and usually goes away within two weeks.

BACK LABOR (See POSTERIOR PRESENTATION)

When most of the pain of labor is felt in a mother's lower back. A baby's facing toward a mother's front instead of toward her back (occiput posterior) may contribute to it as can back problems prior to labor.

BACTERIA

Small microscopic organisms that can cause infection in the body.

BACTERIAL VAGINOSIS (BV)

A common infection of the genital tract that causes vaginal itching and an abnormal fishy-smelling discharge and that may be associated with an increased risk of preterm labor, premature rupture of membranes, preterm birth, and infection of the amniotic sac. (See discussion on page 218.)

BACTERIURIA

The presence of bacteria (germs) in the urine. Usually a sign of infection.

BAGGING

Placing a mask over a newborn's nose and mouth and rhythmically squeezing oxygen from an attached bag to help the baby breathe.

BAG OF WATERS (See AMNION)

BALANCED DIET

Properly nourishing yourself by eating the right amount of nutrients in correct proportions. (See discussion on page 145.)

BETAMETHASONE

A drug given by injection to the mother that helps develop the baby's lungs. Administered when doctors anticipate that the baby may be born prematurely.

BETA-THALASSEMIA

An anemic condition found mainly in persons from Mediterranean countries such as Greece, Italy, or the Middle East that can be passed along genetically to a baby.

β-HUMAN CHORIONIC GONADOTROPIN (β-HCG) (See HUMAN CHORIONIC GONADOTROPIN)

BILILIGHTS

Special fluorescent lights placed above a baby's bed to treat jaundice. Usually, the baby's eyes are covered to protect them from glare.

BILIRUBIN (See JAUNDICE AND KERNICTERUS)

A yellowish-red coloring pigment produced by the body as red blood cells break down. An excess of bilirubin in the bloodstream leads to temporary jaundice (yellowing of the skin and whites of the eyes) in a newborn. Excessive levels may harm the developing baby's brain.

BIOFEEDBACK

The use of sensitive, computer-driven instruments to measure and display the patterns of physical processes such as brain activity, blood pressure, muscle tension, heart rate, and other bodily functions. The feedback from the devices is used to enable individuals to master skills in controlling and managing their body's reactions. Once mastery is achieved, the instruments are no longer needed. Biofeedback training is used to give pregnant women skills in coping with the stress and pain of labor.

BIOPHYSICAL PROFILE (BPP)

A test to assess the health of an unborn baby. The profile measures a series of things: breathing rate, movement rate, muscle tone, the baby's heart rate, and the volume of amniotic fluid in the amniotic sac where the baby floats. It combines the use of a nonstress test together with ultrasound. Not enough amniotic fluid in the uterus is called oligohydramnios.

BIOPSY

The removal of a small piece of tissue from the body to examine it more closely with a microscope.

BIRTH ASSISTANT (labor assistant) (See DOULA and MONITRICE)

Someone who is trained in basic childbirth support skills who attends to a birthing mother's health and comfort needs before, during, and after labor.

BIRTH CANAL

The passage the baby goes through from the uterus (womb) until delivery. It includes the vaginal canal and the bones of the pelvis that the baby passes through.

BIRTH CENTER

A medical facility that serves as an alternative to giving birth at home, or in a traditional hospital setting. Birth centers can be in houses, in medical buildings, or separate rooms inside hospitals. Out-of-hospital birth centers often use midwives. Birth centers try to simulate a home-birth experience while providing additional medical resources. (See discussion on page 164.)

BIRTH DEFECT

A mental or physical problem in a baby caused by an error in how a part of the baby developed. A birth defect may, or may not, be inherited (passed through a parent's genes or chromosomes). According to the American College of Obstetricians and Gynecologists, approximately three percent of babies born in the United States are born with a major birth defect. (See the discussion of genetic factors on pages 179–180, and screening tests on pages 184–185.)

BIRTHING BALL (PT BALL)

A large, sturdy, inflated ball that can be used during labor as a comfort measure. A mother can bounce, rock, sit, or lie on top of it.

BIRTHING ROOM (See BIRTH CENTER)

Rather than moving a mother into a delivery room that resembles an operating theater when birth nears, many hospitals now offer special, homelike rooms where labor and delivery can take place. (See discussion on page 162.)

BIRTH PLAN

A plan created by an expectant mother that expresses her desires for how she would like her labor to be managed, also called Birth Wishes, or Birth Goals. (See discussion on page 90.)

BIRTH TEAM

The people a mother chooses to support her during labor and birth.

BISHOP'S SCORE

A rating system used by healthcare providers to assess how prepared the cervix is for labor. Physicians use it to decide when an induction of labor is most likely to be successful. (See discussion on page 336.)

BLADDER (SEE CATHETER)

The membrane, or sac, inside the body that stores fluid. Sometimes the bladder, which holds urine, can become infected, causing pain. You may be asked to have a full bladder when you go for a sonogram to allow for clearer pictures of the uterus. During some epidurals and a cesarean section, a catheter is inserted in the bladder to protect it by keeping it drained.

BLASTOCYST

What a fertilized ovum (egg) is called once it enters a mother's uterus.

BLIGHTED OVUM (See ANEMBRYONIC GESTATION)

An egg that fails to form into a baby.

BLOOD GLUCOSE (blood sugar, plasma glucose, serum glucose) (See GLUCOSE TOLERANCE TEST)

The amount of glucose (blood sugar) present in the blood. It can be measured by a drop of blood collected from a fingertip or earlobe and placed on a glucometer, a device for measuring glucose levels. Levels are expressed as a number with one hundred considered normal and higher numbers, such as 150 and above, indicating the body's inability to handle glucose.

BLOOD PATCH

The treatment of a severe "spinal" headache that sometimes is the result of the sac surrounding the spinal cord getting punctured during an epidural.

Sterile blood from the mother is injected into the epidural space to form a clot that prevents further leakage of spinal fluid.

BLOOD PRESSURE (See PREECLAMPSIA)

A measurement for the force that the blood exerts against the walls of arteries that enables the blood to flow. Blood pressure is expressed as two numbers. The top number, systolic pressure, is the pressure exerted when the heart contracts. The bottom number, diastolic pressure, is the pressure exerted between heartbeats when the heart is relaxed. It is normal for a pregnant woman's blood pressure to decrease during the second trimester. (See discussion on page 215.)

BLOODY SHOW (See SHOW)

BM

Abbreviation for bowel movement.

BODY MASS INDEX (BMI)

The relationship of a person's height to weight, which is used to determine if a person is underweight, normal, overweight, or obese. The formula is calculated by dividing a person's weight in pounds by height in inches, dividing this figure a second time by height in inches, and then multiplying the figure by 703. Overweight is defined as a BMI of 25 to 29.9, while obesity is defined as a BMI of 30 or above. These calculations do not apply to weight during pregnancy.

BONDING

The feeling of attachment or love between a parent and a baby. Sometimes the feeling emerges soon after birth, but, just as with grown-up relationships, bonding with a baby may be gradual and take more time to grow.

BRACHIAL PLEXUS PALSY
Dysfunction of the nerves that affects the function of a baby's arm. May be caused by an injury to the shoulder during labor and delivery.

**BRADLEY METHOD®
(husband-coached childbirth)**
A childbirth method that encourages natural breathing, husband support, and breastfeeding. (See discussion on page 177.)

BRADYCARDIA (sometimes called a brady spell) (See FETAL HEART RATE)
Excessively slow heartbeat. A newborn's heartbeat is considered too slow when it is measured as fewer than one hundred heartbeats per minute.

BRAXTON-HICKS CONTRACTIONS (false labor) (See CONTRACTIONS)
Contractions of the uterus that occur throughout pregnancy and serve to prepare the uterus for ejecting the baby. During the last weeks of pregnancy, they become more noticeable, but, unlike the contractions of labor, they usually aren't painful or predictable and don't get stronger or closer together over time. (See discussion on pages 57 and 266.)

BREAKING OF WATERS (SEE RUPTURE OF MEMBRANES)

BREECH PRESENTATION (breech birth)
When a baby's buttocks, knees, or feet appear first during birth, instead of the head. The position is rare during labor, occurring in fewer than five percent of births. Labor with a breech baby is more challenging and tends to take longer. Most doctors prefer to deliver breech babies by cesarean, as recent studies suggest that it may be a safer for the baby. Before proceeding with a cesarean, many doctors will first attempt to turn the baby into a headfirst position by external cephalic version (ECV), in which the doctor pushes on the mother's abdomen. (See discussion on pages 261–262.) Frank breech means the baby's hips are flexed and the legs are extended upward toward the baby's face. Complete breech means the baby's legs and arms are folded, Indian-style.

BRETHINE (See TERBUTALINE)

BROWN FAT
A special tissue found in newborn babies that helps to fuel the body's energy and produce body heat.

BROW PRESENTATION
When a baby's head is bent backward during birth, rather than the typical flexed, chin-on-chest position. Presentation is determined by examining the baby's skull using the provider's fingers during a vaginal examination. If the baby's head fails to change to a chin-down position during labor, then an intervention, such as a cesarean section, may be necessary.

BSN
Bachelor of Science in Nursing.

C

CAFÉ-AU-LAIT SPOTS
Light or coffee-colored birthmarks sometimes found on a newborn's arms, legs, or body.

CANDIDA (Candida albicans, Monilia) (See YEAST INFECTION and THRUSH)
A yeast-like fungus that usually grows in the intestinal tract of the body, but can infect other parts of the body causing a variety of symptoms.

CANNULA

A small tube. For example, a small cannula may be inserted into the vein when getting an IV, or into the cervix as part of measuring contraction strength.

CAPPA

Stands for the Childbirth and Postpartum Professionals Association, a professional organization that certifies labor doulas, postpartum doulas, childbirth educators, and lactation educators.

CAPUT SUCCEDANEUM

A lump, or swelling under a newborn's scalp present at birth that is caused by pressure exerted on the baby's head during the birth process. It can be caused by vacuum extraction. The location of the swelling will depend upon the position of the baby's head during birth. It usually disappears within twenty-four to thirty-six hours.

CARDINAL MOVEMENTS

The series of passive movements, such as flexing and rotating, that a baby's body makes in order to be born.

CARDIOMYOPATHY, PERIPARTUM

Rare, pregnancy-related heart failure in women not related to a previous heart condition that occurs during the last month of pregnancy or during the first five months afterward. The cause is unknown, but one-quarter to one-half of women who develop this problem die due to congestive heart failure, irregular heartbeat (arrhythmia), or a blood clot that affects the heart (thromboembolism). Between 1991 and 1997, there were 245 pregnancy-related deaths due to cardiomyopathy or 7.7 percent of all maternal deaths, or a mortality ratio of 0.88 per 100,000 live births. The risk of dying from this condition increases as women age, and African-American mothers are 6.4

times more likely to die from it than Caucasian women.

CARDIOTOCOGRAPH

A machine to measure a baby's heart rate and a mother's contractions. It provides a printout of the information it records.

CARDIOVASCULAR

Pertaining to the heart and blood vessels.

CARPAL TUNNEL SYNDROME (See DEQUERVAIN'S TENDONITIS).

Numbness and/or a pins and needles sensation in the hands and fingers caused by fluid collecting around the wrist joints, which press on the nerves that thread through the narrow channels in the wrist bones leading to the hand. It is thought to affect approximately one out of three pregnant women and disappears within a few weeks following birth.

CASE MANAGER

A person, a nurse or social worker, who is assigned to help parents whose babies have been identified as having specific conditions and who may benefit from counseling and help.

CATARACT

When the lens of the eye is coated with a milky tissue that affects vision.

CATHETER (being catheterized, being cathed)

A small, hollow tube used to flow fluids into, or out of, the body. A catheter is used to help protect the bladder from being bruised or injured. During some epidurals or a c-section, a catheter may be inserted into a mother's urethra, the passage that flows urine out of the body. It will be threaded into the passage until it reaches the bladder. The other end of the catheter empties urine into a plastic bag.

CAUL
A thin, filmy membrane (amnion) that sometimes covers the head of a newborn baby.

CDC
Centers for Disease Control and Prevention

CEPHALIC PRESENTATION
When a baby is proceeding through birth in a head-downward position.

CEPHALOHEMATOMA (cephalhemotoma)
Bleeding under the thick membrane that covers a baby's skull. It can be caused by prolonged pressure of his head against the cervix or a mother's perineum or pubic bones, or from the pressure of vacuum extraction. It can also be caused by the blades of forceps; attempting to rotate a baby's head; or rapid compression and relaxation on the head with precipitous birth or an extremely rapid labor that lasts less than three hours. Swelling and redness may not appear until a few hours after birth, and it may grow larger, and can take six to twelve weeks to disappear.

CEPHALOPELVIC DISPROPORTION (CPD)
When a baby's head is too large to fit through the mother's pelvis.

CERCLAGE
A stitch placed in the mouth of the womb (cervix) to hold it closed in order to help an "incompetent" (weak) cervix to keep a baby inside until birth. (See discussion on page 219.)

CEREBRAL PALSY
A condition that affects a child's ability to move, that is thought to be caused by brain injury. It may result in seizures or mental retardation. Its causes are not completely understood, although infection, injury, or lack of oxygen while the brain is developing may play a part.

CERTIFICATION (CERTIFIED)
When a person or agency has received approval from a professional organization by meeting specific standards. Baby products can also be certified if they have met specific standards set by the juvenile products industry.

CERTIFIED NURSE MIDWIFE (CNM)
A nurse who has completed either a certification program or a master's degree program and has met the certification requirements of the Certification Council (ACC) of the American College of Nurse-Midwives. Certified midwives are able to independently provide pregnancy, childbirth, after birth, and women's reproductive health services.

CERTIFIED REGISTERED NURSE ANESTHETIST (CRNA)
CRNAs are advanced practice nurses with specialized graduate-level education in anesthesiology. During birth, a CRNA may work with your obstetrician or with your anesthesiologist (physician anesthetist) to administer pain management medications to you.

CERVICAL CAP
A flexible contraceptive device designed to tightly fit over the cervix to prevent sperm from entering the uterus and fertilizing the egg.

CERVICAL INCOMPETENCE
When the neck and mouth of the uterus begin to open too soon without contractions before a pregnancy is ready to end. The condition can cause preterm delivery during the second and third trimesters of pregnancy.

CERVICAL OS

The opening in the mouth of the uterus at the tip end of the cervix.

CERVICAL RIPENING (cervix ripening) (See INDUCTION)

The process by which the cervix softens and thins in preparation for labor. It occurs naturally at the end of pregnancy, or it can be accomplished artificially. The cervix may be widened with a balloon-tipped Foley catheter, or softened using medications such as misoprostol or prostaglandin (PGE2).

CERVICOGRAM (partogram)

A way of charting, on an hourly basis, the progress of labor. It is done by using a graph that represents the dilation of the cervix in centimeters and the descent of the baby (station) as measured (in plus or minus centimeters) by the position of the baby's presenting part in relation to the ischial spines over time.

CERVIDIL

A medication used to "ripen" or soften the cervix (mouth of the womb) before labor is induced. Sometimes it can be used to induce labor.

CERVIX

The necklike lower part of a mother's pear-shaped uterus that shortens and thins (effaces) and opens (dilates) during labor to allow a baby to be pushed out of the uterus. The cervix is about one to two inches, or 2.5–4 centimeters long. The center of the cervix is called the cervical canal, which the baby passes through during birth.

CERVIX, RIPE

During the process of birth, the cervix, the mouth of the womb will move from the back of the mother, near her spine, to the front of her abdomen, and it will begin to soften. If a cervix is not ready for artificially starting labor (induction), it will be firm and springy to the touch like the tip of a nose. When the cervix is considered ripe, it will have the texture of lips, soft and mushy, and will spread open more easily to allow the baby out than one that is firm and thick. If the cervix isn't ripe, an induction of labor is more likely to result in a cesarean delivery.

CESAREAN SECTION (c-section, cesarean birth, cesarean delivery, C/S, also spelled Caesarean) (See VAGINAL BIRTH AFTER C-SECTION, VBAC)

Surgically removing a baby from a mother's uterus through an incision (cut) made in her abdominal wall and through the uterus. There are several varieties of c-sections, differing mainly on the location of the incision. The mother is usually given an anesthetic that numbs her lower body, such as an epidural or combined spinal epidural (CSG), and is draped with a curtain between her chest and the surgery. The baby is removed, followed by the placenta.

CHADWICK'S SIGN

Dark blue or purplish discoloration of the cervix (mouth of the womb), or vagina that is one early sign of pregnancy.

CHICKEN POX (varicella, varicella zoster virus [VZV])

A highly contagious virus transmitted by droplets of mucus and the ooze from the itchy skin sores of the disease. Pregnant women who work with children are at risk. In about 2 percent of cases, it can have serious consequences for a fetus during the first twenty weeks of pregnancy. If a person has previously had chicken pox, she will be immune to further outbreaks. Immunity can be detected by a blood test. If a pregnant mother is not immune and is exposed to the virus, she may be treated with zoster immune globulin (ZIG) to protect her baby from congenital varicella syndrome that includes eye, bone, and brain problems, and sometimes early death. Non-pregnant women who have never had chicken pox should be vaccinated against this disease before they become pregnant (the vaccine cannot be given during pregnancy). (See discussion on page 211.)

CHILD HEALTH NURSING

Also called pediatric nursing, it is the field of nursing that focuses on the care of children and their families from birth onward.

CHLAMYDIA (pronounced Clah-MID-i-ah)

The most common sexually transmitted bacterial disease in the United States, it has been labeled "The Silent Epidemic." Women ages fifteen to twenty-four represent seventy percent of all cases. Most victims experience no symptoms. Antibiotics can quickly cure the infection, but left untreated, it can lead to pelvic inflammatory disease (PID), ectopic pregnancy, or chronic pelvic pain. Infected women who deliver a baby may pass the infection on to the baby in the form of severe eye infection or pneumonia. All babies are given antibiotics in their eyes within an hour after birth to protect them against this infection. (See OPTHALMIA NEONATORUM.)

CHLOASMA (chloasma gravidarum, the mask of pregnancy)

Increased skin coloring (pigmentation), brownish-yellow patches that some women develop on their faces during pregnancy. It occurs in the area under each eye and resembles the shape of a butterfly.

CHORIOAMNIONITIS (See AMNIONITIS)

Infection of the amniotic sac and the fluid inside.

CHORIOCARCINOMA (See GESTATIONAL TROPHOBLASTIC DISEASE [GTD])

An extremely rare, highly malignant cancer that grows in the uterus during pregnancy or at the site of an ectopic pregnancy.

CHORION (See AMNION)

The outermost fetal membrane that makes up one layer of the amniotic sac.

CHORIONIC VILLUS SAMPLING

A medical technique that removes a small amount of tissue from a mother's placenta in order to test for chromosomal, metabolic, or DNA abnormalities. The test is generally performed between the tenth and twelfth week of pregnancy. Chorionic villus sampling carries a two to three percent chance risk of miscarriage, and its risks may be higher than for amniocentesis, which is usually done later in pregnancy. (See discussion on page 43.)

CHROMOSOME

A large molecule found in the center (nucleus) of a cell, which carries the genes that determine which parents' characteristics a baby will inherit. Every cell contains forty-six chromosomes except for sperm and egg cells, which each carry twenty-three.

CHRONIC HYPERTENSION (See PREGNANCY-INDUCED HYPERTENSION)

A form of high blood pressure. A mother can have it before she gets pregnant; it can show up before the twentieth week of pregnancy and stays longer than forty-two days after her baby is born.

CIRCUMCISION (See FORESKIN, FRENULUM, GLANS)

The surgical removal of the foreskin covering the end of a newborn male's penis. (See discussion on pages 402–406.)

CLAVICLE, FRACTURED

When a baby's collarbone gets broken during the process of delivery. It requires no treatment and usually heals on its own.

CLEANSING BREATH

A deep, voluntary breath through the nose expelled through the mouth that is used in some comfort management strategies during labor. It is used at the beginning and end of contractions to help restore normal breathing and to help manage stress.

CLEFT LIP (CL)

A malformation found in newborns (approximately one out of eight hundred live births), a groove (cleft) in a baby's upper lip. It can be corrected with surgery.

CLEFT PALATE (CP)

Cleft palate (CP), which is less common than cleft lip (one out of two thousand babies), is a deeper groove that can extend all the way through the lip and into the nose and bony structure at the roof of the mouth. It can be inherited or the result of exposure to harmful drugs or environmental toxins in the womb. It is usually repaired right away by surgery because it can affect a baby's feeding and sucking.

CLINICAL NURSE SPECIALIST (CNS)

A nurse who has completed a master's degree in a specialty, such as neonatal medicine, who can provide expert care to patients, participate in educating and conducting research with other healthcare professionals, and can serve as a special consultant to parents and healthcare providers.

CLUBFOOT (See TALIPES)

CM

Stands for Certified Midwife.

CMV (See CYTOMEGALOVIRUS)

CNM (Certified Nurse-Midwife) (See CERTIFIED NURSE-MIDWIFE)

Signifies a certified nurse-midwife.

COAGULATION

The function of the blood to form clots and scabs.

COCAINE (See NEONATAL ABSTINENCE SYNDROME)

A so-called recreational drug that acts to decrease blood flow to the placenta causing a temporary but dramatic drop in oxygen available to the baby. Cocaine can cause the placenta to tear away from the wall of the uterus causing a life-threatening loss of blood (hemorrhage). Some studies now suggest that babies whose mothers have used cocaine during pregnancy can experience withdrawal after birth, and some may have permanent nervous system (neurological) problems.

COLIC (COLICKY BABY)

Prolonged and frequent crying by a baby with no known cause. It usually appears a few weeks after birth and subsides within the first three months of life.

COLOSTRUM

A thin white or yellowish fluid produced by the breasts of a pregnant mother in the latter months of pregnancy and soon after birth that transfers concentrated protein and specific immunities to the baby. A mother's breasts may secrete tiny amounts of colostrum as early as the sixteenth week of pregnancy.

COMA (in a coma, becoming comatose)

When a person goes into a deep sleeplike state and cannot be awakened. Can be caused by a severe form of preeclampsia.

COMPLETE ABORTION

When all the products of conception (baby and tissues) are expelled from the uterus.

CONCEIVE (getting pregnant)

When a sperm fertilizes an egg.

CONCEPTION (fertilization)

When the sperm succeeds in penetrating the egg.

CONDOM (rubber)

A sheath of rubber that fits over an erect penis to catch semen when a man ejaculates during sex to prevent pregnancy. It is the most effective contraceptive for preventing the transmission of sexually transmitted diseases.

CONDUCTION HEAT LOSS (See CONVECTION HEAT LOSS)

When a baby loses body heat through contact with a cold surface.

CONDYLOMA

A wart near the vagina or rectum.

CONGENITAL CATARACT

Cloudiness of the lens of the eye of a baby that is present at birth.

CONGENITAL DISORDER

A condition present from birth.

CONJOINED TWINS (Siamese Twins)

Twins with joined bodies. Some may share vital organs, which makes surgical separation risky.

CONSTIPATION

Sluggish bowels. Bowel movements may be irregular and are hard, dry, and difficult to push out.

CONTAGIOUS (communicable)

When a disease can be passed from one person to another.

CONTINENCE (See STRESS INCONTINENCE)

Being able to control bladder or bowel function.

CONTRACEPTION

Methods used to prevent a woman from getting pregnant during sex. Could mean the use of a condom (rubber), a specially fitted diaphragm, a contraceptive sponge, or refraining from sex during the times when a woman is fertile and able to conceive. Other methods include contraceptive pills, patches, vaginal rings, intrauterine devices (IUDs), and sterilization.

CONTRACTION (labor pains) (See BRAXTON-HICKS CONTRACTIONS)

Tightening of the abdomen and uterus to expel the baby for birth. They can be strong and regular (happening every three to five minutes), or they can be weak and irregular. Contractions are considered "real" when they work to dilate (stretch) and efface (open) the cervix, or they are sometimes called "false" when they don't cause cervical changes. (See discussion on pages 265–266.)

CONTRACTION STRESS TEST (CST) (See STRESS TEST)

A test used during pregnancy to assess how a baby is doing inside the mother's uterus. It measures a fetus's heart rate in relation to the contraction activity of the uterus. It is rarely used now because of its high rate of "false positives" (suggesting problems when there are none).

CONVECTION HEAT LOSS
(See CONDUCTION HEAT LOSS)
When a newborn loses heat from drafts and cold air. Newborns are quickly wrapped in a blanket or towel to help keep them warm.

CONVULSION (SEIZURE)
A series of spasm-like contractions of the body's muscles. Sometimes babies have convulsions as the result of a rapid rise in temperature from a fever, or a mother may have a convulsion if she has eclampsia.

CORD (See UMBILICAL CORD)

CORD BLOOD BANK
A commercial or public facility that oversees the collection and storage of blood from newborn's umbilical cords for harvesting stem cells for future medical use. Commercial facilities charge fees for the collection, processing, and storage of the blood.

CORD COMPRESSION
When a baby's umbilical cord gets squeezed, usually during birth, so that blood flow is slowed or stopped.

CORDEE (chordee)
An abnormal curvature of the penis most often caused by a congenital abnormality.

CORDIOCENTESIS
A way of getting samples of fetal blood and giving babies blood transfusions in the womb. It can be used for diagnosing hereditary blood disorders such as hemophilia and infections such as rubella, and to assess the levels of oxygen and baby metabolism in intrauterine growth retardation, or fetal anemia in red cell isoimmunization. It is an outpatient technique using local anesthesia.

CORTISOL
Called the stress hormone, cortisol is produced by the adrenal glands in the body. Typically, a woman's cortisol level is significantly higher than normal during pregnancy, more than double her non-pregnant levels. This rise in cortisol is thought to be related to the actions of other hormones, including progesterone. If a mother is under extreme stress, her cortisol can cross the placenta to her baby, but its effects are not completely understood. The baby's own cortisol is critical for the maturation of his lungs, liver, and other organs.

CORD PROLAPSE
(See PROLAPSED CORD)

CORE TEMPERATURE
The temperature deep inside a mother's or baby's body. The normal body temperature as measured by mouth is 98.6 degrees Fahrenheit (37 degrees Celsius). A higher temperature (fever) may indicate the presence of infection in the mother or baby. Sometimes an epidural can also raise a mother's temperature without an infection being present.

CORONA RADIATA
A protective layer of cells surrounding an egg after ovulation that must be penetrated by a sperm to fertilize the egg (ovum).

CORPUS LUTEUM
A structure in the ovary, which develops after an egg has been released, that produces progesterone.

COUVADE SYNDROME
When fathers exhibit the same symptoms as their pregnant partners, including weight gain or loss, digestive disturbances, fatigue, headache, and backaches. (see discussion on pages 64, 244.)

CPD (See CEPHALOPELVIC DISPROPORTION)

CPM (Certified Professional Midwife)

A designation achieved after passing national NARM (North American Registry of Midwives) examination for midwives. (See *Resource Guide,* on page 566.)

CPSC (Consumer Product Safety Commission)

The government regulatory agency that oversees all baby products, except the crashworthiness of children's car seats, which is the responsibility of the National Highway Traffic Safety Administration (NHTSA). (See discussion on page 469, and *Resource Guide* on page 560.)

CRADLE CAP (seborrheic dermatitis)

A skin condition in newborns that causes scaly, yellow patches. It usually appears on the scalp, but sometimes it affects the eyelids, eyebrows, or the genital area. It is common in newborns under three months of age. Your healthcare provider may suggest special cleansing routines, or instruct you simply to leave it alone and wait for it to go away by itself.

CRETINISM

When a baby has insufficient thyroid function. It can lead to mental retardation and other mental and physical changes.

CRNA (See CERTIFIED REGISTERED NURSE ANESTHETIST)

CROWNING (the baby has crowned)

When birth is about to happen because the baby's head has descended so far down into the birth canal that it can be viewed, encircled by the stretched skin of the vagina. Birth typically follows within minutes.

CROWN-TO-RUMP LENGTH

The measurement of a baby's size from the top of the head to the buttocks typically used during ultrasound examinations performed during the first trimester of pregnancy to determine the gestational age of the pregnancy.

C-SECTION (C/S) (See CESAREAN SECTION)

CTX

Shorthand for contractions.

CURETTAGE (See DILATION AND CURETTAGE)

The scraping of the lining of the uterus with an instrument called a curette to remove the products of conception. It is also performed following a miscarriage, in order to remove a polyp, or to obtain a sample for examination in a laboratory. (See discussion on page 31.)

CYSTIC FIBROSIS

An inherited (genetic) disorder that affects a child's lungs and digestive system. It generally occurs among children who are Caucasian and of Northern European descent.

CYSTITIS

Inflammation of the bladder, the saclike organ that stores urine.

CYTOMEGALOVIRUS (CMV)

A herpes-like virus that can cause damage to an unborn baby and also can be caught by the baby during the birthing process if its mother has the infection. In adults, CMV has silent or very mild symptoms similar to mononucleosis, such as fatigue, aches, and fever. About eight thousand babies a year in the United States develop lasting disabilities from being infected by their mothers during pregnancy and birth, including mental retardation, learning disabilities, and hearing or vision loss.

D

D&C (or DNC) (See DILATION AND CURETTAGE)

D ANTIGEN (See: RH FACTOR, and RHESUS ANTI-D GAMMA GLOBULIN INJECTION)

A protein on the surface of red blood cells that is missing for mothers who have Rh negative blood. This condition occurs in about fifteen percent of Caucasians of European ancestry, five percent of African-Americans, and one percent of Asians. If the baby has Rh positive blood, the D antigen could be interpreted as a foreign intruder by the mother's immune system, causing her body to generate antibodies (fighter cells) that cross the placenta and attack the baby's blood cells, resulting in anemia.

DEATH, EARLY NEONATAL

When a baby dies within seven days of being born.

DEATH, LATE FETAL

When a baby dies after the twenty-eighth week of pregnancy.

DECIDUA

The outermost layer of the lining of the uterus (womb). This is the layer of the lining of the uterus (endometrium) into which the pregnancy implants.

DEHYDRATION

A condition caused by the body losing more fluid than it is taking in. In adults, it is signaled by a dry mouth and scant urination. Dehydration can be fatal in babies, and its symptoms are extreme sluggishness and failure to wet diapers.

DEMEROL®

A narcotic commonly used to reduce the sensation of pain during labor and delivery and following birth. Constipation is one potential side effect.

DEOXYRIBONUCLEIC ACID (DNA)

The chemical structure in the body that contains all of the genetic information cells need to duplicate themselves. DNA is the building block of chromosomes.

DEQUERVAIN'S TENDONITIS

A painful hand condition caused by inflammation of the tendons in the thumb that sometimes happens to new mothers. Its causes are not completely understood, although it is thought to be related to post-birth hormonal changes and the stress of lifting the baby. Treatment options include anti-inflammatory medications, splinting the thumb to take pressure off the tendon, and instructing mothers to hold the baby with rigid, rather than flexed wrists.

DEVELOPMENTAL DELAY

When the development of a baby or child is slower than normal.

DIABETES (diabetes mellitus, glucose intolerance) (See GESTATIONAL DIABETES AND GLUCOSE TOLERANCE TEST)

A serious disease that affects the body's ability to absorb glucose from the bloodstream, the body's source of energy. It is caused by the body's not producing enough insulin (a hormone made in the pancreas), or an insensitivity to insulin in the tissues of the body. Diabetes is characterized by high levels of glucose in the blood. Left untreated, this disease can cause dysfunction of various organs in the body, including the heart, kidneys, and blood vessels, and may result in death. During pregnancy, untreated diabetes can cause miscarriage, birth defects, and overly large or very small babies. (See also gestational diabetes, glucose tolerance test, and discussion of diabetes and pregnancy on pages 215 and 407.)

DIAMNIOTIC TWINS

Twins who each have their own separate amniotic sac, but not necessarily their own separate placentas.

DIAPHRAGM

The large muscle in the body that separates the chest cavity from the abdomen involved in inhaling and exhaling. During the latter months of pregnancy, pressure exerted by a baby on a mother's diaphragm can cause the mother a feeling of shortness of breath and episodes of breathlessness. The word also refers to a flexible contraceptive device for women made from a dome-shaped pouch that fits over the mouth of the uterus (cervix) to prevent sperm from entering the uterus to fertilize an egg.

DIASTASIS RECTI

When the muscles running down the center of the abdomen separate and move slightly to the side during late pregnancy. (See exercise recommendations on page 384.)

DIASTASIS SYMPHYSIS PUBIS (DSP) (See SYMPHYSIS PUBIC DYSFUNCTION [SPD])

DIASTOLIC BLOOD PRESSURE

The bottom number in a blood pressure reading, diastolic pressure is the pressure exerted between heartbeats when the heart is relaxed.

DICHORIONIC TWINS

Twins who each have their own separate amniotic sac and their own separate placentas.

DILATION (dilatation)

During pregnancy: the expansion of the opening of the mouth of the womb (cervix) and the passageway in its center (cervical canal) caused by the pressure of the baby's head or body as it descends the birth canal. Dilation is measured as the distance in centimeters from one side of the opening to the other (diameter). One centimeter equals about one-third of an inch. Ten centimeters means the cervix is wide open. This usually signals the onset of the pushing stage. Informally, dilation is measured as fingers, as in three fingers wide. (See discussion on pages 281–284.)

DILATION AND CURETTAGE (D&C, dilatation and curettage)

The stretching of the mouth and neck of the uterus (cervix) and scraping the lining of the uterus (endometrium) with an instrument called a curette. Often performed after a miscarriage in order to prevent an infection caused by incomplete removal of the products of pregnancy.

DILATION AND EVACUATION

A procedure of abortion done during the thirteenth to the twentieth week of pregnancy in which the cervix is gradually stretched open and the fetus is removed using both suction and curettage.

DILATION AND VACUUM CURETTAGE

A procedure used during an abortion that is done prior to thirteen weeks of pregnancy. A mother's cervix is progressively stretched open, and then the contents of the pregnant uterus are suctioned out through a small tube using a vacuum device.

DIRECT-ENTRY MIDWIFE (See CERTIFIED MIDWIFE)

A midwife who learns her skills through self-study, an apprenticeship, or at an independent midwifery school or college. Typically direct-entry midwives deliver babies at home, although some work in birth centers. States differ in the requirements for certification of direct-entry midwives.

DIURETIC

A drug or agent that increases urination.

DIZYGOTIC TWINS (fraternal twins)

Twins derived from two different eggs.

DOMINANT DISORDERS

Genetic (inherited) disorders transmitted from parent to child in which a single altered gene dominates (overrides) a normally functioning gene.

DOPPLER

A handheld ultrasound device that transmits the sounds of a baby's heart rate either through a speaker or into attached earpieces. The device can generally pick up heart tones after twelve weeks' gestation.

DORSAL PENILE NERVE BLOCK (DPNB)

An anesthetic injected into a baby boy's penis to help numb the pain of circumcision.

DOULA (pronounced doola) (See MONITRICE)

The word doula is derived from Greek, meaning trusted servant or woman's servant. A doula (almost always a woman) is a person who provides support and non-medical comfort coaching for mothers and their birth partners during birth. A doula has special training in the natural progression of labor. She may make suggestions on positions to help to move labor along. Many doulas are certified through major childbirth education organizations. (See discussion on page 170.)

DOWN SYNDROME (Down's syndrome, trisomy 21) (See ALPHA-FETO PROTEIN TEST)

The most common type of chromosomal abnormality at birth, it is usually not inherited, but caused by a fetus having an extra copy of chromosome number twenty-one. As a mother's age goes up, her risk for giving birth to a baby with Down syndrome is increased. There are a number of physical characteristics for the syndrome: short stature, special facial structure with an extra fold at the outer corner of the baby's eyelids, and moderate mental retardation. The overall prevalence of the syndrome is one in eight undred babies, but by the time a mother reaches forty-five, its prevalence is one out of every thirty-two babies. It can be detected by specific tests during pregnancy. (See discussion on page 181.)

DTP VACCINATION

A vaccination for babies that protects them against diphtheria, tetanus, and pertussis (whooping cough).

DUCTUS ARTERIOSUS

An artery inside the unborn baby that permits incoming blood to bypass the lungs until they are ready to expand and begin the breathing process immediately after birth. The artery then closes.

DUE DATE (Estimated Date of Delivery [EDD], Estimated Date of Confinement [EDC])

An educated guess for the date your baby can be expected to be born. An average pregnancy lasts 280 days, or about forty weeks measured from the first day of the expectant mother's last menstrual period, but normal pregnancies can last between thirty-seven weeks to forty-two weeks. Only about five of one hundred babies are born on their due date, with most mothers giving birth within two weeks of the date. It is important in measuring the progress of pregnancy, the growth of the baby, and to determine the best timing for testing for fetal abnormalities. Note: First-time mothers (primiparas, primips, or nulliparous women, nullips) are likely to give birth later than mothers who have had more than one child. (See discussion on pages 11–12.)

DYSMATURITY SYNDROME

When a baby is born who appears malnourished with a long and lean body, an alert look on the face, lots of hair, long fingernails, and thin wrinkled skin. Often there can be meconium-stained amniotic fluid. The condition usually occurs in babies born more than one week after their due dates.

DYSPNEA

Difficulty breathing.

DYSTOCIA

A slow and difficult childbirth, which can be due to problems with the baby (unusually large, in the wrong position, stuck shoulders, abnormalities that make birth difficult or impossible, interlocked twins); or problems with the mother (a sluggish or malformed uterus, a small pelvis, a rigid cervix that will not open to allow the baby out). The treatment for dystocia depends upon the condition and can range from simply waiting for delivery to occur naturally, giving medication to stimulate contractions, or performing a cesarean section to remove the baby from the mother's body.

DYSURIA

Pain during urinating.

E

ECLAMPSIA (See PREECLAMPSIA, PREGNANCY-INDUCED HYPERTENSION [PIH], and TOXEMIA)

A rare, life-threatening condition for mothers that can occur at any time between the twentieth week of pregnancy and the first week following birth. It is marked by coma and convulsive seizures, and it can be fatal if not treated. It is estimated that one out of every two hundred mothers who have preeclampsia (toxemia) will develop full-blown eclampsia. Currently, the only cure for eclampsia is giving birth, and the baby of a mother with the more severe form of the illness may have to have her baby delivered early in order to save her life. (See discussion on page 215.)

ECTOPIC PREGNANCY (or tubal pregnancy)

When a fertilized egg implants itself some other place than the mother's uterine wall. The majority of these pregnancies occur in the fallopian tubes that conduct the egg to the uterus, but sometimes the pregnancy can occur in a mother's abdominal cavity, which can lead to life-threatening problems. Symptoms of an ectopic pregnancy include abnormal bleeding, severe abnormal pain, or shoulder pain. Approximately one out of fifty pregnancies is ectopic. (See discussion on page 31.)

ECZEMA (atopic dermatitis)

A broad term for dry, itchy, inflamed skin, which can crack and become oozy. The first symptoms usually appear in babies during the first three months of life. The baby will have red, scaly skin, and red patches may appear on his cheeks that spread to scalp, arms, and legs. Babies with dry, sensitive skin or allergies to ingredients in formula, chemicals in detergents, fabric softeners, pollens, or house dust are more vulnerable to it. Sometimes creams, ointments, lotions, or moisturizers may help, as can steroids, but they should be used only under the guidance of a physician or skin specialist (dermatologist).

EDC (See ESTIMATED DATE OF CONFINEMENT)

EDD (estimated due date) (See DUE DATE)

EDEMA

Swelling of soft tissues as the result of excess fluid retention. Most pregnant women retain more fluid in their lower legs in the latter stages of pregnancy from pressure exerted on their circulatory systems by their babies and hormonal changes. Excess retention of fluid can also be an early sign of toxemia (preeclampsia), especially when it involves the hands and face. (See discussion of edema on page 141, and eclampsia on pages 215 and 355.)

EFFACEMENT

The gradual thinning, shortening, and drawing up of the cervix in preparation for birth. It is expressed in percentages with 100 percent meaning totally thinned. For example, a mother may be told she is "40 percent effaced."

EFFLEURAGE

Light caressing of the abdomen using the fingertips that can be used during labor to help lessen the discomfort of labor contractions.

EGG (ovum)

The reproductive cell produced by the mother that is fertilized by the father's sperm, which forms an embryo that develops into a fetus and then a baby.

EJACULATION

When a man expels a white fluid, semen, from his penis, which contains sperm that seek out and fertilize a mother's egg during the process of sexual intercourse.

ELECTIVE INDUCTION (See INDUCTION)

Choosing to have labor started by drugs rather than on its own.

ELECTRONIC FETAL MONITORING (EFM)

An instrument used to record the baby's heart rate from moment to moment. It can be used as a test during pregnancy of the health of the baby or to monitor the baby during a mother's labor contractions. Monitoring can be continuous or periodic. (See discussion on page 319.)

EMBOLISM

A blood clot that blocks circulation in a blood vessel to a part of the body, such as the lungs. Along with hemorrhage (excessive bleeding), and hypertension (high blood pressure), embolisms are one of the leading causes of maternal death during childbirth. Mothers who have a prolonged labor, a cesarean section, who are significantly overweight, or who have varicose veins are slightly more at risk of having blood clots. Common symptoms are tenderness around a vein, one-sided swelling, and pain in the leg near the ankle.

A pulmonary embolism (pulmonary thrombosis) occurs when the clot travels to the lungs causing sudden breathlessness and chest pain. This can result in respiratory collapse.

EMBRYO

The name for the fetus, or developing baby, up to 10 weeks of menstrual age, menstrual age being calculated from the first day of the mother's last period before pregnancy.

EMBRYONIC STAGE

The second through eighth weeks after conception.

EMLA® CREAM

An anesthetic cream commonly used during circumcision to numb the tip of a baby's penis. It is applied to the skin of the penis in advance of circumcision and contains lidocaine and prilocaine. It may cause swelling and is not advised for use on mucous membranes. (See discussion of circumcision on page 405.)

ENDODERMAL GERM LAYER (endoderm, entoderm)

Area of tissue in early development of the embryo that gives rise to other structures including the digestive tract, respiratory organs, vagina, bladder, and urethra (the tube that flows urine from the kidneys to the bladder).

ENDOMETRIOSIS

When the lining of the uterus (endometrium) is growing in the wrong place in the body such as in the abdominal cavity.

ENDOMETRITIS (See POSTPARTUM ENDOMETRITIS)

ENDOMETRIUM (endometrial tissue)

The lining of the inside wall of the uterus. (This lining sheds and flows out during a period.) The fertilized egg implants itself into this lining and takes early nourishment from it.

ENDORPHIN

Natural, morphine-like hormones made by the body that help to reduce pain and produce a feeling of calmness and peacefulness. Endorphins are secreted by a mother's body during labor.

ENEMA

Fluid flowed into the rectum for the purpose of clearing out the bowels. Enemas were formerly a standard procedure when laboring mothers were admitted to the hospital. They are seldom used now.

ENGAGED (engagement)

A laboring mother may be told that her baby's head has engaged. It means that a baby's head or other body part, such as the buttocks during a breech presentation, has moved down into the bones of the pelvis in preparation for birth. Also known as lightening, a mother will notice that the baby's position is lower and that she is able to breathe easier, but there may also be odd pains and a feeling of increased pressure to her bladder. (See discussion on page 261.)

ENGORGEMENT

Swelling and hardening of a mother's breasts that occurs twenty-four to forty-eight hours after birth, whether or not a mother chooses to breastfeed. Nursing within an hour following birth, and expressing milk can help to treat it. (See breastfeeding discussion on pages 414–419.)

ENTEROVIRUSES

A large family of viruses that live in the intestines and are responsible for many infections in babies and children. There are more than seventy different strains, which include the group A and group B coxsackieviruses, the echoviruses, polio, and Hepatitis A, which can cause paralysis. Most children develop immunity to the most common forms and catch them only once. Typical symptoms include fever sometimes accompanied by stomachache, sore throats, or muscle aches. The viruses can live for days on surfaces at room temperature, and refrigeration and freezing do not kill them, but they are killed by disinfectants. Antibiotics are not useful in treating them. They are most often passed by human contact. Frequent hand washing can help to prevent them.

EPIDURAL (epidural anesthesia) (See BLOOD PATCH, SPINAL HEADACHE, AND WALKING EPIDURAL)

A method for decreasing or eliminating pain during labor. It numbs a mother's body from the lower rib cage downward, but allows a mother to remain alert and awake, so she can watch the birth of her baby. Medication is injected between two vertebrae of the lower backbone and into the epidural space of the spinal column. The tube (catheter) that is used for the procedure remains in place until after delivery. Epidurals are also used

to provide anesthesia for a cesarean delivery. (See discussion on pages 317–322.)

EPISIOTOMY

A surgical incision into the tissue, between the vagina and the rectum done for the purpose of widening a mother's birth outlet for the use of forceps or vacuum extraction or on the premise that it speeds up delivery or allows for better healing than a tear in the tissue. Afterward, your care provider will give an injection of a local anesthetic and stitch up the incision and any lacerations with dissolving stitches. Episiotomies are thought to contribute to more serious tearing and ruptures. (See discussion on page 344.)

ERB'S PALSY (Erb-Duchenne paralysis)

When a newborn is paralyzed due to an injury of the network of nerves in the shoulder and neck that control the arms. The baby's arm will be limp. The condition usually goes away during the first three months of life, but on rare occasions, it can be permanent.

ERYTHEMA TOXICUM

A harmless, red rash with small white bumps on the skin of newborns that happens in about 30–70 percent of babies. It appears within the second or third day of life and fades by the end of the first week.

ERYTHROBLASTOSIS FETALIS (See Rh INCOMPATIBILITY)

A blood disease of newborns characterized by anemia (low blood cell count), jaundice (yellowing of the skin), enlargement of the liver and spleen, and generalized edema (swelling of the tissues). It can happen when a mother with Rh-negative blood carries a baby with Rh-positive blood.

ESTIMATED DATE OF CONFINEMENT (EDC) (See DUE DATE)

Anticipated due date for delivery of the baby. Calculated from the first day of the last menstrual period.

ESTRIOL (SEE ALPHA-FETO PROTEIN TEST)

A hormone related to estrogen that is produced by the placenta. Lower-than-normal levels detected in a pregnant woman's blood may suggest a chromosomal abnormality. (See discussion on page 54.)

ESTROGEN

A female hormone that regulates menstruation. The placenta also produces it during the first trimester of pregnancy to help sustain it.

EVIDENCE-BASED MEDICINE (EBM)

Medical practice based on the careful evaluation of well-designed research studies. (See discussion on page xvi.)

EXCLUSIVE BREASTFEEDING

Breastfeeding a baby without supplemental fluids, such as formula, or glucose water. Babies who are exclusively breast-fed tend to be healthier than formula-fed babies. (See discussion on page 416.)

EXTERNAL VERSION (External Cephalic Version, ECV)

A technique using external hand pressure on a pregnant woman's belly to turn a baby from a head upward (breech) to a head downward (cephalic) position in preparation for birth. Medication may be used to help the mother's uterus relax. (See discussion on page 345.)

EXTRAUTERINE PREGNANCY (EUP) (See ECTOPIC PREGNANCY)

When a fertilized egg (ovum) implants itself in tissue outside of the uterus.

F

FACIAL PARALYSIS

Sometimes a baby may have a face that sags on one side as the result of damage to a nerve during birth, sometimes caused by the use of forceps. The paralysis requires no medical intervention and will usually disappear within a few days to several months. In rare cases, the damage may be permanent.

FACNM (Fellow of the American College of Nurse-Midwives)

FACOG (Fellow of the American College of Obstetricians & Gynecologists)

FAILURE TO PROGRESS (dystocia) (See DYSTOCIA)

A slow or stopped labor, often without a clear-cut reason.

FALLOPIAN TUBES

The tubes that carry eggs (ova) from the ovaries to the uterus. Fertilization often happens in the tubes, then the egg floats down to implant in the uterus. If the egg implants in the tube, it is called an ectopic pregnancy. These are the tubes that are tied (closed off) during female sterilization.

FAMILY-CENTERED CARE

Healthcare based on the philosophy of providing maximum support for the health, security, and well-being of mothers, fathers, and children. In birth centers, or care provider offices, this usually means that the mother can bring her partner and children along for health visits and the birth of her child, with the ability to keep them at her side during labor.

FAMILY PLANNING

The managing of fertility through a variety of options.

FASTING BLOOD SUGAR (See GLUCOSE TOLERANCE TEST)

FDA (Food and Drug Administration)

The FDA is the federal agency that oversees the safety of foods and drugs, including medications used by pregnant women and products used on babies such as baby food, formula, and creams. This agency sometimes recalls products that have been found to be harmful. The FDA currently does not compel any drug manufacturer to test the safety of medications on pregnant women (unless the drug claims specifically to be safe for pregnant women), which is why drug labels often instruct pregnant women to consult with a doctor before taking any medication. (See *Resource Guide*, on page 558.)

FDLMP

First day of last menstrual period. It is used as the starting point for how long pregnancy is expected to last and to calculate a mother's due date using a forty-week time frame.

FECAL INCONTINENCE

The inability to hold in bowel movements (and gas) that can sometimes be the result of tearing during labor usually from having an episiotomy, or deliveries using forceps or vacuum extraction. The condition is often temporary, and most mothers regain control of their bowels between six weeks to four months following birth, but the condition sometimes lasts longer. Kegel exercises may help. In the meantime, adult diapers may be useful. In rare instances, corrective surgery may be needed.

FELLOW

An individual who has completed an M.D. degree as well as a residency in a specialty such as obstetrics or pediatrics, and who is now taking advanced training, such as a fellow in perinatology or neonatology.

FERGUSON'S REFLEX

The release of oxytocin during the second (pushing) stage of labor triggered by the pressure of the baby's head on the tissues of the mother's lower body and mouth of her uterus (cervix). The reflex triggers the mother's urge to bear down. The reflex is more pronounced in labors without painkilling medication.

FERTILITY (BEING FERTILE)

Being able to conceive a baby.

FERTILITY MEDICATIONS

Medicines used to help mothers conceive by manipulating hormone levels and stimulating egg production. Currently, there are drugs approved by the FDA for this purpose, including Clomid®, Gonal-F®, and Pergonal®.

FERTILIZATION

When sperm and egg join together.

FERTILIZATION AGE

Dating pregnancy from the actual date of fertilization (conception), rather than the medical practice of dating pregnancy from the first day of the last period. It is calculated as 266 days or 38 weeks.

FETAL ALCOHOL SYNDROME (FAS)

A series of non-genetic birth defects caused by a mother's drinking of alcohol during pregnancy. Not all children exposed to alcohol in the womb suffer from FAS, although even minimal drinking is now considered a threat to the baby's well-being. Currently, there is no way to predict the effects of alcohol on a baby. (See discussion on page 38.)

FETAL ANOMALY

Fetal malformation or abnormal development.

FETAL BLOOD SAMPLING (percutaneous umbilical blood sampling, PUBS, codiocentesis)

A test for fetal abnormalities in which blood is removed from a baby's umbilical cord while still inside the mother's womb. In less than one percent of cases, it can lead to baby death.

FETAL COMPROMISE (See NONREASSURING FETAL STATUS)

FETAL DEATH IN UTERO (FDIU, intrauterine fetal death, stillbirth) (See STILLBIRTH)

FETAL DIAGNOSTIC TESTING

Tests conducted during pregnancy to ensure that the baby is alive and thriving. Tests include nonstress tests and contraction stress tests, biophysical profiles, amniocentesis, and ultrasound examinations.

FETAL DISTRESS (See NONREASSURING FETAL STATUS)

FETAL GROWTH RETARDATION (intrauterine growth restriction, or IUGR)

Inadequate growth of the fetus during the latter stages of pregnancy.

FETAL HEART RATE (FHR)

A baby's normal heart rate in the womb is between 120–160 beats per minute. The rhythm of a baby's heart rate during labor is considered an important way to measure whether the birthing baby is having a problem. Speeding up is called acceleration, slowing down is called deceleration. If a baby's heart rate slows to less than 100 beats per minute for a period of time, it is called bradycardia, or brady spell, and suggests that the baby may be having problems. It could indicate that the baby should be delivered quickly and receive extra attention after birth.

FETAL HEART TONES (FHT)

The sound made by a baby's heart that can first be detected as early as ten to twelve weeks by ultrasound and between eighteen and twenty weeks by an electronic fetoscope that transmits heart sounds using ear pieces similar to a stethoscope.

FETAL LOSS (fetal death in utero, stillbirth) (See STILLBIRTH)

When a baby dies inside the uterus during pregnancy. (See page 346.)

FETAL MONITOR

Device used to listen to and record a baby's heartbeat during pregnancy or labor. External monitoring uses a device fastened to a mother's abdomen; internal monitoring attaches to the baby's scalp through the mother's vagina.

FETAL MOVEMENT COUNTS (FMCS)

Healthy babies are usually very active inside the uterus. Most mothers don't feel their babies move until around twenty weeks of pregnancy. Beginning the twenty-seventh week of pregnancy, some healthcare providers request that mothers do periodic counts to measure how often their babies move within an hour. Ten times per hour is considered normal. If a mother has not felt her baby move all day (twelve hours), or she becomes aware of a significant change in her baby's activity, then she should contact her healthcare provider.

FETAL PERIOD

The stage in a baby's growth following the first ten weeks of gestation (embryonic period) until birth.

FETAL PULMONARY MATURATION

A baby who is born too soon may have lungs that don't function well. A number of tests are available to tell if a baby's lungs are mature enough for survival after birth which is an issue for preterm (premature) births or when a baby needs to be delivered before thirty-nine weeks of pregnancy for medical reasons. If the baby is suspected of having immature lungs, its mother may be given a course of drugs to help to promote lung maturation.

FETOPELVIC DISPROPORTION (cephalopelvic disproportion)

When a baby is so large that it may not be able to pass through the pelvis of the mother because of its size, when the mother has a smaller-than-normal pelvis, or a combination of these size mismatches. Disproportion is frequently cited as a reason for a cesarean section. A mother's pelvis is usually measured in the weeks prior to birth to detect any potential problems.

FETOSCOPE

A special cone-shaped stethoscope used for listening to a baby's heart. There are many types of fetoscopes available, although a regular stethoscope can also be used. Either type of monitoring device is able to detect a baby's heartbeat after about the eighteenth week of pregnancy.

FETOSCOPY

Passing a tiny tubular-shaped device, an endoscope, through the mother's abdomen into the amniotic cavity in order to take a biopsy of tissue or to perform a surgical intervention on the baby. This is only done when a condition threatens a baby's life, and there is no effective treatment that can be performed after the baby is born.

FETUS

An unborn baby from the end of the eighth week of pregnancy until the moment of birth.

FEVER

When a person's temperature by mouth is elevated above normal: 98.6 degrees Fahrenheit (37 degrees Celsius). Someone's temperature can also be taken rectally, using a thermometer that goes in the ear, or by placing the thermometer in the crease of the underarm, with different numbers indicating what is normal. Fever associated with birth can be a serious sign that could indicate the mother has an infection. The baby may then have to undergo a series of tests to ensure that the infection hasn't been transmitted to him. (Baby fevers are discussed on pages 436–438.)

FEVER, PUERPERAL

When a mother has a fever during or after the process of birth. It could indicate an infection, or it could be one of the effects of an epidural.

FIBROID (myoma)

A non-malignant (non-cancerous) tumor on the uterus that may rarely affect pregnancy, particularly if it is near the amniotic sac or blocking the pathway for birth.

FIVE-POINT HARNESS SYSTEM

A child's car seat feature that refers to the number of straps. The five points refer to two straps for the shoulders, a strap for each side of the baby's waist, and a crotch strap for between the legs. Some rear-facing infant car seats have three-point harness systems (a strap for each shoulder, and for the crotch) which are thought to be less safe than those with five-point systems.

FOCAL POINT

A point of concentration in the room of a birthing mother that helps her to maintain control during contractions.

FOLEY BULB (See FOLEY CATHETER)

FOLEY CATHETHER

A tube with an expanding pocket (balloon) inside that is most often used to drain the bladder, but the Foley catheter is sometimes inserted inside the mother's cervix in order to gradually soften and expand it during labor.

FOLIC ACID (FOLATE)

A member of the vitamin B–complex that increases a mother's metabolism, prevents a rare form of anemia, and is active in the formation of red blood cells and cell structures. Folic acid has also been found to help prevent certain malformations in the fetus including spina bifida. (See discussion on pages 149–150.)

FOLLICLES

Sacs in which eggs develop in a woman's ovaries.

FOLLICLE-STIMULATING HORMONE (FSH)

A hormone that stimulates the development of eggs in a woman's ovaries.

FONTANELS (soft spots)

Spaces between the hard bones of a baby's skull that allow the baby's head to compress during birth. As the skull's bones grow, the size of the fontanels shrinks. Normally, by six months of age, the fontanels become dense and fibrous, and they fuse into hard bone around two years of age.

FORCEPS

A spoon-shaped instrument with two blades and a handle designed to hold onto the sides of a baby's head to aid with delivery. Forceps can cause injury and are less frequently used now than in years past.

FORESKIN (prepuce) (See CIRCUMCISION)

A retractable skin covering that partially or completely covers the glans, or penis head, in a male baby. It is left intact when a baby is not circumcised, but removed by circumcision. In childhood and adulthood, the foreskin acts as a protective cover for a flaccid penis. (See discussion on page 403.)

FORMULA

An artificial substitute for human breast milk usually made from specially processed cow's milk or soy protein and other added components. (See discussion on page 418.)

FRANK BREECH (See BREECH)

When a baby is positioned in the uterus with the buttocks first (nearest to the cervix) and legs stretched upward toward his chest.

FRATERNAL TWINS

Two babies that have developed from two different, separate, fertilized eggs. The opposite of identical twins.

FRENULUM (FRENUM)

A connecting fold of membrane. One type is the elastic band of tissue under the head of a male infant's penis (glans) that connects to the foreskin, which is removed during most circumcision procedures. (See discussion of circumcision starting on page 402.) Another frenulum is the tissue in the center of the underside of baby's tongue, which, if too tight, can interfere with breastfeeding.

FRIEDMAN LABOR CURVE

A widely followed chart for the normal progress of labor that measures cervical dilation over the duration of a mother's labor. The graph estimates that first-time mothers take approximately $6^1/2$ hours to move from the latent to the active phase of labor with active labor lasting approximately $4^1/2$ hours. The second pushing stage is estimated to last about an hour. The latent phase for mothers who have previously had a baby is 4.8 hours, and the active phase lasst about 2.4 hours, with the second, pushing stage taking only about half an hour.[1] (See discussion on page 334.)

FTP (See FAILURE TO PROGRESS)

FULL TERM

A baby is considered full term when he is born between the beginning of the thirty-seventh week and the end of the forty-second week.

FUNDAL HEIGHT (McDonald measurement)

A measurement of the expansion of a pregnant uterus from the edge of the pubic bone to the top of the uterus (the fundus). After the first twenty weeks, the fundal height during pregnancy is generally equal in centimeters to the number of weeks a mother is pregnant, e.g., thirty-two centimeters at thirty-two weeks of gestation.

FUNDUS

The top of the uterus. It can be felt as a firm ridge by pressing downward on a mother's belly.

G

GALACTOCELE (plugged milk duct) (See MASTITIS)

A plugged milk duct inhibits milk flow in the breast. It can feel like a mass or firm nodules in the breast. A too-tight bra can cause it. Nursing a baby can help to dissolve the lump, or it can be suctioned out by a healthcare provider using a syringe.

GBS (See GROUP B STREPTOCOCCUS)

GENERAL ANESTHESIA (general anesthetic)

A drug used for surgery, so the patient is no longer conscious and feels no pain. It sometimes is used during an emergency cesarean, and it can be employed for a planned cesarean or a difficult vaginal birth. The delivery must occur quickly because this type of anesthetic can cross the placenta to the baby and may temporarily depress the baby's breathing. It is primarily used when speed is of the essence, such as when the circulation in a baby's umbilical cord has been blocked and his heart rate has begun to slow down; when there is severe, sudden bleeding that could endanger a mother's life (hemorrhage); or when an epidural or spinal anesthetic would not be safe for the mother.

GENES

A portion of a DNA molecule that is located on a chromosome that carries basic genetic information. Genes are the carriers of traits that are inherited from parents.

GENETIC

Determined by genes, such as inherited conditions.

GENETIC COUNSELING

Counseling for parents whose babies may have defects related to the baby's genetic makeup. (See discussion on page 180.)

GENETIC DISORDER

A mental or physical problem that results from abnormal genes. It can happen by chance or be passed from parent to baby through an error in the parent's genes or chromosomes. (See discussion on page 179.)

GENETIC MARKER

An easily identified piece of DNA that is used to find the gene that may be inherited, whether normal or abnormal.

GENITAL HERPES
(herpes simplex)

A viral infection involving the genital area. It is important to know if a mother has herpes because of the danger of a newborn becoming infected during labor, which can have serious consequences. (See discussion on page 220.)

GENITALS (genitalia)

Male and female sex organs.

GERMAN MEASLES
(See RUBELLA)

GESTATION

Another word for pregnancy: The length of time between the first day of a mother's final menstrual period before conception and delivery of the baby. Typically, the period of gestation is between thirty-seven and forty-one weeks from the first day after the last normal menstrual period, although the calculation of how long a mother has carried a baby is not always very accurate.

GESTATIONAL AGE

Baby's age measured from the first day of the last period: 280 days, or forty weeks. It is two weeks longer than fetal age.

GESTATIONAL DIABETES
(See GLUCOSE TOLERANCE TEST)

A condition that develops during pregnancy when the expectant mother's body does not supply sufficient insulin for the demands of pregnancy. This leaves excessive amounts of glucose in the blood, potentially causing problems for both mother and baby. The increased level of blood sugar (glucose) can be detected in the urine and blood. (See discussion on page 216.)

GESTATIONAL TROPHOBLASTIC DISEASE (GTD)

A rare condition that mimics pregnancy. It occurs when abnormal cells grow in the uterus at the site of the implanted egg. Hydatidiform mole is the most common form, occurring in one out of every fifteen hundred pregnancies. Choriocarcinoma, the cancerous variety, occurs in one of every twenty thousand to forty thousand pregnancies. Symptoms include faster-than-usual abdominal growth, severe nausea and vomiting, non-menstrual vaginal bleeding, fatigue and shortness of breath from anemia, and blood clots or watery brown discharge. Dislodged pieces of the tumor that resemble a bunch of grapes. GTD most often happens with very young (less than seventeen years) or older women (thirty to forty years). It is treatable even in its late stage and has a ninety percent survival rate, although a medical specialist may be required.

GLANS

The bulbous, soft tip of the penis that is covered by the foreskin in an uncircumcised baby.

GLUCOSE

A form of sugar present in the blood that serves as the main fuel of the body. (See discussion of diabetes on page 215.)

GLUCOSE TOLERANCE TEST (fasting blood sugar test) (See GESTATIONAL DIABETES)

A blood test that measures the level of glucose in the bloodstream. The test is usually performed around twenty-eight weeks of pregnancy. First, a fasting blood sugar reading is taken from a small blood sample. The pregnant woman is then asked to drink a heavily sweetened beverage. An hour later, blood is drawn to measure blood sugar levels. There may be additional tests in the hours that follow. High blood sugar levels may be a sign of diabetes mellitus, or gestational diabetes. (See discussion on pages 81 and 193.)

GLUCOSURIA

Glucose in the urine. (See discussion of diabetes on pages 215–216.)

GONORRHEA

A highly contagious infection of the reproductive organs of men and women that is transmitted primarily through sexual intercourse. The incidence of gonorrhea during pregnancy is low, but it has been associated with miscarriages, low birthweight babies, premature rupture of the amniotic sac, chorioamnionitis, and pelvic infections following birth. (See discussion on page 222.)

GRAV 1 (gravida 1, gravida one)

First pregnancy (pregnancy number one).

GRAVIDA (See MULTIGRAVIDA and PRIMIGRAVIDA)

Number of pregnancies.

GRIEF, STAGES OF

First identified by Dr. John Bowlby, a British researcher, it refers to stages that parents go through that are a part of the natural grieving process. The series of feelings, called phases, include numbness, yearning and searching, despair, and disorganization, followed eventually by hope and rebuilding.

GROUP-B STREPTOCOCCUS (GBS)

A bacterium found in the intestines and on the genitals of approximately one out of five pregnant women, who may not show any outward symptoms of colonization by the bacterium. It is the leading cause of serious neonatal infection of newborns and can affect the blood, spinal fluid, and lungs. It can be passed from mother to infant during delivery. Although only a small portion of exposed babies develops serious complications, the infection can be fatal. You will likely be screened for GBS late in your pregnancy (See RVC [Rectal/Vaginal Culture]), and given an antibiotic such as penicillin during labor if you are found to carry the organism. (See discussion on page 188.)

GROUP PRACTICE

A group of physicians and/or midwives who practice together in order to provide better around-the-clock coverage for their pregnant patients.

G.Y.N. OR GYN

Abbreviations for gynecologist.

H

HABITUAL ABORTION

Three or more consecutive, spontaneous miscarriages.

HEARTBURN (indigestion, sour stomach, gastroesophageal reflux, gastric reflux)

A burning sensation in the upper chest or throat caused by gastric juices being released upwards into the esophagus. Heartburn during pregnancy is thought to be caused by crowding of a mother's stomach by the growing baby, hormonal changes in the body, and eating excessive fat, caffeine, or spicy foods. (See discussion on page 132.)

HEAT RASH (prickly heat, milaria rubra)

Pink bumps that appear on a baby's forehead under caps or visors, in body folds, or on the upper back, chest, and arms that are caused by the pores of sweat glands becoming plugged. The tiny pink bumps may form water blisters and can become itchy. Although heat rash is more common in warm weather, it can also occur when babies are over-dressed in winter. Skin oils, lotions, and ointments can aggravate the condition. If the rash is accompanied by a fever, it may be a sign of chicken pox or a reaction to chicken pox vaccine. A healthcare provider may recommend a cleansing routine.

HEEL STICK

Pricking a baby's heel to obtain small amounts of blood for testing. The baby may have a big bandage on his heel afterward.

HEGAR'S SIGN

The softening of the area between the cervix and the body of the uterus that is a sign of pregnancy.

HELLP SYNDROME

A severe form of preeclampsia associated with significant risks for both mother and baby. HELLP stands for hemolysis (H), elevated liver enzymes (EL), and low platelet count (LP), which are measured by blood tests. Babies of mothers with HELLP Syndrome are more likely to be small for gestational age (SGA). Potential HELLP symptoms include pain in the upper right-hand side of the chest or stomach area, sometimes accompanied by nausea and vomiting. Mothers with HELLP are more likely to have anemia and cesarean deliveries, and are more at risk for heavy bleeding.

HEMATOCRIT (Hct, blood count)

The percent of blood cells in the total blood volume in a blood test. Important in diagnosing anemia.

HEMOGLOBIN

Pigment in red blood cell that carries oxygen to body tissues.

HEMOPHILIA

A genetically inherited blood disorder that disrupts the ability of the blood to clot. Persons having hemophilia may be labeled bleeders.

HEMORRHAGE, POSTPARTUM

Life-threatening bleeding from the uterus. If the bleeding doesn't stop, it may require a blood transfusion or other medical or surgical interventions, and, more rarely, a hysterectomy. Primary hemorrhage occurs within the first twenty-four hours after birth, secondary hemorrhage refers to excessive blood loss from the vagina between twenty-four hours and six weeks after birth. (See discussion on page 356.)

HEMORRHOIDS (PILES)

Swollen blood vessels around the anus that can become inflamed and painful. Sometimes they bleed. They can be caused by constipation during pregnancy, lightening when the baby settles more deeply into the pelvis, or the pressure of the baby or childbirth on the veins of the rectum. (See discussion on page 133.)

HEPARIN LOCK

A capped-off intravenous (IV) line usually placed on the back of a mother's hand or forearm that can be used later should medications or fluids be needed.

HEPATITIS B

A serious infection of the liver caused by a virus that typically is transmitted through sexual intercourse or exposure to an infected person's blood. It can be transmitted from mother to baby during the process of birth, unless the baby receives preventive medication following delivery and is then vaccinated against it. People at high risk for contracting this disease, including expectant mothers, should be vaccinated against hepatitis B, and it is currently recommended that all newborns be vaccinated too.

HERNIA

A protrusion of an organ or part of an organ into surrounding tissues.

HERPES SIMPLEX (See GENITAL HERPES)

HIP DYSPLASIA

When the top of a baby's thigh bone (the femoral head) is badly positioned in or is dislocated from the socket of the pelvis (acetabulum).

HIV (HUMAN IMMUNODEFICIENCY VIRUS)

HIV is a sexually transmitted disease that causes AIDS (Acquired Immunodeficiency Syndrome). The virus attacks the body's immune system, causing a loss of resistance to various infections. HIV may circulate in the bloodstream many years before the symptoms of AIDS appear. It is transmitted through contact with blood, semen, vaginal secretions, and, more rarely, through human breast milk. Mothers with HIV are most often infected through heterosexual contact with an infected partner or through drug use. Twenty to thirty percent of babies born to untreated mothers with HIV will get the infection during pregnancy or during labor and delivery, but with therapy, only one to two percent of infants who are born to an infected mother will acquire HIV from the mother.

HOMAN'S SIGN

When a mother feels pain in her calf when her foot is flexed upward. The sign, along with swelling and tenderness in one leg following birth, may indicate a mother could have thrombosis, a clot forming in her leg.

HORMONE

A chemical secretion produced in the body to stimulate or slow down the function of various organs or body systems.

HUMAN CHORIONIC GONADOTROPIN (hCG) (β-Human Chorionic Gonadotropin, β-hCG)

A hormone produced by the embryo as measured in pregnancy tests. It stimulates the secretion of estrogen and progesterone for maintaining pregnancy. It doesn't appear to play a role in the second and third trimesters of pregnancy but is thought to be related to nausea and vomiting during early pregnancy.

HUMAN GENOME

An individual's entire collection of genes.

HUMAN PLACENTAL LACTOGEN
Hormone of pregnancy produced by the placenta found in a mother's bloodstream. It plays a role in the body's processing of blood sugar (glucose).

HYALINE MEMBRANE DISEASE (See RESPIRATORY DISTRESS SYNDROME [RDS])

HYDATIDIFORM MOLE (See GESTATIONAL TROPHOBLASTIC DISEASE [GTD])
An abnormal pregnancy in which there is no fetus, only the abnormal growth of the placenta.

HYDRAMNIOS (See AMNIOTIC SAC)
Greater than normal amount of fluid in the amniotic sac.

HYDROCEPHALUS (hydrocephaly)
The collection of an abnormal amount of fluid in the brain, causing an enlargement of a baby's skull. It can be caused by spina bifida. Putting a small tube, called a shunt, inside the baby's head after birth will allow the fluid to be drained.

HYPERBILIRUBINEMIA (jaundice) (See BILIRUBIN and JAUNDICE)
An excess of bilirubin in the blood.

HYPEREMISIS GRAVIDARIUM (See MORNING SICKNESS)
Ongoing, extreme nausea and vomiting during pregnancy that can lead to serious dehydration in mothers. It requires medical intervention. (See discussion on pages 40 and 129.)

HYPERGLYCEMIA (See DIABETES MELLITUS, GESTATIONAL DIABETES, and GLUCOSE TOLERANCE TEST)
Having too much blood sugar (glucose) in the blood. Usually a sign of diabetes or gestational diabetes. (See discussion on page 215.)

HYPERKALEMIA
Greater-than-normal levels of potassium in the blood that can be caused by the excessive vomiting of hyperemesis gravidarium.

HYPERPIGMENTATION
The darkening of skin color. During pregnancy, this is most common in the nipples and areola of the breasts, the vagina, and the area surrounding the rectum. It is thought to be a side effect of pregnancy hormones, which make the body's skin cells produce more pigment.

HYPERTENSION (See PREGNANCY INDUCED HYPERTENSION)
High blood pressure. If it occurs for the first time in the second half of pregnancy, it is called pregnancy-induced hypertension. Hypertension is a significant cause of problems in both mothers and babies, complicating about ten percent of all pregnancies. (See discussion on page 214.)

HYPERTHYROIDISM
Elevation of the thyroid hormone in the bloodstream.

HYPERVENTILATION
When a mother breathes too fast and too many times per minute. It can cause symptoms of tingling, dizziness, and numbness in the hands.

HYPOTENSION

Low blood pressure. It can affect the delivery of oxygen to the baby through the placenta. Sometimes it occurs with epidural analgesia.

HYPOTHYROIDISM

Low or inadequate levels of thyroid hormone in the bloodstream. (See discussion on page 121.)

HYPOVOLEMIA
(See HEMORRHAGE)

Lower than normal blood volume often due to bleeding.

HYPOXIA

A lack of sufficient oxygen. A baby may suffer hypoxia during labor if his mother's blood pressure falls, or his umbilical cord gets compressed.

HYSTERECTOMY, PERIPARTUM
(See HEMORRHAGE)

The removal of the uterus. It may done during the period surrounding birth in order to save a mother's life when there is uncontrollable bleeding.

I

ICEA

Stands for a nonprofit childbirth education organization, the International Childbirth Education Association. (See description on page 176, and *Resource Guide* on page 557 for contact information.)

IDENTICAL TWINS
(monozygotic twins)

Twins formed from the division of a single egg into two separate fetuses.

IMMUNE SYSTEM

The protective system of the body that fights the invasion of what it interprets as foreign substances such as bacteria, viruses, or fungi.

IMMUNIZATION

An injection that makes the body resistant to a certain virus or bacteria, such as hepatitis or the flu. When a body is exposed to a virus, its immune system will create fighters (antibodies) to eliminate the germ. If the body is exposed again, disease-fighting cells will recognize the bug and destroy it. Vaccines are made from killed, weakened, or genetically altered forms of a virus or bacteria, which activate the immune system to protect the body should it be exposed to virus later on. (See discussions on pages 204 and 435.)

INCISION

The cut made to open the body during surgery using a sharp knife (a scalpel).

INCOMPETENT CERVIX
(See CERCLAGE)

A cervix that dilates painlessly, without contractions, and may not be able to hold a baby inside. (See discussion on page 218.)

INCOMPLETE ABORTION
(See DILATION & CURETTAGE)

A miscarriage (losing the pregnancy naturally or through medical intervention) in which part, but not all, of the uterine contents are expelled. The remaining tissue can lead to infection or bleeding and needs to be removed.

INCONTINENCE
(See STRESS INCONTINENCE and URINARY INCONTINENCE)

The body's inability to hold in urine or feces. Sometimes incontinence is related to vaginal births, although many women who have it have never given birth.

INCUBATOR (ISOLETTE)

A small bed often made out of clear plastic for newborns that maintains an even temperature to keep the baby warm. Incubators are often used with vulnerable premature and low-birth-weight babies.

INDUCTION
(Induction of Labor, IOL)

Using artificial means to start labor. Medical induction is the use of drugs to cause the uterus to contract. Amniotomy is a form of induction by the breaking of the bag of waters in order to trigger labor. Sweeping the membranes induces labor by stimulating the release of hormones from the cervix. (See discussion on page 339.)

INEVITABLE ABORTION
(See MISCARRIAGE)

Pregnancy complicated with bleeding and cramping in which a miscarriage, the loss of the pregnancy, cannot be prevented.

INFANTICIDE

The purposeful killing of a baby.

INFECTION

An illness caused by the invasion of bacteria, viruses, or fungi. Infections often are signaled by a fever.

INFORMED CONSENT

Being given full information about a medical procedure or medication including benefits and known risks to enable a patient to make a decision about whether or not to agree to undergo it. In some cases, a patient may be asked to sign a form to provide a record that she has been fully informed of the potential consequences of a decision. Informed consent ensures that a patient is given adequate information by a healthcare provider and to protect the healthcare provider from a potential legal action should a patient later claim she was not properly informed about the risks or side effects of procedures or medications. (See discussion on page 274.)

INFUSION

The injection of a substance into a vein.

INHALATIONAL PNEUMONITIS

A rare and serious lung infection resulting from an unconscious patient inhaling stomach contents or acids during general anesthesia. The reason why, as a precaution, some healthcare providers feel mothers should not drink or eat during labor.

INSULIN

A hormone made by the pancreas that enables the body to use glucose in order to create energy for the body.

INTESTINAL MOTILITY

Movements of the intestines that force food from the stomach to the rectum. Increased levels of progesterone and other hormones during pregnancy can slow down the speed with which food moves through the stomach and intestines. This may contribute to nausea, vomiting, heartburn, and constipation.

INTRACRANIAL HEMORRHAGE
(ICH)

Bleeding inside or on the surface of the brain. In newborns, it can be related to trauma during birth, infection, prematurity, and many other factors.

INTRAPARTUM FEVER
(puerperal fever)

Fever occurring in a mother during labor and delivery. It can be caused by an infection of the lining of the uterus, the fluid surrounding the baby, a urinary tract infection, an oncoming cold, or viral or other infectious illness. It may also be caused by epidural analgesia during labor.

INTRAUTERINE GROWTH RETARDATION (IUGR, intrauterine growth restriction)

When a baby grows more slowly than normal during pregnancy.

INTRAVENOUS CATHETER (IV) (See IV)

A small needle or hollow tube (catheter) inserted into a vein in order to administer fluids or medications.

INTRAVENTRICULAR HEMORRHAGE (IVH)

Bleeding inside the brain, in the ventricles of the brain. In babies, usually related to prematurity.

IN UTERO

Within the uterus.

IN VITRO FERTILIZATION

The fertilization of an egg by a sperm conducted outside of the uterus and then implanted back into the body to grow.

INVERTED NIPPLES (flat nipples)

Normal nipples stick out from the areola, particularly when they are stimulated or become cold. Inverted nipples do not protrude out of the areola or become erect. Partially inverted nipples (dimpled or folded) will not protrude when stimulated but can be pulled out manually by the fingers, while a severely inverted nipple will retract more deeply into the areola when it is squeezed, making it level or recessed from the areola. The condition may affect a baby's latching on for breastfeeding, but correct positioning of the baby to the breast may help. (See breastfeeding positioning information on page 124.)

INVOLUTION

The process of the uterus returning to its normal size after birth.

IRON DEFICIENCY ANEMIA

A common condition of pregnancy, it is produced by not getting enough iron in the diet and can be treated with iron supplements, usually pills. (See discussion on page 218.)

ISCHIAL SPINES (See STATION)

Two bony knobs on the inside of the pelvis that are located at its narrowest point. The spines can be felt by hand and are used to gauge how far down a baby's head has moved during birth.

ISOIMMUNIZATION (See Rh FACTOR)

The development of immune fighters (antibodies) in a mother's body most commonly when she has Rh-negative blood cells and her baby has Rh-positive blood cells. It can be prevented with the administration of Rh Immunoglobulin.

ISOLETTE (incubator)

A small, enclosed bassinet used for extremely premature babies to help supply them with oxygen, keep them warm, and protect them from outside germs.

IUD (Intrauterine Device)

A small contraceptive device made of plastic or metal that is implanted in a woman's uterus to interfere with the passage of sperm reaching an egg. It may also discourage the implantation of a fertilized egg, if fertilization has managed to occur.

IV (Intravenous) (See INTRAVENOUS CATHETER)

Intravenous literally means "into a vein," and it is a method for providing fluid or infusing drugs into the body. Fluid is injected or dripped from a plastic bag suspended from a stand through a long tube and into a catheter inserted and taped onto the back of one hand, or along the forearm. IVs are used during labor and birth to prevent dehydration and can also be used to administer Pitocin®, a drug that strengthens and increases the number of contractions. IV risks include fluid overload in the mother, or redness and swelling at the insertion site.

IV SITE (SEE IV)
The place where an IV enters the skin, usually the back of the hand or in the forearm.

J

JAUNDICE (neonatal jaundice, icterus neonatorum)
In the first few days after birth, more than half of full-term babies and about 80 percent of premature babies who are otherwise healthy develop a yellowish discoloration of their skin and the whites of their eyes, called jaundice. While some babies are jaundiced at birth, most develop it during the second or third day of life. It is not a disease, and in most cases, means a baby's liver simply isn't mature enough to process a substance called bilirubin, which is created as the body recycles old or damaged red blood cells. It is not painful for the baby, but should the levels of bilirubin become too high (see kernicterus), it can cause brain damage. Usually jaundice disappears within one to two weeks. Your health-care practitioner may want to monitor your baby and may recommend the use of special treatment lights or sunlight to help the body break down the excess bilirubin. (See discussion on page 429.)

JPMA (Juvenile Products Manufacturers Association)
The trade organization for the makers of products for babies and young children. Products certified by the JPMA will have a sticker showing they adhere to voluntary safety standards that require testing of their product lines for safety and durability.

K

KANGAROO CARE (wearing your baby)
Modeled after how a mother kangaroo holds her baby (a joey) next to her bare chest in her pouch, it is the practice of giving babies skin-to-skin contact to help in soothing and nurturing them.

KAROTYPE
A picture of chromosomes from a cell that is enlarged and grouped for study.

KEGEL EXERCISES (Kegels)
Named after Dr. Arnold Kegel, these are a form of exercise that calls for the repeated contracting and releasing of the muscles that surround the anus and vagina and those used to stop urination. It's done to tone up the pelvic floor during pregnancy, to strengthen these muscles for childbirth, and to help control post-birth urine leaks (urinary incontinence) some mothers experience after giving birth.

KERNICTERUS (See JAUNDICE)
A rare complication of jaundice in which the base of the baby's brain and portions of the spine become invaded by excess bilirubin during the second to eighth day of life with serious consequences.

KETONES (KETOSIS)
Ketones are substances in the body produced by the body's fat processing (metabolism). Ketosis is the incomplete metabolism of fatty acids that can be caused by a lack of sufficient carbohydrates in the body or by diabetes mellitus. Ketosis can be tested in the urine.

L

LABIA

Literally means lips and refers to the two sets of skin folds that protect a woman's genitals. The outer set has pubic hair, the inner set does not.

LABOR

The act of giving birth beginning with the onset of periodic, rhythmical contractions, through the dilation of the cervix, the emergence of the baby, and the expelling of the placenta (afterbirth).

LABOR, BACK
(see BACK LABOR)

LABOR, LATENT (latent phase)

The early stage of labor that is characterized by regular contractions and slow dilation and effacement of the cervix that lasts about eight hours for first-time mothers, but is shorter for mothers who have given birth before. Typically, it ends when the cervix is approximately four centimeters dilated and has reached complete (100 percent) effacement. (See centimeter chart on page 284.)

LABOR, OBSTRUCTED

When labor slows or stops, and delivery may not be achieved without medical intervention, such as a cesarean delivery.

LABOR SUPPORT PERSON
(See DOULA)

Sometimes refers to a doula, or it can mean an inexperienced, untrained friend or relative whom you have chosen to accompany you through labor.

LABORING DOWN

A medical practice that allows a mother with an epidural to hold back from pushing until she has the urge to do so, or until certain signs of readiness appear, such as the position of the baby low in her body (at least one centimeter below the ischial spines), his head rotation, and the pulling back of the mouth of the uterus (cervix) during contractions.

LACERATIONS

A laceration is any sort of tear. In pregnancy, lacerations refer to tears in the opening of the vagina that occur during birth. The seriousness of the tear is usually expressed in degrees. A first-degree laceration is minor, involving only the superficial layers of skin. A fourth-degree laceration is the most serious, involving several layers of flesh to the rectum. It is more likely to occur with the use of episiotomies, forceps deliveries, and vacuum extractions.

LACTATION

Another word for breastfeeding or milk making.

LACTATION CONSULTANT

A person trained in advising mothers and medical personnel about breastfeeding.

LACTOSE INTOLERANCE

Some people, especially non-Caucasians, have symptoms such as bloating, diarrhea, gas, and indigestion after drinking milk or eating dairy products due to a lack of sufficient amounts of a certain digestive enzyme. (If you have this problem, note that milk is not the only source of calcium during pregnancy.)

LA LECHE LEAGUE (LLLI)

An international, nonprofit organization that provides information and support for expectant and breastfeeding mothers through trained leaders and monthly in-home group meetings, state level conferences, and bi-annual international conferences. It also provides a Web site and a national, toll-free information line. (See *Resource Guide* on page 547.)

LAMAZE INTERNATIONAL

An international organization to help parents preparing for childbirth. Its theories were initially developed by Dr. Ferdinand Lamaze based on the concept that the body and breathing control could help to control the experience of pain during labor and delivery. Lamaze has moved far beyond breathing instructions. Trained instructors teach mothers and supporting partners about the processes of pregnancy, birth, and baby care, and offer a variety of relaxation techniques to help allay fear and cope with discomfort during the different stages of labor.

LAMINARIA

Small rod-shaped pieces of dried seaweed, which, when placed within the mouth of the uterus (cervix), gradually cause it to widen for birth (dilate).

LANUGO

Soft, downy hair that covers the body of a baby in the uterus. Some babies are born with the hair.

LAPAROSCOPY

The viewing of the inside of the abdomen, such as the ovaries and fallopian tubes, using a viewing instrument (laparoscope) inserted through a small incision in the belly.

LARGE FOR GESTATIONAL AGE (LGA) (See MACROSOMIA)

A newborn weighing more than 90 percent of babies that are the same gestational age—approximately $9^{3}/_{4}$ pounds or more for a full-term newborn.

LCSW (See GRIEF, STAGES OF)

Stands for licensed clinical social worker. The skills of a social worker may be used to assist parents in planning for their baby's special needs or to help them in coping with the shock and grief of baby loss.

L&D (or LD)

Stands for labor and delivery. An L&D nurse specializes in helping mothers during the process of labor and delivery.

LDR (labor and delivery room)

Refers to the room where mothers labor and give birth in a hospital. They may then be transferred to a private or semi-private room until discharge.

LDPR (Labor Delivery Postpartum Room)

Refers to a room where mothers labor, give birth and stay until they are discharged from the hospital.

LENGTH OF STAY (LOS)

How long a patient stays in the hospital before going home. Current insurance practices usually allow a mother giving birth vaginally a two-day stay, and those having cesarean sections, three to four days.

LEOPOLD MANEUVERS

The way a midwife or obstetrician positions his hands to tell the position of a baby inside the mother's abdomen. The baby's head will feel hard and round and will move in response to a gentle push. The baby's rump feels larger than the head and bulkier and does not move much in response to pressure. The practitioner will then press in with his hands on the sides of the abdomen to tell the direction of the baby. The back of the baby will feel smooth and hard. The front will have both soft and hard bumps that move in response to pressure. Fingers are used to locate the baby's brow to determine if the head is well flexed and how low the baby has dropped into the pelvis.

LETDOWN (let-down reflex, milk-ejection reflex)

A letdown happens when the stimulation of a baby's sucking, the action of a breast pump, or a mother's images of breast-feeding cause hormones in a mother's body to stimulate her breasts to flow milk into ducts inside the breast so it flows toward the nipple. Sometimes milk will drip from the nipples, or even spew out in a steady stream.

LEUKORRHEA

White or yellowish discharge from the vagina that does not itch. (See discussion on page 137.)

LEVATOR ANI

The major muscle that helps to hold up a mother's pelvic floor and prevent loss of stool from the rectum.

LIE

Position of a baby during labor in relation to the mother's body. Longitudinal lie refers to a baby's body being parallel to the mother's spine. Transverse lie refers to a baby's lying crosswise.

LIGHTENING

When a baby moves lower and deeper into the pelvis in the weeks prior to the onset of labor.

LINEA NIGRA

A brownish or blackish line that runs from the top of the pubic bone to the belly button during pregnancy. It becomes more noticeable during the latter part of pregnancy.

LISTERIOSIS

A rare illness (only about four hundred cases of listeria are reported for pregnant women each year in the United States), listeriosis is caused by bacteria that may be found in certain foods such as unpasteurized milk products, undercooked poultry, and prepared meats, including hot dogs and sandwich meats, soft cheeses, raw vegetables, and shellfish. Its symptoms are similar

to the flu and can include fever, chills, headache, aches and pains, and sore throat. Samples of fluids from a mother's vagina, cervix, and blood and the baby's amniotic fluid may be checked if a provider is concerned a mother may have the disease. Listeriosis can also be transmitted during the baby's travel down the birth canal. It can lead to life-threatening blood infections and meningitis in the newborn.

LITHOTOMY POSITION

A position traditionally used in labor which places a woman on her back with her legs and feet spread apart with her knees bent. While it gives easy access for the provider to the head of the baby as it delivers, it can be an uncomfortable and ineffective position during the pushing (second) stage of labor. Patients can ask to try other positions, such as squatting, or lying on the left side. (See discussion of labor positions on pages 308–310.)

LMP (also LNMP)

Stands for last menstrual period or last normal menstrual period. It's shorthand term for the way pregnancy is dated, which is from the first day of normal menstrual bleeding prior to getting pregnant.

LOBI

Stands for low birthweight infant.

LOCAL ANESTHESIA (a local)

Any anesthetic injected to numb a small area on the body, usually lidocaine or novocaine. If a mother is given an episiotomy, she may be given a local while the incision is stitched up.

LOCHIA

Vaginal discharge after delivery. It resembles a heavy period that lasts for about six weeks after birth. (See discussion on page 377.)

LOW BIRTHWEIGHT BABY (LOW BIRTHWEIGHT INFANT, LBWI)

A baby weighing less than five pounds, eight ounces at birth. These babies have a greater chance of health problems. A very tiny, premature baby is referred to as an extremely low birthweight baby (ELBW). (See discussion of premature delivery on pages 217–218.)

LYMPHATIC SYSTEM

A series of glands, nodes, and vessels in the body that filter a clear or milky fluid called lymph. The body uses the lymphatic system to carry waste products away from the tissues and back into general circulation for removal from the body.

M

MACROSOMIA

When a baby is larger than average (e.g., $9\frac{3}{4}$ pounds). Sometimes a very large baby is related to a mother's having diabetes or a baby's being born later than its due date. A large newborn may also result from having a large parent. Sometimes a baby's size in relation to its mother can cause problems during and after delivery.

MAGNESIUM SULFATE

A medication sometimes used in an attempt to prevent premature birth. Also used for women with preeclampsia to decrease their chance of having a seizure (eclampsia).

MAGNETIC RESONANCE IMAGING (MRI)

A diagnostic tool, an MRI can be used to obtain a closer and clearer image of the baby (or a mother) than ultrasound. The procedure is non-invasive and is similar to getting an X-ray, but it uses a magnetic field and radio waves to create an image.

MALPOSITION (MALPRESENTATION)

When a baby's head or body is in an abnormal position during birth.

MAMMARY GLANDS

Milk-producing glands of the breast.

MANA (Midwives Alliance of North America)

An organization of midwives, student/ apprentice midwives, and persons supportive of midwifery that works to promote basic competency in midwives, and develops guidelines for their education. MANA offers legal, legislative, and political information and resource referrals for midwives. (See *Resource Guide* on page 565.)

MANEUVERS OF LEOPOLD (See LEOPOLD MANEUVERS)

MARIJUANA (cannabis, joint, or weed)

Like alcohol and tobacco, marijuana use during pregnancy has been linked to low birthweight and premature babies. Studies have shown that it can be associated with slow embryo growth and spontaneous abortion in the early stages of pregnancy. Symptoms such as excessive trembling and withdrawal-like irritability in newborns have also been associated with heavy marijuana use by the mother.

MASK OF PREGNANCY (See CHLOASMA)

MASTITIS

Inflammation of the breast with redness and tenderness in an area of the breast accompanied by fever, mastitis is usually caused by bacterial infection. It most often occurs to breastfeeding mothers. Sometimes there may be a discharge of pus. Treatment includes gentle massage, moist, warm compresses, nursing heavily on the affected side, and rest. In some instances, antibiotics may be recommended.

MATERNAL AND CHILD HEALTH NURSING

A field in nursing that specializes in the health of women, their partners, and their babies and children. It focuses on the problems associated with giving birth and rearing children.

MATERNAL-FETAL MEDICINE

A medical subspecialty of obstetrics that offers training in advanced fetal diagnosis, such as targeted ultrasound, skills in special surgeries, and interventions for fetuses prior to birth, such as transfusions, genetic counseling for parents, and management of severe pregnancy complications.

MATERNAL-FETAL MEDICINE SPECIALIST (MFM, perinatologist)

A fully trained medical doctor and obstetrician/gynecologist who has undergone three additional years of training in the management of special conditions during pregnancy such as high-risk pregnancies. He or she also cares for pregnant women that had medical conditions prior to their pregnancies, who develop medical or surgical problems during their pregnancies, or who carry a fetus with a problem.

MATERNAL MORTALITY RATE

The number of mothers who die during pregnancy or within forty-two days after birth in the United States, expressed as the number of deaths per 100,000 live births. The cause of death must be related to or aggravated by the pregnancy or its management. The rate excludes accidental, or non-pregnancy-related causes of death. The most common causes for maternal death are hemorrhage, embolism, and pregnancy-induced hypertension (eclampsia). The overall maternal mortality rate for 2000 was 9.8 deaths per 100,000 live births. The mortality rate for African-American mothers was 22 per 100,000, or roughly three times higher than for Caucasian mothers (7.5 per 100,000).

MATERNITY NURSING (perinatal nursing)

The field of nursing that focuses on the care of childbearing women and their families during pregnancy, childbirth, and the first four weeks afterward.

M.D.

Medical Doctor, Doctor of Medicine.

MEATUS

The outer opening of the urethra through which urine passes.

MECONIUM

The first bowel movements of a newborn. The BM can be dark green or yellow in color and tarry in consistency, consisting of cells, mucus, and bile. Once meconium has cleared the baby's system, its bowels will become softer and turn to green, and then to yellow, custardy stools if the baby is breastfed. The appearance of heavy meconium staining during the process of birth may indicate that a baby is in distress.

MECONIUM ASPIRATION (See ASPIRATION)

MECONIUM STAINING

When meconium stains the amniotic fluid. It sometimes indicates a baby is in trouble (non-reassuring status fetal distress).

MEDICAL GENETICIST

A physician who specializes in genetic disorders.

MEMBRANES

Refers to amnion and chorion that make up the amniotic sac, which contains the fluid in which a fetus floats inside the uterus.

MENINGITIS

A serious infection of the membranes of the brain or spinal cord that can result in disability or death, especially in infants and children.

MENINGOMYELOCELE

A congenital defect of the central nervous system of the baby. The covering of the spinal cord and sometimes the spinal cord itself protrude through an opening or defect in the vertebral column.

MENSTRUAL CYCLE

The monthly change in a woman's reproductive organs as they prepare the uterus for implantation if the egg is fertilized by a man's semen. A typical cycle lasts twenty-eight days and is counted from the first day of a woman's period to the first day of her next period. The ovaries usually release an egg approximately two weeks into the cycle.

MERCURY

A toxic substance that can harm an unborn baby's brain or nervous system. Found in high concentrations in certain fish, including shark, swordfish, king mackerel, or tilefish. Current recommendations include limiting the ingestion of these fish to two servings a week and taking a DHA (fish oil) supplement as an alternative source for omega-3 fatty acids thought to play a role in fetal brain development.

MFM (see MATERNAL-FETAL MEDICINE)

MICROCEPHALY

A birth defect in which the baby's brain fails to develop to a normal size.

MIDWIFE

A person with professional experience and/or training to provide health services and care for pregnant women during pregnancy, labor, birth, and immediately after birth. Midwives also assist in family planning.

MILIA

Harmless, tiny white spots on a newborn's nose, forehead, and cheeks that originate in the oil glands that disappear in the first few weeks of life. No treatment is needed.

MISCARRIAGE (spontaneous abortion)

The spontaneous loss of a pregnancy before the fetus can survive outside the uterus. Most miscarriages occur in the first trimester of pregnancy. They happen in 15–20 percent of all pregnancies. The causes of miscarriage are not completely known, but more than half of those that occur during the first trimester of pregnancy are caused by problems with the fetus' chromosomes. Other causes may be an infection in the uterus; the mother's hormonal imbalance; chronic disease, such as poorly controlled diabetes; or the chronic and heavy use of cigarettes, alcohol, or certain recreational drugs.

MISOPROSTOL (Cytotec®)

A drug used to soften the cervix and to induce labor. (See discussion on pages 336–337.)

MISSED ABORTION

During the first twenty weeks of pregnancy when an embryo or fetus dies but stays in a mother's uterus for four weeks or more afterward. Eventually, the mother will have a heavy, long period that releases the products of the pregnancy. Some women choose to have a dilation and curettage or to take medications in order to avoid heavy bleeding by encouraging the total expulsion of the products of the pregnancy.

MM (MILLIMETERS)
A measurement of size used, for example, in measuring the embryo or fetus during sonograms. There are ten millimeters in a centimeter and 25.4 millimeters in an inch.

MN
Master of Nursing.

MOHEL
A person of the Jewish faith who is legally certified and religiously ordained to perform circumcisions.

MOLAR PREGNANCY (See GESTATIONAL TROPHOBLASTIC DISEASE)

MOLDING
The temporary reshaping of a baby's head in order to pass through the birth canal.

MONGOLIAN SPOTS (blue-gray macules)
A birthmark of slate-blue discolorations resembling bruises that are commonly found on the lower back of newborns, particularly those of African, Indian, Asian, or Mediterranean descent. These marks are not signs of abuse, nor are they associated with mental retardation as some people believe. They usually, but not always, fade during the preschool years, and no treatment is required.

MONILIA (moniliasis) (See YEAST INFECTION)
A yeast infection. (See discussions on pages 138–139.)

MONITOR
In medical terminology, a machine to record vital body signs such as heart rate, breathing, and body temperature, or the length of contractions. Monitors can also be devices used to listen to baby sounds at home (nursery monitor) or to keep tabs on baby breathing (apnea monitor).

MONITRICE
A specially trained nurse who is usually hired by a doctor, a woman, or couple, to provide support, nursing care, and assessment during labor.

MONOZYGOTIC TWINS (See IDENTICAL TWINS)
Twins conceived from the splitting of one egg into two eggs.

MONS PUBIS (hairy mound)
The hair-covered, fatty pad over the top of a woman's pubic bone.

MONTGOMERY'S TUBERCLES (Montgomery's glands)
The small, goose pimple–like gland openings that supply lubrication to the areola (dark part) of the breast and alter the pH of the skin to discourage growth of bacteria.

MORNING SICKNESS (See HYPEREMESIS GRAVIDARIUM)
Nausea and vomiting, usually occurring during the first thirteen weeks of pregnancy. Although this is called morning sickness, it can strike any time during the day or night. Severe morning sickness, called hyperemesis gravidarium, when a mother can't keep down liquids or food, can cause serious dehydration and requires medical intervention. (See discussion on pages 40 and 129.)

MORO REFLEX
A primitive, preprogrammed reaction (reflex) seen in newborn babies, usually in response to noise or movement, such as tilting the baby's head backward. The baby will react by flinging its arms and legs wide open and will stiffen, usually

followed by crying. The reflex normally disappears spontaneously by four months of age. (See page 390.)

MORULA
A fertilized egg about three days following conception that consists of a cluster of thirteen to thirty-two cells. It moves down the fallopian tube to implant in the uterus.

MOTOR DEVELOPMENT
The way in which a baby's muscle skills become more sophisticated over time.

MOXIBUSTION
A traditional Chinese treatment to promote a baby's changing position near the time of birth from a head up (breech) position to a head down position. Herbs are burned to stimulate acupuncture points on the mother's body.

MSAFP (maternal serum alpha fetoprotein) (See ALPHA-FETO PROTEIN TEST)

MSCN (MSN)
Master of Science in Nursing.

MSD (mean sac diameter)
The size of the amniotic sac (bag of waters) that is usually measured by ultrasound during the early first trimester before the fetus is visible.

MSW (See SOCIAL WORKER)
The letters after a person's name signify that he has a master's degree in social work.

MUCOUS MEMBRANES
The moist surfaces lining the vagina, rectum, mouth, nose, and throat.

MUCUS PLUG (See SHOW)
A jellylike plug that serves to seal off the neck of the uterus (cervix) during pregnancy. It is chunky and can be pinkish, white, or clear. When it is discharged, it indicates that the cervix is starting to efface (pull up and become thinner) and dilate (spread open). Usually mothers discover it within hours or days of starting labor, but sometimes labor may not start for as long as several weeks after it appears. (See discussion of labor signs on pages 262–265.)

MULTIGRAVIDA
A person who has previously been pregnant. She may have aborted or delivered a viable baby.

MULTIPARA (multip)
A woman who has had more than one baby in the past weighing at least five hundred grams or twenty weeks old, regardless of whether the baby has lived or not. Sometimes written as para II, or para III, depending upon the number of births. A grandmultipara is a woman who has delivered five or more times. (See discussion on page 212.)

MULTIPLE PREGNANCY (multiple gestation)
When a mother is carrying more than one baby inside. Babies will initially be labeled as Twin A, Twin B, etc., depending upon which baby is anticipated to be born first.

MUTATION
A non-inherited genetic disorder that happens when an egg, sperm, or embryo undergo spontaneous changes.

MYOMETRIUM
The muscle layer of the uterus that does much of the work of labor.

N

NAEGELE'S RULE

A simple method for estimating a mother's expected due date. It works best if the mother has regular twenty-eight-day cycles with ovulation on day fourteen. From the mother's first day of her last period, add seven days, subtract three months, and add one year.

NARCOTICS

Drugs that reduce pain and anxiety by acting on the central nervous system. Common brand names are Nubain® and Demerol®. These drugs are sometimes used during birth, though they're not sufficiently powerful to totally eliminate pain. They are often used to "take the edge off" pain. Narcotics can be administered by mouth, as an injection, by inhalation, or through an IV. They may cross the placenta, and rarely, temporarily depress a baby's breathing after birth, which is treated by medication. Note that narcotic drugs can cause constipation, which can be very uncomfortable after birth.

NASW

National Association of Social Workers. It is used to signify that the social worker has been approved for practice by the national organization.

NATURAL ALIGNMENT PLATEAU

A period of time during labor when the cervix stops dilating although contractions continue. It often ends with a rapid dilation of the cervix.

NATURAL CHILDBIRTH (normal childbirth)

Childbirth without medical interventions, such as the use of analgesics, sedatives, or anesthesia. Mothers who choose natural childbirth rely more on personal encouragement and support during labor and birth than medical technology and obstetrical interventions. Bradley® and Lamaze, for instance, are considered natural, or normal childbirth methods. Proponents of natural birth use the term hospital birth to denote the opposite.

NAUSEA (See MORNING SICKNESS and HYPEREMESIS GRAVIDARIUM)

NEONATAL

Means near the time of birth—the period from the time the baby is born until it reaches four weeks of age. The term may also be used in titles of nurses and physicians specializing in dealing with problems of babies around the time of birth, i.e. neonatal nurses who specialize in the care of sick babies in the neonatal intensive care unit (NICU—sometimes pronounced nick'-ewe); neonatal nurse practitioners who specialize in training in the management of newborns and can perform some procedures usually done by physicians; and neonatologists, physicians who specialize in the care of premature babies and those with medical or surgical problems.

NEONATAL ABSTINENCE SYNDROME (baby drug withdrawal)

Babies whose mothers are addicted to heroin, barbiturates, amphetamines, or other drugs inherit their mothers' drug dependence. A baby may appear normal at birth but begin to show extreme irritability, constant crying, poor feeding, vomiting, diarrhea, respiratory problems, tremors, hyperactivity, and seizures within eight to ten hours after birth. The baby may be medicated temporarily and placed in a dim room to help it weather the withdrawal.

NEONATAL CLINICAL NURSE SPECIALIST

A registered nurse with a master's degree who is a specialist through study and supervised practice in care of newborns.

NEONATAL DEATH

Death of a live-born infant any time between birth and twenty-eight days.

NEONATAL INTENSIVE CARE UNIT (NICU, pronounced nick´-ewe)

An intensive care unit just for newborns where babies who are born too early or have special medical needs are taken after birth. Babies in NICU may have been premature or show signs of physical problems, such as breathing problems or fever. NICUs are staffed with specialists trained to care for babies with special needs. Some hospitals also have step-down units for babies needing long-term care who are not well enough for regular nursery care.

NEONATAL MORTALITY RATIO

The number of deaths of babies prior to twenty-eight days of life per 1,000 babies. The primary causes of neonatal mortality are prematurity, low birth-weight, and birth defects. In the year 2000, the U.S. neonatal mortality rate was 4.6 per 1,000 live births.

NEONATAL NURSE PRACTITIONER (NNP)

A registered nurse with clinical expertise in the nursing care of newborns. He can conduct assessments and diagnoses and manage caseloads of newborn patients in collaboration with physicians.

NEONATE

Another word for newborn.

NEONATOLOGIST

A physician specializing in pediatrics with advanced training in the care of sick newborns. Neonatologists often head neonatal intensive care units.

NEONATOLOGY (See PEDIATRIC NEONATOLOGY)

A specialty field in medicine and nursing for the care of premature and sick newborns that have special medical needs.

NESTING INSTINCT (nesting)

Many pregnant mothers feel a strong urge to prepare for their new babies as the time to go into labor nears. A nesting mother-to-be may feel an uncharacteristic surge of energy that she spends cleaning the house or organizing things. It's important, though, to consider conserving energy for the upcoming work of giving birth.

NEURAL TUBE DEFECT (NTD) (See ANENCEPHALY, HYDROCEPHALUS, and SPINA BIFIDA)

Any of a group of birth defects related to the fetal brain and spine. (See discussion on page 179.)

NEWBORN

Another name for a baby between birth and one month of age.

NFTD

Stands for normal full term delivery.

NICOTINE

A substance found in tobacco that can be potentially harmful to the fetus.

NICU (pronounced nick-ewe) (See NEONATAL INTENSIVE CARE UNIT)

NIPPLE CONFUSION

When newborns drink formula from an artificial nipple, they may adapt sucking patterns that interfere with suckling at their mothers' breasts.

NIPPLES, INVERTED (See INVERTED NIPPLES)

NONREASSURING FETAL STATUS (fetal distress)

A term that indicates concern that a baby is not receiving sufficient oxygen from the placenta. The baby may not move for a period of time or have a slower-than-normal heartbeat (60–80 beats per minute instead of a heart rate greater than 140).

NONSTRESS TEST (NST)

A way of measuring fetal activity in the uterus when there is a concern that the baby may not be thriving. An instrument strapped around a pregnant mother's abdomen measures the fetal heart rate. The mother is directed to push a button each time she feels the baby move, which is recorded on a paper. The fetus's heart rate is expected to rise when the mother senses movement.

NOTOCHORD

A rod of cells that appears in the sixth week of gestation that will eventually become your baby's spinal cord.

NPO (*Nil* per *Oram* [Latin])

Literally translated as nothing by mouth, the term refers to a medical order that restricts someone from eating and drinking to protect from vomiting and aspirating regurgitated matter into the lungs during general anesthesia (being put to sleep for surgery). The policy of preventing pregnant women from eating and drinking during labor is now no longer universally accepted unless there is a problem during labor. (See discussion on page 288.)

NUCHAL TRANSLUCENCY

In the first fifteen weeks after conception, fetal skin is very thin and semi-transparent from the fluid that gathers between the fetus's skin and underlying structures. When the baby has a chromosomal disorder, fluid tends to be increased. Excessive fluid is detected by ultrasound of the baby's neck (nuchal) area.

NULLIPARA (nullip, nulliparous [adj.])

A woman who has never delivered a viable baby.

NURSE-MIDWIFE

A nurse with special training and/or certification for assisting with birth (labor and delivery). Nurse-midwives can perform most of the same tasks as physicians including delivering a baby and most have a backup physician in the event of an emergency requiring surgical intervention, such as a cesarean delivery.

NURSE PRACTITIONER

A nurse who has completed a master's degree or post-master's degree program in a specialty and is certified to practice by the appropriate professional organization, such as obstetrics or neonatal medicine. Nurse practitioners can diagnose medical conditions, treat them, prescribe medications, and offer medical advice to families, but they do not deliver babies.

O

OB/GYN (Obstetrics & Gynecology)

Stands for obstetrics and gynecology (pronounced guy-nuh-kology).

OBSTETRIC EMERGENCY

A rare, severe, life-threatening condition related to pregnancy or delivery that requires urgent medical intervention to prevent the likely death of the mother or baby. Major signs of an obstetric emergency during pregnancy, birth, or within six weeks after giving birth include the following: heavy bleeding, high fever, convulsions, loss of consciousness, or severe blood loss (hemorrhage).

OBSTETRICIAN (An OB or an OB/GYN, an obstetrician gynecologist)

A physician with special training in providing medical care for women who are pregnant and giving birth. An OB can perform surgery, such as c-sections, if needed, or operative vaginal deliveries using forceps or vacuum extraction. Often, obstetricians also specialize in the reproductive health of women of all ages. In that case, they are often called by the initials of their specialty: an OB/GYN.

OBSTETRICS
(See OBSTETRICIAN)

The branch of medicine dealing with the management of pregnancy, labor, and the postpartum period (the first forty-two days after birth).

OBSTRUCTED LABOR
(See DYSTOCIA)

When labor doesn't progress at a normal, steady pace. The formal, medical term is dystocia. (See discussion on page 352.)

OLIGOHYDRAMNIOS

Abnormally low amount of fluid in the baby's amniotic sac during pregnancy.

OMPHALOCELE

A birth defect involving a failure of the abdominal wall to form at the place where the umbilical cord attaches to a baby's belly. If this occurs, the baby's intestines are usually protruding out of its belly into a sac. It can be repaired surgically after delivery.

OPERATIVE VAGINAL DELIVERY

Assisting the process of birth with the use of forceps or vacuum extraction when a mother's or baby's health is compromised during the process of labor or if the mother is having difficulty pushing the baby out. Medical terms are used to describe how deeply inside the mother forceps or vacuum extraction are applied. High or midpelvis refers to reaching into the highest point in the mother, followed by low, and outlet forceps deliveries when the baby is lower in the mother's birth canal or its scalp is already visible.

OPHTHALMIA NEONATORUM

A severe newborn eye infection of the lining of the eye and eyelids that occurs within the first ten days of life acquired by an infection of a mother's birth canal at the time of delivery. Gonorrhea is responsible for the great majority of cases, but it can also be caused by a staph infection, strep, and chlamydia. All states in the United States require that babies receive eye medication soon after birth to protect them from the blindness that may result from these infections.

OTITIS MEDIA

The medical name for a middle ear infection, an infection behind the eardrum.

OVARIAN CYST

A swelling of the ovary from fluid. It is most common in women after they start having periods and before they go through menopause. Most ovarian cysts are harmless.

OVARIES

The part of a woman's reproductive system that produces and releases eggs and secretes the hormones estrogen and progesterone into the bloodstream.

OVULATION

The release of an ovum (egg) from the ovary, which usually occurs around the middle of the menstrual cycle, or 14 days from beginning of the last period.

OVUM

A human egg.

OXYTOCIN (PITOCIN®)

A natural, and sometimes synthetic (manmade) hormone used to artificially start labor (called induction) by making the uterus contractions stronger. Its natural form in the body causes the uterus to contract and is involved in the let-down of breast milk.

OZ (OUNCE)
A measure of weight. There are sixteen ounces in a pound.

P

PA (Physician's Assistant)
Stands for physician's assistant, a person certified to provide basic medical services under the supervision of a licensed physician.

PALPATION
To feel with the hand, as in pressing down upon or massaging a mother's belly in order to determine the baby's position.

PARACERVICAL BLOCK
Local anesthetic for the cervix (the mouth of the womb).

PARTURITION
The giving of birth. Birthing mothers are sometimes called parturients.

PATENT DUCTUS ARTERIOSUS
A heart defect in newborns in which a part of the heart, the ductus arteriosus, stays open, causing excess blood flow into the lungs and potential heart failure.

PATIENT-CONTROLLED ANALGESIA (PCA)
A mechanical pump used to allow a mother to control the administration of pain-killing medication (analgesia) according to her need for pain relief. The pump regulates the amount of analgesia a mother receives over a period of time to prevent overdosing.

PCA (SEE PATIENT-CONTROLLED ANALGESIA)
Stands for patient-controlled analgesia.

PEDIATRICIAN
A physician with special training in the care of healthy and sick infants and children.

PELVIC FLOOR MUSCLES
A group of muscles inside the base of the pelvic bones that help to support the vagina, uterus, bladder, urethra, and rectum. These muscles also help to prevent leaking urine or bowel movements (incontinence). (See KEGEL EXERCISES.)

PELVIMETRY (See PELVIS, CONTRACTED)
Measurements taken by a healthcare provider using hands, an X-ray, or CT scan to determine the dimensions and proportions of a pregnant woman's pelvic bones in order determine if there is adequate space for a baby to pass through during labor and delivery.

PELVIS
The basin-shaped bones at the bottom the spinal column that connect the hip bones to the body. A baby must journey through the narrowest portion of the pelvis in order to be safely born. The size and shape of the pelvis are important measurements taken prior to birth. The pelvis bones are joined by ligaments that can stretch the pelvis by as much as one-third during birth, especially when a squatting position is used, or the mother is in an upright position.

PELVIS, CONTRACTED
Narrow pelvic bones in a mother that could conceivably interfere with the birth process. In severe cases, a cesarean delivery may be advised.

PERCUTANEOUS UMBILICAL BLOOD SAMPLING (PUBS)

A test for fetal problems in which blood is removed from the umbilical cord while the baby is still inside the mother's womb.

PERINATAL

The period shortly before and after birth. It is defined by various sources as beginning with the completion of the twentieth to the twenty-eighth week of pregnancy and ending anywhere between the seventh and twenty-eighth days following delivery.

PERINATAL DEATH

Death of a fetus occurring after the birth of a live baby between the time it weighs at least five hundred grams, or between the twentieth and twenty-eighth completed weeks of gestation and up through the seventh to twenty-eighth day after delivery.

PERINATOLOGIST (MFM, Maternal-Fetal Medicine Specialist)

A fully-trained medical doctor and obstetrician/gynecologist who has undergone three additional years of training in the management of special conditions during pregnancy such as high-risk pregnancies. He, or she, cares for pregnant women who had medical conditions prior to their pregnancies; who develop medical or surgical problems during their pregnancies; or who carry a fetus with a problem.

PERINEAL SUTURE

Stitches used to sew up tears or cuts made in a woman's perineum. (See episiotomy and discussion on pages 375–379.)

PERINEUM

The tissues and muscular structures that surround the vagina.

P.G. (Preggo, Preggers)

Slang for being pregnant. "I'm P.G.," or "I'm preggo."

PHENYLKETONURIA (PKU)

A condition in babies found at birth in which the body lacks a specific enzyme that can lead to abnormal metabolism and, when untreated, could result in brain damage.

PHOSPHATIDYL GYLCEROL

A substance in the family of chemicals called surfactants that is present when fetal lungs are mature. If a baby's lungs are immature (prior to thirty-eight weeks of pregnancy), surfactants may not present in sufficient quantities, which will affect a baby's ability to breathe after birth.

PHOTOTHERAPY

A treatment for babies with jaundice. These bright lights, called bililights, help babies breakdown bilirubin in their blood. Excessive levels of bilirubin are the cause of neonatal jaundice.

PHYSIOLOGIC ANEMIA OF PREGNANCY (See ANEMIA)

Anemia during pregnancy caused by an increase in the amount of plasma (fluid) in the blood compared with the number of cells in the blood.

P.I.

Stands for premature infant.

PICA (pronounced pye-ka)

The strong urge by some pregnant women to eat nonfood items such as clay, ice, laundry starch, cornstarch, plaster, or dirt. It is thought to be related to anemia.

PITOCIN (See OXYTOCIN)

A synthetic form of oxytocin.

PITUITARY GLAND (See SHEEHAN'S SYNDROME)

A gland located in the center of the front of the brain that produces a variety of hormones that have many jobs, including signaling the breasts to produce milk in a mother. A mother's pituitary gland may be affected by hemorrhage.

PLACENTA

A red, round fleshy organ resembling a large piece of liver about six to seven inches in diameter at birth. It forms and grows alongside the baby inside and is fastened to the side of one wall of the uterus with tiny, fingerlike projections called villi. The placenta extracts oxygen and nutrition from the mother's blood and transfers it to the fetus's blood. The expelling of the placenta after a baby is born is known as the third stage of labor. (See AFTERBIRTH.)

PLACENTA ACCRETA

When the placenta slightly invades the muscles of the uterus during pregnancy making it difficult to remove after birth. Sometimes with the condition, the placenta will not separate, and a removal of the uterus is necessary after delivery of the baby in order to stop the mother from bleeding.

PLACENTA INCRETA (See PLACENTA ACCRETA)

When the villi of the placenta penetrate deep into uterine muscles.

PLACENTAL ABRUPTION (placenta abruption)

When the placenta separates from the uterus wall prior to the delivery of the baby.

PLACENTAMEGALY

When the placenta undergoes abnormally large growth during pregnancy.

PLACENTA PERCRETA (See PLACENTA ACCRETA)

When the villi of the placenta penetrate completely through uterine muscles.

PLACENTA PREVIA

When the placenta is abnormally positioned over the mouth of the uterus (cervix), it can result in serious bleeding during mid- or late pregnancy. Even though placenta previa may be noted on an ultrasound during the first two trimesters of pregnancy, it may not actually cover the cervix by the time labor begins. If it doesn't move out of the way, a cesarean delivery may be necessary.

PNEUMONITIS, INHALATIONAL (See INHALATIONAL PNEUMONITIS)

POLYCYTHEMIA

When a newborn's red blood cell count (hematocrit) reaches such a mass that the blood is too thick to flow through an individual's body. In newborns it may be associated with low blood sugar, sluggishness, poor feeding, jitteriness, possibly seizures, respiratory distress, and blood clots. The baby's blood may be thinned through a special transfusion. Potential causes are intrauterine growth restriction, a mother's diabetes mellitus, asphyxia, some medications taken by mothers, smoking, and pregnancy at a high altitude. The blood condition can result in neonatal jaundice.

POLYDACTYLY

When a baby is born with extra fingers or toes.

POLYHYDRAMNIOS

An excessive amount of amniotic fluid during pregnancy.

POLYP
A small growth of tissue in the lining of the uterus or the intestines. It is usually harmless during pregnancy.

PORT WINE STAIN
A birthmark that appears as a patch of reddish-blue skin. Your healthcare provider should evaluate it since it is sometimes associated with genetic problems.

POSITIONAL APNEA
Refers to interrupted breathing that may occur in a premature or low–birthweight baby as the result of being placed in a sharply angled, nearly upright position, such as that provided by a rear-facing infant seat. If a baby is suspected of having positional apnea, a healthcare practitioner may suggest ways to pad the car seat, or recommend that a flat infant bed be used that is designed specifically for restraining a small baby in a fully reclined position while riding in the car.

POSTDATE PREGNANCY
(See POSTTERM PREGNANCY)
A pregnancy that lasts longer than forty-two weeks of gestation.

POSTDURAL HEADACHE
(spinal headache)
A headache that results when the needle used to place an epidural catheter for epidural analgesia accidentally punctures the covering of the spinal cord, causing seepage of spinal fluid into the epidural space. It is less common due to the increased sophistication of the procedure including the use of better needles for the injection of painkilling liquid into the epidural space (the space outside the sac that covers the spinal cord).

POSTERIOR PRESENTATION
(occiput posterior)
When the back of the head of the baby presses on the back of the mother. A baby's being in this position can play a part in back labor and may make it more difficult for the mother to push the baby out.

POSTMATURE PREGNANCY
A pregnancy that lasts longer than forty-two weeks.

POSTNATAL PERIOD
The time following delivery, usually between birth and ten to twenty-eight days, when mothers and babies are carefully watched for complications.

POSTPARTUM
After delivery.

POSTPARTUM DEPRESSION
(PPD)
PPD can set in any time during the year after a baby is born. It affects ten to fifteen percent of new mothers and is more serious and prolonged than baby blues. It requires professional help.

POSTPARTUM ENDOMETRITIS
(See INTRAPARTUM FEVER)
Swelling and infection in the inner layer of the uterus following birth. Its symptoms are a fever, a uterus that is tender to the touch, discharge from the vagina that is foul-smelling, and a change in blood cells due to infection. It is treated with a strong course of antibiotics. The infection occurs in approximately one to three percent of women who have given birth vaginally and between ten to thirty percent of women following cesarean sections. It remains one of the leading causes of death from cesarean

section, although the aggressive use of antibiotics has made that occurrence extremely rare.

POSTPARTUM HEMORRHAGE (See HEMORRHAGE)

POSTPARTUM PSYCHOSIS

Mental illness that is precipitated by pregnancy and birth. It is rare and affects approximately 0.1 percent of new mothers (or about one out of one thousand women). It can happen any time during the first year after childbirth and is marked by a break with reality that resembles bipolar disorder. Symptoms may include hallucinations (seeing things that aren't there) and delusions (believing things that aren't true). Professional intervention is needed.

POSTPARTUM THYROIDITIS

Fluctuating thyroid function after childbirth. Symptoms may include fatigue, anxiety, emotional ups and downs, and feelings of weakness and tiredness. It is not usually associated with a painful or tender thyroid gland, which is located in the center of the neck. (See discussion on page 385.)

POST-TERM GESTATION (See POST-TERM PREGNANCY)

POST-TERM PREGNANCY (post-mature pregnancy, post-term gestation)

A pregnancy that lasts beyond forty-two weeks from the first day of the mother's last period. About 95 percent of babies born after forty-two weeks are normal, though the risk of a poor pregnancy outcome increases the longer a woman's pregnancy extends beyond this time. Between 3 and 12 percent of all pregnancies last beyond the forty-second week of gestation, or 294 days. Many cases of post-term pregnancy are simply the result of inaccurate estimations about

a baby's age, but when pregnancy is prolonged, labor may be induced.

POST-TRAUMATIC BIRTH DISORDER (post-traumatic stress disorder)

Severe emotional turmoil following birth experienced by some women whose births were complicated, or who have perceived that mistakes were made during their deliveries. It is more common in women who had previous emotional vulnerabilities prior to giving birth, such as a history of emotional, physical, or sexual abuse. Symptoms include feelings of panic when nearing the place where the birth occurred; obsessive thoughts about the birth; feelings of numbness and detachment; disturbing memories of the birth experience; nightmares; flashbacks; and unexplainable sadness, fearfulness, anxiety, or irritability.

PRECIPITOUS BIRTH

Labor and delivery that lasts less than three hours.

PREECLAMPSIA (toxemia) (See ECLAMPSIA)

A complication of pregnancy that occurs after the 20th week of pregnancy. Sometimes it can be silent with no outward symptoms, but a mother will have protein in her urine and high blood pressure. Physical symptoms include rapid weight gain and swelling in fingers, face, and ankles from fluid retention. A mother may also experience odd vision problems such as blurring or headaches. The causes of preeclampsia are not completely understood, but poor nutrition and genetic predisposition are thought to be contributors. Preeclampsia (toxemia) left untreated can turn into seizures (eclampsia) and could lead to coma and possibly death. (See discussion on pages 215 and 355.)

PREGNANCY GINGIVITIS

Pregnant women often have swollen red gums that are tender to the touch and bleed easily. This condition is thought to be caused by hormonal changes in the body plus the buildup of a bacterial film on the teeth. Swelling generally starts during the second month of pregnancy and reaches a peak during the last month and a half before birth. The condition can last from three to six months after delivery and can be mild or severe depending upon the condition of gums prior to pregnancy. Effective dental hygiene, including frequent brushing and flossing, and having the teeth cleaned are thought to be important treatments for the condition.

PREGNANCY-INDUCED HYPERTENSION (PIH)

A condition of pregnancy marked by high blood pressure that occurs after twenty weeks of pregnancy.

PREMATURE BABY (PREEMIE)

A baby that comes early, that is, one that is born before thirty-seven weeks of gestation.

PREMATURE LABOR (See PRETERM LABOR)

PREMATURE RUPTURE OF MEMBRANES (PROM) (See AMNIOTOMY)

When the bag of waters ruptures prior to going into labor so that fluid drains from the vagina. Often labor soon ensues after this happens, but if it doesn't, there is a risk of complications or infection that may be controlled using antibiotics and delivery of the baby. (See discussion on page 353.)

PRENATAL

Means before birth. Prenatal checkups refer to a mother getting regular exams throughout her pregnancy.

PRENATAL CARE

Medical care during pregnancy that includes assessing a mother's risk and interventions to help reduce the risk of a poor pregnancy outcome.

PREPUCE

The foreskin, the fold of skin that naturally covers the tip (glans) of the penis. Circumcision surgically removes it.

PRESENTATION

The part of the baby that will deliver first. Cephalic presentation is head first; breech presentation is the buttocks or leg.

PRESENTING PART

The part of the baby's anatomy that delivers first, usually the skull, but it could be an arm, or the buttocks or a leg in a breech presentation.

PRETERM BABY (premature baby)

A baby born before thirty-seven weeks of pregnancy, regardless of weight.

PRETERM DELIVERY (PTD, preterm birth)

Delivery of a baby prior to thirty-seven weeks of completed pregnancy that happens in five to sixteen percent of all deliveries. Currently, PTD can rarely be predicted, prevented, or effectively treated. Some factors thought to contribute to preterm delivery include infection, abnormalities in the baby or uterus, problems with the placenta, bleeding caused by pregnancy, multiple gestation (twins, etc.), premature rupture of the amniotic sac (bag of waters), and hydramnios (too much fluid in the amniotic sac). But in one-third to one-half of the cases, there is no known cause for PTD.

PRETERM LABOR
Labor that happens after twenty weeks of pregnancy, but before the end of the thirty-seventh week. It includes regular contractions occurring at intervals ten minutes apart or less for at least an hour, accompanied by changes in the cervix.

**PRICKLY HEAT
(See HEAT RASH)**

**PRIMAGRAVIDA
(pronounced pry-me-grav-ida)**
A woman who is pregnant for the first time.

PRIMIPARA (PRIMIP, PRIMY)
A woman who has given birth for the first time to a baby or babies, alive or dead, weighing at least five hundred grams from a pregnancy that has lasted at least twenty weeks.

**PRODROMAL LABOR
(false labor) (See FALSE LABOR)**
Another term for Braxton–Hicks contractions or any contractions that happen before actual labor sets in. Sometimes it is called false labor, though it is a legitimate form of preparation that the uterus goes through prior to giving birth. (See discussion on page 266.)

PROGESTERONE
A hormone that keeps the uterus from contracting and promotes the growth of blood vessels in the wall of the uterus.

PROGNOSIS
A prediction about the course of a disease and its outcome. A poor prognosis means that a mother, or baby, may not be expected to do well (or survive).

PROLACTIN
A hormone that is involved in the production of breast milk. Called the mothering hormone, prolactin together with oxytocin are thought to be partly responsible for the strong feelings of attachment that mothers have toward their babies. During pregnancy, prolactin speeds the growth of breast tissues in preparation for breastfeeding.

PROLAPSED CORD (prolapse)
When a loop of a baby's umbilical cord slips down below the body and into the birth canal during birth.

PROLONGED LABOR
A labor lasting more than eighteen to twenty-four hours.

PROLONGED PREGNANCY
A pregnancy that lasts longer than forty weeks of gestation.

PROMETHAZINE
An antihistamine given by injection, often with a narcotic, to counteract nausea and relieve pain during the early stages of labor.

PROSTAGLANDINS (PGE-2)
A hormone sometimes used as a drug, to ripen and soften an unready cervix in order to induce labor. It is not recommended for use with mothers who have certain forms of heart disease or severe asthma.

PROTEIN
Proteins are chains of amino acids that are required to repair and build the body tissue especially needed for fetal growth. Common sources of protein for pregnancy are milk, eggs, cheese, fish, meat, beans, tofu, and some vegetables. (See dietary recommendations on page 382.)

PROTEINURIA
When protein is found in the urine. Sometimes a sign of preeclampsia.

**PROTRACTED LABOR
(See LABOR, OBSTRUCTED)**
A labor that lasts longer than expected.

PRURITIS GRAVIDARIUM
Itching during pregnancy.

PUBIC SYMPHYSIS
The front part of the pelvis. The bony ridge at the top of the pubic symphysis is used for measuring the growth of the uterus up into the abdominal area.

PUBOCOCCYGEUS MUSCLE (PC)
One of the muscles of the pelvic floor. This muscle is tightened when doing Kegel exercises.

PUDENDAL BLOCK
A type of pain relief frequently used just prior to delivery. It is injected through the walls of the vagina to numb the vaginal area.

PUERPERAL FEVER (See PUERPERAL SEPSIS)

PUERPERAL SEPSIS (puerperal fever, puerperal infection) (See INTRAPARTUM FEVER)
A maternal infection around the time of childbirth that can be a cause of maternal death if it is not treated in time.

PUERPERIUM
A period of time following delivery that lasts about six to eight weeks when a mother's reproductive organs and body gradually return to the prepregnancy state. The uterus undergoes involution, a remarkable reduction in size. There is also a discharge of blood and other fluids, called lochia, for four to six weeks following pregnancy.

Q

QUICKENING
The moment a mother first feels her baby move. The sensation is similar to a slight flutter or gas bubbles in the belly. While ultrasound can often pick up fetal movement around the eighth week of menstrual age, most mothers don't detect it until about the eighteenth to the twenty-second week. If the placenta has attached to the front of the uterus, a mother may not experience a baby's movement until the fetus is larger.

R

RDS (See RESPIRATORY DISTRESS SYNDROME)

RECALL
Baby products routinely undergo federally mandated recalls or corrective actions when serious safety flaws are discovered. Unsafe products may be removed from the marketplace, or they may simply be furnished with new components to make them safer. Cribs, strollers, toys, and other baby products are recalled by the U.S. Consumer Product Safety Commission (CPSC), car seats by the National Highway Traffic Safety Administration (NHTSA), and baby formula and cosmetics by the Food and Drug Administration (FDA). (See *Resource Guide*, on page 560, and discussion on pages 469 and 472 of the *Baby Gear Guide*.)

RECESSIVE DISORDER
A genetic disorder that is transmitted to a child when both parents are carriers of defective genes.

RECTUM

Lower part of the large intestine about five inches (12.7 cm) in length that connects from the colon to the anus, the outward opening for bowel movements.

RECTUS ABDOMINUS

The two muscles that run parallel to one another down the front of the abdominal wall, on each side of the belly button to the pubic bone. During pregnancy, the muscles and the tissues that connect them stretch to accommodate a mother's expanding belly, sometimes causing the muscles to draw apart. (See DIASTASIS RECTI.)

RECURRENT ABORTION

When a mother has lost two or more babies to miscarriages.

RED BLOOD CELLS

Cells in the blood that carry oxygen and carbon dioxide to and from the tissues of the body.

REGIONAL ANESTHESIA

Numbing of just the lower part of a mother's body during labor, in contrast to general anesthesia, which puts the mother totally to sleep.

RELAXIN

A hormone produced by a pregnant mother's ovaries and uterus during the latter months of pregnancy. It is thought to play a part in the loosening of the ligaments holding the joints together and may play a part in the ability of the pelvic bones to expand during birth.

RESIDENT

A physician who has completed an M.D. degree and is in the process of training in a specialty under the supervision of experienced specialists, such as obstetricians or pediatricians.

RESPIRATORY DEPRESSION

Slowed or shallow breathing that can be caused by medications that a mother is taking. It may occur temporarily when a mother hyperventilates (breathes too fast) during birth.

RESPIRATORY DISTRESS SYNDROME (RDS, hyaline membrane disease)

A lung condition occurring in some premature babies when their lungs don't completely expand or expand imperfectly. It can be caused by the lack of a surfactant in the airway. Treatments include giving the baby oxygen and administering a surfactant.

RETAINED PLACENTA

When the placenta (afterbirth) remains in the uterus for thirty minutes or more after birth. Action is usually taken to remove the placenta at that time to help lower the risk of infection and heavy bleeding (hemorrhage).

RETINOPATHY OF PREMATURITY (ROP, retrolental fibroplasia)

An eye condition that can develop in very premature newborns. In milder cases, a premature baby's eyes will recover, but if the baby is very immature, the blood vessels within the retina may not have had adequate time to grow, and the baby may be visually impaired or blind.

RETRACTION

The unique muscle process in the uterus by which its muscle fibers shorten after each contraction.

RETROLENTAL FIBROPLASIA (See RETINOPATHY OF PREMATURITY)

RETROVERTED UTERUS
(tipped uterus, tilted uterus)

Normally the uterus is suspended in a straight up-and-down position, or it tips slightly forward toward the abdomen. A retroverted uterus tips or tilts backward, pointing toward the spine. The condition is usually inherited, but pregnancy can also cause the uterus to tilt backward when the ligaments holding the uterus stretch, or relax. In most cases, the uterus will return to a forward-facing position after childbirth. The condition can sometimes result in painful sex.

RHESUS ANTI-D GAMMA GLOBULIN INJECTION
(Rh IMMUNOGLOBULIN [Rhlg], Rhogam)

An injection given to Rh negative pregnant woman at twenty-eight weeks of pregnancy, or at the time of an amniocentesis, to prevent the development of antibodies that could be harmful to the baby. If the baby is Rh-positive, the injection will be given again within seventy-two hours following birth.

Rh FACTOR (Rh blood factor)

A protein found in the blood serum. If a mother has this substance, she is considered Rh-positive; if she does not have it, she is Rh-negative. (Rh stands for rhesus.) An Rh-negative mother carrying an Rh-positive baby may produce antibodies against the fetus that attack the fetus's blood. Rh incompatibility requires special care during pregnancy. (See discussion on page 188.)

Rh IMMUNOGLOBULIN (Rhlg)
(See RHESUS ANTI-D GAMMA GLOBULIN INJECTION)

Rhogam (See RHESUS ANTI-D GAMMA GLOBULIN INJECTION)

RINGER'S LACTATE SOLUTION

A special salt solution used in an IV (intravenous tube) designed to replace the body's fluid loss. Its main ingredients are sodium, potassium, and calcium balanced with chloride and lactate.

ROOTING

Instinctive head and mouth movements of a baby (reflexes) that help it in finding its mother's nipple. A baby will turn his head toward the nipple, open his mouth, and extend his tongue to enclose the nipple for nursing.

ROUND-LIGAMENT PAIN

Pain caused by ligaments stretching on the sides of the uterus during pregnancy.

RSV DISEASE
(Respiratory Syncytial Virus)

RSV infects nearly all children by the time they reach two. It usually causes mild coldlike symptoms, but in premature babies with vulnerable lungs, the infection can be serious and potentially fatal. Babies are more at risk of catching RSV if they are in child care, have school-age siblings, or are exposed to tobacco smoke.

RUBELLA (German measles, 3-day measles)

A highly contagious form of measles causing a red rash that is usually mild, which can cause severe damage to a fetus if contracted during the early months of pregnancy.

RUPTURE OF MEMBRANES
(breaking of waters, amniotomy)
(See ARTIFICIAL RUPTURE OF MEMBRANES)

The membranes make up the amniotic sac, the tissue-like balloon where the fetus floats inside the uterus during pregnancy. It will rupture naturally

during the process of labor, or sometimes earlier, or it may be intentionally
ruptured to start labor. If the waters
rupture, and labor doesn't start right
away, the baby's umbilical cord could
come out first, cutting off his oxygen
supply. Also, mother and baby may be
more vulnerable to infection.

RVC (Rectal/Vaginal Culture) (See GROUP B STREPTOCOCCUS)

A test to determine if a mother is carrying Group B Strep during pregnancy or
labor.

S

SAC (See AMNIOTIC SAC, MEMBRANES)

SCAN (See ULTRASOUND)

Another term for an ultrasound examination or a sonogram. (See discussion on
pages 191–192.)

SCIATIC NERVE

The largest nerve in the body, it is the
diameter of the little finger. It runs from
the spinal column down the legs and
provides sensation and movement to
the back of the thighs, the lower parts
of the leg, and the soles of the feet.

SCIATICA (pinched nerve) (See SCIATIC NERVE)

During pregnancy, pressure from the
baby or inflammation to the sciatic
nerve can cause pain, burning, tingling,
numbness, or electric shock–like, shooting sensations that follow the path of the
nerve. The mother's changing positions,
such as lying on the opposite side from
the pain, doing gentle stretching exercises, or elevating one leg can sometimes
bring relief.

SCM (State Certified Midwife)

SDMS

Member of the Society of Diagnostic
Medical Sonographers, persons trained
to perform ultrasound tests.

SEMEN

White fluid containing sperm from a
man's penis that fertilize an egg (ovum),
which causes pregnancy. Semen is
ejaculated (spewed out) during sex.

SEPSIS

The presence of infection in the blood.

SEXUALLY TRANSMITTED DISEASE (STD)

An infection transmitted primarily
through sexual contact between a man
and a woman. Syphilis and gonorrhea
are two STDs that can seriously harm
unborn babies. (See discussion on pages
219–222.)

SHEEHAN'S SYNDROME (postpartum pituitary necrosis)

When a mother's pituitary gland dies
as the result of severe bleeding (hemorrhage) following childbirth. Symptoms
are a cessation of periods, shrinking of
the genitals, and premature aging.

SHOULDER DYSTOCIA

When a baby's shoulders become
entrapped in the bones of the mother's
pelvis following the delivery of his head.
It is rare and can be life-threatening for
the baby.

SHOW (bloody show)

A discharge from the vagina of a jelly-
like mucus plug that serves to seal off
the neck of the uterus (cervix) during
pregnancy. It is chunky and can be
pinkish, white, or clear. Show indicates
that the cervix is starting to efface
(get thinner) and dilate (open). Usually

mothers discover show within hours or days of starting labor, but sometimes labor may not begin for as long as several weeks after it appears.

SICKLE-CELL ANEMIA

A genetic disorder that occurs in families of African descent that causes red blood cells to be crescent shaped, rather than round, and to clump in small capillaries so that the body has trouble getting adequate oxygen from the blood. The result is anemia, fatigue, delayed growth, and development and episodes of severe, debilitating pain.

SICKLE-CELL TRAIT

A disorder in which a mother carries the trait of sickle-cell anemia, but her red blood cells have a normal lifespan. Presence of the trait for sickle-cell anemia is not sickle-cell disease itself.

SKIN-TO-SKIN CONTACT

Allowing a newborn to lie chest-to-chest on its mother's body in order to help with mother/baby bonding, breastfeeding, and maintaining the baby's body temperature.

SLEEP APNEA (Obstructive Sleep Apnea—OSA) (See also APNEA and POSITIONAL APNEA)

Some pregnant women develop breathing problems as the result of physical changes during pregnancy, such as changes in the upper airway, increased nasal congestion, and pressure from the baby on the mother's lower chest. Symptoms can be breathing irregularity, snoring and restlessness during sleep, and exhaustion after awakening. Treatment includes adequate hydration, nasal strips, adopting a semi-upright position, and, for serious cases, the use of a mask attached to a ventilation machine to offer a continuous air supply. Some premature babies also suffer from sleep apnea.

SLIUP (SINGLE LIVING INTRAUTERINE PREGNANCY)

A single, live pregnancy in the womb.

SMALL FOR GESTATIONAL AGE (SGA)

A newborn that is less than the smallest ten percent of babies of a similar gestational age. It may mean that the baby is not growing as well as it should; that a mother's due date hasn't been calculated accurately, or simply that a baby is taking after his small parents.

SMEGMA

A white, curdlike substance that forms under the folds of an uncircumcised boy's foreskin and in the folds of a girl's vagina. It serves to moisturize and lubricate delicate genital tissues. Smegma has antibacterial and antiviral properties to protect from infection, so there is no need to try to wash or wipe it off.

SMFM

An abbreviation for the organization Society of Maternal-Fetal Medicine.

SONOGRAM (See ULTRASOUND)

An ultrasound image of your baby inside your uterus. (See discussion on pages 191–192.)

SONOGRAPHER (ultrasound technologist, scanner)

The person who performs an ultrasound (sonogram) examination.

SONOLOGIST

A physician specifically trained to perform ultrasound examinations and to interpret their findings.

SPECULUM

A plastic or metal device used to spread a woman's vaginal opening in order to make viewing the mouth of the womb (cervix) easier.

SPIDER VEINS (spider nevi, telangiectasias, angioma)

Small, red or blue blood vessels that appear close to the surface of the skin during pregnancy. They resemble the branching pattern of a tree or a spider web with short jagged lines and appear on the nose or cheeks, or sometimes on the back, chest, or arms. They usually disappear by six weeks after delivery.

SPINA BIFIDA

A defect in the spine of a fetus that results in the failure of the vertebra to fuse. It can occur anywhere along the spine, but most often the condition happens at the base of the back or lower spine. In some cases, folic acid deficiencies in the mother can result in this condition.

SPINAL BLOCK (spinal anesthesia) (See EPIDURAL)

A spinal block is similar to an epidural. An anesthetic injected into the spaces surrounding the spinal cord to numb the lower half of the body. After the numbing medicine is put in the mother's back, an anesthetic medicine is injected; however, the tube is not left in place as in an epidural. The spinal lasts for a limited time, and it is usually done shortly before birth. Sometimes it may cause a mother's blood pressure to drop, and this may be treated with intravenous (IV) fluids and medication.

SPINAL HEADACHE (See BLOOD PATCH)

SPONTANEOUS ABORTION

Another name for miscarriage, the loss of a baby during the first twenty weeks of pregnancy.

SPONTANEOUS LABOR

Labor that starts on its own without the use of medical augmentation, such as drugs that cause the uterus to contract (induction) or the artificial rupture of the membranes.

SPONTANEOUS MISCARRIAGE (spontaneous abortion)

When the body discharges a baby before the baby is ready to be born.

STAGES OF LABOR

Labor is divided into three stages. The first stage is from the onset of labor until the cervix, the mouth of the uterus, is completely thinned (effaced) and stretched open (dilated). The second stage is the pushing stage during which the baby is ejected from the uterus. It lasts from full dilation of the cervix until the baby is born. The third stage lasts from the birth of the baby until the placenta and membranes have been expelled. (Stages of labor are discussed starting on page 281.)

STATION

The location of a birthing baby's head in relation to the ischial spines, small bony knobs inside the pelvis. The location of the baby's presenting part is measured in centimeters. A baby above the ischial spines is said to be at a minus station using numbers to indicate the exact location (-3, -2, -1). The baby is said to be at the 0 (zero) station if the presenting part is level with the spines. Positive numbers (+1, +2, +3) indicate that the baby's head is below the ischial spines and therefore closer to being born.

STEM CELLS

A basic blood cell, or mother cell, found in a baby's umbilical cord blood that can reproduce and give rise to different blood cell lines of distinct characteristics and appearance. Cord blood stem cells make red blood cells for carrying oxygen, white blood cells for fighting infections, and platelets for clotting blood. Stem cells have been used experimentally to help in treating patients with leukemia and other blood disorders.

STEP-DOWN NURSERY

Where babies are sometimes sent after being discharged from the neonatal intensive care unit (NICU), but before they are moved to a standard nursery. The care in a step-down nursery is less intensive than in the NICU, but more specialized than nurseries for healthy newborns.

STILLBIRTH (intrauterine death, intrauterine stillbirth, intrapartum death, or intrapartum stillbirth)

When a baby dies inside its mother or during the process of being born. The exact cause of a baby's dying is often difficult to pinpoint, although research shows that stillbirth happens more often in pregnancies with multiple babies, to mothers who smoke, those with previous cesarean sections, and to those who are over thirty-five years of age. (See discussion on page 346.)

STILLBORN (STILLB.)

Born dead.

STORK BITE

A red birthmark that is flat and whitens on touch. It usually appears on the back of the neck, but can also appear on the face. The mark may gradually fade, or it may be permanent but only show up when a person blushes, becomes excited, or gets hot.

STRAWBERRY MARK (nevus vaculosus)

A raised, red birthmark with a rough surface that may be present at birth or not appear until days or weeks later. The mark usually goes away on its own, but if constant chafing irritates it, surgical removal may be recommended.

STREPTOCOCCUS, GROUP B (See GROUP-B STREPTOCOCCUS)

STRESS INCONTINENCE

Being unable to hold in urine (urinary incontinence) or bowel movements (fecal incontinence) when sneezing or coughing. Pelvic floor exercises (Kegel exercises) can sometimes help to alleviate this problem. Some mothers may experience these conditions after forceps or a vacuum delivery. The condition may be temporary, or surgery may be required to correct it.

STRETCH MARKS (STRIAE)

Areas of the skin that are stretched by rapid weight gain during pregnancy often found on the abdomen, breasts, buttocks, and legs. They resemble rippled stripes that are lighter than normal skin, and usually disappear after pregnancy.

SUDDEN INFANT DEATH SYNDROME (SIDS, pronounced sids, like kids)

A sudden, unexplained death of a baby less than one year of age, and the leading cause of death in babies after one month of age. Most deaths occur between two and four months of age, and more happen in colder months. Babies placed to sleep on their stomachs are much more likely to die than those placed on their backs. African-American babies are twice as likely to die of SIDS than white babies, and Native-American babies nearly three times more likely to die from it. The U.S. Consumer Product Safety Commission recommends that all babies be placed on their backs for sleep. (See SIDS warning on page 398.)

SUPINE HYPOTENSION (supine hypotensive syndrome)

When the pressure of the pregnant uterus compresses a large blood vessel, the inferior vena cava, impeding the return of blood to the heart, which results in a drop in blood pressure (hypotension), a speeding up of the heart rate (tachycardia), and, possibly, fainting. A mother's upper body should always be kept at a raised angle, or she should be placed on her left side to allow the weight of the uterus to move away from the great vein.

SURFACTANT

A slippery substance covering the inner lining of the air sacs inside the lungs so they can expand normally during breathing. Premature babies may need to be given a surfactant to enable their lungs to function.

SWEEPING OF THE MEMBRANES

Inserting a gloved finger up into the rim of a mother's cervix in order to free the baby's membranes from their attachment at the rim of cervix. It is used to encourage the onset of labor. The procedure can be painful and cause minor bleeding.

SYMPHYSIS PUBIC DYSFUNCTION (SPD)

Pain in the pubic area during pregnancy or following birth caused by a misalignment of the pelvis or gaps in the alignment of the front pubic bones caused by their stretching apart during pregnancy or

after birth. Diastasis Symphysis Pubis (DSP) is the name for the problem in its most severe form when the bones of the pelvis actually separate or tear apart. Lifting one leg at a time or parting the legs can be extremely painful and interfere with putting on clothes, getting out of a car, climbing stairs, and other everyday activities. Using pillows and supports and gentle stretching exercises using an exercise ball may be of some help.

SYNDACTYLY (syndactylism)

When a baby is born with webbed fingers or toes.

SYPHILIS

A sexually transmitted disease (STD) that can affect an unborn baby. (See discussion on page 221.)

SYSTOLIC BLOOD PRESSURE (See BLOOD PRESSURE)

The first number in a blood pressure reading, it is the highest blood pressure produced by the contraction of your heart.

T

TACHYCARDIA

Rapid heartbeat. For an unborn baby, that can mean 160 bpm (beats per minute) or more. Causes include oxygen starvation (hypoxia), maternal fever, maternal hyperthyroidism (hyperactive thyroid), and certain drugs that affect the nervous system.

TACHYPNIA (transient tachypnia)

Abnormally fast breathing.

TALIPES (CLUBFOOT)

A foot deformity that affects babies in one out of one thousand births and is more common in boys than girls. The baby's foot is held in a drawn-up, turned-in position that will require orthopedic correction at some point. Positional clubfoot is when a newborn's feet are turned inward because of pressure inside the uterus. It goes away without treatment.

TAY-SACHS DISEASE

One of a series of inherited genetic disorders common among Ashkenazi Jews. The enzyme needed to break down certain lipid fats is absent, resulting in physical and mental retardation, enlargement of the head, and eventually death.

TENS (Transcutaneous Electrical Nerve Stimulation)

A device that applies low-level electrical stimulation to the nerves in a mother's back that can help to mask her sensation of pain. (See discussion on page 312.)

TERATOGEN

A drug or agent that can cause abnormal fetal development or physical deformities when a woman is exposed to it during pregnancy.

TERATOLOGY

The study of the effects that drugs, medications, chemicals, and other exposures may have on babies during pregnancy. A drug will be termed teratogenic if it is known to cause changes in a baby's body during pregnancy.

TERBUTALINE SULFATE (Brethine)

An asthma medication sometimes used to slow down or stop labor contractions during preterm labor by relaxing the smooth muscles of the body (the uterus contains smooth muscle).

TERM (See FULL TERM)

The length of pregnancy, usually measured in weeks.

TERMINATION

Another word for abortion, or the purposeful ending of a pregnancy, perhaps because of detected abnormalities.

THALASSEMIA

Group of inherited disorders of hemoglobin formation, which result in a decrease in the amount of hemoglobin formed. This can cause severe anemia and require blood transfusions.

THREATENED. ABORTION

When symptoms show that a pregnancy may not be able to continue because of bleeding or other problems. A threatened abortion may go on to become a miscarriage (spontaneous abortion).

THROMBOPHLEBITIS (thrombosis) (See EMBOLISM)

Inflammation of a vein associated with a blood clot (thrombus).

THRUSH

Monilial or yeast infection occurring in the mouth or mucous membranes of a newborn infant. It appears as milky, white patches on a baby's tongue that cannot be wiped off.

TLC (Tender Loving Care)

Refers to giving babies gentle, loving attention. Example: "All babies need lots of TLC."

TOCOLYSIS (See TOCOLYTICS)

When contractions are stopped during premature labor with the use of medication.

TOCOLYTICS (See TOCOLYSIS)

Drugs, including magnesium sulfate and beta-mimetic agents designed to reduce involuntary contractions in smooth muscles, such as the uterus. A mother who has gone into premature labor may be given a tocolytic by injection in an attempt to make her uterus stop contracting (tocolysis) so pregnancy can continue. There is little evidence to demonstrate that these drugs have succeeded in reducing the rate of preterm births or the death of premature babies, but they may succeed in stopping labor for a short period of time, at least forty-eight hours. Their use is not recommended after thirty-four weeks of pregnancy, and many tocolytics have side effects that may affect mothers with serious physical problems, such as heart or kidney disease.

TOL (See TRIAL OF LABOR)

TONIC NECK REFLEX

A built-in baby behavior (reflex). During sleep, the baby's head is turned to one side with one arm bent behind the head and the other arm extends in front of the face in a fencing position.

TOP

Stands for medical termination of pregnancy, an abortion.

TORSION

Twisting.

TORTICOLLIS (wryneck)

When a baby's neck is stiff on one side as the result of birth trauma so that his head is pulled to one side of the neck and his chin to the opposite side. Although the problem may not show up at birth, within two weeks a small lump can be felt in a muscle of the neck. Parents may be given exercises to help stretch the baby's neck, and physical therapy may be recommended. Rarely, surgery may be required.

TOXEMIA (See PREECLAMPSIA)

TOXOPLASMOSIS

An airborne protozoa (Toxoplasma gondii) found in cat feces that can also be caught from contaminated, raw, or rare meat, and unwashed fruits and vegetables or from gardening without gloves. The infection can affect unborn babies, but most mothers have already developed immunity to it from prior infection. The disease is not serious unless a mother catches it for the first time during pregnancy. Exposure can cause blindness, mild retardation, and hearing loss in unborn babies. Some children may develop brain or eye problems years after birth. Most healthcare providers routinely test to see if a mother is at risk.

TRANSITION STAGE

The period of time at the end of the first stage of labor when the cervix dilates from eight to ten centimeters prior to the second stage of labor. It is often a short but challenging time marked by irritability or confusion for the mother.

TRANSVERSE LIE (See EXTERNAL VERSION)

When a baby lies crosswise in the uterus prior to birth, which can cause the shoulder to present first. A healthcare provider may attempt to turn the baby externally by applying pressure to put it in a more favorable position for birth. (See discussion on page 88.)

TRAUMA

An injury or a wound. Birth trauma can refer to physical injury to the baby as a result of delivery, or the term is sometimes used to refer to profound psychological damage from the birth experience that remains a part of a person's deep, but repressed, memories even into adulthood.

TRIAL OF LABOR (TOL, trial of labor after cesarean section) (See VBAC)

Choosing to enter into labor after having had a prior cesarean in an attempt to have a vaginal birth, rather than undergoing a second (or subsequent) cesarean prior to the start of labor, called an elective cesarean.

TRICHOMONAS VAGINITIS

Inflammation of the vagina caused by a parasitic protozoan that causes itching and a profuse, bubbly, yellow discharge.

TRIMESTER

Pregnancy is divided into three parts: up to fourteen weeks for the first trimester, fourteen to twenty-seven weeks for the second trimester, and twenty-eight weeks until delivery, the third trimester. Stated as: "I am in my second trimester of pregnancy."

TUBAL PREGNANCY (See ECTOPIC PREGNANCY)

When a fertilized egg stays in the fallopian tube instead of traveling down to the uterus to implant. (See "Ectopic Pregnancy.")

U

ULTRASOUND (ultrasonography)

A device that uses high-frequency sound waves to produce a picture of a baby's body. It shows the position and size of the baby and the placenta, the baby's heartbeat, breathing, and body movements. It can also be used to measure the amount of amniotic fluid. Level II ultrasound is a closer look at the fetus in search of structural and anatomic abnormalities. (See discussion on pages 191–192.)

UMBILICAL CORD

The flexible, cordlike structure that connects a baby at the navel with the placenta, which, in turn, is attached to the uterus. It contains two umbilical arteries and one vein that transport blood, oxygen, and nutrients to the baby and carry away waste products and carbon dioxide.

UMBILICAL CORD BLOOD BANKING (See CORD BLOOD)

Harvesting and storing stem cells from the blood of a baby's umbilical cord following birth, usually for a fee. It may offer promising therapies in the future, especially for family members who may need a transplant of stem cells in order to overcome serious diseases, such as leukemia, but at this time the procedure and the uses for stem cells are still in the experimental phase.

UMBILICAL STUMP

The leftover portion of a baby's umbilical cord that dries up and falls off a few weeks after birth. Sometimes the stump can get infected, causing the belly button area to turn red and ooze pus. Antibiotics may be necessary to prevent the spread of infection (umbilical sepsis).

UMBILICUS (NAVEL)

Another word for belly button.

UNDESCENDED TESTICLES (cryptorchidism)

Failure of a baby boy's testicles to descend into the scrotum through the small, inguinal canal at the time of birth. More common in premature boys. It usually resolves itself in time.

UNRIPE CERVIX (See CERVICAL RIPENING and CERVIX, RIPE)

UPT

Urine Pregnancy Test.

URETER

The tube that transports urine from the kidneys to the bladder.

URETHRA

The tube that transports urine from the bladder to the outside of the body.

URGE TO PUSH

An inborn body reaction (reflex) at the end of labor that gives the mother an overwhelming urge to bear down in order to push the baby out.

URINARY INCONTINENCE (UI) (See CONTINENCE and INCONTINENCE)

When a woman accidentally urinates while sneezing or coughing. Pelvic floor exercises can help alleviate this problem, and usually healthcare providers will give instructions. (Some mothers may experience fecal incontinence, the inability to hold in a bowel movement following childbirth.) (See KEGEL EXERCISES.)

URINARY SPHINCTER (See URINARY INCONTINENCE)

A tight ring of muscle at the neck of the bladder that helps to hold in urine and support the muscles of the pelvic floor.

URINARY TRACT INFECTION (UTI)

Urinary tract infections (UTIs) occur when bacteria or other infectious organisms invade the organs that produce urine and transport it out of the body—the urethra, bladder, ureter, or kidneys. There may be no symptoms, or symptoms could include a frequent and urgent need to urinate (every thirty to sixty minutes); burning or painful urination; or blood in the urine. UTIs are more common during pregnancy, and untreated, they can lead to a kidney infection that could contribute to early labor. (See discussion on page 140.)

US

Ultrasound.

USCPSC (or CPSC)

Stands for the U.S. Consumer Product Safety Commission, a federal agency that oversees the safety of baby products and issues recalls for dangerous products. (See *Resource Guide*, on page 560, and page 469 in the *Baby Gear Guide*.)

UTERINE ATONY

When the uterus becomes flaccid and soft, lacking in normal tone and strength. When this occurs after the birth of the baby, there is a danger of heavy blood loss to the mother at the site where the placenta was attached.

UTERINE HYPERSTIMULATION (TACHYSYTOLE)

Defined as more than five uterus contractions per ten minutes, and sometimes as more than seven contractions over fifteen minutes. Although it can sometimes happen during non-medicated (spontaneous) labor, it is more common during the induction or augmentation of labor, such as with the use of oxytocin (Pitocin®) or misoprostol (Cytotec®).

UTERINE INERTIA

When contractions become sluggish or come to a stop during labor.

UTERINE INVERSION

When a mother's placenta fails to separate from the wall of the uterus during the third stage of labor so that part of the uterus comes out of the vagina. Women who have had several babies, who have had long labors, or who have been given magnesium sulfate, a drug that lowers blood pressure and acts as a muscle relaxer, are more at risk for the problem. Pulling on the baby's umbilical cord in an attempt to delivery the placenta can also cause inversion. An attempt may be made to manually reposition the uterus back in the body, or, in more serious cases, surgery may be required to put it back in place.

UTERINE INVOLUTION

The return of the uterus to normal size following birth.

UTERINE RUPTURE

When scar tissue from previous obstetrical surgery, such as a cesarean section, ruptures during the process of birth. The most common sign of rupture is a slowing down of the baby's heartbeat, or an undetectable heart rate accompanied by a labor that fails to progress. A uterine rupture can be life threatening.

UTERUS

A hollow, muscular, pear-shaped organ where a fertilized egg implants, it serves to nurture a growing baby during pregnancy. Its muscular walls help push the baby out during birth. While a nonpregnant uterus is about three to four inches long and weighs about three ounces, at the time of birth it will weigh approximately two pounds.

UTI

Urinary tract infection.

V

VACCINATION (immunization, shots) (See IMMUNIZATION and VACCINE)

Another word for immunization to help prevent diseases. (See discussion on pages 204 and 435.)

VACCINE (See IMMUNIZATION and VACCINATION)

A preparation containing killed or weakened living microorganisms that cause the body to form protective fighter (antibodies) against that type

of organism. Once that happens, the person is protected from catching the disease, either permanently, or for a period of time. (See discussion on pages 204 and 435.)

VACUUM EXTRACTION (vacuum-assisted birth) (See CAPUT)

A procedure using a device similar to a suction cup that attaches to the baby's head, guiding it through the birth canal during delivery. It causes temporary swelling on the baby's scalp. (See discussion on page 342.)

VAGINA

The canal, or birth canal, that leads from the uterus to the opening between the labia.

VAGINAL BIRTH

Birth of the baby through the birth canal, versus a c-section, which is the birth of the baby through an opening in the abdomen.

VAGINITIS (See BACTERIAL VAGINOSIS)

A vaginal infection with a number of causes. Symptoms may include unusual discharge that may be green, yellow, or strong smelling; redness; soreness; or itching around the vagina.

VALSALVA MANEUVER

Encouraging a mother in her second (bearing down) stage of labor to hold her breath while pushing down with the diaphragm. The maneuver is thought by some healthcare providers to be outdated and potentially harmful to the baby, because of the potential for decreasing a mother's heart output and lowering her blood pressure, which could diminish blood flow and oxygen to the baby. (See discussion on page 289.)

VARICOSE VEINS

Blood vessels (veins) that are dilated or enlarged, most often in the calves of the legs.

VBAC (pronounced vee back) (See TRIAL OF LABOR)

Stands for vaginal birth after cesarean section, and refers to giving birth through the birth canal (vagina) after having undergone one or more cesarean sections with previous babies. Pre-VBAC, or trial of labor (TOL) after a cesarean, allows a mother to enter into normal labor with close monitoring to see whether it is safe for her to deliver vaginally rather than having to undergo another cesarean. There is a rare risk of a life-threatening uterine rupture during a VBAC from the scar of a prior cesarean.

VENEREAL DISEASE (See SEXUALLY TRANSMITTED DISEASE)

VENTRAL WALL HERNIA

A protrusion of the contents of the body of the fetus, usually its abdominal organs, sometimes discovered during an ultrasound examination.

VERNIX (vernix caseosa)

A thick, protective white or yellowish cream produced by an unborn baby's skin that protects the skin while the baby floats in the amniotic fluid. It is often wiped off immediately after birth, but can also be gently massaged into the baby's skin. It contains antibacterial properties.

VERSION (See EXTERNAL VERSION)

VERTEX PRESENTATION (See PRESENTATION)

The typical, chin-against-the-chest position of a baby being born headfirst.

VIABLE

Able to live. A baby mature enough to survive outside the womb.

VILLI (chorionic villi)

The villi attach the placenta to the mucous lining of the uterus so that nutrients from the mother's blood can be flowed to it and the baby.

VITAMIN K

All newborns routinely receive injections of vitamin K, which encourages the liver to produce blood-clotting agents to assist a baby's immature liver and to prevent excessive bleeding. Excessive vitamin K in a baby's bloodstream can lead to jaundice.

VULVA

A woman's external genital organs. The vulva includes the labia (the lips around the opening of the vagina) and the clitoris (a small knob of tissue at the opening of the vagina that helps a woman achieve orgasm during sexual intercourse).

W

WALKING EPIDURAL

The administration of an epidural that allows a mother to maintain sensation in her legs so that she is able to stand for periods of time although she may be asked to wear monitors for herself and her baby.

WEIGHT GAIN DURING PREGNANCY

A steady pattern of weight gain is important for a baby's growth. Unusual weight gain, more than two pounds in one week, may be an early sign of preeclampsia. Failure to gain weight, on the other hand, may signal growth problems for the baby. At the time of birth, a baby weighs only about 7.5 pounds of the 24–28 pounds that a mother typically gains. The placenta weighs one pound; amniotic fluid, two pounds; the uterus, 2.5 pounds; breast tissue, three pounds; increased blood volume, four pounds; a mother's fat stores, four to eight pounds. (See weight discussion on page 154.)

WHARTON JELLY

A jellylike substance on the umbilical cord that is thought to protect the vessels of the cord and to prevent kinking.

WIC

Women, Infants, and Children Supplemental Nutrition Program that provides counseling, formula, and food supplementation for low-income mothers and children.

WITCHES' MILK

Small amounts of white, milky discharge from a newborn's swollen nipples due to stimulation of the male or female baby's breast tissue by high levels of female hormones. The swollen nipples should not be massaged, which may introduce infection. The swelling will disappear within two weeks as the hormonal levels drop.

WOMB

Another name for the uterus.

Y

YEAST INFECTION (Candida infection, Monilia, moniliasis)

A vaginal infection common during pregnancy, its symptoms are intense itching, bright red coloration, and a white discharge that smells like baking bread. Consult your healthcare provider before undertaking any over-the-counter treatment. Babies can also have yeast infections. If it occurs in a baby's mouth, it is called thrush and is a white, milky patch that cannot be rubbed off.

YOGA, PRENATAL

A form of stretching exercises designed to help mothers remain limber.

Z

ZINC OXIDE

A thick, white cream used in diaper rash products to protect baby's skin and aid in healing.

ZYGOTE

A fertilized egg from the union of sperm and ovum that will soon begin to divide and grow.

Calculate Your Baby's Due Date

The length of an average pregnancy is about 266 days from the day the baby is conceived until delivery, but calculations for a woman's due date and her baby's weight are famous for being wrong. Conception usually happens 14 days after your last period. Add extra or subtract extra days per month if your periods are longer or shorter. Healthcare providers typically calculate your length of pregnancy from the first day

JAN	1	2	3	4	5	6	7	8	9	10	11	12	13	14	15
	OCT 8	OCT 9	OCT 10	OCT 11	OCT 12	OCT 13	OCT 14	OCT 15	OCT 16	OCT 17	OCT 18	OCT 19	OCT 20	OCT 21	OCT 22
FEB	1	2	3	4	5	6	7	8	9	10	11	12	13	14	15
	NOV 8	NOV 9	NOV 10	NOV 11	NOV 12	NOV 13	NOV 14	NOV 15	NOV 16	NOV 17	NOV 18	NOV 19	NOV 20	NOV 21	NOV 22
MAR	1	2	3	4	5	6	7	8	9	10	11	12	13	14	15
	DEC 6	DEC 7	DEC 8	DEC 9	DEC 10	DEC 11	DEC 12	DEC 13	DEC 14	DEC 15	DEC 16	DEC 17	DEC 18	DEC 19	DEC 20
APR	1	2	3	4	5	6	7	8	9	10	11	12	13	14	15
	JAN 6	JAN 7	JAN 8	JAN 9	JAN 10	JAN 11	JAN 12	JAN 13	JAN 14	JAN 15	JAN 16	JAN 17	JAN 18	JAN 19	JAN 20
MAY	1	2	3	4	5	6	7	8	9	10	11	12	13	14	15
	FEB 5	FEB 6	FEB 7	FEB 8	FEB 9	FEB 10	FEB 11	FEB 12	FEB 13	FEB 14	FEB 15	FEB 16	FEB 17	FEB 18	FEB 19
JUN	1	2	3	4	5	6	7	8	9	10	11	12	13	14	15
	MAR 8	MAR 9	MAR 10	MAR 11	MAR 12	MAR 13	MAR 14	MAR 15	MAR 16	MAR 17	MAR 18	MAR 19	MAR 20	MAR 21	MAR 22
JUL	1	2	3	4	5	6	7	8	9	10	11	12	13	14	15
	APR 7	APR 8	APR 9	APR 10	APR 11	APR 12	APR 13	APR 14	APR 15	APR 16	APR 17	APR 18	APR 19	APR 20	APR 21
AUG	1	2	3	4	5	6	7	8	9	10	11	12	13	14	15
	MAY 8	MAY 9	MAY 10	MAY 11	MAY 12	MAY 13	MAY 14	MAY 15	MAY 16	MAY 17	MAY 18	MAY 19	MAY 20	MAY 21	MAY 22
SEP	1	2	3	4	5	6	7	8	9	10	11	12	13	14	15
	JUN 8	JUN 9	JUN 10	JUN 11	JUN 12	JUN 13	JUN 14	JUN 15	JUN 16	JUN 17	JUN 18	JUN 19	JUN 20	JUN 21	JUN 22
OCT	1	2	3	4	5	6	7	8	9	10	11	12	13	14	15
	JUL 8	JUL 9	JUL 10	JUL 11	JUL 12	JUL 13	JUL 14	JUL 15	JUL 16	JUL 17	JUL 18	JUL 19	JUL 20	JUL 21	JUL 22
NOV	1	2	3	4	5	6	7	8	9	10	11	12	13	14	15
	AUG 8	AUG 9	AUG 10	AUG 11	AUG 12	AUG 13	AUG 14	AUG 15	AUG 16	AUG 17	AUG 18	AUG 19	AUG 20	AUG 21	AUG 22
DEC	1	2	3	4	5	6	7	8	9	10	11	12	13	14	15
	SEP 7	SEP 8	SEP 9	SEP 10	SEP 11	SEP 12	SEP 13	SEP 14	SEP 15	SEP 16	SEP 17	SEP 18	SEP 19	SEP 20	SEP 21

of your last period. To that, they add 280 days (or 40 weeks), but there can be 3 weeks' leeway (37–42 weeks) for a pregnancy to still be considered normal. Use this handy calendar to figure out your baby's "due date." The date of your last menstrual period (LMP) is in bold; your anticipated due date is below. You most likely conceived between 13 to 15 days after the date in bold.

16	17	18	19	20	21	22	23	24	25	26	27	28	29	30	31
OCT 23	OCT 24	OCT 25	OCT 26	OCT 27	OCT 28	OCT 29	OCT 30	OCT 31	NOV 1	NOV 2	NOV 3	NOV 4	NOV 5	NOV 6	NOV 7

16	17	18	19	20	21	22	23	24	25	26	27	28	X	X	X
NOV 23	NOV 24	NOV 25	NOV 26	NOV 27	NOV 28	NOV 29	NOV 30	DEC 1	DEC 2	DEC 3	DEC 4	DEC 5			

16	17	18	19	20	21	22	23	24	25	26	27	28	29	30	31
DEC 21	DEC 22	DEC 23	DEC 24	DEC 25	DEC 26	DEC 27	DEC 28	DEC 29	DEC 30	DEC 31	JAN 1	JAN 2	JAN 3	JAN 4	JAN 5

16	17	18	19	20	21	22	23	24	25	26	27	28	29	30	X
JAN 21	JAN 22	JAN 23	JAN 24	JAN 25	JAN 26	JAN 27	JAN 28	JAN 29	JAN 30	JAN 31	FEB 1	FEB 2	FEB 3	FEB 4	

16	17	18	19	20	21	22	23	24	25	26	27	28	29	30	31
FEB 20	FEB 21	FEB 22	FEB 23	FEB 24	FEB 25	FEB 26	FEB 27	FEB 28	MAR 1	MAR 2	MAR 3	MAR 4	MAR 5	MAR 6	MAR 7

16	17	18	19	20	21	22	23	24	25	26	27	28	29	30	X
MAR 23	MAR 24	MAR 25	MAR 26	MAR 27	MAR 28	MAR 29	MAR 30	MAR 31	APR 1	APR 2	APR 3	APR 4	APR 5	APR 6	

16	17	18	19	20	21	22	23	24	25	26	27	28	29	30	31
APR 22	APR 23	APR 24	APR 25	APR 26	APR 27	APR 28	APR 29	APR 30	MAY 1	MAY 2	MAY 3	MAY 4	MAY 5	MAY 6	MAY 7

16	17	18	19	20	21	22	23	24	25	26	27	28	29	30	31
MAY 23	MAY 24	MAY 25	MAY 26	MAY 27	MAY 28	MAY 29	MAY 30	MAY 31	JUN 1	JUN 2	JUN 3	JUN 4	JUN 5	JUN 6	JUN 7

16	17	18	19	20	21	22	23	24	25	26	27	28	29	30	X
JUN 23	JUN 24	JUN 25	JUN 26	JUN 27	JUN 28	JUN 29	JUN 30	JUL 1	JUL 2	JUL 3	JUL 4	JUL 5	JUL 6	JUL 7	

16	17	18	19	20	21	22	23	24	25	26	27	28	29	30	31
JUL 23	JUL 24	JUL 25	JUL 26	JUL 27	JUL 28	JUL 29	JUL 30	JUL 31	AUG 1	AUG 2	AUG 3	AUG 4	AUG 5	AUG 6	AUG 7

16	17	18	19	20	21	22	23	24	25	26	27	28	29	30	X
AUG 23	AUG 24	AUG 25	AUG 26	AUG 27	AUG 28	AUG 29	AUG 30	AUG 31	SEP 1	SEP 2	SEP 3	SEP 4	SEP 5	SEP 6	

16	17	18	19	20	21	22	23	24	25	26	27	28	29	30	31
SEP 22	SEP 23	SEP 24	SEP 25	SEP 26	SEP 27	SEP 28	SEP 29	SEP 30	OCT 1	OCT 2	OCT 3	OCT 4	OCT 5	OCT 6	OCT 7

Endnotes

1. Your Pregnancy Week-by-Week

1 Reported in a meeting of the American Association for the Advancement of Science by Dr. John W. Olney, a brain researcher at Washington University in St. Louis, MO. The findings are based on mouse studies. See *The New York Times*: "Two Drinks Can Kill Brain Cells in a Fetus, Studies Suggest," February 15, 2004.

2 Scientists such as Robin Baker of the University of Manchester in England have theorized that some of the funnier-looking sperm may exist specifically to sacrifice themselves in attacks.

3 From the Center for Disease Control report, "Preventing Smoking During Pregnancy," National Center for Health Statistics, 2001.

4 From studies cited by the National Institute on Drug Abuse (NIDA). See: http://www.drugabuse.gov/NIDA_Notes/NNVol15N5/DrugAbuse.html. Also see: Kotimaa, AJ, Moilanen, I, et al. "Maternal smoking and hyperactivity in 8-year-old children." *Journal of the American Academy of Child and Adolescent Psychiatry*. 2003. 42(7). Pages 826-33.

5 National Health Service (UK). See: http://www.cancerresearchuk.org/aboutus/publications/ pubmisc/pdfs/leaflet_smoking_sept03.pdf.

6 Anderson, A-MN, Wohlfahrt, J, et al. "Maternal age and fetal loss: population based register linkage study." *British Medical Journal*. 2000. 320 Pages 1708–12.

7 Kieler, H, Cnattingius, S, et al. "Sinistrality—a side-effect of prenatal sonography: A comparative study of young men." *Epidemiology*. 2001. 12. Pages 618–23.

8 Fryer, RG, and Levitt, SD. "The causes and consequences of distinctively black names." National Bureau of Economic Research Working Paper No. W9938. Sept., 2003. See: http://www.ssrn.com/abstract=439619.

9 American College of Obstetricians and Gynecologists (ACOG). "What to expect after your due date." Patient education pamphlet, 1999.

10 Nathanielsz, PW. "A time to be born," in *Life Before Birth and A Time To Be Born*. (Promethean, 1992.) Pages 162–81.

2. Managing Your Pregnancy

1 A.D.A.M., Inc. "How serious are migraines?" University of Maryland Patient Education Posting, 2002. See: http://www.umm.edu/patiented/articles/how_serious_migraines_000097_2.htm.

2 Peikert, A, Wilimzig C, and Kohne-Volland, R. "Prophylaxis of migraine with oral magnesium: results from a prospective, multi-center, placebo-controlled and double-blind randomized study." *Cephalalgia*. 1996.16(4). Page 257.

3 Thompson Micromedex. Medline "Plus. Zolmitriptan (Systemic)." Revised 2001. See: http://www.nlm.nih.gov/medlineplus/druginfo/uspdi/203425.html.

4 U.S. Food and Drug Administration. "Accutane risk management program strengthened." *FDA Consumer.* 2002. 36(1). See: http://www.fda.gov/fdac/features/2002/102_acne.html.

5 Li, K, Liu, L, and Odouli, R. "Exposure to non-steroidal anti-inflammatory drugs during pregnancy and risk of miscarriage: a population based cohort study." *British Medical Journal.* 2003. 327. Page 368.

6 "Pregnancy-related carpal tunnel syndrome." *Journal of Hand Surgery [Br].* 1998. 23 (1). Pages 98–101.

7 Consumer Reports. "Preventing and relieving carpal-tunnel syndrome." *Consumer Reports on Health.* 1998. 10(3). Page 8.

8 National Institutes of Health. "Urinary Tract Infections in Adults." (NIH publication no. 04-2097.) 2003. See: http://kidney.niddk.nih.gov/kudiseases/pubs/utiadult/index.htm.

9 U. S. Food and Drug Administration. "Recommended daily dietary allowances for women." *FDA Consumer.* April 1990 (revised). See: http://www.cfsan.fda.gov/~dms/wh-rda.html.

10 Clinical Nutrition Service, Warren Grant Magnuson Clinical Center Office of Dietary Supplements. "Facts about dietary supplements." 2002. See: http://www.cc.nih.gov/ccc/supplements/vitb12.html#veg.

11 Roan, S. "Getting your body back after the baby." *Parenting.* 2004 (Feb). Page 92.

12 Watkins, ML, et al. "Maternal obesity and risk for birth defects." *Pediatrics.* 2003.111(5), Part 2. Pages 1152–58. Comments on a study conducted by Leena Hilakivi-Clarke, Ph.D., professor of oncology at Georgetown University, in collaboration with Finnish epidemiologist Riitta Luoto, MD.

13 Clapp, JT III. *Exercising Through Your Pregnancy.* (Addicus Books, 2002.) Page 87.

14 Clapp, JT III. Loc. cit.

15 Lavine, M. "Feeling stressed? Try yoga." News release of the Endocrine Society. June 19, 2003.

16 George Brainard. Center for Integrative Medicine, Thomas Jefferson University Hospital, Philadelphia. See: http://www.endo-society.org/pubrelations/pressReleases/archives/2003/yoga_endo.cfm.

17 Williams, L, et al. "Surveillance for selected maternal behaviors and experiences before, during, and after pregnancy: Pregnancy Risk Assessment Monitoring System (PRAMS), 2000. Surveillance Summaries." *Morbidity and Mortality Weekly Report (MMWR).* 2003. 52(SS11). Pages 1–14.

18 Evans, J. "Induction rate doubled in the US from 1990 to 1998." *OB/GYN News.* 2002. 37 (9). See: http://www.findarticles.com/cf_dls/m0CYD/9_37/85591457/p1/article.jhtml.

19 Jones, C. *Alternative Birth: The Complete Guide.* (Tarcher, 1990.)

20 Mehl, L, et al. "Outcomes of elective home births: a series of 1146 cases." *Journal of Reproductive Medicine.* 1977.19(5). Pages 281–90; Olsen, O. "Meta-analysis of the safety of home birth." *Birth.* 1997. 24(1). Pages 4–13, and discussion pages 14–16.

21 Centers for Disease Control and Prevention (2002). *Births: Final data for 2000.* National Vital Statistics Reports, 50(5): 1–24.

22 Centers for Disease Control (CDC). "National Vital Statistics Report for 2002." Dec. 2003. 52 (10).

23 The risk is .5 percent. See: Wren, C, Birrell, G, Hawthorne, G. "Cardiovascular malformations in infants of diabetic mothers." *Heart*. 2003. 89(10). Pages 1217–20.

24 The March of Dimes. "Clubfoot and Other Foot Deformities." (Fact Sheet.) 2001. See: http://www.marchofdimes.com/professionals/681_1211.asp.

25 The March of Dimes. "Down Syndrome." (Fact Sheet.) 2001. See: http://www.marchofdimes.com/professionals/681_1214.asp.

26 Alfirevic, Z, Sundberg K, Brigham, S. "Amniocentesis and chorionic villus sampling for prenatal diagnosis." Cochrane Review. *The Cochrane Library*, Issue 2, 2004.

27 National Institutes of Health (NIH*)*. *Medical Encyclopedia*. See: http://www.nlm.nih.gov/medlineplus/ency/article/003935.htm.

28 Boyd, PA, Chamberlain, P, and Hicks, NR. "Six-year experience of prenatal diagnosis in an unselected population in Oxford, UK." *Lancet*. 1998. 352. Pages 1577–81.

29 Kieler, H. Interviewed in Sample, I. "Ultrasound scans may disrupt fetal brain development." *NewScientist.com*. 2001. 17(56). Based on findings reported in: Kieler, H. "First trimester ultrasound scans and left-handedness." *Epidemiology*. 2002.13(3). Page 370.

30 Werler, MM, Mitchell, AA, and Shapiro, S. "First trimester maternal medication use in relation to gastroschisis." *Teratology*. 1992. 45. Pages 361–67. See also: American College of Obstetricians and Gynecologists (ACOG) and the American College of Allergy, Asthma, and Immunology (ACAAI). "The use of newer asthma and allergy medications during pregnancy." *Annals of Allergy, Asthma, and Immunology*. 84. Pages 475–80.

31 Briggs, GG, Freeman, RK, and Yaffe, SJ (Eds). *Drugs in Pregnancy and Lactation: A Reference Guide to Fetal and Neonatal Risk (5th Ed)*. (Williams & Wilkins, 1998.) Pages 577–78 and 627–28.

32 "Green tea may fight allergies." (News release.) Sept. 18, 2002. Based on Fujimura, Y, et al. *Journal of Agricultural and Food Chemistry*. 2002. 50(20). Pages 5729–34.

33 Briggs, GG, loc. cit.

34 See: http://www.RxList.com, an online source for drug information and pregnancy use warnings.

35 Tarkan, Laurie. "Dealing with Depression and the Perils of Pregnancy." *The New York Times*, January 13, 2004, F5 (col. 2).

36 Hendrick, V, Smith, LM, et al. "Birth outcomes after prenatal exposure to antidepressant medication." *American Journal of Obstetrics and Gynecology*. 2003. 188(3). Pages 812–15.

37 Chambers, CD, et al. "Birth outcomes in pregnant women taking fluoxetine." *New England Journal of Medicine*. 1996. 335. Pages 1010–15. Cited by California Teratogen Information Service, University of California at San Diego in UPI Science News (1996).

38 Lagace, E. "Safety of first trimester exposure to H2 blockers." *Journal of Family Practice*. 1996. 43(4) 342–43. Czeizel AE, Toth, M, Rockenbauer, M. "No teratogenic effect after clotrimazole therapy during pregnancy." *Epidemiology*. 1999. 10. Pages 437–40.

39 Collins, E. "Maternal and fetal effects of acetaminophen and salicylates in pregnancy." *Obstetrics and Gynecology.* 1981. 58(5) (Suppl). Pages 57S–62S. Macones, GA, et al. "The controversy surrounding indomethacin for tocolysis." *American Journal of Obstetrics and Gynecology.* 2001. 184. Pages 264–72.

40 Nagourney, E. "When Coffee Puts Fetus at Risk." *The New York Times,* March 4, 2003, F6 (col. 1).

41 Center for Science and the Public Interest Nutrition Action Newsletter, December 1996. See: http://www.cspinet.org/nah/caffeine/caffeine_corner.htm.

42 Center for the Evaluation of Risks to Human Reproduction of the National Institute of Environmental Health Sciences (CEHR). "Caffeine." October 13, 2003.

43 National Institute on Drug Abuse. "Rat study shows exposure to ecstasy early in pregnancy induces brain, behavior changes." Aug. 29, 2003. (News release based on the research of Lipton, JW and Koprich, J, at Rush Presbyterian St. Luke's Medical Center.) See: http://www.drugabuse.gov/Newsroom/03/NR8-29.html.

44 Turner, S. "Nicotine changes newborn behavior in ways similar to heroin and crack." See: http://www.brown.edu/Administration/News_Bureau/2002-03/02-143.html. Based on research published as: Koprich, JB, Campbell, NG, and Lipton, JW. "Neonatal 3,4-methylene-dioxymethamphetamine (ecstasy) alters dopamine and serotonin neurochemistry and increases brain-derived neurotrophic factor in the forebrain and brainstem of the rat." *Developmental Brain Research.* 2003, 147(1–2). Pages 177–82.

45 Meis, PJ, Klebanoff, M, et al. "Prevention of recurrent preterm delivery by 17 alpha-hydroxyprogesterone caproate." *New England Journal of Medicine.* 2003. 348(24). Pages 2379–85.

46 Drakeley, AJ, Roberts, D, and Alfirevic, Z. "Cervical stitch (cerclage) for preventing pregnancy loss in women." Cochrane Review. In *The Cochrane Library,* Issue 2, 2004.

47 Reuters, "Drug Found to Protect Babies Born Prematurely." *The New York Times.* November 26, 2003. A16 (col. 4).

48 Watts, DH, et al. "A double-blind, randomized, placebo-controlled trial of acyclovir in late pregnancy for the reduction of herpes simplex virus shedding and cesarean delivery." *American Journal of Obstetrics and Gynecology.* 2003.188(3). Pages 836–43.

49 Brody, S, Potterat, JJ. "Autoinoculation of human papillomavirus and vaginal transmission of human immunodeficiency virus: an appeal for rigorous verification." *Sexually Transmitted Diseases.* 2004. 31(1). Pages 65–66.

50 Gray, RH, Pardthaisong, T. "In utero exposure to steroid contraceptives and survival during infancy." *American Journal of Epidemiology.* 1991.134(8). Pages 804–11.

51 Lippman, SA, et al. "Uterine fibroids and gynecologic pain symptoms in a population-based study." *Fertility and Sterility.* 2003. 80(6). Pages 1488–94.

52 Vilos, GA. "Uterine fibroids: relationships to reproduction." *Minerva Ginecologica.* 2003. 55(5). Pages 417–23.

53 Nagourney, E. "On the Scales: New Babies Add to Fathers' Girth." *The New York Times*, March 9, 2004. F6 (col. 1).

54 Martin, JA, Hamilton, B, et al. "Births: final data for 2002." *National Vital Statistics Reports*. 2003. 52 (10). See: http://www.cdc.gov.

3. Guide to Giving Birth

1 Russell JGB. "Moulding of the pelvic outlet." *Journal of Obstetrics and Gynecology of the British Commonwealth*. 1969; 76:817–20.

2 Schlenzka, PF. "Safety of alternative approaches to childbirth." Stanford University Dissertation. 1999. See: http://www.home.i-plus.net/scochran/doc/safety.rtf.

3 Centers for Disease Control and Prevention (CDC), National Center for Health Statistics, National Vital Statistics System. "Table 19: Infant, neonatal, and postneonatal mortality rates." See: http://www.cdc.gov/nchs/data/hus/tables/2003/03hus019.pdf.

4 Jackson, DJ, et al. "Impact of collaborative management and early admission in labor on method of delivery." *Journal of Obstetric, Gynecologic and Neonatal Nursing (JOGNN)*. 2003. 32, pages 147–57. Albers, L. Commentary. Loc. cit., pages 158–60. McNiven, PS, Williams, JI, et al. "An early labor assessment program: A randomized, controlled trial." *Birth*, 1998. 25, pages 5–10.

5 Murray, M. "Maternal or fetal heart rate? Avoiding intrapartum misidentification." *Journal of Obstetric, Gynecologic and Neonatal Nursing (JOGNN)*. 2004. 32. Pages 93–104.

6 Achiron, R, Zakut, H. "Misinterpretation of fetal heart rate monitoring in case of intrauterine death." *Clinical and Experimental Obstetrics and Gynecology*. 1984. 11(4). Pages 126–29.

7 American College of Obstetricians and Gynecologists. "ACOG Committee Opinion on Ethical Dimensions of Informed Consent." Number 108, May 1992.

8 Based on Kozak, L, et al. "National hospital discharge survey 2000: annual summary with detailed diagnosis and procedure data." *National Center for Health Statistics*. 2000. 13 (153). Pages 1–203.

9 Gupta, JK, and Nikodem, VC. "Women's position during second stage of labour." Cochrane Review. *The Cochrane Library*, Issue 4, 2003.

10 Ng, A, and Smith, G. "Gastroesophageal reflux and aspiration of gastric contents in anesthetic practice." *Anesthesiology and Analgesia*. 2001. 93. Pages 494–513.

11 Fraser,W, Marcoux, S, Krauss, I, Douglas, J, Gaulet C, et al. "Multicenter randomized controlled trial of delayed pushing for nulliparous women in second stage labor with continuous analgesia." *American Journal of Obstetrics and Gynecology*. 2000. 182. Pages 1165–72.

12 Simkin, P, and Ancheta, R. "Drive angle" in *The Labor Progress Handbook*. (Blackwell Publishing, 2000.) Page 17.

13 AWHONN, Cesario, S, Longacre, S, et al. *Evidence-Based Clinical Practice Guideline: Nursing Management of the Second Stage of Labor*. The Association of Women's Health, Obstetric, and Neonatal Nurses (Washington, DC, 2000).

14 Wiswell, TE, Gannon, CM, et al. "Delivery room management of the apparently vigorous meconium-stained neonate: results of the multicenter, international collaborative trial." *Pediatrics.* 2000.105(1 Pt 1). Pages 1–7.

15 Kuszkowski, KM. "Ambulatory labor analgesia: what does an obstetrician need to know?" *Acta Obstetricia et Gynecologica Scandinavica.* 2004. 83 (5). Page 415.

16 Melzak, R, Taenzer, P, Feldman, Kinch, RA. "Labour is still painful after prepared childbirth training." *Canadian Association Medical Journal.* 1981, 124: 357.

17 Hodnett, ED, Gates, S, et al. "Continuous support for women during childbirth." Cochrane Review. *The Cochrane Library,* 2004.

18 For a detailed discussion of breathing techniques for labor, see: Kitzinger, S. *The Complete Book of Pregnancy and Childbirth.* (Knopf, 1996.) Pages 201–08.

19 Smith, CA, Collins, CT, et al. "Complementary and alternative therapies for pain management in labour." Cochrane Review. *The Cochrane Library.* Issue 2, 2004.

20 Simkin, P, and Ancheta, R. "Drive angle" in *The Labor Progress Handbook.* (Blackwell Publishing, 2000.) Page 17.

21 Trolle, B, Moller, M, et al. The effect of sterile water blocks on low back labor pain. *American Journal of Obstetrics and Gynecology.* 1991. 164 (5 Pt 1). Pages 1277–81.

22 Balaskas, J. "Waterbirth." Presentation at the 2001 Lamaze Annual Conference. (Minneapolis, Minnesota. October 2001.)

23 Haire, D. "FDA approved obstetrics drugs: their effects on mother and baby." Published on the Alliance for the Improvement of Maternity Services. 2001. See: http:/www.aimusa.org.

24 IUPCs are estimated to be used in 15 to 20 percent (600,000–800,000) of the four-million-plus deliveries each year in the U.S. The catheter's readings are converted into Montevideo units (MVUs), which are scores created by multiplying millimeters of mercury measured by the catheter minus the baseline pressures measured over a ten-minute period. If a mother's cervix remains unchanged even though she is in active labor (more than three to four centimeters of dilation), and her contraction pattern exceeds 200 MVUs for at least two hours, then her labor is thought to be arrested, and drugs to augment labor will be suggested.

25 DeMott, K. "Acetaminophen didn't prevent epidural-associated fever in study: inflammation may be the culprit." *OB/GYN News.* July 1, 2002.

26 Gabbe, SG, Niebyl, JR, Simpson, JL. *Obstetrics: Normal and Problem Pregnancies.* (Churchill Livingstone, 2002.) Pages 441–46.

27 Law, YY, Lam, KY. "A randomized controlled trial comparing midwife-managed care and obstetrician-managed care for women assessed to be at low-risk in the initial intrapartum period." *Journal of Obstetric and Gynecology Research.* 1999. 25(2). Pages 107–12.

28 Olsen, O. "Meta-analysis of safety of home birth." *Birth.* 1997. 24(1). Pages 4–16.

29 Based on Friedman, EA. "Normal and dysfunctional labor," in *Management of Labor (2nd Ed.).* (Aspen, 1989.) Pages 1–18.

30 Cammu, H, Martens, G, et al. "Outcome after elective labor induction in nulliparous women: a matched cohort study." *American Journal of Obstetrics and Gynecology.* 2002. 186. Pages 240–44; Seyb, ST, et al. "Risk of cesarean delivery with elective induction of labor at term in nulliparous women." *Obstetrics and Gynecology.* 1999. 94. Pages 600–07. Yeast, JD, et al. "Induction of labor and the relationship to cesarean delivery: a review of 7001 consecutive inductions." *American Journal of Obstetrics and Gynecology.* 1999. 180 (3 pt 1). Pages 628–33. Maslow AS, Sweeny, AL. "Elective induction of labor as a risk factor for cesarean delivery among low-risk women at term." *Obstetrics and Gynecology.* 2000; 95 (6 pt 1). Pages 917–22.

31 Bishop, EH. "Pelvic scoring for elective induction." *Obstetrics and Gynecology.* 1964. 24. Pages 266–68.

32 The Bishop Score was not developed using first-time mothers, who are more likely to have their inductions fail and to subsequently undergo cesarean sections. See: Cammu, H, Martens, G, Ruyssinck, G, Amy, JJ. "Outcome after elective labor induction in nulliparous women: a matched cohort study." *American Journal of Obstetrics and Gynecology.* 2002. 186. Pages 240–44.

33 Sanchez-Ramos, L, Bernstein, S, et al. "Expectant management versus labor induction for suspected fetal macrosomia: a systematic review." *Obstetrics and Gynecology.* 2003 Jun; 101(6):1312–18. Nov. 2002, 100:5. Pages 997–1002. Also see: Gifford DS, et al. "Lack of progress in labor as a reason for a cesarean." *Obstetrics and Gynecology.* 2000. 95:4. Pages 589–95.

34 Alfirevic Z. "Oral misoprostol for induction of labour." Cochrane Review. *The Cochrane Library.* Carlan, SJ, et al. "Safety and efficacy of misoprostol orally and vaginally: a randomized trial." *Obstetrics and Gynecology.* 2001. 98. Pages 107–12. Adair, CD, et al. "Oral or vaginal misoprostol administration for induction of labor: a randomized, double-blind trial." *Obstetrics and Gynecology.* 1998. 92. Pages 810–13. Sanchez-Ramos, L, et al. "Misoprostol for cervical ripening and labor induction: a meta-analysis." *Obstetrics and Gynecology.* 1997. 89. Pages 633–42.

35 American College of Obstetricians and Gynecologists. "Committee Opinion 248 (In response to Searle's [the manufacturer's] warning on the drug)." December 2000.

36 Heffner LJ, Elkin,E, and Fretts, RC. "Impact of labor induction, gestational age, and maternal age on cesarean delivery rates." *Obstetrics and Gynecology.* 2003. 102:2. Pages 287–93.

37 Fraser, W, et al. "Amniotomy for shortening spontaneous labor." Cochrane Review. *The Cochrane Library.* Issue 3, 2004.

38 Cunningham, FG, et al. *Williams Obstetrics (21st Ed.)* (McGraw-Hill, 2001). Page 538.

39 Smith, GCS, Pell, J, and Dobbie, R. "Caesarean section and risk of unexplained stillbirth in subsequent pregnancy." *Lancet.* 2003. 362. Pages 1779–84.

40 Normand, MC, Damato, EG. "Postcesarean infection." *Journal of Obstetric, Gynecologic and Neonatal Nursing (JOGNN).* 2001. 30. Pages 642–648.

41 Lydon-Rochelle, M, et al. "Risk of uterine rupture during labor among women with a prior cesarean delivery." *New England Journal of Medicine*. 2001. 345(1), pages 3–8.

42 Parker, WH, Rosenman, AE, and Parker, R. *The Incontinence Solution: Answers for Women of All Ages*. (Simon & Schuster Fireside, 2002.)

43 Curran, C. "Intrapartum emergencies." *Journal of Obstetric, Gynecologic and Neonatal Nursing (JOGNN)*. 2003. 32(6). Pages 802–13.

44 International Perinatal HIV Group. "The mode of delivery and the risk of vertical transmission of human immunodeficiency virus Type 1— a meta-analysis of 15 prospective cohort studies." *New England Journal of Medicine*. 1999. 340 (10). Page 34.

45 Hirozawa, A. "Preeclampsia and eclampsia, while often preventable, are among top causes of pregnancy-related deaths." *Family Planning Perspectives*. Jul/Aug 2001. 33 (4). Page 182.

46 Roman, AS, and Rebarber, A. "Seven ways to control postpartum hemorrhage." *Contemporary OB/GYN*. 2003. 48(3). Pages 34–53.

4. You and Your Baby

1 For a list of citations regarding intelligence and breastfeeding, see: http://www.lalecheleague.org/cbi/bibborn.html.

2 Cronenwett, L, et al. "Single daily bottle use in the early weeks post-partum and breast-feeding outcomes." *Pediatrics*. 1992. 90(5). Pages 760–66.

3 Detailed information on storing breastmilk can be found in Mohrbacher, N, and Stock, J. *The Breast-Feeding Answer Book (3rd Ed.)*. (La Leche League International, 2003.)

7. Pregnancy Dictionary

1 Friedman, EA. *Labor: Clinical Evaluation and Management (2nd Edition)*. (Appleton-Century-Crofts, 1979.)

Index

A

abdominal muscles, postpartum training for, 384
abortion, previous, 230
abruptio placentae, 135–136, 215
abuse, during pregnancy, 245
accidents, 226
Accutane, 119
acetaminophen (Tylenol®), 114, 203, 206–207, 225
  for baby, 438
acne, 119–120
acupressure
  for labor pain relief, 304
  for nausea and vomiting, 131
acupuncture, for labor pain relief, 304
advice
  baby-care, 370
  unsolicited, 238–239
aftercare, 164
after pains, 365–366
age
  and multiples, 212
  over thirty-five, 211–212
    and pre-term labor, 217
AIDS, 219–220, 354–355
air travel, 231–232
  with baby, 445–447
alcohol, 16, 205
  abuse, 211

allergy medications, 199–200
alpha-fetoprotein, 54, 190
altitude, high, 226
aluminum hydroxide, magnesium hydroxide (Maalox®), 198–199, 200
American Academy of Husband-Coached Childbirth, 177
amniocentesis, 61, 184–185, 193–194
amnioinfusion, 353
amnionitis, 353–354
amniotic fluid, 83
amniotic fluid embolism, 356
amniotic sac, 264
amniotomy, 280, 336, 341
  and cesarean delivery, 342
  percentage of mothers having, 276
amphetamine abuse, 211
analgesia, 313, 315. See also epidural
anembryonic gestation, 30
anemia, 10, 115
  fatigue in, 118
  postpartum, 367
  and preterm labor, 218
anencephaly, 179
anesthesia, 315. See also general anesthesia; local anesthesia
antacids, 132, 198–199, 200
antibiotics, 200–201, 226
antidepressants, 201–203, 235
antidiarrheal drugs, 200–201
antifungal drugs, vaginal, 202–203

B

C

café-au-lait spots, 396
caffeine, 16, 131, 132, 141, 205–207
caffeine habit, breaking, 208
calcium
    dietary sources of, 146, 148
    for leg cramps, 141
    requirements, in pregnancy, 146
calcium carbonate (Tums®),
        198–199, 200
calories
    intake of, in pregnancy, 155, 156
    requirements, in breastfeeding,
        155
camcorders, 515–516
carbohydrates, avoiding, 235
cardiopulmonary resuscitation
        (CPR), for baby, 440–442
care provider, 41, 172–175
    changing, 63
    interviewing, 165–166
    for multifetal pregnancy, 213
    options for, 166–169
    selecting, 165–166
carpal tunnel syndrome, 81
    pregnancy-related, 126–127
carrier, baby, 457, 464–465
soft, 524–526
car seat, 96, 329, 456, 462–463,
        491–498
flaws in, 470–471
preemies and, 490–491
castor oil, 272
cat litter, 16
Centering Pregnancy and Parenting
        Association (CPPA), 178
cephalic position, 88
cephalohematoma, 343
cephalopelvic disproportion, 352

cerclage, cervical, 219
Certified Nurse Midwives, 6, 162,
        167–168, 172–173
Certified Professional Midwife,
        168–169
cervix, 11
    dilation of, 273–274, 281–284
        mechanical devices for, 341
        rate of, 335
    effacement, 263, 273, 281–284
    incompetent, 138, 218–219
    ripening of, 262
cesarean delivery, 343–344
    avoiding, 344–345
    discomfort after, 366–367
    epidural and, 321
    herpes and, 221
    hospital policy and, 163
    for lack of progress in labor, 337
    for multiples, 351–352
    percentage of mothers having,
        276
    procedure for, 347–349
    recovery after, 346, 347, 349–350,
        376–379
    risk for
        with amniotomy, 342
        with artificial induction of
            labor, 340, 345
    risks of, 346–347
changing table, 498–500
childbirth
    emergency, 332–333
    in nonhospital setting, 331–333
    sensations after, 328
childbirth classes, 53, 171–179
    online, 178–179
childcare, 252, 442–445
    caregiver for, characteristics of,
        444
    commercial, 444–445
    in-home, 443

D

E

F

G

H

Q

R

S

T

U

V

NOTES

NOTES

NOTES

NOTES

NOTES

NOTES